Foundations of Nursing Practice

4th Edition

Foundations of Nursing Practice

Themes, Concepts and Frameworks

Edited by

RICHARD HOGSTON &
BARBARA MARJORAM

palgrave
macmillan

The Publisher and the Author make no representation, express or implied, with regard to the accuracy of the information contained in this book and connate accept any legal responsibility or liability for any errors or omissions that may be made.

First edition 1999
Reprinted three times
Second edition 2002
Reprinted six times
Third edition 2007
Fourth Edition 2011

1006412284

Published by
PALGRAVE MACMILLAN

Palgrave Macmillan in the UK is an imprint of Macmillan Publishers Limited, registered in England, company number 785998, of Houndmills, Basingstoke, Hampshire RG21 6XS.

Palgrave Macmillan in the US is a division of St Martin's Press LLC, 175 Fifth Avenue, New York, NY 10010.

Palgrave Macmillan is the global academic imprint of the above companies and has companies and representatives throughout the world.

Palgrave® and Macmillan® are registered trademarks in the United States, the United Kingdom, Europe and other countries

ISBN 978-0-230-23274-7

This book is printed on paper suitable for recycling and made from fully managed and sustained forest sources. Logging, pulping and manufacturing processes are expected to conform to the environmental regulations of the country of origin.

A catalogue record for this book is available from the British Library.

10 9 8 7 6 5 4 3 2 1
20 19 18 17 16 15 14 13 12 11

Printed in China

Contents

List of Figures, Tables and Charts

Figures

Tables

Charts

Notes on Contributors

WAYNE ARNETT BN (Hons), RGN, Cert Mang, is a Lecturer at the University of Southampton, UK and the lead for Moving and Handling in the Faculty of Health Sciences.

SID CARTER PhD, MSc, BA, RN (LD), PGCEA, AdvCert (Human Sexuality) is a Lecturer in Learning Disabilities at the School of Health and Social Care, Bournemouth University, UK.

NADIA CHAMBERS RGN, BSc (Hons), PgDipEd, MA, PhD is a Consultant Nurse for Older People at Southampton University Hospitals NHS Trust.

YVETTE COX Dip N Ed, MBA is a Lecturer, teaching leadership and management subjects to undergraduate, postgraduate and master's programmes at the University of Southampton, UK.

JAN DEAN BA (Hons), DipN, RGN is a Lecturer in adult nursing at University of Southampton with an interest in respiratory nursing.

PAM DIGGENS BSc (Hons), MA, RN is a Lecturer at the University of Southampton, UK, with a specific interest in physical assessment and history taking.

ANITA GREEN D. Nursing, MA, BA (Hons), RCNT, RGN, RMN is a Dual Diagnosis Nurse Consultant working for Sussex Partnership NHS Foundation Trust and a visiting fellow with the School of Nursing and Midwifery at the University of Brighton.

SUE M. GREEN RN, BSc, MMedSci, PhD, PGCert has a BSc and Master's degree in science subjects and a PhD in biopsychology. She is currently a Senior Lecturer at the Faculty of Health Sciences, University of Southampton, UK.

ROB HAYWOOD MSc, PGCE, RN is a Lecturer at the University of Southampton with a specific interest in critical care and advanced life support.

RICHARD HOGSTON MSc (Nurs)., PGDipEd., BA (Hons) RN, is Professor of Healthcare Education and Regulation and Dean of the Faculty of Health at Leeds Metropolitan University, UK.

NEIL HOSKER MSc (health informatics), BA (Hons) nursing, PGDip, DPSN, RN is a Senior Lecturer in the Faculty of Health & Social Care, University of Chester, teaching on the pre-registration nursing programme and Foundation Degree in Health Informatics.

KEVIN HUMPHRYS RNLD. Cert Ed. MSc Applied Psychology (Learning Disabilities) is a Lecturer in Learning Disabilities at the University of Southampton and supports the lead for Moving and Handling in the Faculty of Health Sciences.

PAM JACKSON MPhil, BSc (Hons), RGN, RHV, RNT, is Senior Lecturer and Academic Lead for Interprofessional Learning at the Universities of Southampton and Portsmouth.

ADAM KEEN MEd, MSc, Dip HE, RN is a Senior Lecturer within the Faculty of Health & Social Care at the University of Chester, UK.

MELANIE JASPER PhD, MSc, BNurs, BA, PGCEA, RGN, RHV, RM, NDNcert is a Professor and Head of the School of Health Science at Swansea University, UK. She is also the Editor of the *Journal of Nursing Management*.

JANET McCRAY PhD, MSc, BSc (Hons), RNT, RN (LD) Cert Ed, is a Principal Lecturer in Health and Social Care Leadership at the University of Chichester, UK.

BARBARA MARJORAM TD, MA, RN(A), Cert Ed was formerly Senior Lecturer and Associate Director for Pre-Registration Nursing and Midwifery, at the Faculty of Health Sciences, University of Southampton. Her previous publications have included the use of information technology in nursing, enquiry-based learning and elimination.

SOMDUTH PARBOTEEAH PhD, MSc, SRN, RCNT, Cert Ed, Dip N (London) is Principal Lecturer in the Faculty of Health and Life Sciences at De Montfort University, UK. He is also Programme Leader for the MSc Advanced Health and Professional Practice.

DELIA POGSON RN (LD), FETC, Cert.Ed., RNT, M.Sc., M.Phil. is Senior Lecturer in the Faculty of Health Sciences, University of Southampton, UK, and is a member of the Network of Educators for the NHS Genetics Education and Development Centre.

ELIZABETH PORTER BA, MPhil, PGCEA, RN, RM, RHV, FWT is currently a Senior Lecturer at the University of Southampton where she is programme leader for the MSc and BSc (Hons) public health practice degrees.

PHIL RUSSELL MSc, MA, BA (Hons), DipEd is a Lecturer Practitioner and Bereavement Service Co-ordinator at the Rowans Hospice.

LYNN TAYLOR PGC, BSc (Hons) RN, RM is the Lead Clinical Nurse Specialist in Tissue Viability. Lynn initiated the Tissue Viability service in Portsmouth before moving to Southampton to set up the service there. She lectures for the university and the Trust.

STEVE TEE DClinP, MA, PGCEA, BA, DipPSN, RMN has worked within health-care practice and education for 25 years with research activity focusing on ethical decision-making and professionalism in clinical practice.

CHRIS WALKER MSc, BSc (Hons), DipHE, RN is a Consultant Nurse working in the Emergency Department of Queen Alexandra Hospital, Portsmouth.

Acknowledgements

Many thanks to all the authors and publishers for their support in the production of this 4th edition. This edition is dedicated to Ian Douglas, a valued colleague, who contributed to the first three editions but sadly lost his fight against cancer before this edition was started.

Barbara A Marjoram

The editors and publishers would also like to thank the past contributors who have helped to develop this book over the past three editions: Ian Douglas, Debra Elliot, Ruth Sadik, Penelope Simpson and Graham Watkinson. They also wish to thank the following for permission to use copyright material: Nursing and Midwifery Council for Chart 3.1 from NMC (2008) *The Code*; Department of Health for Fig 3.1 from DoH (2003) *The NHS Confidentiality Code of Practice*, Chart 3.2 from DoH (2001) *Consent – What You Have a Right to Expect: A Guide for Adults*, and Chart 18.2 from DH (2008) *Involving People and communities: A Brief guide to NHS Duties to involve and report on consultation*, London: DH licensed under the Open Government Licence v1.0; Elsevier Ltd for Table 3.1 published in *Evidence-based Healthcare*, by Muir Gray (pg 37) © Churchill Livingstone (2001) and Table 18.2 in Public Health and Health Visiting in Robotham, A. and Frost, M. (eds) *Health Visiting: Specialist Community Public Health Nursing*, © Elsevier (2005); National Audit Office for Fig 3.3 from *Improving quality & safety – Progress in implementing clinical governance in primary care: lessons for the New Primary Care Trusts*, Health Services Management Centre, University of Birmingham, © 2007; Nelson Thornes for Fig 4.1 from Jasper (2003) *Beginning Reflective Practice*, Nelson Thornes, Cheltenham; Environment Agency for Table 5.1 from Environment Agency (2004) *Guidance for the recovery and disposal of hazardous and non-hazardous waste* licensed under the Open Government Licence v1.0; Food Standards Agency for Fig 7.1 and Chart 7.1 originally from www.food.gov.uk (2009) licensed under the Open Government Licence v1.0; Norgine Pharmaceuticals for Figs

8.2 and 8.3 © 2000, 2005 Norgine Pharmaceuticals Ltd; Nursing Times for Fig 8.9 from Haslam, J. (1997) Floor plan. *Nursing Times* 93(15): 67–70; Wiley Blackwell for Chart 10.1, Table 10.1 and Table 10.4 from Mackway-Jones et al (2005) *Advanced Paediatric Life Support 4th edition*, BMJ Books, Blackwell Publishing Limited; Edward Arnold (Publishers) Limited for Table 10.2 from *Trauma Care Manual* by I. Greaves, K. Porter and J. Ryan published by Hodder Arnold Copyright © 2001; National Pressure Ulcer Advisory Panel for Chart 11.2 from European Pressure Ulcer Advisory Panel and National Pressure Ulcer Advisory Panel (2009) *Prevention and treatment of pressure ulcers: quick reference guide*; Judy Waterlow for Table 11.4(a) Waterlow Risk Assessment Tool © 1985, 2005; Barbara Braden and Nancy Bergstrom for Table 11.4 (b) Braden Scale (www.bradenscale. com); Health and Safety Executive for Chart 12.1 from *ALARP at a Glance*. hwww.hse.gov.uk/risk/theory/alarpglance.htm, (HSE, 2009), licensed under the Open Government Licence v1.0; Drinkaware for Fig 14.1 from www.drinkaware.co.uk; Skills for Health and Public Health Resource Unit for Table 18.1 from *Multidisciplinary/multi-agency/ multi-Professional Public Health Skills and Career Framework*. Public Health Resource Unit, Oxford, licensed under the Open Government Licence v1.0; Institute of Futures Studies for Fig 18.1 from Dahlgren, G & Whitehead, M (1991) *Policies and Strategies to Promote Social Equity in Health*, Stockholm, Sweden: Institute for Futures Studies; Information Commissioners Office for Chart 19.3 for information from Data Protection Act Fact Sheet; April Brooks and National Back Exchange for Chart 12.4 from Brooks. (2008) *Manual Handling Questions*. The Column, Severnprint, Gloucestershire. Every effort has been made to trace all the copyright holders, but if any have been inadvertently overlooked the publishers will be pleased to make the necessary arrangements at the first opportunity.

Introduction

This text is designed to be used as a study guide to support many of the theoretical aspects of the Nursing and Midwifery Council (NMC) Essential Skills Clusters (NMC, 2007) that were introduced as compulsory elements, from 2008, to pre-registration nursing programmes. There is a map of how the Essential Skills Clusters match the chapters on the companion website (see www.palgrave.com/nursinghealth/hogston). Students on other programmes may also find the text very useful, for example, those undertaking the Return to Practice, Foundation Degree programmes. This edition has been designed to develop the readers' theoretical skills throughout their nursing programmes and therefore is not solely based on the theory required for first-year student nurses. Nurses reading for a degree need to be able to apply theoretical perspectives within their clinical area.

Using, as a backdrop the NHS Next Stage Review by Lord Darzi, *High Quality Care for All* (DoH, 2008), the book reflects on the multidisciplinary care needed to fulfil quality care for all. Each chapter has been written by subject specialists and we hope that their enthusiasm for their topic areas is evident when you read them. The chapters are not designed to be read in any particular order and should be tackled when you feel they are relevant to your learning.

About the Book

The interactive style of the chapters is intended to make you think, explore further and reflect on your learning. The learning outcomes give you an idea of what you can achieve when you are working through the chapters, and a glossary of terms used, within each chapter, will enhance your understanding and vocabulary. The cross referencing or 'Links' between each chapter, increases the coherence of the text and illustrates the expanse of knowledge available. The client case studies in the Caseboxes draw on all four fields of nursing as well as featuring a range of settings; these are designed to encourage reflection and how what you are reading about can apply in practice. Each chapter also includes a variety of activities that will allow you to develop your learning and explore the topics further for yourself. At the end of each chapter there are a number of 'Test Yourself' questions so that you can check your understanding. Answers and feedback to these can be found in Chapter 21.

Chapter Guide

The book is divided into three sections: Nursing Skills and Concepts, Nursing Interventions and Professional Issues. Chapter 1 introduces the nursing process and provides examples of managing care, situating these within the responsibilities of autonomous practice governed by the NMC's Code – *Standards of Conduct, Performance and Ethics for Nurses and Midwives* (NMC, 2008).

Communication and the skill of working effectively in a team is a key part of nursing at all levels. Chapter 2 introduces these topics, helping you to develop your skills. Clearly focusing on the future, challenges to professional practice are explored in Chapter 3. The image of nursing that you started out with is likely to change as you progress throughout your career, and reflective practice, which is explained in Chapter 4, will be one tool to help you with this.

In Part II, Chapters 5 and 6 will identify some of the safeguards, legal and otherwise, available to protect you and your clients within the care setting involving infection control and medicines management. Eating and drinking can pose particular problems for clients, so you will be encouraged in Chapter 7 to review your own knowledge and habits, aiming to help clients to achieve optimum nourishment for their changing needs. Elimination is a logical progression and therefore Chapter 8 will help to dispel some taboos and myths, with a healthy emphasis on achieving and attaining relative normality across a life span. Respiration in Chapter 9 and circulation in Chapter 10, explores the nurse's role in assessing and implementing the care of clients with difficulties of breathing and maintenance of circulation. Chapter 11 explores issues related to wound management and how our clients' lifestyles can have an impact on the healing process. Movement and mobility affects not only the client, across many areas of care, but also has an impact on you and how you aid and handle clients; these important areas of study are explored within Chapter 12. Nurses cover the life span from the cradle to the grave and therefore Chapter 13 explores loss and bereavement. It also considers how changes to health can make clients question or confirm their beliefs, particularly when life is limited. Chapter 14 is a brand new chapter and explores the ever-increasing contemporary issue of substance misuse.

In Part III, Chapter 15 explores body image and sexuality which can be markedly affected by problems of diminished health, this area demands sensitive and thoughtful care and hence is a key professional issue to be considered. Chapter 16 uses the topic of genetics and the developments in this area of science to pose some thoughts for the future of health care within an ethical and legal framework.

Chapter 17 considers the importance of working within the inter-professional context, while Chapter 18 gives an insight into the public health approach to nursing practice. Access to and distribution of accurate information affects our everyday life and no more so than in health care; Chapter 19 therefore explores how this impacts across all health-care provision. And finally, Chapter 20 explores the management and leadership skills required, even from an early stage, to develop into a registered autonomous practitioner.

Note to reader

Terminology – throughout this book we have used words that are interchangeable, for example patient/client/service user. You will come across all these in various settings and therefore to reflect this, no one word is used. Likewise the terms 'practitioner', 'health professional' are used as not all aspects of care are only within the nurse's remit and you will be working within the multidisciplinary team (MDT).

References

DoH (Department of Health) (2008) *High Quality Care for All: NHS Next Stage Review by Lord Darzi*. DoH, London.

NMC (Nursing and Midwifery Council) (2007) *Essential Skills Clusters*, NMC Circular 07(2007) Annexe 2. NMC, London.

Guide to the book

Foundations of Nursing Practice is a feature-rich textbook that has been created to help you understand and reflect on the key elements of your course.

As you work through the text you'll find:

Contents listed at the beginning of each chapter for clear identification of what the chapter covers.

Learning outcomes which give you a clear indication of the aims and objectives of the chapter.

Caseboxes offering practice examples drawn from all fours branches of nursing, in a range of settings, to help you reflect and apply what you've read to practice.

Links providing cross-references within and between chapters to enable you to navigate the text, connect key pieces of learning and extend your knowledge.

Activities of many different types, encouraging reading, writing, discussion and reflection, helping you to engage with the text and draw upon personal and placement experiences.

Term **Key term definitions** to aid your understanding of specialist terminology. Found in the margin to minimize disruption to your reading, they'll ensure the text remains accessible throughout. (A searchable glossary can also be found on the companion website: www.palgrave.com/nursinghealth/hogston.)

Test yourself! questions at the end of each chapter for you to check your understanding. They're also useful tools for revision. (See chapter 21 for answers).

Further reading boxes offer suggested resources to kick-start further study. Live link web-based resources for all chapters can also be found on the companion website.

Nursing Skills and Concepts

1

Managing Nursing Care

📖 Contents

☑ Learning outcomes

The purpose of this chapter is to explore how nurses manage care; it will take you through a five-stage problem-solving approach known as the nursing process. At the end of the chapter, you should be able to:

- Define the stages of the nursing process
- Undertake a nursing assessment
- Identify nursing diagnoses from the assessment data
- Devise and implement a plan of care
- Evaluate your actions
- Consider the link between evaluation and quality of care.

Throughout the chapter, a working example using a client who is experiencing pain will be used to demonstrate how each of the stages of the nursing process is applied. The chapter also provides an opportunity for you to undertake some exercises that will assist you with your care-planning skills.

What Is the Nursing Process?

The **nursing process** is a problem-solving framework that enables the nurse to plan care for a client on an individual basis. The nursing process is not undertaken once only, because the client's needs frequently change and the nurse must respond appropriately. It is thus a cyclical process consisting of the five stages shown in Figure 1.1.

nursing process
a five-stage problem-solving framework enabling the nurse to plan individualised care for a client

The nurse is an autonomous practitioner whose responsibilities are now governed by *The Code: Standards of Conduct, Performance and Ethics for Nurses and Midwives*, devised by the Nursing and Midwifery Council (NMC, 2008). This requires nurses to be accountable for the care that they prescribe and deliver and to 'keep clear and accurate records of the discussions [they] have, the assessments [they] make' (NMC, 2008). Today, one's ability to use the nursing process is governed by the standards for pre-registration nursing education (NMC, 2010) as outlined by the statutory body, the NMC, and embedded in parliamentary statute (DoH, 2000). The standards state that conditional to registration is the ability to:

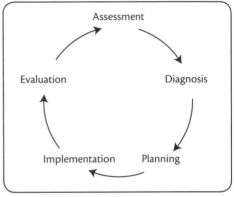

Figure 1.1 The nursing process

> Make a holistic person centred and systematic assessment of physical, emotional, psychological, social, cultural and spiritual needs, including risk and develops a comprehensive personalised plan of nursing care. (NMC, 2010)

Failure to keep a record of nursing care or to use the nursing process can lead to a breakdown in the quality of care that is provided. The Clothier Report (DoH, 1994), which was published following the inquiry into Beverley Allitt (the nurse who was convicted of the murder of children in a hospital in Grantham, Lincolnshire), noted how:

> Despite the availability of a nurse with responsibility for quality management, there were no explicit nursing standards set for ward four. In addition the nursing records were of poor quality and showed little understanding of the nursing process.

High Quality Care for All (Darzi, 2008) states that clinicians' first and primary duty will always be their clinical practice or service, delivering high quality care to patients based on patients' individual needs. Therefore, the importance of understanding and using a systematic patient-centred approach (such as the nursing process) to the provision of nursing care cannot be overestimated.

There has been some debate within the profession over the number of stages needed in the nursing process, some suggesting four and others five. With a four-stage approach, the nurse does not have time to reflect on the assessment data that have been collected and instead moves from assessment to planning. The five-stage process enables the nurse to identify the client's **nursing diagnosis** in order to plan the appropriate care.

nursing diagnosis
the second stage of the nursing process, often described as a 'nursing problem', for which the nurse can independently prescribe care

The nursing process should not be seen as a linear process: it is a dynamic and ongoing cyclical process (Figure 1.1). Assessment, for example, is not a 'one-off' activity but a continuous one. Take the example of the individual who is in pain – it is not enough to make a pain assessment that may warrant an intervention; the nurse then needs to make a reassessment after having evaluated whether the pain-relieving intervention has been successful.

The nursing process is a problem-solving activity. Problem-solving approaches to decision-making are not unique to nursing. The medical profession uses a specific format based upon an assessment of the body's systems. A number of questions are asked in a systematic manner to enable the doctor to make a diagnosis based upon the information that has been collected. Problem-solving approaches are also taken outside the health-care field. Car mechanics undertake a sequence of activities in order to diagnose what is wrong with your car when you tell them that there is a squeak or a rattle.

Stage 1: Assessment

Sources of assessment data

> **✴ Activity 1.1**
>
> Think about the client and other sources that you may be able to consult to assist you when conducting a comprehensive assessment. Write them down in a list.

Before beginning to consider what sort of information you might need to collect, we need to look at the skills that are necessary to ensure that the data analysed are comprehensive. Assessment is not an easy process as it includes collecting information from a variety of sources. The quality of the assessment will, however, depend on one's ability to put together all the sources at one's disposal. Spend a few minutes on Activity 1.1.

The sources that you have listed in Activity 1.1 have probably included the following:

- Your client
- Relatives, friends and significant others
- Current and previous nursing records
- The records of other health professionals such as doctors and physiotherapists
- Statements and information from the police, ambulance personnel, witnesses at an accident scene and others.

Your client

The first and most important source for data collection is from the individual whom you are assessing. It will not, however, always be possible to obtain all the information you require, for a number of reasons, so you will also need to consult other people.

Relatives, friends and significant others

If you are assessing a baby, most of the verbal information you require will be obtained from his or her parent(s) or guardian(s). With a child, you will need to qualify some of your information through the same source. In the case of an adult who is unconscious or is having difficulty breathing, you will again need to obtain data from friends, relatives, ambulance personnel, the police and so on. The same applies if the client has difficulty understanding as a result of dementia or severe learning disabilities.

Nursing, medical and other records

It will not always be possible to have immediate access to existing records, especially in an emergency or with a first consultation, but these sources hold valuable information that you need to analyse. They provide details that may assist and prompt you. If the client has been admitted to a hospital, you may have a letter from the GP, district nurse, health visitor or community psychiatric nurse. Similarly, on discharge from hospital, you will provide discharge information if community-based professionals need to be involved. Telephone calls to these professionals, visits and case conferences may also feature. As the roll out of the national programme for IT within the NHS occurs the use of electronic patient records should enable much faster access to a range of data (www.connecting-forhealth.nhs.uk).

> **∞ Link**
> Chapter 19 has more information on IT initiatives.

Skills

Having considered some of the sources at your disposal, we now need to think about what other factors have a bearing on a successful assessment. Spend a few minutes on Activity 1.2.

As we are beginning to see, the process of assessment is a complex one. Although we have identified some of the sources of information, the quality of the information collected depends upon a number of other factors. In your list from Activity 1.2, you may have included:

- Listening
- Observing
- The use of verbal and non-verbal communication and open and closed questions
- Physical examination
- Measurements.

> **✷ Activity 1.2**
> Spend a little while thinking about what kinds of skills you need in order to conduct your assessment. Write them down in list form.

> **∞ Link**
> Chapter 2 contains a detailed examination of how the nurse can most effectively use some of these skills. You may wish to consult this before reading on.

Listening

One of the most important features of an assessment interview is the nurse's ability to listen to the client. This means giving the client time to answer questions. You will appreciate from your own life experience that when you are asked a question, you want time to think and then answer without interruption. A premature interruption may lead to clients withholding information or not feeling that you are really interested in what they have to say. Although it is important for you to focus on the information you require and not digress, the fact that Mrs Jones has been admitted as an emergency and is meant to be on the school run in an hour will be the only thing of interest to her until you are able to contact someone who can collect her children.

Observation

Observation can in itself provide the nurse with a great deal of information. The bluish tinge (cyanosis) seen around the mouths, nailbeds and faces of some breathless patients may be indicative of respiratory distress and will be an indication of how little oxygen is circulating in their blood. A yellowish tinge to the skin (jaundice) may be indicative of biliary disease. Similarly, facial and other body expressions may give you an indication of pain.

Open and closed questioning

Both these methods of communication need to be used when collecting information. The use of **closed questions** allows the client who is, for example, breathless, anxious, in pain or depressed to answer with a simple 'yes' or 'no'. **Open questions**, however, will allow you to provide your clients with a full opportunity to tell you the history of their illness or pain.

Chapter 2 discusses open and closed questions in more detail.

Physical examination

The physical examination of clients allows you to observe and make a judgement about their symptoms. You will be able to determine the integrity (state) of the skin, which is an important consideration in an immobile client. Physical damage such as wounds can be seen, as can even the small puncture marks left by an intravenous drug abuser. Skin that feels very warm and moist to the touch may be a sign of **pyrexia**.

Measurements

Measurements come in many forms, for example the taking of a blood pressure, pulse or temperature. Also included here is the use of other assessment tools such as a nutritional analysis, a pressure ulcer risk calculator (use the tool used in your locality, for example Braden or Waterlow) or a pain chart.

Data collection

As we have seen, nurses must, in order to be able to plan care for their clients, be able to gather information that will enable them to make informed decisions. But what information do nurses need to gather, what questions should they ask and how much do they need to know? The answer is determined on an individual basis, the nurse collecting both subjective and objective information. Before looking in detail at what information should be collected, undertake Activity 1.3.

From the activity, in addition to name, age and date of birth, you may have collected some of the following information:

Physical health information
- Current and past health problems
- Nutritional and dietary information
- Patterns of activity and rest
- Stamina

Link

Chapters 9 and 10 explain some causes of cyanosis and identify the difference between central and peripheral cyanosis.

closed questions

those designed to elicit a simple 'yes' or 'no' answer

open questions

those in which clients can express their answers in as many words as they choose

pyrexia

fever, body temperature elevated from normal

Link

Chapter 11 has a section on wound assessment.

Link

Chapter 10 explores blood pressure and explains how to take an arterial blood pressure reading.

✹ Activity 1.3

Select a friend or relative and ask them if you can spend about 20 minutes undertaking a health assessment. Now take a blank piece of paper and collect the information that you feel is important when making some decisions about your chosen person's health status.

- Physical parameters
- Factors affecting health (cigarettes, alcohol and so on)

Psychological information

- How does the client react to stress, challenge and so on?
- What are the person's hopes, expectations, demands?

Social health information

- What is the person's lifestyle?
- Employment/unemployment details
- Family or other responsibilities

- Dental, hearing, vision and so on
- Elimination patterns
- Sexual history.

- Communication
- Values and beliefs.

- Leisure
- Exercise
- Social environment/networks.

How did you decide what you needed to ask, how did you decide to word the questions, and did you collect everything to enable you to feel that you had conducted a thorough assessment?

Framework for assessment

One way of organising the information that you need to collect is by using a nursing framework. The 'activities of living' framework devised by Roper et al. (2008) uses a list of the client's activities of living (Chart 1.1) as a framework for assessment, the nurse systematically collecting the physical, psychological, sociocultural and economic aspects of these activities.

✺ Activity 1.4

Read Holland et al. (2008) for further reading related to the activities of living.

Chart 1.1 The activities of living

- Maintaining a safe environment
- Communicating
- Breathing
- Eating and drinking
- Eliminating
- Personal cleansing and dressing
- Controlling body temperature
- Mobilising
- Working and playing
- Expressing sexuality
- Sleeping
- Dying

Breathing, one of the activities of living, will now be used as a framework to demonstrate the type of information that the nurse needs to collect during an assessment. At any given time during the assessment process, it may be necessary to concentrate more on one activity than another.

Breathing

The information that the nurse needs to collect about this and any other activity of living depends on the answers to certain trigger questions. You may, for example, start off by asking your client whether she has any problems with breathing. Even though the answer may be 'no', you would, as a professional, need to investigate further. The client whom you are assessing may not feel that she has a problem with breathing, but consider the following questions:

⌾ Link

Chapter 9 provides methods of respiratory assessment.

1   'Do you smoke?' The answer here may be 'yes' even though the client has said she has no problems with breathing. Indeed, she may still feel that she does not have any problems. This is, however, a trigger for further questioning.

2   'Do you suffer from any breathlessness?' The answer at the outset may again be 'no', but if you ask about running up the stairs or running for a bus, the client may admit that, yes she does then, but this is because she does not usually do any exercise.

3   Taking this one step further allows the nurse to extract even more information about the status of the client's breathing: 'Do you cough?' The answer may be 'no', but when prompted the client may admit to coughing for a little while in the morning, although this clears rapidly and she thinks nothing of it.

If the client is a normal healthy young adult, the nurse may at this stage still perceive that the client does not actually have a problem with breathing in the short term even though she is partaking in health-damaging behaviour. In the long term, however, the consequences of smoking could be fatal. At this stage in the assessment process, it may be sufficient to make a note of the information gathered so far; when it comes to planning care, the action that will be prescribed will then include health education about smoking. This will be expanded on in the section on planning and implementation below.

Summary and worked example

✴ Activity 1.5

Read the client profiles in Casebox 1.1. Choose one of the profiles and, for any two of the activities of living, write down the information that you would need to collect during a nursing assessment.

This section has introduced you to the nursing process and looked in some detail at assessment. The activities should have enabled you to experience some of the issues that you need to consider when undertaking a nursing assessment. We have examined the skills that the nurse needs to use when assessing clients, and we have been introduced to one assessment framework that may assist the nurse during the process. By way of a summary of the information that needs to be gained when undertaking an assessment, the following section takes pain as an example and outlines the questions and methods that can be employed when assessing a client's pain. This will be revisited as we consider the other four stages of the nursing process later in the chapter. Having read this summary, you may like to return to the client profile you chose and identify the information you feel would be important for your chosen profile. Alternatively, you might like to take the opportunity to participate in the assessment process during your practice placements in the common foundation programme.

Pain assessment

∞ Link

Chapter 10 deals with pain arising from circulatory problems.

The assessment of pain is a complex activity that involves a consideration of the physical, psychological and cultural aspects of the individual. Because pain is a subjective experience, the nurse needs to be able to summarise the information gained against some objective criteria. This is essential for diagnosis and for evaluating the effectiveness of interventions. Only the person experiencing the

Casebox 1.1

Joan Harris is a 69-year-old lady who tripped and fell over a protruding pavement slab this morning while out shopping. She has been admitted to the orthopaedic ward of her local NHS Foundation Trust hospital suffering from a fractured neck of femur. Mrs Harris is pale and is anxious about who will look after her cat while she is in hospital. She is complaining of severe pain in her hip and knee, and has grazes and cuts to her lower leg.

Amanda Cohen is 29 years old and has profound learning disabilities. She lives in staffed residential accommodation with two other young women. For two weeks, Amanda has been showing signs of distress – hitting her face, lifting her jumper and crying. At first it was thought that this might be because of premenstrual tension. After a while, however, someone thought to arrange a dental inspection under anaesthetic: the dentist found a particularly nasty dental abscess (adapted from NHSE, 1993).

Andrew Holly is 5 years old and has been admitted to the accident and emergency department of the local NHS Trust hospital. He is complaining of a very sore and painful arm, is withdrawn and is sobbing. He is accompanied by his mother, his 2-year-old sister and their newborn baby brother.

Alison Simpson, 21 years old, lives in a hostel for people with mental health problems. She has no close family, having left home at 18. She finds it difficult to develop relationships and is suspicious of people who try to befriend her. Alison is very withdrawn and has on two occasions attempted to take her own life through an unsuccessful paracetamol overdose. She was found this morning slumped in a corner, covered in blood and complaining of extreme pain in her left hand. On the floor nearby was a razor blade, and on examination she had severe lacerations to her left forearm.

pain knows its nature, intensity, location and what it means to them. One of the most seminal, widely used and accepted definitions of pain was put forward by McCaffery and Beebe (1999), who suggest that pain is 'what the person says it is existing when and where the person says it does'.

Assessments of the patient's pain experience

To begin with, it is essential to identify the characteristics of the client's pain. This means that the nurse should consider:

- *The type of pain:* is it crampy, stabbing, sharp? How the client describes the pain may help in diagnosing its cause. Myocardial (heart) pain is often described as stabbing, but biliary pain as cramping or aching.

  biliary
  pertaining to bile, bile ducts or gall bladder

- *Its intensity:* is it mild, severe or excruciating? Pain assessment scales are helpful here. The nurse can ask the patient to rate the pain on a scale of 0 to 10, zero being no pain and 10 intolerable pain. With children, a range of pictures showing a child changing from happy to sad can be used. Colour 'mood' charts, with a series of colours from black through grey to yellow and orange, have also been used and are very useful for clients who have difficulty grasping numbers or articulating exactly what their pain is like.
- *The onset:* was it sudden or gradual? Find out when it started and in what circumstances. What makes it worse? What makes it better? What was the patient doing immediately before it happened?
- *Its duration:* is it persistent, constant or intermittent?
- *Changes in the site:* there may be tenderness, swelling, discolouration, firmness or rigidity. With appendicitis, a classic sign is the movement of pain from the umbilicus to the right iliac fossa. In a myocardial infarction (a heart

attack), pain classically radiates down the arm, and with biliary pain it can radiate to the shoulder.

- *Its location:* ask the patient to be as specific as possible, for example indicating the site by pointing.
- *Any associated symptoms:* Chart 1.2 shows some of the common symptoms of disease that can influence the response to pain.
- *Signs such as redness, swelling or heat.*

Chart 1.2 Common symptoms of disease that influence the response to pain

• Anorexia	• Nausea and	• Oedema
• Malaise and	vomiting	• Immobility
lassitude	• Cough	• Anxiety and fear
• Constipation	• Dyspnoea	• Depression
• Diarrhoea	• Inflammation	• Dryness of the mouth

Summary

Table 1.1 provides a summary of some of the issues to consider when assessing pain. In essence, this section demonstrates how much detail the nurse needs to collect when making a full assessment of the client's pain. Consider your own experiences of pain, both personally and from clients you have nursed in clinical practice, and reflect on how comprehensive the assessment was then.

Stage 2: Nursing Diagnosis

The second stage of the nursing process is making a nursing diagnosis. This enables the nurse to translate the information gained during the assessment and identify the nursing problems. In order to avoid confusion, it is worth noting that 'diagnosis' is not a concept unique to medicine: car mechanics diagnose mechanical problems, teachers diagnose learning difficulties, and consequently

Table 1.1 Assessment of pain

Initial sympathetic responses to pain of low-to-moderate intensity	Parasympathetic responses to intense or chronic pain	Verbal responses	Muscular and postural responses
Increased blood pressure	Decreased blood pressure	Crying	Increased muscle tone
Increased heart rate	Decreased heart rate	Gasping	Immobilisation of the affected area
Increased respiratory rate	Weak pulse	Screaming	Rubbing movements
Decreased salivation and Gastrointestinal activity	Increased gastrointestinal activity	Silence	Rocking movement
Dilated pupils	Nausea and vomiting		Drawing up of the knees
Increased perspiration	Weakness		Pacing the floor
Pallor	Decreased alertness		Thrashing and restlessness
Cool, clammy skin	Shock		Facial grimaces
Dry lips and mouth			Removal of the offending object

nurses diagnose nursing problems. The language of nursing diagnosis originated in North America in an effort to move the art, science and theoretical basis of nursing forward and readers are advised to visit the informative website at www.nanda.org.

Nursing diagnosis is a critical step in the nursing process; it depends on an accurate and comprehensive nursing assessment and forms the basis of nursing care-planning. Nursing diagnosis is the end-product of nursing assessment, a clear statement of the patient's problems as ascertained from the nursing assessment (Roper et al., 2008). Furthermore, the International Council of Nurses has, for the purposes of the International Classification for Nursing Practice, defined a nursing diagnosis as 'a label given by a nurse to the decision about a phenomenon which is the focus of nursing intervention' (ICN, 1999). A visit to the website at www.icn.ch is recommended for more detailed information and to appreciate the collaborative work on nursing diagnosis and the International Classification for Nursing Practice is progressing.

The key components of what constitutes a nursing diagnosis are outlined in Chart 1.3.

Chart 1.3 Key components of a nursing diagnosis

- A nursing diagnosis:
- Is a statement of a client's problem
- Refers to a health problem
- Is based on objective and subjective assessment data
- Is a statement of nursing judgement
- Is a short concise statement
- Consists of a two-part statement
- Is a condition for which a nurse can independently prescribe care
- Can be validated with the client

Source: Adapted from Shoemaker (1984); Bellack and Edlund (1992); Iyer et al. (1995).

Making a nursing diagnosis

Nursing diagnoses can be actual or potential. Actual diagnoses are those which are evident from the assessment, for example pain caused by a fractured neck of femur. Potential diagnoses, on the other hand, are those which could or will arise as a consequence of the actual diagnoses. For example, an individual who is normally active but is confined to bed is at risk of becoming constipated or developing a pressure sore. In this instance, two potential diagnoses arise:

- a potential risk of constipation as a result of enforced bedrest
- a potential risk of pressure sore development from enforced bedrest.

Stage 3: Planning Nursing Care

There are two steps to the planning stage:

- Setting goals
- Identifying actions.

⚭ Link

Chapter 8 considers the causes, diagnosis and treatment of constipation.

✷ Activity 1.6

Return to the two activities of living that you assessed during Activity 1.5. Try to identify one actual and one potential nursing diagnosis. Use the guidelines in Chart 1.3 to ensure that your diagnoses meet the criteria.

✷ Activity 1.7

For the diagnoses that you identified during Activity 1.5, try to identify one short-term and one long-term goal for your chosen client. Remember to ensure that they meet the MACROS criteria (see below for description).

goal
the intended outcome of a nursing intervention, sometimes referred to as an objective

A **goal** is a statement of what the nurse expects the client to achieve and is sometimes referred to as an objective. In other words, goals are the intended outcomes and can be short or long term. Goals are client centred and must be realistic, being stated in objective and measurable language. They help both nurse and client to define how the nursing diagnosis will be addressed. Goals serve as the standard by which the nurse can evaluate the effectiveness of the nursing actions.

When writing goals, they need to conform to the MACROS criteria; they should be:

- Measurable and observable so that the outcome can be evaluated
- Achievable and time limited
- Client centred
- Realistic
- Outcome written
- Short.

Using the example of pain, the short-term goal will be that the client will state that he is comfortable and pain free within 20 minutes. The long-term goal, however, is that the client will state within 12 hours that he feels in control of his pain. (It is important to remember to take account of the non-verbal clues discussed earlier – is the client really pain free?) With the move to shorter hospital stays and the emphasis on care in the community, it may not always be necessary to formulate both long- and short-term goals for all problems. It is, however, always better to have a number of short-term goals that are reached so that new goals can be set rather than having a long-term goal that takes weeks to achieve. With Mrs Harris (see Casebox 1.1 above), who will have surgery for her hip, this will be a series of goals that progress her towards full mobility following her operation, for example: 'Mrs Harris will walk one way to the toilet unaided by [enter date]. Mrs Harris will be able to climb one set of stairs by [enter date].' This avoids a long-term goal that reads 'Mrs Harris will be fully mobile by [enter date].'

Action planning

The next stage is to plan the nursing care that will ensure that clients achieve their goals. This is where the nurse prescribes nursing actions that can then be implemented and evaluated. In 'care-planning' language, these are the nursing actions – the prescribed interventions that are put into effect in order to solve the problem and reach the goal. It is against these actions that the nurse may, when evaluating care, have to make some adjustments if the actions have not been effective. In today's NHS, when we are seeing a decreasing number of registered nurses against an increase in those of bank and agency nurses and unqualified health-care support workers, documenting the prescribed nursing care ensures a degree of continuity. In this way, the care plan can be seen as the diary of the client's nursing care. When planning nursing care, use the REEPIG criteria, which will ensure that your plan of care is:

- *Realistic:* it is important that the care can be given within the available resources, otherwise it will not be achievable.

- *Explicit:* ensure that statements are qualified. If you suggest that a dressing needs changing, state exactly when. This will ensure that there is no room for misinterpretation.
- *Evidence based:* nursing is a research-based profession. When planning nursing care, the research findings that underpin the rationale for care must be considered.
- *Prioritised:* start with the most pressing diagnosis. Given that time is of the essence, the first priority may be, for example, to plan care for the client's pain.
- *Involved:* the plan of care should involve not only the client, so that he or she is aware of why such care is needed, but also the other members of the health-care team who have a stake in helping the client back to health, for example physiotherapists and dietitians.
- *Goal centred:* ensure that the care planned meets the set goals.

Returning now to the example of pain, the nurse needs to make decisions about what sorts of intervention will most effectively relieve Mrs Harris's pain. This involves not only decisions about prescribed medications, but also other considerations such as how often the pain assessment tool should be used and what alternative non-pharmacological methods, such as comfort through pillows, the use of skin traction for the leg and distraction therapy, can be implemented. The nursing care plan for Mrs Harris may therefore detail the following nursing actions:

- Give the prescribed analgesic and monitor its effects; record them on the pain chart
- Apply skin traction (if appropriate)
- Nurse on a bed equipped with pressure-relieving equipment
- Ensure regular changes of position and assessment of equipment needs to achieve this while encouraging independence; encourage Mrs Harris to change her position regularly
- Ensure that Mrs Harris has a supply of chosen reading/writing materials and access to the television/radio/MP3 player.

> **⊂⊃ Link**
> Chapter 11 examines pressure ulcer grading and risk assessment

> **✷ Activity 1.8**
> Return to the client for whom you chose to identify nursing diagnoses and goals. Consider what nursing care you would need to plan in order to achieve those goals.

Stage 4: Implementation

Implementation is the 'doing' phase of the nursing process. This is where the nurse puts into action the nursing care that will be delivered and addresses each of the diagnoses and their goals. The nurse will undertake the instructions written in the care plan in order to assist the client in reaching these goal(s). This will involve a process of teaching and helping clients to make decisions about their health. It also involves deciding upon the most appropriate method for providing nursing care, and the liaison and involvement of other health professionals. Look at the list of health professionals in Chart 1.4. Do you know what their primary roles and functions are and when you might need to involve them?

Chart 1.4 Other members of the health-care team

• Physiotherapist	• Health visitor	• Occupational therapist
• Community psychiatric nurse	• District nurse	• Dietitian
	• Podiatrist GP	• Key worker
• Speech therapist	• Social worker	• School nurse

Managing Nursing Care in the Clinical Environment

A number of different approaches to the delivery of nursing care are available to nurses. These include task allocation, patient allocation, team nursing, primary nursing, the key worker and caseload management. The benefits or otherwise of each of these methods need to be considered in the light of the skill mix of available staff (that is, the number and grade of qualified and unqualified staff) and what it is that the nursing team wants to achieve. It is difficult to evaluate the right approach without considering the benefits or drawbacks of each of these methods. The published reports of clinical governance reviews by the Care Quality Commission (www.cqc.org.uk) considers the management and organisation of nursing care as well as the quality of care and record keeping.

Task allocation

task allocation
the provision of nursing care that centres on a range of tasks allocated to nurses/support workers

Task allocation (also known as functional nursing) is a highly ritualistic method of organising care that centres on nurses and support workers being assigned tasks. With this system, one nurse will be assigned to undertake the observations of temperature, pulse, blood pressure and respiration. Another nurse undertakes all the dressings, whereas another takes care of the drugs. This is a fragmented method of providing nursing care that will ensure that the client receives aspects of care from a multiplicity of nurses and support workers, akin to a production line process. The emphasis on tasks naturally removes the notion of individualised client care and as such is incompatible with the nursing process.

Client allocation

client allocation
individualised care provided by a named nurse, often assisted by a support worker

Client allocation is where the total care for a number of clients is undertaken by one nurse, often assisted by a support worker. Although this system means that there is an emphasis on total client care being delivered by an individual nurse for a designated period of time, continuity of care may become compromised if the same clients are not cared for on a regular basis by the same nurse. With this system, extra attention needs to be paid to the detail in the nursing care plan because of the number of nurses who may have contact with a client.

Team nursing

team nursing
care provided by a team of nurses/support workers led by a 'team leader'

Team nursing occurs where a designated group of clients is cared for by a team of two or more nurses (at least one of whom is a registered nurse) who accept collective responsibility for the assessment, planning, implementation and evaluation of the clients' care. Although each team will be headed by a team leader, each registered nurse is accountable for his or her actions in accordance with the Code (NMC, 2008). This is important to remember in an effort to counteract any criticism surrounding who is ultimately responsible under a system of collective responsibility.

Walsh and Ford (1989) have described how team nursing and client allocation evolved as the successor to task allocation on the premise that being cared for by a team rather than an array of nurses led to more holistic care. They suggested that team nursing really resembles a small-scale version of task allocation, especially if there is a lack of continuity between shifts when the same team may not be on duty, leading to fragmentation of care. Consequently, there has to be a commitment to ensure that tasks are not assigned to each team member.

Team nursing has received a positive press from student nurses. Lidbetter's (1990) small-scale study describes how students working in a hospital ward practising team nursing spent more time working alongside a qualified nurse and rated their skill acquisition and their evaluation of the effectiveness of client care higher than did those from a ward practising primary nursing. Students were also, as a learning experience, afforded the opportunity to assume the role of team leader, under supervision.

Primary nursing

Primary nursing has been described as a professional patient-centred practice (Manley, 1990). In this approach, the primary nurse accepts full responsibility and accountability for his or her clients during their stay. In its purest form, the implication is that the primary nurse has 24-hour responsibility 7 days a week (Manthey, 1992). In reality, a team of associate nurses continues to provide nursing care under the direction of the primary nurse and in his or her absence. Again, accountability and autonomy rest with the individual registered nurse under the Code of Conduct (NMC, 2008). Positive effects of a move to primary nursing can be seen in the literature (Laakso and Routasalo, 2001; Drach-Zahavy, 2004).

primary nursing
care provided on an individual basis by a named nurse who, in its purest form, holds 24 hour accountability for the package of care

Person-centred planning

Popular in the field of learning disabilities, a person-centred approach to planning care is advocated in the White Paper *Valuing People Now* (DoH, 2009a). Person-centred planning starts with the individual, and is at the heart of enabling people with highly complex needs to lead fulfilling lives.

Care programme approach

Focusing on personalised planning supporting individuals with severe mental illness, DoH (2008) provides comprehensive guidance on the care programme approach. Useful links are signposted with other assessment and planning frameworks, such as person-centred planning highlighted above.

Caseload management

⊂⊃ Link

Chapter 18 has more information on how teams interface between hospital, home and other community settings.

This is the most popular method of organising nursing care in the community setting. It revolves around the designated named nurse with extended qualifications in health visiting/district nursing who acts as the caseload manager. Caseloads are normally organised either geographically or by GP attachment, each caseload manager leading a team of qualified nurses and health-care support workers. Continuity of care is maintained because the teams are organised to ensure that a member of the team is available every day of the week; as such, it is less affected by the demands of the shift system. Each registered nurse is accountable for his or her own actions (NMC, 2008), the caseload manager being responsible for ensuring that the skill mix and resources are adequate. Given the shift of care from the secondary to primary setting and the role of the community matron, keeping patients out of hospital by managing long-term conditions in the community will see this method of managing care increase (DoH, 2009).

✳ Activity 1.9

From your own experiences in clinical practice, what method(s) of care organisation have you experienced? Write down two positive aspects and then consider whether one of the other methods described above would have been suitable and why.

Stage 5: Evaluation

At the beginning of this chapter, it was noted that the stages of the nursing process need to be seen as ongoing rather than as once-only activities. This means that the final stage, evaluation, is in reality the end of the beginning and where the process in essence restarts. One of the key components of quality nursing practice is the nurse's ability to make a clinical judgement based upon a sound knowledge base. Evaluation is about reviewing the effectiveness of the care that has been given, and it serves two purposes. First, the nurse is able to ascertain whether the desired outcomes for the client have been achieved. Second, evaluation acts as an opportunity to review the entire process and determine whether the assessment was accurate and complete, the diagnosis correct, the goals realistic and achievable, and the prescribed actions appropriate.

Increased health-care costs require managers throughout the professions to reduce expenditure and seek the most cost-effective options. The population at large are also more informed about health-care matters and are arguably less passive recipients of health care, demanding a detailed and open explanation for their care (Hogston, 1997). It is therefore the responsibility of each nurse to ensure that the prescribed care takes account of these issues. Given that nursing records are legal documents that could be used in a court of law, extreme care and accuracy are essential when completing the care plan to which the registered nurse puts her signature. In its guidance on record keeping the NMC states that 'good record keeping is a mark of a skilled and safe practitioner, while careless or incomplete record keeping often highlights wider problems with that individual's practice' (NMC, 2007b).

In order to raise standards of care, and in keeping with the clinical governance agenda, the government has published benchmarks in fundamental aspects of care (DoH, 2010a), one of which focuses on record-keeping. Readers should familiarise themselves with this particular benchmark. It is important to note that the document stresses that the best interests of *people* are maintained throughout the assessment, planning, implementation, evaluation and revision of care and development of services and when a system for continuous improvement of quality of care is in place.

Methods of evaluating nursing care

Having discussed the importance of evaluation and the place it has in maintaining quality, it is important to consider some of the methods that nurses can use. First of all, undertake Activity 1.10.

Your list, from Activity 1.10 may have included some of the following:

- Nursing handover
- Reflection
- Patient satisfaction or complaint
- Reviewing the nursing care plan.

✴ **Activity 1.10**

How do you think that nursing care is evaluated? You may have witnessed some methods in your own clinical placements; write them down as a list. If you have not, try to think generally about how you evaluate any service you have received – buying a meal or an item from a shop, for example.

Nursing handover

You may have had experience of a nursing handover, which is where a team of nurses hand over information about the nursing care of clients to another group of nurses, usually at the end of a shift, for example from day care to night care. Using the nursing care plan as the focus, nurses share information about the clients and their planned care. This serves as a valuable forum for evaluating care through a discussion of its effectiveness. The variety of experiences and professional expertise held by a number of nurses allows a sharing of that information. The importance of nursing handover was stated by the Audit Commission (1992) as being critical for maintaining continuity of client care.

Reflection

The role of reflection in quality and evaluation has been discussed in some detail in the literature, and Chapter 4 discusses the concept in more detail. Reflection can, however, be both formal and informal. You probably reflect on your experiences both socially with other friends who are nurses and more formally in lecturer-led tutorials. This leads to an analysis of your actions and some of the ways in which you could have done things differently or which you would want to repeat. The use of critical incident analysis, for example, enables nurses to evaluate a given situation or event; this is a tool that is used by qualified nurses in their personal portfolios, which must be kept in order for the nurses to be eligible for triennial re-registration.

∞ Link

Chapter 4 reviews types of reflection, thoughtful practice and reflection in practice settings.

Patient satisfaction

The appreciation that is sometimes offered by clients through, for example, a letter, is an indicator of how satisfied individuals have been with their nursing care. In contrast, a letter of complaint may lead to an investigation into the reasons why a client has not been satisfied with the care received. Although the number of letters of complaint appears to be on the increase, this is probably the result of a culture comprising a more informed public. In many ways, such letters lead to an analysis of what went wrong; this may not necessarily be a result of poor nursing care but of other environmental factors. Hopefully, however, such publicity allows those who have control over resources to evaluate the priorities.

Health-care providers are now required to publish statistics on indicators of quality ranging from, for example, how long clients have to wait in accident and emergency departments to the number of clients who receive a visit from the community nurse within the two-hour appointment time. In the same vein, letters and cards of satisfaction should be closely monitored.

Reviewing the nursing care plan

This is where the nurse evaluates the effectiveness of the care that has been given against the set goals and writes an evaluation statement. When evaluating care, it is useful to ask yourself a series of questions about each of the stages of the nursing process, which will provide you with answers about your plan of care:

- Have the short-term goals been met?
- If the answer is 'yes', has the diagnosis been resolved? If so, it no longer needs to be addressed.
- If the answer is 'no', why have the goals not been met? Did they meet the MACROS criteria?
- Was the planned care realistic? Did it meet the REEPIG criteria?
- Has a new diagnosis arisen or a potential diagnosis become an actual one?
- Was the method of care delivery appropriate?
- Was there effective communication within and between the nursing staff and other members of the multidisciplinary team?
- How satisfied was the client with the care?

Finally, take a look at the completed care plan for Mrs Harris outlined in Table 1.2 and compare it with your own completed care plan.

Table 1.2 Worked example of a care plan for Mrs Harris

Nursing diagnosis	Pain due to fractured femur
Short-term goal	Mrs Harris states that she is comfortable with a pain scale rating below 2 within 15 minutes
Long-term goal	Mrs Harris feels that she is in control of her pain and that it is no longer a major concern for her within 24 hours
Nursing actions	Give the prescribed analgesic and monitor its effects Apply skin traction Nurse on a bed equipped with a pressure-relieving mattress Ensure two-hourly changes of position by attaching a trapeze pole to the bed, and encourage Mrs Harris to change her position regularly Ensure that Mrs Harris has a supply of chosen reading/writing materials and access to the television and radio
Evaluation	Mrs Harris states that she is comfortable and her pain scale rating remains below 2.

Information Technology and Care-planning

The input of information technology to health care is having a significant impact on the NHS as advanced computerised information systems record and evaluate everything from finance to personal records. From your own experiences, you may already have seen laptop/palm-top and office-based computers that can record client details and an analysis of nurses' workload. As the NHS network expands, all health-care workers are able to access electronic records, email and increasingly the World Wide Web. This will provide nurses with rapid access to client data such as previous nursing records. There are also currently a number of care-planning computer packages used by different NHS Trusts.

Computerised care-planning offers the nurse a number of advantages. It is quick, because there are a number of templates for common nursing diagnoses. Although these are sometimes criticised for moving towards a more communal rather than an individualised approach to nursing care, each of the templates has a menu of options that can be tailored to the individual client. The ability to raise at the push of a button a client's previous records is also an advantage and generally allows a more rapid search than does a paper-based system.

Computerised care-planning is, however, only as effective as the person who operates the system and generates the care plan. The skills of assessment, identifying nursing diagnoses and goal-setting, and the required nursing actions, can only be effective if the nurse has a sound knowledge base and uses the skills outlined within this chapter. The profession should, and indeed does, welcome the move to more electronic-based systems, if only because the approach is fast and usually efficient. The government has published its national programme for IT; a visit to its interactive website at www.connecting forhealth.nhs.uk is recommended in order to view the implementation plan and appreciate the rapid advances in this area. However, following the publication of the Coalition Government's White Paper (DoH, 2010) the future of a national approach to IT is under consideration.

> **✴ Activity 1.11**
>
> Review the assessment, nursing diagnosis, goal(s), planned care and method of implementation for your chosen client and then write an evaluation statement. Remember to ask the questions outlined in the text.

> **∞ Link**
>
> Chapter 19 has more information on computerised care planning and the use of IT in health care.

Chapter Summary

This chapter has introduced you to a systematic method for delivering nursing care through the framework known as the nursing process. You have been introduced to the five basic stages of assessment, diagnosis, planning, implementation and evaluation. Using the vehicle of structured activities, you have been offered the opportunity to develop a care plan for a chosen client.

At this stage, you may feel that the nursing process is a complex activity that demands a great deal of thought and practice, but your skills and experiences will continue to grow and develop as your professional career continues. Working through a structured chapter such as this is no substitute for practice and experience, but the principles of care-planning and the issues you need to consider are offered as the basis of accountable nursing practice. You may, for example, have been surprised at how complex and comprehensive the process of assessment is. The depth of material that you needed to collate when undertaking your assessment may have led you to reflect on the importance of probing and accurate questioning. As you progress in your chosen professional career, you will find that your ability to plan care will become greater. The important point to remember is that the whole practice and process of nursing is ever changing, new strategies, treatments and knowledge arriving almost daily. New research informs nursing practice and must be incorporated into one's professional repertoire. The process of nursing, like the process of learning, is an ongoing rather than a once-only activity.

? Test yourself!

1   Name the stages of the nursing process.
2   Give two reasons for using the nursing process.
3   What sort of information needs to be collected during a nursing assessment?
4   How many types of nursing diagnosis are there?
5   What are the two stages of the planning phase?
6   What criteria should goals conform to?
7   How can the nursing care plan be evaluated?

References

Audit Commission (1992) *Making Time for Patients: A Handbook for Ward Sisters*. HMSO, London.

Bellack, J.P. and Edlund, B.J. (1992) *Nursing Assessment and Diagnosis*, 2nd edn. Jones & Bartlett, London.

Darzi, Lord A. (2008) *High Quality Care for All* (Cm. 7432, 2008) [Internet], Department of Health, London. http://www.dh.gov.uk/en/Publicationsandstatistics/Publications/PublicationsPolicyAndGuidance/DH_085825 (accessed 29 June 2009).

DoH (Department of Health) (1994) *The Allitt Inquiry: Independent Inquiry Relating to Deaths and Injuries on the Children's Ward at Grantham and Kesteven Hospital during the Period February–April 1991* (Clothier Report). HMSO, London.

DoH (Department of Health) (2000) *Nurses, Midwives and Health Visitors (Training) Amendment Rules Approval Order 2000*. Stationery Office, London.

DoH (Department of Health) (2001) *Valuing People: A New Strategy for Learning Disability for the 21st Century*. Stationery Office, London. www.valuingpeople.gov.uk/dynamic/valuing-people136.jsp

DoH (Department of Health) (2008) *Refocusing the Care Programme Approach: Policy and Positive Practice Guidance*. DoH, London. http://www.dh.gov.uk/en/Publicationsandstatistics/Publications/PublicationsPolicyAndGuidance/DH_083647 (accessed 29 2009).

DoH (Department of Health) (2009) *Supporting People with Long-term Conditions: Commisioning Personalised Care Planning: A Guide for Commissioners*. DoH, London. http://www.dh.gov.uk/en/Publicationsandstatistics/Publications/PublicationsPolicyAndGuidance/DH_093354 (accessed 29 June 2009).

DoH (Department of Health) (2009a) *Valuing people now: a new three year strategy for people with learning disabilities*. DoH, London. http://www.dh.gov.uk/prod_consum_dh/groups/dh_digitalassets/documents/digitalasset/dh_093375.pdf (accessed 6 October 2010)

DoH (Department of Health) (2010). *Equity and Excellence: Liberating the NHS*. Cm 7881. London: Department of Health. Available at: www.dh.gov.uk/en/Publicationsandstatistics/Publications/PublicationsPolicyAndGuidance/DH_117353 (accessed on 5 October 2010).

DoH (Department of Health) (2010a) *Essence of Care 2010: Benchmarks for the fundamental*

aspects of care. DoH, London. http://www.
dh.gov.uk/prod_consum_dh/groups/
dh_digitalassets/@dh/@en/@ps/documents/
digitalasset/dh_119978.pdf (accessed 6
October 2010)

Drach-Zahavy, A. (2004) Primary nurses'
performance: role of supportive management.
Journal of Advanced Nursing 45(1): 7–16.

Hogston, R. (1997) Nursing diagnosis: a position
paper. Journal of Advanced Nursing 26:
496–500.

Holland, K., Jenkins, J., Solomon, J. and Whittam, S.
(2008) Applying the Roper-Logan-Tierney Model
in Practice, 2nd edn. Churchill Livingstone,
Edinburgh.

ICN (International Council of Nurses) (1999)
International Classification for Nursing Practice.
ICN, Geneva.

Iyer, P.W., Taptich, B.J. and Bernocchi-Losey, D.
(1995) Nursing Process and Nursing Diagnosis,
3rd edn. W.B. Saunders, Philadelphia.

Laakso, S. and Routasalo, P. (2001) Changing to
primary nursing in a nursing home in Finland:
experiences of residents, their family members,
and nurses. Journal of Advanced Nursing 33:
475–83.

Lidbetter, J. (1990) A better way to learn? Nursing
Times 86(29): 61–4.

McCaffery, M. and Beebe, A. (1999) Pain: Clinical
Manual for Nursing Practice, 2nd edn. Mosby,
St Louis.

Manley, K. (1990) Intensive care nursing. Nursing
Times 86(19): 67–9.

Manthey, M. (1992) The Practice of Primary
Nursing. King's Fund, London.

NHSE (National Health Service Executive) (1993)
Learning Disabilities. DoH, London.

NMC (Nursing and Midwifery Council) (2007)
Record Keeping. NMC, London. http://
www.nmc-uk.org/aDisplayDocument.
aspx?documentID=4008 (accessed 29 June
2009).

NMC (Nursing and Midwifery Council) (2008) The
Code: Standards of Conduct, Performance and
Ethics for Nurses and Midwives. NMC, London.
www.nmc-uk.org

NMC (Nursing and Midwifery Council) (2010)
Standards for pre-registration nursing education.
NMC. London. http://standards.nmc-uk.org/
Pages/Downloads.aspx (accessed 6 October
2010)

Roper, N., Logan, W. and Tierney, A. (2008) The
Roper-Logan-Tierney Model of Nursing Based
on Activities of Living. Churchill Livingstone,
Edinburgh.

Shoemaker, J. (1984) Essential Features of a Nursing
Diagnosis. In Kim, M.J., McFarland, G. and
McLane, A. (eds) Classification of Nursing
Diagnoses. C.V. Mosby, St Louis.

Walsh, M. and Ford, P. (1989) Nursing Rituals:
Research and Rational Actions. Butterworth
Heinemann, Oxford.

2

Social Behaviour and Professional Interactions

📖 Contents

- Therapeutic Communication
- Core Qualities
- Therapeutic Skills
- Working Together: People in Groups
- Being in Control Rather than Controlling
- Non-verbal Communication
- Chapter Summary
- Test Yourself!
- Further Reading
- References

☑ Learning outcomes

This chapter, concerned with one-to-one and group interactions, is divided into three sections. After reading through it, you should be able to:

- Describe the core qualities of therapeutic communication
- Identify six therapeutic interventions and suggest ways in which these might be implemented in your practice
- Describe the difference between primary and secondary groups
- Describe the interdependence of team, task and individual needs
- Discuss the importance of assertiveness to nursing practice
- Describe the process for refusing requests and handling criticism
- Reflect on further areas of study to enhance your own therapeutic communication skills.

The first section of this chapter examines **therapeutic communication**, or the **therapeutic** use of self. It will start by exploring the meaning of these terms before asking what qualities are required to enhance communication beyond just conveying information. The last part of this section will examine in more detail some of the tools available to start the process of developing good therapeutic skills that can be used with patients, families and colleagues.

Nurses seldom work in isolation but are more usually part of a specific group or team. Groups tend to have their own dynamics, and an understanding of how groups function can help in developing happier and more efficient teamwork. Nurses may work with a variety of diverse groups, for example support groups for patients, therapy groups, commonly found in mental health settings, and families, which form a special kind of group. The second section will examine some of the issues important to group dynamics. What constitutes a group? What sort of group are you likely to encounter? What is the role of nurses as group members? What makes effective teams and good leaders?

The third part of this chapter will examine a more specific aspect of interaction, building on some of the issues raised in the first section. Nurses are at the forefront of care and have an important role in liaising with an extremely wide range of people. In doing so, they sometimes have to deal with difficult situations. This section will examine how, through developing assertiveness, nurses can develop greater self-confidence and work more effectively towards positive working relationships and patient outcomes.

Throughout this chapter, the term 'nurse' will be used for the person who is the provider of the therapeutic communication. The nurse may be from any branch – mental health, learning difficulties or adult nursing. The terms 'client' and 'patient' are often used interchangeably, some branches using the term 'client' more freely than others. To avoid any confusion, the recipient of the therapeutic exchange will be referred to here as the client.

Finally, this chapter is not intended to be a training manual or a comprehensive guide to social interactions. Instead, it offers some signposts on which to base further study, investigation and development.

Therapeutic Communication

The term 'therapeutic communication' has been chosen rather than 'interpersonal skills' or 'counselling'. We all use interpersonal skills all the time whenever we are relating to another person, sometimes constructively, sometimes destructively. To be therapeutic, however, means to aid the well-being of an individual; thus, therapeutic communication has the intention of assisting or helping others.

There is evidence to suggest that the communication exchange between health-care professionals and clients, including relatives, is not always as good as it might be (Farrell et al., 2005; Healthcare Commission, 2007). There are many diverse and complex reasons for this. Perhaps the fact that we are all communicating all the time results in a feeling that we do not need to learn how to

therapeutic
aiding an individual's well-being

therapeutic communication
purposeful communication aimed at enhancing an individual's well-being

do something we have been doing all our lives: it seems to be common sense. Perhaps nurses have become complacent about communication. Furthermore, there is a tendency for some nurses to see themselves as people of action rather than words. Many nurses are not comfortable unless they are 'doing', a stance influenced by the ethos of today's clinical environment and the pressures of work. Hewison (1995) found support for the fact that many nurse–client interactions continue to be task oriented, routine and often superficial.

Nevertheless, nurses do express a desire to communicate well with clients; Buckroyd (1987) found that paediatric nurses wanted to be able to help children in distress but often felt ill-equipped to deal with these emotional and difficult interactions. Skilled therapeutic interventions can, as Wilkinson et al. (2008) point out, minimise the psychological morbidity associated with ill-health, and nurses are ideally placed to provide this kind of care to clients. Therapeutic communication is an essential and central aspect of nursing, whichever branch nurses specialise in.

The NHS Knowledge and Skills Framework (NHS KSF) sets communication as its first core dimension (DoH, 2004). The purpose of the NHS KSF is to define and describe the essential components of communication that NHS staff need to apply in their work if they are to deliver quality care. Within the communication dimension there are four levels:

1 Communicate with a limited range of people on day-to-day matters.
2 Communicate with a range of people on a range of matters.
3 Develop and maintain communication with people about difficult matters and/or in difficult situations.
4 Develop and maintain communication with people on complex matters, issues and ideas and/or in complex situations. (DoH, 2004)

Some of these will be explored in this chapter but the next section will focus primarily on the core qualities that underpin therapeutic communication and some of the skills that can assist in the process and practice of therapeutic communication.

> ✴ Activity 2.1
>
> Try to think of some scenarios that would be applicable to each of the levels of the communication core dimension.

Core Qualities

Three particular qualities have been identified as playing an important part in any therapeutic alliance:

1 Empathic understanding
2 Genuineness, or **congruence**
3 Unconditional acceptance.

> **congruence**
> a matching of inner feelings and outer behaviour

The requirement for these attributes was first identified in the context of counselling by Carl Rogers, the father of person-centred therapy. Rogers identified these three qualities as being necessary and sufficient to enable constructive personality change (Rogers, 1957). In other words, no other forms of therapeutic intervention are needed. This approach has had a considerable influence on nursing because of the control it gives back to clients, empowering them to make their own decisions and enabling their psychological growth. Nurses, however, do need many other communication strategies as usually nursing has a broader function than counselling alone. Nevertheless, these three core qualities are considered to be important components in the therapeutic relationship and lay the foundation on which other skills and strategies can be built. They are thus worthy of further explanation.

Empathic understanding

Empathic understanding is essentially a sensitivity for *what* another person is feeling but not for *how* he or she is feeling. You can never feel exactly the same as other people as their construction of the world will always differ from yours in some way. You can, however, be sensitive to what they are feeling and convey this to them in a way that helps them to feel someone has a valid insight into their world: they feel understood. Rogers (1980) describes empathy as 'a way of being with another person, entering into their world, communicating their sensings'. Nevertheless, it remains a difficult concept to understand and practise as it is more than just a communication process.

Egan (2004) defines two types of empathy: 'primary empathy' and 'advanced empathy'. The former is much more straightforward, although not necessarily simple. It involves listening carefully to what clients are saying and responding in a way that indicates an understanding of what they are saying from their perspective. The latter is a deeper kind of empathy more akin to reading between the lines, picking up not only what the client says, but also what lies behind it. As Rogers (1980) suggests, it is 'sensing meanings of which the client is scarcely aware'. This might usefully be compared with being a musician. Some musicians can read the score and play the notes in the correct sequence, but the highly skilled musician sees behind and beyond the notes, understanding the full expression of the music as intended by the composer. Developing these sensitivities appears to come more easily to some than others, but empathic understanding can be enriched with careful reflection on how you respond to clients. What is not required is some sort of phoney understanding. It is important to be genuine.

Genuineness

Genuineness is about being open and honest, and is sometimes referred to as congruence or authenticity. This is not to suggest that carers are being dishonest, but it is possible to be deceived about your feelings towards others. The professional mask often worn by nurses can distort the way of being with a client. Genuineness is less to do with telling untruths and more to do with having an openness, an attitude that conveys congruence between what you are thinking and feeling, and what you are saying. It is not hiding behind a uniform or a professional role: the very process of professionalisation can result in taking on a role that hides the self. Unfortunately, such a lack of genuineness often shines through to clients like a bright light, causing them to withdraw into themselves. Egan (2004) offers some guidance on developing an attitude of genuineness:

✱ Activity 2.2

Think of someone you know well and, in your mind, try to become that person. As that person, write a character sketch of yourself. In other words, try to see yourself through someone else's eyes.

empathic understanding
the ability to perceive accurately the feelings of another person and to communicate this understanding to him or her

genuineness
the ability to show oneself without putting on a façade

- *Not overemphasising the helping role:* and thus avoiding being patronising and condescending.
- *Being spontaneous:* this is not the same as overtly expressing all your current feelings, but it does mean not being afraid to express them when appropriate.
- *Not being defensive:* as a nurse, you will not always find that you are able to help, but getting to know your own strengths and weaknesses will enable you to be less defensive.
- *Being open:* when appropriate, do not be afraid to use your own life experience (see Nelson-Jones, 2005, for guidance on appropriate self-disclosure).

Much of being genuine is about having a better understanding of ourselves. Activity 2.3 and Figure 2.1 will give you some insight into your own experiences. If, for example, you have experienced a loss, this might help you to understand a client better, but it might also make you less tolerant of an angry client who reminds you of your own undealt-with anger.

Unconditional acceptance

Unconditional acceptance or unconditional positive regard is a frequently misunderstood quality. It can appear as if you must like everyone, regardless of what they have or have not done or who they are. Indeed, if you accept the statements above about genuineness, pretending that you like everyone means

POSITIVE
Start school (5)   Sister born (6)   Happy holiday (11)   Passes A levels (16)

Mum in hospital (7)   Had big argument with Dad (12)   Grandparent died (17)
NEGATIVE

Figure 2.1 Example of a life line (with age brackets)

that you are not being genuine. Unconditional acceptance, however, is about accepting clients as fellow humans entitled to care and respect, which is not the same as liking them as you do your friends or accepting their behaviour and value systems, which may be at odds with your own. As Mearns (2002) comments, 'Don't confuse unconditional positive regard with liking'. You may not like certain individuals, or their behaviour, but it is not for you to judge them, especially from your position as a carer. Developing the skill of acceptance depends very much on your ability to accept yourself. These are not easy qualities to cultivate or execute, although some nurses will find this easier than others. What is of concern is the way in which individuals often assume that they possess these qualities just because they have read about them, as if they develop through some osmotic process. These are qualities that take time to develop and must be practised. In reality, they are never fully available to us, so

---

Activity 2.3

Draw a life line similar to the one in Figure 2.1 and identify the positive and negative influences in your life. Think about how these events have helped to mould and create you, and how they might influence your relationship with your clients.

---

unconditional acceptance

an attitude that values the worth of another person

Link

Chapter 4 provides some guidelines on how to reflect on your practice.

we can only aspire to them. One way to start the process of developing them is to begin reflecting on our interactions with clients and colleagues.

These core qualities form an important element in developing a person-centred approach to care. This approach is one that holds the needs of the individual central and represents a shift in the view we hold of caring practices (Ford and McCormack, 2000). Talerico (2003) suggests that the key features of a person-centred approach are:

- Knowing the person as an individual and being responsive to individuals and family characteristics
- Providing care that is meaningful to the person in ways that respect the individual's values, preferences, and needs
- Viewing care recipients as biopsychosocial human beings
- Fostering development of consistent and trusting care-giving relationships
- Emphasising freedom of choice and individually-defined, reasonable risk taking
- Promoting physical and emotional comfort
- Appropriately involving the person's family, friends and social network.

These key features represent a whole philosophy of care and do not only relate to communication, but communication itself must adopt an approach that puts the patient and family at the centre of care. The following framework provides a valuable toolkit and is based on a humanistic approach that values a person's unique needs and preferences.

Therapeutic Skills

Heron (2001) has devised a simple but comprehensive model for therapeutic communication that is referred to as six-category intervention analysis. Within the six primary categories lie a wide range of more specific interventions; although the categories are considered to be exhaustive, the interventions are not and have the capacity for great flexibility. Heron (2001) emphasises that the categories are not a model of counselling but instead a set of analytical and behavioural tools. Many of the interventions are not uniquely identified by Heron, but he provides an effective framework, within which all six interventions, including those related to giving information and advice, can be used in one-to-one interactions. Figure 2.2 illustrates the six categories.

The first three categories – confronting, informative and prescriptive – are authoritative in that the nurse is taking greater responsibility for guiding the client's responses. The other three interventions are catalytic, cathartic and supportive, with facilitative interventions, the authority remains primarily with the client.

No single intervention is more important than any other, and none of the interventions seeks to control or take autonomy away from the client. Instead the emphasis is on developing an enabling relationship in which clients can explore their own worlds and make appropriate decisions for themselves.

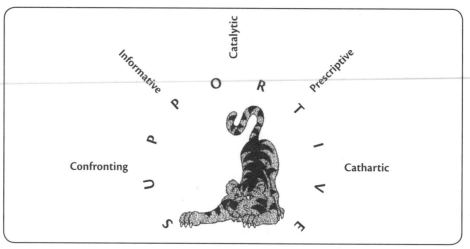

Figure 2.2 Six-category intervention analysis
Source: Adapted from Heron (2001).

Catalytic category

catalytic interventions
a set of basic
interventions that assist
the client with self-
discovery and learning

Although there is no hierarchy to the six categories, the **catalytic** category will be outlined first because it probably contains the most frequently used interventions. Heron describes catalytic interventions in terms of learning and problem-solving. These interventions enable clients to explore their thoughts and feelings, thus gaining insight and enabling them to be in a better position to make decisions about their future. The skill lies in effective listening and responding in ways that help clients to move on, but at their own pace and with their own agenda. This category requires the nurse to identify which intervention from the toolkit is most appropriate for assisting clients in this exploration. The following interventions will be outlined here: listening; simple and selective reflection; paraphrasing; open and closed questions; logical and empathic building; and checking for understanding.

Listening

Before you can listen to others, it is important to give the individuals concerned your full and free attention. This can be difficult if there is much going on in the immediate environment and your mind is focused on other issues. Heyes-Moore (2009) suggests that we have three modes of awareness; a *process mode*, an *inner awareness* and an *outer awareness*. When your awareness is on process, you are conscious of your thoughts and images; for example, you may be trying to interpret what the person has just said or thinking about your own past or future agendas. When your awareness is inside, you are aware of your own inner sensation: as you sit reading this book, you may be aware of your eyes straining to read the words on the page. If your awareness lies outside, you are focused on external events, what is going on outside you, such as listening to a client with your attention fully focused on him or her. If you can learn to distinguish between these zones of awareness, it is possible to use them more effectively, thus keeping your focus out and with the client, fleetingly changing the focus to fantasy to check out your own thoughts and occasionally being aware of your own internal sensations.

One way in which you can demonstrate your attention and interest in clients is by giving them quality time. Even if this is only a couple of minutes, it can be devoted to the client as quality time rather than being a rushed and haphazard event with you distracted by your surroundings and what is going on in your head. This, of course, takes practice, but giving quality time to others is one of the most important skills you can offer. In addition, your body language should convey the message that you are listening with interest to the client. Maintaining good eye contact, a relaxed open posture and a friendly and interested facial expression invites the client to talk to you. The occasional appropriate nod of the head indicates that you are listening and interested. Once you are giving clients your full attention, it is necessary to demonstrate that you are trying to understand their world from their frame of reference. In other words, you are being empathic rather than imposing your world, values, beliefs or judgements on the client.

Simple and selective reflection

Simple reflection, sometimes known as echoing, is helpful when the client appears stuck. It involves repeating the last word or few words back to the client with the same intensity of expression used by the client. The client may, for example, end the sentence saying, 'and I feel very unhappy'; you respond, 'You feel very unhappy', and the client is encouraged to continue the story, 'Yes, ever since…'. The difficulty in using this intervention is in deciding when it is appropriate and beneficial, as inappropriate use will simply annoy the client.

Selective reflection is similar, involving listening carefully for issues that seem to stand out as being significant and then feeding them back to the client without changing the content: 'You commented a moment ago about how angry you were with your mother.' This gives the client the opportunity to continue to develop this theme. Care must be taken not to direct the client down avenues of your own choosing rather than of the client's choice. It is easy to think that you know what the client's problem is, but in reality you will often be misguided in your assumption. In both simple and selective reflection, you should be listening for the emotionally charged words the client uses.

Paraphrasing

Paraphrasing is one way of conveying to clients that you have listened to them and have tried to grasp an understanding of what they are saying to you. When paraphrasing, you rephrase what the client has said in your own words. An example of this type of intervention might be:

Client: I'm very worried about my daughter. This problem has been going on for so long, I wonder if she will ever be the same again.

Nurse: It seems like there is no end to your daughter's problem and you're worried she will never be the little girl you used to know.

Open and closed questions

dichotomous
divided into two
separate groups

These **dichotomous** interventions are relatively simple but take practice to master. Open questions invite an open answer, whereas a closed question invites a closed answer. As an example of a closed question, 'Do you have pain?', invites a yes or no response, whereas 'How are you feeling?' invites a response much more of the client's choosing. Although it is rather simplistic, the 'who', 'what', 'where', 'when' and 'how' questions tend to elicit a more open response. The important word to be remembered here is 'invites': a closed question may instead receive an open response and an open question a closed one.

These questions are more appropriately seen as lying on a continuum of being more or less open; the more open they are, the greater the opportunity for client self-direction. The compulsive helper who tends to try to maintain control of the interaction more frequently asks closed questions. They can, however, be useful in eliciting specific information such as a name or telephone number. 'Why' questions should be used cautiously as they may alienate clients by forcing them to introspect inappropriately. After all, if they knew 'why', they would very often not need help.

Logical and empathic building

Logical building helps to develop a scaffolding for the client by bringing together salient points from the dialogue. Clients are often confused and appear to be rambling as they try to express their feelings; the nurse can assist by periodically marshalling the various points into some coherent order. For example, you might say, 'It seems as if these are your main concerns, Mr Jones. You are worried about how you will cope if you return to work and about who will take care of the children.'

Empathic building is rather like reading between the lines. As you carefully listen to what the client is saying, you are attempting to understand the feeling behind the words. It is important to use other cues such as tone of voice, eye contact and facial expression to help you to understand what the client might be experiencing. Your empathic understanding is then relayed to the client in the form of a statement: 'It sounds as if you are really hurting about…' or 'You are really frightened because…'.

Checking for understanding

It is very important to check periodically that you are, as fully as possible, understanding what the client is saying. This is especially important if you feel that you are becoming confused or if the client is giving contradictory messages. Clarifying the situation can prevent much misunderstanding and helps you to stay within the client's frame of reference.

Cathartic category

As a baby and during infancy, the tendency is to spontaneously give vent to emotions, be they of joy, grief, anger or fear. As you grow older, the responses become modified through modelling, learning or choice as you decide the best way to master life. You learn perhaps that it is wrong to cry and bad to express anger, that to be fearful might show weakness, or even that it is *not OK* to have fun and enjoy yourself. This may make it difficult to express yourself, particularly at times of crisis. The difficulty with helping others with their emotions is that you may not yet have come to understand your own repressed emotional world. It is one thing to intellectualise and say to the client that it is OK to cry, but if you are sitting there feeling uncomfortable with your own emotions, this may well be conveyed to the client. It is also unhelpful to coerce someone into expressing emotions, such as insisting on a bereaved person crying. Given time, space and permission, clients can choose when and how they want to express their emotions.

Working with emotions can be difficult and often requires specific training, but becoming more responsive to people's emotional needs does not require in-depth training. What it does require, however, is for you to become sensitive to your own emotions and those of your clients. The angry client may awaken memories of an angry parent in your life, or a dying client may provoke memories of an earlier loss. What makes you laugh, cry or get angry? Do you close down your emotions because it is easier that way and you stand less chance of getting hurt? The best way to help clients with their emotions is to be accepting of them and give them permission – permission to be angry parents when they find that their new baby has learning difficulties, permission to be afraid when they find out they have multiple sclerosis or cancer, permission to cry when old hurts are uncovered in a group therapy session, permission to feel relief when someone they love dies as their loved one has been released from suffering and they themselves from the burden of caring.

Touching, eye contact, listening, being with someone and giving permission are all ways of using **cathartic interventions**, but it is also important to be conscious of the cultural perspective. Touch may not be acceptable in some cultures, and eye contact may offend. Do not be afraid to check these things out. Does your eye contact cause the client to withdraw or become more responsive? Ask whether clients would like you to hold their hand.

cathartic interventions
interventions that seek to enable clients to let go of painful emotions including anger, fear, love and grief, thus releasing tension that has built up within them

Confronting category

Confronting interventions are involved with informing clients of what they are unaware of. Because of the nature of confrontation, the intervention may be received by clients with some degree of shock as they come face to face with issues that they were either not aware of or not acknowledging. For the nurse, the process of confrontation can also be uncomfortable. He or she is to some extent making an informed judgement that the client will benefit from the confrontation, but the nurse's fear of being wrong or managing the confrontation poorly can lead to anxiety about how to deliver the information. Furthermore, the nurse may become aware of feelings related to previous confrontations in his or her own life. These anxieties can lead the nurse to avoid the issue and 'beat around the bush' or alternatively take a very direct and heavy-handed approach. A more appropriate approach is to take control of these inner feelings

confronting interventions
interventions that directly challenge and heighten the client's awareness of restrictive attitudes, beliefs or behaviours of which he or she may be unaware

and get the confrontation right in order to convey the confrontation clearly and supportively.

What sorts of issue might be seen as confrontations? There are many potential examples, such as breaking bad news or raising awareness of attitudes and behaviours. The examples below give some indication of how confrontations can be used.

Breaking significant news is an example of a confronting intervention. Wilkinson et al. (2005) found considerable benefits to patients and practitioners when significant news was provided honestly and skilfully. However, you cannot alter the bad news as it remains bad news however it is broken, but you can break the news in a way that is supportive and gives the client a chance to absorb what is happening. Baile et al. (2000) provide a good description of Buckman's six-stage protocol for breaking bad news, called SPIKES:

⊂∞ Link

Chapter 13 discusses end-of-life issues.

- *Setting*: prepare clients for the news, offer them privacy and ensure that they are sitting down.
- *Perception*: assess what the patient already knows and understands.
- *Invitation*: find out what it is the patient wants to know. It is always best in these situations to 'lead from behind', allowing the patient to be in control of what information they want and at what depth.
- *Knowledge*: start by reinforcing the information the patient already knows and then build on this by giving the information in a simple, informative and unambiguous manner.
- *Emotions*: acknowledge the patient's response and provide appropriate support through touch, sensitive reflection and silence. Allow them time to take the news in, and as appropriate give them the choice of being alone or having someone remain with them.
- *Strategy and summary*: summarise the main points inculing any anxieties identified. Check if there are any remaining questions and prepare the patient for the next step and any help that may be available.

While giving significant news clearly confronts patients with news they were probably unaware of it also contains information giving and this is the next intevention we will explore.

Casebox 2.1

- In a group session, John appears to avoid talking about his feelings:
  'You have explained what you were thinking John, but what is it you are feeling?'
- Mr Patel does not appear to be taking responsibility for looking after his recently fashioned colostomy:
  'I notice you are always asking nurse Radley to change your colostomy bag'
- Fasia is a young woman with Down's syndrome who is preparing for her first job:
  'Fasia, are you aware that whenever someone speaks to you, you look away?'
  (The nurse demonstrates what Fasia may be unaware of)
- You notice that the parents of three-month-old Stephanie, admitted with a chest infection, are irregular visitors:
  'It seems you are unable to visit Stephanie very often.'

Informative category

Why do you need to give information? Clients clearly require information so that they can understand their illness or health problem. Without information, they are left groundless and are not in a position to make reasoned decisions about their care. It is important that information is given to help clients to understand and maintain control rather than this just being a duty of the health-care professional. It appears that most people want information about their illness, even if it is bad news (Meredith et al., 1996; Ley, 1988). It also seems that clients are reluctant to seek out information in health-care settings, often being afraid of wasting nurses' time, being unsure of whom or what to ask, or sometimes not being sure whether they *can* ask for information. It therefore falls to the health-care professional to ensure that quality information is delivered appropriately and in the client's best interest.

Informative interventions are often seen as the easiest to master. Most people feel that they are capable of providing information, but it is perhaps this confidence itself that results in a poor delivery of information. Although clients want and need information, it must be delivered at the right level in the right quantity and at the right time. Too many clients fail to understand the information given to them or forget what they have been told, especially if this is bad news (Ley, 1988). You may be able to remember occasions on which a lecture has been overloaded with information or delivered at a depth or in a manner that leaves you confused. The good lecture provides the right information at the right depth and at the right time in the course, perhaps leaving you to find something out for yourself. This last aspect is often important in mental health nursing, where you may wish to encourage clients to find out some information for themselves and take responsibility for doing so.

Prescriptive category

Prescriptive interventions are suggestions that might help in choosing a course of action from a number of options. One pitfall of this intervention is that it can be too prescriptive, thus removing control from the client. What health-care professionals believe is in the clients' best interests does not always relate to how clients themselves see the situation. Nevertheless, the nurse is in possession of much knowledge and may feel in some situations it is important to be more directive than in other situations such as stopping a diabetic client accidentally overdosing with an insulin injection. There will be times when clients make choices that seem eccentric but if they have mental capacity then they have every right to make such choices.

Supportive category

Supportive interventions underpin the use of all other interventions. Whatever intervention is being used, it should be used in such a way that supports the individual and is not in any way destructive. Heron (2001) identifies three ways

informative interventions
interventions that seek to impart new knowledge, information and meaning that are relevant to the client's needs

✱ Activity 2.5

For each of the six categories discussed above, give two or three examples of how you might constructively use them when interacting with actual clients or colleagues with whom you have worked.

∞ Link

Chapters 5 and 6 discuss safety issues. Chapters 3 and 13 outline the main features of the Mental Capacity Act.

prescriptive interventions
interventions that seek to suggest, advise or propose ideas to the client

supportive interventions
interventions encompassing an attitude of mind that unconditionally affirms the worth and value of the client

of using interventions. The first is a valid way that is appropriate to the needs of the client. In other words, it is the correct intervention delivered in the right way at the right time and in the correct manner. The second interventional style is degenerative, in which, despite good intention, intervention is used poorly because of a lack of skill, experience, self-awareness or a combination of all three. Finally comes a perverted intervention in which the intervention is used in a deliberately perverse way, to the detriment of the client.

Although the supportive category underpins all other categories, it is also a category in its own right. The interventions it encompasses involve the affirmation of others, being with them and demonstrating in a genuine way a care and concern for them. It may involve appropriate touch or appropriate self-disclosure. You demonstrate support for your clients when you willingly do things for them, when you greet them welcomingly and celebrate their achievements, however small these may appear to be. This should be conveyed in an unpatronising manner, and you must resist becoming overly nurturing, which may deny clients their independence. The three core conditions of empathy, being genuine and offering unconditional acceptance are central to the supportive category.

✸ Activity 2.6

Think of all the groups you belong to, both in and out of work. Choose two or three of these and consider what role you play in the group.

The above interventions provide a useful framework within which therapeutic communication can be developed. What has been presented here is an outline on which you can build. All the interventions can be developed and extended, requiring practitioners to research their use and practise their application if they are to be successfully employed.

Make a list of all the people that might go to make up an interdisciplinary team in your area of practice.

Working Together: People in Groups

As social animals, people tend to live in groups or be members of a group. There are a whole variety of different groups to which you might belong: you probably belong to a family, have a group of friends, perhaps belong to a club and maybe are a member of an organisation such as the Royal College of Nursing. You will belong to a large group called 'nurses', you may be a committee member, you are part of a work group in your clinical area and, as a student, you are part of a particular intake. Other groups you may come across may be study groups, rehabilitation groups and therapy groups. Nursing often involves working with a specific group or 'team' of nurses. They also form part of a larger group of health-care professionals that work together as the interdisciplinary team. A team is a group of people that have a common goal and need to work cooperatively to achieve that goal. The more effective the teamwork, the better the client care and the greater the satisfaction with your work role.

Belonging to a group has many benefits, such as a feeling of belonging, having a shared identity and the benefits of the support you receive from the group. There is a degree of security from being part of a group in which attitudes and values are similar and in which learning can take place. There is, however, also some cost to belonging to a group. You are expected to conform, and you may feel that you are surrendering some of your own personal identity.

The study of groups has interested psychologists and sociologists for a long time and has generated considerable research. This section will confine itself to some of the core issues of groups as a platform for further study.

What is a group?

Most people have a common concept of what a group is, and few of the examples above will be difficult for readers to identify as groups. It should also be evident that groups are very diverse and can vary considerably in their size and function, some being more formal than others. Because of this, definitions are not always helpful, and it is more productive to focus on some of the central characteristics of groups than on definitions. A principal feature of a group is that individuals believe themselves to be members of the group, there being some degree of interdependence and interaction.

Groups can be divided into primary and secondary groups. Secondary groups are usually considered to be larger, and their members have less direct contact. The hospital in which you work is a larger group, and you may never have contact with many of its members. Nursing as a profession is a large secondary group, as is a political party.

Primary groups tend to be closer and more intimate, all the members having face-to-face contact. Such groups might be family groups, friendship groups or small work groups. If you belong to a group, you probably have some expectations of that group, for example the way in which members are likely to behave, some of the attitudes you might expect them to hold and perhaps a code of conduct, be it explicit or implied. Nurses will be expected to have an attitude of caring and working in a manner that is in the best interests of the client. These expectations are known as **norms** and are attained through observation, experience and learning. Although there is invariably a degree of flexibility, it is also expected that all members of the group will more or less conform to these norms. Without some conformity, it would be very difficult to operate in a social world. We would be left with a sense of '**anomie**', bewilderment, with no frame of reference. Imagine what would happen if, each time you came to work, your group of nursing colleagues behaved radically differently, one day caring, the next not, sometimes wearing a uniform and sometimes casual clothes.

The group you work with in your clinical area is a formal primary group, and this group will have established a set of informal norms and expectations related to the group's behaviour. The degree to which members of the group uphold these norms is an indication of the cohesiveness of the group. The hierarchy may impose other, more formal norms, and it would be expected that these would be adhered to. Needless to say, these two sets of norms may on occasions clash, causing some discontent.

> ✷ **Activity 2.7**
>
> Make a list of the norms for your clinical area. A simple example may be whether or not you wear a uniform. What might be the consequences if the group ignored these norms?

norm
a shared way of behaving and thinking

anomie
lack of the usual social and ethical standards

Leadership of groups

Various research studies have identified different styles of leadership and their effectiveness (Lewin et al., 1939; Sayles, 1966; Fielder, 1971). These styles reflect the divide between being autocratic, when one person makes the decisions; democratic, when a consensus of opinion is sought; person-centred, in which the leader places greatest emphasis on people; and task-centred, in which the focus is on completing the task. These dimensions are probably best viewed as a continuum rather than as definitive styles of leadership. Good leaders, although they may have a predominant style, will adjust their leadership according to the situation (Bass, 1990). It is, for example, often important to be autocratic in a cardiac arrest situation, everyone needing to know exactly who is in charge and what needs to be done. On other occasions, such as when deciding on a new policy, a more democratic, person-centred style may be more productive, allowing for open discussion and the sharing of ideas.

Leaders may be emergent, elected or appointed. Emergent leaders are common in crisis situations or when no leader has previously been identified; elected leaders are common in political situations or on committees. In the case of a clinical area, there is usually an appointed leader, someone given the position because of his or her skills and qualifications. Although you may currently be a student, you will in due course become a staff nurse and will be expected to have some responsibility as an appointed leader.

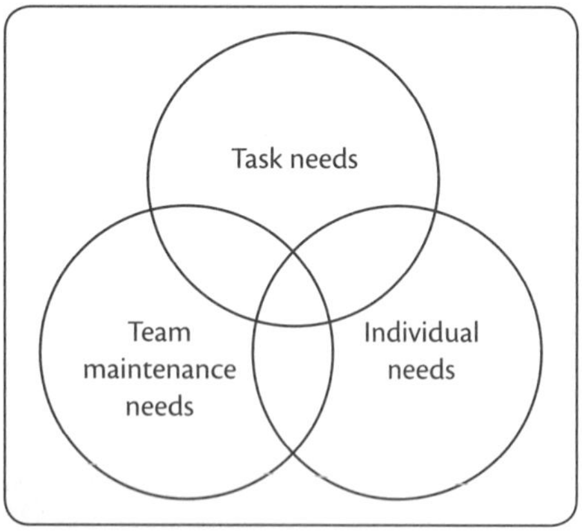

When a group comes together to achieve a common goal they are usually referred to as a team and Adair (2009), identifies three broad areas of need to be considered by the leader in order to maintain good teamwork. These are the 'team', the 'task' and the 'individual', each being equally important and interrelated, as shown in Figure 2.3. These three areas are now discussed in more detail.

> **Link**
>
> Chapter 20 discusses leadership skills.

Figure 2.3 Three circles model
Source: Adapted from Adair (2009).

Maintaining the team

A team is made up of individuals and as such takes on its own personality distinct from that of its individual members. One of the responsibilities of the leader is to form a cohesive team that will go forward together to meet the agreed objective without diminishing the individuality of its members. One of the difficulties often expressed by new staff nurses is how to manage an appropriate distance from the team, one that is neither over familiar nor too distant. One suggestion is that distance should be emphasised if the nurse was known to the staff before adopting the new position, if the nurse feels that staff are becoming over familiar and taking advantage of the situation, or when the leader is responsible for implementing unpopular decisions. Distance should be minimised when trying to establish and build trust, and if all members are roughly equal in knowledge and experience. The assertiveness skills referred to in the next section of this chapter should help in this respect.

Groups or teams take time to establish, and Tuckman (1965) suggests that, as groups develop, they pass through a series of stages. Being aware of these stages can help in understanding the progress of a group, and you may be able to identify some of these stages in relation to your group of students and how they have changed since commencing training. The four stages of forming, storming, norming and performing are shown in Chart 2.1.

Chart 2.1 Tuckman's four-stage group process

Forming	Storming	Norming	Performing
• The group meets • Trust is low • Little productive activity	• Alienation between members • Relationships are explored • Tension between individual and group needs	• The group settles down • Rules and roles established • The group begins productive work	• Acceptance and trust of group members • Cooperation between members • Productive work

Source: Adapted from Tuckman (1965).

This process is most clearly seen in the smaller groups that come together to achieve a given purpose, the groups and subgroups formed during nurse training being good examples of these. However, many other groups, such as the group you work with in the clinical area, go through similar stages, and this is often cyclical in nature as the environment and personalities change.

Maintaining the task

The task is the objective to be achieved by the group. Such objectives may be very varied, from the day-to-day care of individuals to establishing new **protocols** for working practices. The success of such endeavours may depend heavily on the team working together and will require clearly defined objectives. Imagine working with a team and trying to achieve some ill-defined goal. This will be not only inefficient, but also frustrating for the team members. When all the team members understand what is required of them and what their role is in achieving the aim, morale and enthusiasm for the task will remain high.

protocols
regulations or patterns of working

Maintaining the individual

All groups consist of individuals and as such have individual needs and individual skills. The leader must be careful not to undermine these needs but to encompass them; in this way, individuals can be valued and their skills used to maximum effect within the group. Meeting members' needs may be as simple as ensuring regular meal breaks or valuing them as individuals, providing security, trust and a sense of autonomy.

Leaders do not always of course select their own team members, and some members will need more support than others. Harkins (1987) has identified a phenomenon called social loafing in which some members of the group may do as little work as they can get away with. It is a bit like one member of a tug-of-war team appearing to pull but in fact not exerting any effort at all, the task then becoming far harder for the other members. By identifying each person's role, encouraging and monitoring progress, and encouraging group support, social loafing can be minimised.

✷ Activity 2.8

Think of a particular task you might want to achieve as a team, such as implementing a new ward procedure. Using Figure 2.3 above, blank out the Task area of the three circles. How will this influence achieving your objective? Now blank out the Team circle. How will this influence reaching your goal? Finally, blank out the Individual circle and carry out the same exercise.

Being in Control Rather than Controlling

assertiveness

a positive way of behaving in relationships that is based on honesty, openness and a respect for all parties

Assertiveness is sometimes confused with aggressiveness, arrogance and getting one's own way. It is not, however, about controlling others but about being in control of yourself. It is about respecting yourself and others, recognising that you have rights, including the right to be listened to, while remembering that others also have the same rights. It is about good, positive and equitable communication and negotiation so that both people in the interaction feel respected. It is working towards a win–win situation rather than a win–lose or lose–lose scenario. Some people find that being assertive comes quite naturally to them, others feel less confident and sometimes intimidated, whereas others become aggressive.

There are many reasons why people behave in the way they do, often related to learned behaviour during childhood. Some of the gendered messages commonly conveyed by parents, teachers and the media are shown in Table 2.1.

Table 2.1 Gendered behaviour messages

Male	Female
Be strong	Be gentle
Be successful at any cost	Be kind
Don't let people walk over you	Don't argue
Don't be weak	It is wrong to be angry
Stand up for yourself	It is selfish to think of yourself
Be in control	

⊘ Link

Chapter 15 explores gender issues.

Those in the first column have traditionally been the messages conveyed to boys and those in the second column the messages to girls. Men traditionally strive to win and see compromise or giving in as weakness and failure. Women have tended to acquiesce, being afraid to speak out, especially on their own behalf. The young are often told not to answer back, to have respect for authority, but although this may be valid, what they are not told is how to be heard while still being respectful to others, whoever the others may be. The messages in either of the columns may of course apply to either sex, and not all women become passive or all men aggressive.

transactional analysis

a theory of personality and an approach to communication that promotes personal growth and change

The 'I'm OK, you're OK quadrangle', taken from **transactional analysis** and shown in Figure 2.4, gives us a picture of the different ways in which people may have learned to respond as a result of childhood experiences. In quadrant 1, the aggressive person does not really care about the rights or feelings of the other person: the 'I'm all right Jack' syndrome. In quadrant 2, the person puts himself down; he may be fearful of hurting or offending others and tends to believe that others are better, echoing the 'children should be seen and not heard' approach. This person may be liked but not respected, or may be seen as weak and used by others. In the third quadrant, the person is deceitful. He may be complimentary to others or full of excuses and apologies; before you know where you are, you are doing something for him that you did not really want to do. You suddenly

1 AGGRESSIVE I'm OK but you are not OK	2 SUBMISSIVE/PASSIVE I'm not OK but you are OK
3 MANIPULATIVE I'm OK and I'll let you think you're OK but really I don't believe you are	4 ASSERTIVE I'm OK and you're OK

Figure 2.4 The 'I'm OK, you're OK' quadrangle

feel cheated and not quite sure how you got into that situation. The assertive person, shown in quadrant 4, cares both about himself and about others. He speaks clearly about his wants and needs in an unambiguous way but also listens to the needs and wants of others. Although some people's behaviour very obviously matches one of these quadrants, it is more common to take something from each of the four quadrants. It is more usual for us to be able to be assertive in some situations and not others. Some people are assertive at home or with their friends and relations but not assertive at work. Others may be assertive at work but struggle to be assertive in their private lives.

Why assertiveness?

Although assertiveness is important for any group, nurses have been identified as a group that finds being assertive difficult (McCartan and Hargie, 1990). This might be attributable to being a profession whose principal purpose is to care for others. Furthermore, nursing has historically had a tradition of duty and subservience. Becoming more assertive is, however, important for two main reasons. The first is to promote mental health in that non-assertive behaviour can lead to being pushed aside and not listened to, or to being labelled aggressive. Indeed, these have been some of the common stereotypical portrayals of nurses: the submissive, dutiful carer or the dominant, matronly figure. Both these approaches can lead to increased stress and loss of confidence for the nurse, whereas being assertive earns respect from others and an increase in self-confidence.

Second, being assertive is important for the sake of those for whom the nurse is caring and for colleagues and staff working alongside the nurse. It enables the nurse to be in a position to be an advocate for the client, whether in relation to a client's direct care or indirectly by challenging working practices. Staff working relationships can be one of the greatest stresses for health-care workers, but by caring for one another, by being open and respectful, working relationships will be enhanced. Hargie et al. (1994, p. 273) identify seven functions of assertiveness that will help individuals to:

- Ensure that their personal rights are not violated
- Withstand unreasonable requests from others

✴ Activity 2.9

Try to identify situations in which you find it easy to be assertive and ones in which you find it difficult. Ask yourself what it is about these situations that makes it easier or harder.

- Make reasonable requests of others
- Deal effectively with unreasonable refusals from others
- Change the behaviour of others towards them
- Avoid unnecessary aggressive conflicts
- Confidently, and openly, communicate their position on any issue.

Enhancing your assertiveness skills

There are five principles central to being assertive:

1 *Listen carefully to what the other person has to say:* this immediately shows some respect for the other person's opinion and feelings. Furthermore, you have the information you need rather than defensively jumping to conclusions.
2 *Say what you think and feel:* your feelings and thoughts are as important and relevant as anyone else's. You have the right to be heard.
3 *If appropriate, say what you want to happen:* without this, the other person is left guessing what you want. It is important here to be specific.
4 *Be persistent:* do not be side-tracked or wrong-footed but stay with the issue in hand, repeating it if necessary until the issue has been satisfactorily addressed.
5 *Be prepared to compromise:* this must be done from a position of choice to bring about a satisfactory conclusion for all involved rather than because of coercion or 'just for a quiet life'.

Non-verbal Communication

non-verbal communication
communicating without the use of spoken language, for example by gestures, body posture and facial expression

In addition to these central aspects, it is important to project yourself in a positive manner using your body language and **non-verbal communication**. It is no good saying the right things if your body language does not complement your words. Birdwhistell (1970) estimates that up to 70 per cent of social interactions are conveyed via a non-verbal channel; therefore, if your non-verbal communication conveys aggression or passivity, that is what the receiver will be aware of no matter what you are saying.

Positive communication requires positive non-verbal communication. It is of course important to take into account cultural differences in body language, in which eye contact, proximity and touch may be very different. In principle, eye contact should be direct and appropriate rather than aggressive staring or passive avoidance. Good eye contact demonstrates that you are interested in the other person and have nothing to hide. An individual's personal space is also important. We usually stand closest to those with whom we are most intimate and furthest away during normal social encounters (Hall, 1966). Standing inappropriately close can be threatening, whereas standing too far off can be interpreted as withdrawing. Your posture should be upright and open, with an absence of any gestures that could be interpreted as being aggressive, such as finger-pointing, folded arms or the hands on the hips. The tone of voice should be firm but relaxed and gentle. A good understanding of non-verbal communication can enhance interactions, and it is worthwhile taking the time to consider how you use non-verbal communication and to observe how others use it.

Assertiveness techniques

Two aspects of assertiveness will be outlined here – saying no to a demand and managing critism – both of which can be potentially difficult to manage.

Saying no

Saying no can be particularly difficult for some people. It often raises old anxieties, reminders of when people have said no to us, particularly as children. There is often an underlying fear of hurting or offending others. Furthermore, if you say no, they may not like you, and the feeling of rejection can be painful and frightening. Simply agreeing to a request when you do not want to can, however, mean being taken for granted and used by others. It can also mean not respecting the other person's ability to accept the refusal. Remember that you have the right to say no without feeling guilty. It is the request rather than the person that is being turned down. Nevertheless, some people do seem to have difficulty in understanding that no means no, so unfortunately it is sometimes necessary to be persistent and explicit in saying no.

Before saying no, take time to consider the request. You may, for example, say, 'Can I come back to you in five minutes?' or 'Can I consult my diary before I give you an answer?' If you really do want to say no, say it clearly and unambiguously. You do not have to give a reason, but if it helps then do so, providing that it does not undermine your decision. Remember that it is your choice whether to say yes or no. It is the act of choosing that is so important; you do not then feel that you have been railroaded into a decision or have backed down when you really wanted to say no. Once you have made your decision, you must stick to it; two techniques can help in sticking to the point.

- *The broken record*. This really is just repeating what you have already said. If, for example, your manager asks you to do an extra shift but you already have a prior appointment, you may, after careful consideration, say, 'No, I can't do that shift; I have already made other arrangements.' But your manager persists. You can respond by saying, 'As I said, I have made other arrangements and I am not able to do that shift.' Remember that this should not be conveyed in an aggressive manner but in a firm and respectful one. In some cases, it may be necessary to repeat yourself several times to reinforce the message, and you should try to use some of the same words each time so that you do not become diverted.
- *Fielding the response*. This is in some ways similar to the above, but it involves a summarising technique as well as sticking to and repeating your statement. This summarising can be important because it conveys to others that you have heard them and understand their point of view. In the following example, you acknowledge the other person's difficulty and indicate that you would be willing to help if you could, but you also make it clear that

> ✳ Activity **2.10**
>
> If you find it difficult to use your voice assertively, choose a range of scenarios and try verbalising your response to yourself until you get a feel for the right manner and tone of voice. If possible, stand up and speak into a tape-recorder.

you have needs of your own and these, too, should be respected: 'No, I can't work that shift. I realise that you are short of nurses for this shift and if I could help I would, but as I have said, I have made other arrangements.'

Managing criticism

Managing criticism is included here because nurses, along with many other professionals, receive criticism as part of their everyday lives. Criticism can be positive if handled well but a source of hurt and anger if it is not constructively imparted. Given constructively, criticism can help you to reflect on your practice and, if appropriate, modify and enhance it.

There are basically three possible responses to criticism. First, the criticism may be *invalid*, in which case you can reject it. Second, it can be *valid*, in which case you can accept it. Third, it can be *partly valid*, in which case you can accept the valid aspects and reject the invalid ones (Bond, 1986). Before any judgement can be made, you must, however, listen to the criticism. Do not reject it immediately; if necessary, ask for time to think about what you have been told.

Some examples may help to illustrate the three responses.

1 **Invalid**
   Staff nurse to student: 'You don't attend any of the ward rounds.'
   Student: 'I do; in fact I have been on every ward round that has taken place when I have been on duty.'

2 **Valid**
   Staff nurse to student: 'Nurse Kahn, you have forgotten to attend to Mrs Walmsley's dressing.'
   Student: 'Yes I have, I'm sorry. I will go and do it as soon as I have finished this.'

3 **Partially valid**
   Staff nurse to student: 'Nurse Reid, you're always late for these meetings.'
   Student: 'I am late for this meeting and I apologise, but in fact I have been here on time for all the other meetings.'

Fogging

A useful technique to use when you feel that you are being attacked is that of fogging. Fogging tends to slow the other person down and gives you time to formulate a response. There is often an expectation on the part of the person attacking you that you will immediately disagree, but if you agree in part with what they are saying, this tends to draw them from their critical parental stance to a more adult one. An example may help to illustrate this. After you have been in the difficult situation of breaking bad news to a client, the charge nurse sees the client crying and appears to blame you: 'What have you said to Ms Bland? You have obviously upset her.' You might respond by saying, 'Yes, she is very upset; I have just explained to her …'. Here, you are not agreeing that it is your fault, but you do agree that Ms Bland is upset. The scene is then set for more constructive dialogue to take place between you and the charge nurse.

Conclusion

The very notion of assertiveness can alienate some people. This may be because of their misunderstanding of assertiveness or because of their observations of people who claim to have been on an assertiveness course. It is, in essence, just good, caring communication, communication that respects one's autonomy and the autonomy of others. The techniques involved in being assertive are relatively straightforward, but changing your behaviour may be less easy. Assertiveness training rarely addresses the archaic reasons why you as an individual communicate the way you do. This is not to say that you cannot improve your communication skills through being assertive, but this needs to be carried out alongside developing your own self-awareness. It may, however, take time and practice to adjust the way in which you present yourself. Taking small steps in situations you can cope with will be more rewarding than trying to change overnight. Use your reflective practice to examine your own behaviour, and consider situations in which you were assertive and in which you wish you had been more assertive.

> **⊂⊃ Link**
>
> Chapter 4 discusses reflective practice.

Chapter Summary

Despite the research suggesting most complaints in the NHS are about poor communication there are many examples of good communication and excellent care. But your ability to be with people who are suffering needs to be nurtured and your communication skills developed. Clients need more than scientific intervention as part of their care, they need compassionate caring and need to be heard. Whatever your chosen branch, your skills must include an expertise in open and caring communication with clients, families and colleagues. It is possible to enhance your communication style and develop good therapeutic communication skills supported by research-based theory. This chapter has only allowed a glimpse into the world of social and professional interactions but provides a basis for further study, reflective practice.

? Test yourself!

1 Name the three core qualities that are necessary for personal growth and change.

2 Name the six categories of Heron's six-category intervention analysis and give examples of how these may be used in your area of practice.

3 Give five interventions that could be used in the catalytic category.

4 What does the acronym SPIKES stand for in breaking bad news?

5 List seven members of the interdisciplinary team in your area of practice.

6 Describe what is meant by a 'primary group' and a 'secondary group'. Give two examples of each.

7 Describe the elements of the Three Circles model.

8 What are the four stages that Tuckman suggests groups move through as they establish themselves?

9 There are four ways to respond in an interaction, one of which is by being manipulative. What are the other three?

10 What are the five principal ways of being assertive?

11 How are you going to develop the themes described in this chapter?

The following books will help to develop the themes referred to in this chapter.

The core conditions

Mearns, D. and Thorne, B. (2007) *Person-centred Counselling in Action,* 3rd edn. Sage, London.
Rogers, C.R. (1980) *A Way of Being* Houghton Mifflin, New York.

Therapeutic interventions

Communication Skills for Nursing Practice
Culley, S. and Bond, T. (2004) *Integrative Counselling Skills,* 2nd edn. Sage, London.
Heron, J. (2001) *Helping the Client: A Creative Practical Guide.* Sage, London.
Adair, J. (2009) *Effective Leadership*: *How to Be a Successful Leader.* Pan Books, London.
Niven, N. (ed) (2006) *The Psychology of Nursing Care,* 2nd edn. Palgrave Macmillan, Basingstoke.
Assertiveness
Back, K. and Back, K. (2005) *Assertiveness at Work: A Practical Guide to Handling Awkward Situations.*
   McGraw-Hill, Berkshire.

Further Reading

For live links to useful websites see: www.palgrave.com/nursinghealth/hogston

References

Adair, J. (2009) *Effective Leadership: How to Be a Successful Leader.* Pan Books, London.

Baile, W.F., Buckman, R., Lenzi, R., Glober, G., Beale, E.A., and Kudelka, A. P. (2000) SPIKES: a six-step protocol for delivering bad news: application to the patient with cancer. *Oncologist* **5**: 302–31.

Bass, B.M. (1990) *Handbook of Leadership: Theory, Research and Managerial Applications*, 3rd edn. Collier-Macmillan, London.

Birdwhistell, R.L. (1970) *Kinesics and Context.* University of Pennsylvania Press, Philadelphia.

Bond, M. (1986) *Stress and Self-awareness: A Guide for Nurses.* Heinemann Nursing, London.

Buckroyd, J. (1987) The nurse as counsellor. *Nursing Times* **83**: 42–4.

DoH (Department of Health) (2004) Agenda for Change Project Team, *The NHS Knowledge and Skills Framework and the Development Review Process.* Appendix 2. Core Dimension 1: Communication: Department of Health, London.

Egan, G. (2004) *Skilled Helper: A Problem Management and Opportunity Development Approach to Helping,* 7th edn. Wadsworth Publishing, Kentucky.

Farrell, C., Heaven, C., Beaver, K. and Maguire, P. (2005). Identifying the concerns of women undergoing chemotherapy. *Patient Education and Counseling* **56**: 72–7.

Fielder, F.E. (1971) Validation and extension of the contingency model of leadership effectiveness: a review of empirical findings. *Psychological Bulletin* **76**: 128–48.

Ford, P. and McCormack, B. (2000) Keeping the person in the centre of nursing. *Nursing Standard* **14**(46): 40–4.

Hall, E.T. (1966) *The Silent Language.* Doubleday, New York.

Hargie, O., Saunders, C. and Dickson, D. (1994) *Social Skills in Interpersonal Communication.* 3rd edn. Routledge, London.

Harkins, S. (1987) Social loafing and social facilitation. *Journal of Experimental Social Psychology* **23**: 1–18.

Healthcare Commission (2007) *Spolight on Compliant.* Commission for Healthcare Audit and Inspection, London.

Heron, J. (2001) *Helping the Client: A Creative Practical Guide.* Sage, London.

Hewison, A. (1995) Nurses' power in interaction with patients. *Journal of Advanced Nursing* **21**: 75–82.

Heyes-Moore, L. (2009) *Speaking of Dying: A Practical Guide to Using Counselling Skills in Palliative Care.* Jessica Kingsley, London.

Lewin, K., Lippitt, R. and White, R. (1939) Patterns of aggressive behaviour in experimentally created 'social climates'. *Journal of Social Psychology* **10**: 271–99.

Ley, P. (1988) *Communicating with Patients.* Croom Helm, London.

McCartan, P.J. and Hargie, O.D.W. (1990) Assessing assertive behaviour in student nurses: a comparison of assertion measures. *Journal of Advanced Nursing* **15**: 1370–76.

Mearns, D. (2002) *Developing Person-centred Counselling*, 2nd edn. Sage, London.

Meredith, C., Symond, P., Webster, L., Lamont, D., Pyper, E., Gillis, C.R. and Fallowfield, L. (1996) Information needs of cancer patients in West Scotland: cross sectional survey of patients' views. *British Medical Journal* **313**: 724–6.

Nelson-Jones, R. (2005) *Practical Counselling and Helping Skills*, 5th edn. Sage, London.

Rogers, C.R. (1957) The necessary and sufficient conditions of therapeutic personality change. *Journal of Consulting Psychology* **21**(2): 95–103.

Rogers, C.R. (1980) *A Way of Being*. Houghton Mifflin, New York.

Sayles, S.M. (1966) Supervisory style and productivity: review and theory. *Personnel Psychology* **19**(3): 275–86.

Talerico, K.M. (2003) Person-centered care: An important approach for 21st century health care. *Journal of Psychosocial Nursing & Mental Health Services* **41**(11): 12–16.

Tuckman, B.W. (1965) Development sequence in small groups. *Psychological Bulletin* **63**(6): 384–99.

Wilkinson, S.M., Fellowes, D. and Leliopoulou, C. (2005) Does truth-telling influence patient's psychological distress? *European Journal of Palliative Care* **12**(3): 124–6.

Wilkinson, S., Perry, R. and Blanchard, K. (2008) Effectiveness of a three-day communication skills course in changing nurses communication skills with cancer/palliative care patients: a randomised controlled trial. *Palliative Medicine* **22**: 365–75.

3

Challenges to Professional Practice

📖 Contents

- Introduction
- The Professional Context of Nursing Practice
- The Responsibilities of Professional Practice
- Confidentiality
- Consent
- Working with Others
- Professional Accountability
- Evidence-based Practice
- Reflective Practice
- Caring with Integrity

- Cultural Competence in Health Care
- Quality, Performance and Choice
- The NHS Constitution for England
- Clinical Governance
- Chapter Summary
- Test Yourself!
- Further Reading
- References

☑ Learning outcomes

At the end of the chapter, you should be able to:

- Define professional practice and explore the responsibilities involved
- Describe the professional context of practice as detailed in the NMC Code
- Describe the role that personal values play in underpinning practice and decision-making
- Appreciate how the nurse's role as caregiver takes place within a dynamic system of health-care delivery
- Describe how standards of practice are maintained through the codes that guide nursing practice, governance and choice
- Identify sources of information on patients' rights.

Introduction

The title of this chapter, 'challenges to professional practice' has been chosen to reflect the realities of modern professional practice. When nurses undertake their roles and responsibilities they will encounter situations that are both intellectually and practically demanding. Each situation will often require immediate and well-considered professional judgements to be made.

The aim of this chapter is to enable the nurse to understand and navigate through the many professional, statutory and policy considerations that impact on their decision-making. Commencing with an analysis of the meaning of professionalism and professional practice, the chapter explores the philosophical principles that underpin the Nursing and Midwifery Council (NMC) Code of conduct, known as *The Code: Standards of Conduct, Performance and Ethics for Nurses and Midwives* (NMC, 2008). Particular reference is made to consent, confidentiality and capacity and the implications for nurses' professional accountability.

Drawing on contemporary professional and policy initiatives, examination is made of such concepts as evidence-based and values-based practice, standards, quality and choice, multi-professional practice and governance. Reference to the policy origins of these ideas will be made, along with consideration of key legislation that shapes the landscape of practice which includes the laws on consent, freedom of information and data protection.

While no single chapter can capture all the challenges that the nurse might face in practice, through clearly stated learning outcomes and a selection of reflective activities, the reader is at least armed with a greater awareness and deeper appreciation of the context of modern health-care practice and thus more prepared for the challenges they will encounter.

The Professional Context of Nursing Practice

The practice-based discipline of nursing, conducted within a modern health-care environment, is an exciting and hugely rewarding experience for the practitioner. Delivering effective nursing care, however, in a professional and thoughtful way, within an increasingly complex and diverse practice environment, requires considerable personal awareness as well as extensive discipline, knowledge and skill. The process of nursing is guided and influenced by many professional, statutory and policy factors that can have a direct and immediate impact on the outcomes for clients and their families or carers. The effective nurse needs to understand what it means to deliver professional practice within this constantly changing environment.

What Is Professional Practice?

To be a professional is to be engaged in activities that are guided by a body of knowledge and evidence. The growing body of 'evidence' for nursing practice blends knowledge from a wide range of disciplines, across the life and social sciences, to develop unique research questions focused on nursing practice problems. The nurse's role is to exercise professional judgement in the application of this knowledge to situations encountered in practice.

The Responsibilities of Professional Practice

The regulatory body overseeing nursing and midwifery is the Nursing and Midwifery Council (NMC), which was established in 2002. The NMC's stated purpose is to 'safeguard the health and well-being of the public' (www.nmc-uk. org). The core functions are to:

1   Register nurses and midwives and ensure that they are properly qualified and competent to work in the UK.
2   Set the standards of education, training and conduct that nurses and midwives need to deliver high-quality health care consistently throughout their careers.
3   Ensure that nurses and midwives keep their skills and knowledge up to date and uphold the standards of their professional Code.
4   Establish fair processes to investigate allegations made against nurses and midwives who may not have followed the Code.

The full NMC remit is set out in the Nursing and Midwifery Order 2001.

In order to meet these functions the NMC publishes a wide range of guidance for professionals, employers and the public, explaining the standards nurses are expected to achieve. The focus of this next section is to consider in more detail the third item, namely to uphold the standards of the professional Code.

> **✴ Activity 3.1**
>
> Access and explore the NMC Code at the NMC website, www.nmc-uk.org. Discuss your findings with your mentor in practice.

Philosophy of practice

In order to carry out their practice effectively the judgements, exercised by the nurse, need to be informed by an explicit set of professional values that unify practice around a common set of behaviours. It is also important for nurses to appreciate the philosophical underpinnings of their profession and be conversant with the values and performance expectations to which all nurses subscribe. Being familiar with these expectations will enable the nurse to practise confidently and navigate their way through challenging situations.

In this context, the term 'philosophy' is used as it relates to certain knowledge, thought, and meaning that in turn relates to a particular system of beliefs or values. For the nurse it concerns the ideas or beliefs that underpin everyday nursing practice. A particularly relevant branch of philosophy is ethics. Ethics seek to address questions of morality. In other words how the right decisions can be made to achieve the right outcomes for patients.

Practice ethics are concerned with doing the right thing for the patient and their families, which on the face of it, sounds straightforward. So often nurses are faced with decisions that result in having to choose between two or more equally valid options. Ethical practice requires the nurse to consider the benefits or risks of taking decisions within their particular field of practice. To illustrate this dilemma let's consider the following simple but common scenario within Activity 3.2.

The NMC (2008) Code adopts what is known as a deontological perspective. This means it is based on the rights of the individual, which are often legal rights, and the responsibilities or duties of the nurse, in other words those behaviours expected of a professional nurse. The Code uses the ethical principles of respect for the person (autonomy), the obligation to maximise benefit (beneficence), to avoid harm and keep people safe (non-maleficence) and the responsibility to treat everyone equally and ensure that they are informed of their rights (justice).

The Code (NMC, 2008), as currently configured, is broadly divided into four sections concerned with care for the individual, working with others, standards of practice and professional behaviour. As we go through the chapter the implications of each of these will be considered in turn. However, as you will see, each section should not be viewed in isolation as so often nursing decisions require us to take account of several factors simultaneously.

The first part of the Code, outlined in Chart 3.1, states that the nurse must 'Make the care of people your first concern, treating them as individuals and respecting their dignity'.

Chart 3.1 Make the care of people your first concern, treating them as individuals and respecting their dignity

• Treat people as individuals	• Ensure you gain consent
• Respect people's confidentiality	• Maintain clear professional boundaries
• Collaborate with those in your care	

Source: NMC (2008) *The Code*. Reproduced with kind permission of the NMC.

So how does the Code help to resolve the dilemma arising from the scenario in Activity 3.2? The clinical principles outlined above make it very clear that the first concern is to the individual receiving care and that the nurse must, among other things, respect their right to confidentiality. Therefore it is clear that the nurse should not disclose confidential information about the patient concerning diagnosis, treatment or prognosis, even if it is to a close family member. It also indicates that the nurse would need to obtain consent and ensure that the individual who lacks capacity, in this case Emily, is at the centre of decision making about their care. However, bluntly responding to Dora stating that the nurse cannot divulge any information would not be a satisfactory outcome for Dora or indeed potentially Emily's future care. Let's consider confidentiality and consent in more detail.

Confidentiality

Out of concern for patient confidentiality the Department of Health (DoH, 2003, p. 7) published clear guidance in the form of a code of practice for anyone who works in the National Health Service. The duty of confidence is where any persons shares information with another in a situation where it is 'reasonable to expect' the information will remain confidential. The DoH (2003) further outlines four components of a confidential service as outlined in the model (Figure 3.1).

✹ Activity 3.1

Scenario: You are a nurse looking after Emily who is an 88-year-old lady. She is a widow with one very close relative, Dora, her 82-year-old sister. Emily has been admitted recently having had a stroke and is not currently conscious. You receive a phone call from Dora, who is very caring and concerned, asking how her sister has been. She asks what is wrong with Emily and the likely prognosis, as she wants to make appropriate plans.

You are faced with the dilemma of supporting Dora, who is clearly concerned and distressed, but at the same time you are required to protect Emily's right to privacy and dignity. What would you do and why?

The answer is in the main text of this chapter.

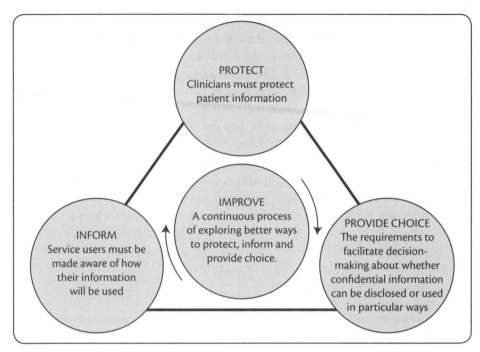

Figure 3.1 The confidentiality model

Source: DoH (2003). Reproduced with kind permission of the Department of Health.

English common law also protects the individual's right to confidentiality although there are two exceptions to this. First, public interest – for example, a health professional passing information to the police if the patient is felt to be a danger to the public. Secondly, where a disclosure of confidential information is required by court order. In Scotland national guidance has been issued to NHS board's Healthcare Policy and Strategy Directorate (2008), which outlines the arrangements to follow where a patient is suspected of a criminal act. Other legislation that concerns the protection of personal information is the Data Protection Act 1998 and the Freedom of Information Act 2000.

Data Protection Act

To emphasise the importance of the protection of personal data, the Data Protection Act 1998 established rules that prohibit the misuse of personal information by any organisation. The eight Data Protection Principles, listed below, provide essential protection personal data.

The Data Protection Principles require personal information to be:

- fairly and lawfully processed
- processed for limited purposes
- adequate, relevant and not excessive
- accurate
- not kept longer than necessary
- processed in accordance with the individual's rights

🔗 Link

Chapter 19 also discusses the Data Protection Act 1998 and Freedom of Information Act 2000.

- kept secure
- not transferred abroad without adequate protection. (adapted from http://www.direct.gov.uk/en/RightsAndResponsibilities/DG_10028507)

The Freedom of Information Act 2000

The Freedom of Information Act 2000 actually came into force in 2005. Importantly it provides the right for any citizen to ask public bodies for information held on any subject. The organisation must provide the information within a month. This means patients may also ask for copies of all personal information that public bodies may hold on them. The overall purpose of this legislation is to foster openness and accountability. Scotland has a similar Act to England, Wales and Northern Ireland. It is therefore important for the nurse to understand how to respond to a member of public who makes such a request in order to avoid any breach of the law. More information can be found at: www.direct.gov.uk.

Consent

Understanding the principles of consent, in particular the need for informed consent, when providing any form of care or treatment, is an essential component of practice. The Royal College of Nursing (RCN, 2005) provide a helpful definition of informed consent:

> an ongoing agreement by a person to receive treatment, undergo procedures or participate in research, after risks, benefits and alternatives have been adequately explained to them. (RCN, 2005, p. 3)

In principle this seems fairly straightforward but it becomes particularly challenging when caring for vulnerable individuals, adults or children, whose cognitive ability may be impaired developmentally due to a learning difficulty or illnesses such as dementia.

Informed consent is only achieved when the person has been given full information and understands the procedures they are due to undergo. Therefore the patient needs to have time to process the information. The concept of informed consent is a legal term reflecting an individual's right to receive information prior to receiving treatment. There is now considerable information available online to the public which explains what consent means. The example in Chart 3.2 is taken from the Department of Health website and is intended for patients (www.dh.gov.uk).

As it states above English law assumes adults can make their own decisions. However, the challenge for the nurse is how to manage situations where consent cannot be freely given. There are a number of specific instances where patients may be examined and given treatment without consent, for example patients who have a notifiable disease, those detained under certain elements of mental health legislation, where life is in danger or where the individual is unconscious and unable to indicate their wishes (Citizens Advice, 2009). Although these

Chart 3.2 Consent – What you have a right to expect: A guide for adults

Before any doctor, nurse or therapist examines or treats you, they must seek your consent or permission. This could simply mean following their suggestions, such as your GP asking to have a look at your throat and you showing your consent by opening your mouth. Sometimes they will ask you to sign a form, depending on the seriousness of what they're proposing or whether it carries risks as well as benefits. It does not matter so much how you show your consent: whether you sign or say you agree. What is important is that your consent is genuine or valid. That means:

- you must be able to give your consent
- you must be given enough information to enable you to make a decision
- you must be acting under your own free will and not, say, under the strong influence of another person.

English law assumes that if you're an adult you are able to make your own decisions, unless it's proved otherwise. As long as you can understand and weigh up the information you need to make the decision, you should be able to make it.

Source: DoH (2001). Reproduced with kind permission of the Department of Health.

circumstances may at times be obvious, in many instances the way forward may not be clear-cut and it is therefore vital that the nurse remains vigilant to the situation and takes every opportunity to determine the capacity of the patient before proceeding with any procedure.

The Mental Capacity Act 2005

Capacity in this context simply refers to the mental ability of the individual. In 2007 the Mental Capacity Act 2005 came into force with the aim of protecting people who cannot make decisions for themselves due to a learning disability, a mental health condition, stroke or head injury. The Act generally only affects people aged 16 or over and provides a statutory framework to empower and protect people.

The Act is underpinned by a set of five key principles, which are important considerations for nursing practice:

1   Every adult has the right to make his or her own decisions and must be assumed to have capacity to do so unless it is proved otherwise;

2   A person must be given all practicable help before anyone treats them as not being able to make their own decisions;

3   Just because an individual makes what might be seen as an unwise decision, they should not be treated as lacking capacity to make that decision;

4   An act done or decision made under the Act for or on behalf of a person who lacks capacity must be done in their best interests; and

5   Anything done for or on behalf of a person who lacks capacity should consider options that are less restrictive of their basic rights and freedoms.

(Office of the Public Guardian, 2009)

Carefully considering these principles of consent, alongside those of capacity, the nurse will then need to use effective communication skills that avoid the use of jargon, to ensure understanding so that the patient is fully informed of the nature of the procedure, the risks and potential consequences. Without this, consent could be deemed invalid leaving the nurse professionally vulnerable.

While consent may be obtained verbally it is good practice to ask the patient to sign a consent form. This is particularly important in procedures where there is high risk to the patient. Where consent has been obtained this will need to be recorded in the patients' notes. However, consent needs to be seen as an ongoing requirement, sometimes known as continued consent, where the patient is kept informed of any changes to the original information and is given further opportunity to consent or refuse the treatment. A further, less robust aspect of consent is 'implied' consent. This is where through the patients' response and actions, consent is assumed. For example, a person attending for a blood test and offering up their arm to the nurse could, through their behaviour, be implying consent. However, to be fully compliant with the expectations of the law, the nurse should still explain procedures and determine that the patient understands what is happening.

Children and consent

In the case of children and adolescents similar principles operate for children between 16 and 18 unless the child refuses, in which case the parents or guardian may be asked to be involved. For younger children the same procedure will be adopted depending on such issues as the age of the child, their ability to understand and the seriousness of the condition or procedure to be undertaken.

Again, situations may exist where a child or young person may be examined and given treatment without their consent, such as a child who is a ward of court and the court decides that a specific treatment is in the child's interests or where a court or someone who has parental responsibility authorises treatment (Citizens Advice, 2009).

Working with Others

Having explored issues of confidentiality, consent and capacity it seems appropriate to recognise at this point that nurses never work as the sole health-care practitioner providing care and treatment. There are always other people involved within the care team, with whom the nurse will be expected to cooperate, collaborate or delegate.

The second part of the Code (NMC, 2008) provides further guidance on how we are expected to work with others to protect the health and wellbeing of those receiving care, their families and carers and the wider community (see Chart 3.3).

If considered in the context of the scenario in Activity 3.1, discussed earlier, the nurse would be operating under the Mental Capacity Act 2005 using the principle of best interests. While concern is for the patient, Emily, it is clear that the Code (NMC, 2008) expects the nurse to consider the broader picture, including the role of others such as health-care colleagues as well as the wellbeing of family members.

Link

Chapters 6 and 13 also discuss the Mental Capacity Act.

Activity 3.4

You are required to administer some medication to a patient in your care. List the issues to be considered when obtaining informed consent.

Chart 3.3 Work with others to protect and promote the health and well-being of those in your care, their families and carers, and the wider community

• Share information with your colleagues	• Delegate effectively
• Work effectively as part of a team	• Manage risk.

The judgement to be exercised here is to consider how best to support Dora while preserving Emily's right to privacy. While we cannot assume that all family members have the best interests of their kin in mind, to respond in a dismissive 'work to the rule-book' manner may add to Dora's anxieties and may not ultimately improve the situation for all parties. This scenario in many ways captures the essence of professional practice in that it highlights the need to consider different dimensions of an issue and make professional judgements about the holistic care of an individual, rather than taking a task-oriented, rule-bound approach.

In essence, a way forward may be to share the matter with medical colleagues, ascertain Dora's current understanding of the situation, facilitate a conversation between the Responsible Medical Officer and Dora, and keep clear and accurate records of information exchanged so that all team members are aware of the situation. While these actions do not abdicate responsibility for maintaining confidentiality, they do at least facilitate a way forward which will potentially lead to beneficial outcomes for all.

Multi-professional practice

From one perspective multi-professional practice would appear to be a straightforward process of well-meaning professionals working together in harmony pursuing a common purpose of caring for the patient. However, the issue of professional values also plays an important role in the delivery of effective care. As an illustration of this in a study undertaken by Colombo et al. (2003) showed that within a multidisciplinary team of psychiatrists, social workers and nurses who thought they shared the same values, there were in fact very different values at work which impacted on their effectiveness as a team. The psychiatrists were often more concerned with medication whereas the social workers focused on risk. While the team remained unaware of these differences they became the origins of problematic communication patterns. Importantly, however, when the values were made more explicit they could become the vehicles for discussion and common agreement, thus making the team more effective.

Link

Chapter 17 explores multi-professional practice in more depth.

Supporting the function of teams and that of multi-professional practice is another key element reflected in the Nurses' Code (as already highlighted in Charts 3.1 and 3.2) (NMC 2008). As McCray (2009) points out, working with other health and social care professionals is, for many, part of everyday practice and it is clear from the Code (NMC, 2008) that there are high expectations on nurses to cooperate, liaise and collaborate. The term 'multi-professional', as opposed to 'inter-professional', is used to reflect practice across a wide range of groups and agencies. However, as discussed by McCray (2009) there are different terms used in the literature to denote working collaboratively, across and between agencies, through formal and informal networks. What ever the choice of terminology they are all linked by the common view that such multi-professional models of practice are a positive and essential means to achieving effective outcomes for patients. The policy drive toward multi-professional practice can often be linked to the outcomes of public inquiries into the care of vulnerable people such as Clunis (Ritchie et al., 1994), Climbié (Laming, 2003) and Shipman (Smith, 2005) that consistently cite failures in communication between agencies.

While there is clearly a responsibility to work collaboratively and coopera-tively with colleagues, and the nurse will encounter numerous situations where this is the case, the need to take appropriate and rational decisions within the context of multi-disciplinary approaches does not in any way mean the nurse can abdicate responsibility for their own decision. Nurses are professionally accountable for the decisions they take and so they must ensure the care pro-vided is based on the best available evidence thus ensuring the highest standards of care possible.

Professional Accountability

Professional accountability is an important dimension of decision-making. It means nurses being answerable for the decisions they have taken, particularly when problems arise. Nurses may be accountable to several different bodies simultaneously: namely an employer, under a contract of employment; the patient under existing legal provision; and to the profession under the terms of the Nursing and Midwifery Order 2001.

In the context of professional accountability, nurses, registered with the NMC, are legally accountable for their work and can be removed from the register for behaviour that breaches the NMC Code (2008). Therefore it is vital that nurses understand that they are assumed to be competent in their area of practice, should be able to justify the basis on which their decisions have been made and explain how the decisions taken are in the best interests of the patient. This means keeping clear and accurate records of the decisions taken and the care or treatment provided.

Record keeping

Record keeping is acknowledged as essential to safe and effective care (NMC, 2009). It helps to improve accountability and demonstrates how patient care decisions were made. Effective record keeping supports the process of com-munication and facilitates greater continuity of care among members of the multi-professional team. It will also support in addressing any complaints or legal action that may arise in the course of patients' treatment. The guidance details the principles underpinning good practice in record keeping and also makes important links with legislation in this crucial area of practice.

> ✸ **Activity 3.5**
>
> Identify a patient who receives care from a team of different professionals and identify the role of each team member. What are the potential benefits and challenges of the multi-professional approach for the patient?

> ✸ **Activity 3.6**
>
> You should access and read the guidance for nurses which can be found at the NMC website, www.nmc-uk.org/and then search for 'record keeping guidance', which emphasises the importance of record keeping

Student nurse accountability

NMC (2005) makes it clear that pre-registration student nurses are not professionally accountable to the NMC. Student nurses cannot therefore be called by the NMC to account for any actions and omissions. The NMC is concerned with registered practitioners, with whom the student may be working, who are professionally responsible for the consequences of the student nurses' actions and omissions. This is the reason why students must always work under the direct supervision of their mentor in practice. This does not mean, however, that student nurses can never be called to account by their university, the NHS or by the law for the consequences of their actions or omissions as a pre-registration student (see also NMC, 2005).

Delivering high standards of care

Being accountable for practice requires an appreciation of notions of evidence, skills, knowledge and standards of practice and nurses are required to provide care based on the best available evidence (see Chart 3.4). The challenge for the nurse is to locate, retrieve, appraise and understand the evidence before adopting it in practice, which is not always as straightforward as it sounds.

Chart 3.4 Provide a high standard of practice and care at all times

- Use the best available evidence
- Keep your skills and knowledge up to date
- Keep clear and accurate records.

Let us consider Casebox 3.1.

In Casebox 3.1 the nurse, while doing the right thing in terms of seeking evidence, is not sure of the reliability of the evidence found. Examining what constitutes the best available evidence requires an understanding of the nature of evidence-based practice (EBP).

> **Casebox 3.1**
>
> You are working in an emergency department and have been caring for Phillip, aged 70, who has dementia. He has at times become aggressive toward staff and has been difficult to manage. You are uncertain how to manage the aggression and you have been reading textbooks to look for effective techniques which protect Phillip, yourself, colleagues and other patients in the department. The evidence contained in the textbook is helpful but you are not sure if it is based on current best practice.

Evidence-based Practice

A commonly used definition comes from Sackett and colleagues who define EBP as:

Activity 3.7

Consider a nursing decision you have recently taken and explain to your mentor in practice the rationale for your decision. Make reference to any relevant clinical guidelines, evidence-based practice and sections of the NMC Code (2008).

the conscientious, explicit, and judicious use of current best evidence in making decisions about the care of individual patients . . . [by] integrating individual clinical expertise with the best available external clinical evidence from systematic research (Sackett et al,, 1996, pp. 71–2).

Once again we can see an emphasis on exercising professional judgment in carrying out care. In other words having the skills to discern between good and poor quality evidence and the applicability of that evidence to the context in which the nurse is working. Importantly this definition refers to two key elements of EBP, namely clinical expertise and systematic research. A number of hierarchies have been constructed to help us make an initial evaluation of 'evidence'. The hierarchy in Table 3.1 (Muir Gray, 2001, p. 37), illustrates the relative strengths in terms of the design and methods used for obtaining the 'evidence'.

As you can see in Table 3.1 the evidence available ranges from type 1, systematic reviews, which are considered the strongest form of evidence, down to type 5 which involves expert opinion. The implication is that wherever possible nurses should aim to use evidence from high up the hierarchy to support their decisions. Therefore the skills of searching and acquisition of 'evidence' are important tools for the effective nurse.

✴ Activity 3.8

Read the Study Guide to accompany *Essentials of Nursing Research: Methods, Appraisal and Utilization* by Polit, Beck and Hungler (2006) for further discussion of research methods.

Table 3.1 Hierarchy of evidence

Type	Evidence
I	Strong evidence from at least one systematic review of multiple, well-designed, randomised control trials.
II	Strong evidence from at least one properly designed, randomised controlled trial of appropriate size.
III	Evidence from well-designed trials without randomisation, single group pre-post cohort, time series or matched case-control studies.
IV	Evidence from well-designed non-experimental studies from more than one centre or research group.
V	Opinions of respected authorities, based on clinical evidence, descriptive studies or reports of expert committees.

Source: Muir Gray (2001, p. 37), published with kind permission of Elsevier Ltd Publishers.

Acquiring the best evidence

Obtaining the best evidence and using best practice demands the skills of identification, selection and appraisal of the evidence. This can be potentially time consuming and so Sackett et al. (2000) suggest limiting searches for evidence from 'high-yield' sources which are directly relevant to clinical practice. They also suggest avoiding dated sources which are difficult to rapidly update, such as textbooks. In order to appraise evidence in an effective manner a number of critical appraisal tools have been developed, such as those that can be found at the Public Health Resources Unit website (PHRU, 2009).

Another important point made by Dollaghan (2004) is to be judicious about the use of basic science findings as they may not be directly relevant to clinical practice. They argue that the focus and design of such studies will be quite different to those studies attempting to answer questions about practice. While such basic science studies may provide insights they often need to be followed up by studies designed to address questions about clinical practice.

In the example in Casebox 3.1 the Code (NMC, 2008) requires the nurse to question the evidence on which practice is based and perhaps source more contemporary sources of evidence. One of the problems this evidence reveals is that 'textbook' evidence can be quickly out of date due to changes in legislation, clinical guidelines and empirical evidence. It is therefore important for the nurse to develop skills of information retrieval and appraisal in order to keep skills and knowledge up to date. One good source of evidence is the National Institute for Health and Clinical Excellence (NICE: http://www.nice.org.uk) which provides up-to-date guidance and best practice on a whole range of clinical problems.

However the hierarchy of evidence does have its critics. Writers such as Dollaghan (2004) make the important observation that the available external clinical evidence from systematic research often gets more attention in the literature than that of individual clinical experience. Dollaghan (2004) further argues that evidence from systematic research should not be considered the only basis for clinical decision-making, but that the experiences, values and preferences of clients or patients must also contribute to clinical decisions. This is an important point for those working in areas such as mental health and learning disability services, where systematic reviews may not be possible and other forms of evidence may be required to inform practice decisions.

Therefore nurses need to develop techniques that can assimilate findings from research, clinical guidelines, expert opinion and patient preferences and incorporate these into their decision-making. A helpful strategy is to foster a reflective approach to practice.

Reflective Practice

Link

Chapter 4 explores reflection in more depth.

Reflective practice is considered an essential skill for nurses, entailing the ability to use reflection to learn from and develop their practice. Although Chapter 4 explores this issue in greater depth it is worth mentioning it briefly here in the context of assimilating evidence into decision making.

Writers such as Dewey (1933) considered reflection as a reasoning process having the function of identifying and challenging beliefs or knowledge:

Active, persistent and careful consideration of any belief or supposed form of knowledge in the light of the grounds that support it and the further conclusions to which it tends. (Dewey, 1933, p. 9)

Importantly for nurses more recent writers such as Clarke and Graham (1996) have emphasised the value of reflection when faced with complex decisions. They suggest that reflection is the key tool for making sense of a situation and moving toward resolution:

Faced with complex decisions, thinking it through (reflecting) allows the individual to separate out the various influencing factors and come to a reasoned decision or course of action. (Clarke and Graham 1996, p. 26)

Other influential writers such as Schön (1983) have written extensively on the value of reflecting on action and reflection in action. Reflection on action involves retrospective critical thinking in order to reconstruct events and learn from experience. Reflection in action is seen as what distinguishes an expert practitioner in that they reflect in the midst of action in order to reshape action. While these may seem rather abstract concepts they are important in that they imply the dynamic nature of practice and the interrelationship between the practitioner and the environment in which they are working.

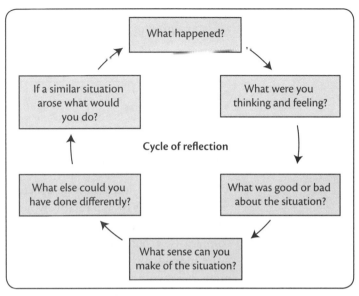

Figure 3.2 Cycle of reflection

Gibbs (1988, 1998) outlined a cycle of reflection and while others – Smyth (1989), Johns (1995) – have developed similar models, they all have common features represented in Figure 3.2. Essentially the model (Figure 3.2) illustrates a process which enables the nurse to reflect on their decision making following an event.

Reflecting on and learning from experience is a mechanism for developing insight into one's values and behaviour which are important processes for practising with integrity, which brings us onto the next section of the Code (NMC, 2008).

✸ Activity **3.9**

Think of a recent event and work through the above cycle to determine what you have learnt from the situation and what you would do differently in the future.

Caring with Integrity

The process of reflection helps us to develop our decision-making ability and to make appropriate decisions based on sound evidence. The process of reflection will also help to identify the values from which we practise, which is an important dimension of decision making. As a nurse we are expected to behave with integrity. This means being honest, reliable and trustworthy. The Code (NMC, 2008) clearly indicates that registered nurses are expected to behave in ways that do not bring the profession into disrepute. This means adhering to the code of conduct at all times and upholding the reputation of the profession. Chart 3.5 provides greater detail of the expectations of professional behaviour.

On the face of it these look straightforward considerations and entirely consistent with notions of integrity. However, what happens when we are caring for someone whose values and beliefs are not consistent with our own or the service we are attempting to provide? Demonstrating personal and professional commitment to equality and diversity demands a high level of insight into the nature of diversity and awareness of how our own values and beliefs can influence our decisions. An approach to help us navigate through such eventualities is the 'sister' to EBP, known as values-based practice (VBP)

Chart 3.5 Be open and honest, act with integrity and uphold the reputation of your profession

• Act with integrity	• Uphold the reputation of your
• Deal with problems	profession.
• Be impartial	

Values-based practice

VBP provides an important perspective that links the issues of EBP and integrity (Fulford 2004). VBP is a relatively new way of working positively with difference and is seen as the close relative of EBP, developed in response to the increasing complexity around clinical decision-making. VBP seeks to make health care more individualised by understanding a person's values and attempting to integrate them within the process of decision-making. It attempts to enable common ground to be found on which ideas and actions can be exchanged.

VBP, as discussed by Fulford (2004), provides the theory and related skills for decision-making in circumstances where there is potentially conflicting values. It emphasises effective processes for managing conflicting issues and requires engagement with the patient's values in order to bring about improved health outcomes. The underpinning philosophy is that if evidence is used to bring about health-improving decisions in a manner that recognises and respects the individual's values then there is a greater likelihood that the decision will be shared, owned and acted upon. Casebox 3.2 provides a vehicle for exploring this further.

Casebox 3.2 illustrates how values and assumptions can be at odds with that of the client. On the face of it, the nurse was acting with the best of intentions, but did she pick up on all the available cues, did she attempt to explore more deeply and go beyond the obvious outward signs, were there other indications of distress that were not immediately apparent?

While well intentioned, the nurse may assume that the potential benefits of the intervention are shared by the young girl. It may have been difficult to ascertain the underlying causes of this girl's behaviour due to the sensitivity of the issue or that the girl was overwhelmed by the 'power' differential in the

Casebox 3.2

You are referred a young girl who attends a practice clinic for a health check. She is generally quiet and uncommunicative and rather obese. She reports that she has been over-eating for the last year. You believe strongly that her health is at risk and provide clear evidence-based health education about healthy eating and exercise.

After the girl has left you subsequently learn that, earlier in the year, she was sexually abused by a family member.

relationship between the patient and nurse. On the other hand it may have been the nurse who was overwhelmed by the situation, because it conflicted with her own values and beliefs and unconsciously avoided raising the topic or probing too deeply.

In order to adopt a VBP approach, Woodbridge and Fulford (2004) suggest there are four essential skills that the nurse needs to foster, namely:

1   To become more aware of own beliefs and values and how these impact on decisions taken.
2   To understand the four ethical principles (autonomy, beneficence, non-maleficence, justice).
3   To have knowledge of the personal accounts of clients through studies that explore peoples experience of health problems.
4   To be effective communicators to ensure that the values and evidence which inform care decisions are brought together.

Adopting this approach in their practice will enable the nurse to acquire the skills required to provide services that are sensitive to the diversity of patients encountered within a multicultural society. Therefore, linked to VBP is the broader aim of developing culturally competent services

Cultural Competence in Health Care

The need to be able to work across increasingly diverse practice environments demands services that can adapt to the needs of its service users, in other words to be culturally responsive and competent. Betancourt et al. (2002) have defined cultural competence as:

> the ability of systems to provide care to patients with diverse values, beliefs and behaviours, including tailoring delivery to meet patients' social, cultural, and linguistic needs. (p. 5)

It is suggested that services that develop greater cultural competence lead to reductions in differences in health-care outcomes among minority and diverse populations. In Betancourt et al.'s (2002) study they found links between cultural competence, quality improvement, and the elimination of racial or ethnic difference. However, they argued that to achieve greater culturally competent health-care delivery, further quality improvement was required at the level of service design as well as the more immediate clinical interface with patients.

A helpful framework developed by Seeleman et al. (2009) identifies the competencies that health professionals need to develop and specifies the attitudes, knowledge and skills required for effective practice. In many ways this links to the previous section on values-based practice in that they suggest that the important attitudinal competencies are awareness of one's own prejudices as well as understanding cultural impacts on behaviour and patients' social contexts. They further highlight the importance of gaining knowledge of the epidemiology and manifestations of disease as well as the different effects of treatment on individuals from different ethnic groups. Examples include the culturally specific presentation of symptoms and the genetic differences that can influence metabolisation of drugs. While Seelemen et al. (2009) emphasise the importance of communication skills, again an area we have touched on in earlier sections, they specifically highlight the issue of transferring information in an understandable and accessible manner which often requires both flexibility and creativity in working with diverse groups.

It is evident that cultural competence, which Luquis and Perez (2003) suggest is the ability to both understand and respect difference, is a vital component of effective nursing care. As Mahabeer (2009) points out, rapidly changing demographics requires health-care providers to develop these competencies or risk facing legal challenge. The risks of physical harm or worse, due to a nurse's lack of cultural understanding and inability to provide appropriate intervention, are a very real concern in the modern health-care context.

Barriers to the development of culturally competent care include health-care systems that are poorly designed to meet the diverse needs of patients and poor communication skills of practitioners. The implication for nurses is to find ways in which people from different racial, ethnic and cultural backgrounds can inform the development of services and decisions about the care being provided. An important challenge, highlighted by Olavarria et al. (2009) is the distinction between treating everyone the same, which may be described as 'equitable' treatment, and the cultural competent approach whereby different clients require different services, which is described as 'equity' in treatment. Therefore the objective, as Olavarria et al. (2009) indicates, is to tailor services in an efficient and effective manner. This brings us onto the issue of the quality of services and providing choice for patients.

Quality, Performance and Choice

The term quality implies a standard of care and while we may all view high and low quality of care differently, writers such as Sutherland and Coyle (2009) indicate that:

> Quality in healthcare is a multifaceted concept that is not amenable to a single performance measure or simple metric. (p. 16)

For instance, a patient may view a good quality service as one which responds quickly to their needs and provides a high level of comfort, whereas someone from a Primary Care Trust who commissions services on behalf of a whole population may judge a quality service as one with the highest levels of activity at the lowest possible cost.

In other words the quality of care provided can be measured in a number of different ways. Sutherland and Coyle (2009) have helpfully identified the key domains for determining quality which are:

- Effectiveness
- Access and timeliness
- Capacity
- Safety
- Patient centredness
- Equity.

Against each of these domains will be a series of performance indicators or metrics, which can be used to determine whether an organisation is effective. Key performance indicators (KPIs) are considered to be both financial and non financial measures (or metrics) used to help organisations define and evaluate how successful they are in achieving their goals. For example, if we choose the quality domain of effectiveness the underlying principle will be that:

> Healthcare services should be based, as far as possible, on relevant rigorous science and research evidence (Sutherland and Coyle, 2009, p. 17).

The measures that may be used to determine performance could include the mortality rates of patients and how compliant the service is with adopting evidence-based guidelines. If we take the safety domain the principle would be that the service does not cause harm or expose patients to unnecessary risk. Measurements against this domain could include infection rates, medication errors and the number of falls.

This approach to judging quality will be an important consideration for nurses and will have an increasing impact on nursing practice. In fact we know that in 2008 the UK Government announced plans to develop measures specific to the quality of nursing care in areas such as compassion, safety and effectiveness (DoH, 2008a). If we adopt the principles outlined by Sutherland and Coyle (2009) that health care should be based on a partnership between nurses and their patients and delivered with compassion, empathy and responsiveness to individual needs, then it is clear that this could easily be measured through evaluation of care and surveys of patient experience.

The increasing need for nurses to be able to clearly define what they do and demonstrate achievement of KPIs are an important reality of modern health-care delivery within the NHS. They may at times appear to conflict with professional judgements concerning priorities, but within the context of services being open to ever-increasing scrutiny they highlight a cultural shift in which services are expected to be highly responsive to the needs and choices of the people that use them.

Choice

The shift toward providing increasing opportunities for patients to make choices about different elements of their care and treatment has been a central plank of successive governments' health-care policy in recent years (DoH, 2008a; NHS, 2009b). They have cited surveys that they claim demonstrate that patients want greater choice. An example of this was the 2005 British Social Attitudes Survey (National Centre for Social Research, 2005) which revealed that 65 per cent of patients wanted choice of treatment, 63 per cent wanted choice of hospital and 53 per cent welcomed a choice of appointment time.

The UK Government, in 2008, attempted to expand patient choice in the NHS. An example of this includes the principle of free choice, which allows patients referred to a specialist to choose where they will be treated. This means that any hospital that meets NHS standards, including some private providers.

The NHS has established a website at www.nhs.uk (NHS, 2009a) which provides accessible information about the choices available and how other patients have rated their experiences. While unfortunately the choice does not currently extend to mental health and maternity services, these still represent significant developments in the way the NHS, and those working within it, will be expected to function.

The changing landscape of service delivery

In the UK a great deal of health care continues to take place within the National Health Service. In 2008 the NHS celebrated its 60th anniversary and in preparation for this in England in 2007, Lord Darzi was asked by the Government to lead a 60th year review of the National Health Service (DoH, 2008b).

The emerging priorities are already shaping the landscape of service delivery and are likely to be the impetus for change over the next ten years. The key priorities included a much stronger focus on public health, with a drive toward healthier lifestyles; improved and more straightforward pathways to the right care any time of the day or night; care to be delivered closer to home and increases in specialist centres for major trauma, stroke and coronary care; a greater focus on long-term conditions including self-management strategies; increased information and choice and improving awareness of the rights of patients; greater focus on strategies for patient safety and finally a drive toward speeding up the process of translating new developments derived from innovation, into patient treatment and care (DoH, 2008b). As a result, traditional models of service delivery are very likely to change.

One of the key recommendations in Lord Darzi's report *High Quality Care for All* (DoH, 2008b) was the publication of an NHS Constitution that outlines what key stakeholders (staff, patients and the public) can expect from the NHS.

The NHS Constitution for England

The NHS Constitution is a key development in the context of health-care policy in that it outlines the purpose, principles and values of the NHS. It also brings together the rights, pledges and responsibilities for staff and patients. The rights and responsibilities were the result of extensive discussions and consultations with staff, patients and public. From the perspective of the nurse a useful resource is the Handbook to the NHS Constitution (see www.dh.gov.uk/) which provides important information about:

✷ Activity 3.10

Access the four UK country websites (see above) and locate information on patients' rights. How easy was it to find the material? Compare and contrast each country's commitment to patients' rights and choice.

- Access to health services
- Quality of care and environment
- Nationally approved treatments, drugs and programmes
- Respect, consent and confidentiality
- Informed choice
- Involvement in your health care and in the NHS
- Complaint and redress
- Patient and public responsibilities.

The introduction of the NHS Constitution arguably reflects an ongoing shift in the culture of the NHS from one which was professionally focused to one which is increasingly outward looking, engaging more directly with the needs and preferences of its patients. It is important to note that the NHS Constitution focuses on NHS services in England alone. As a result of devolution Scotland (www. show.scot.nhs.uk), Wales (www.wales.nhs.uk) and Northern Ireland (www. hscni.net) have evolved their own health systems and consequent accountabilities. However, each has detailed, in various forms, their commitments to patients and what can be expected from their respective health-care systems.

Wherever nurses work in the UK, within all good quality health-care organisations there are likely to be in place structures necessary to determine the quality of care being provided and mechanisms that can make continuous improvements should the quality fall short of the expectations and the commitments made to patients and the public. Ongoing scrutiny of an organisation's performance demands robust reporting mechanisms and the system currently in place for ensuring this happens is clinical governance.

Clinical Governance

Governance is simply a method of identifying potential causes of failures in any system of service delivery and ensuring that preventive action is taken to avoid potential damage. Within health care the term 'governance' was, according to Storey et al. (2008) a key component of the Labour Government's modernisation of the NHS. Similar to the introduction of the NHS Constitution, it represents a cultural shift from services that are provider oriented to services that are service-user oriented.

Principally the aim of governance in the clinical setting is to provide:

A framework through which NHS organisations are accountable for continually improving the quality of their services and safeguarding high standards of care by creating an environment in which excellence in clinical care will flourish. (Scally and Donaldson, 1998)

Therefore the main aim of clinical governance is continuous quality improvement achieved through the following principles:

- Clear lines of responsibility and accountability for the overall quality of clinical care.
- A comprehensive programme of quality improvement systems (including clinical audit, supporting and applying evidence-based practice, implementing clinical standards and guidelines, workforce planning and development).
- Education and training plans.
- Clear policies aimed at managing risk.
- Integrated procedures for all professional groups to identify and remedy poor performance.

It is evident that no one system or task represents clinical governance. Rather there is a series of processes which, when undertaken individually, build up a more accurate picture of the quality of the service provided by the organisation. These processes include:

- Accountability
- Audit
- Clinical effectiveness
- Continuing professional development
- Patient and public involvement
- Remedying underperformance
- Risk management
- Staff management.

✹ **Activity 3.11**

Identify the processes within your practice setting that contribute to clinical governance.

More information on clinical governance can be found at www.doh.gov.uk.

The components outlined in Figure 3.3 provide important considerations for nurses who will be expected to make a significant contribution to each clinical governance component. As indicated earlier in the chapter, when considering accountability nurses will have dual responsibilities and accountabilities both to their professional body and their employer. The system of clinical governance highlights those aspects that will ensure the nurse is making an effective contribution to the quality of care within the employing organisation.

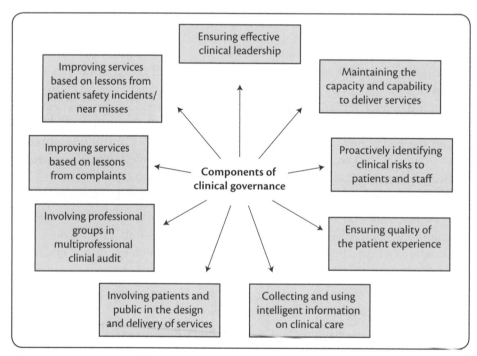

Figure 3.3 Components of clinical governance
Source: National Audit Office (2007), reproduced with kind permission of NAO.

Chapter Summary

While the practice of nursing and the bulk of care delivery largely will take place at the level of the immediate interface between the nurse and their patient, this chapter has highlighted the practice challenges for nurses who need to be aware of their wider accountabilities, as well as professional and legal responsibilities. As we have discussed, the effective nurse often needs to balance the expectations of the profession, which are clearly articulated in the professional code, with their accountabilities to their employer, under the contract of employment.

This chapter has also demonstrated the impact of the wider context in which they practise, including local and national policy initiatives which shape the contemporary landscape of practice and which impact directly on outcomes for patients.

Modern nursing takes place within increasingly independent, target-driven organisations that will be judged on their success using a wide range of measures. These measures will include the quality of care provided, the number of complaints, the throughput of patients, length of waiting lists, the involvement of service users in decisions about the shape and function of services and the support given to staff. Therefore to be effective the nurse must be able to navigate these competing demands in order to deliver the most effective care to their patients as well as contribute to the success of their employing organisation.

❓ Test yourself!

1 What is meant by the term 'professional practice'?

2 What ethical principles underpin the NMC's Code?

3 Describe how nurses display professional accountability.

4 What are the key components of evidence-based practice?

5 What are the key skills required to adopt a values-based practice approach?

6 What is the NHS constitution and how does it help patients?

Dimond, B. (2008) *Legal Aspects of Nursing,* 5th edn. Pearson Education Ltd, Harlow.

Thompson, I.E., Melia, K.M., Boyd, K.M. and Horsburgh, D. (2006) *Nursing Ethics,* 5th edn, Churchill Livingstone, Elsevier, Oxford.

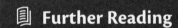 **Further Reading**

For live links to useful websites see: www.palgrave.com/nursinghealth/hogston

References

Betancourt, J.R., Green, A.R. and Carrillo, J.E. (2002) *Cultural Competence in Health Care: Emerging Frameworks and Practical Approaches.* The Commonwealth Fund. www.cmwf.org

Citizens Advice (2009) *Consent, Advice Guide.* Citizens Advice Bureau. www.adviceguide.org.uk/index/family_parent/health/nhs_patients_rights.htm#Consent

Clarke, D.J. and Graham, M. (1996) Reflective practice: the use of reflective diaries by experienced registered nurses. *Nursing Review* **15**(1): 26–9.

Colombo, A., Bendelow, G., Fulford, K.W.M. and Williams, S. (2003) Evaluating the influence of implicit models of mental disorder on processes of shared decision making within community-based multidisciplinary teams, *Social Science and Medicine* **56**: 1557–70.

Dewey, J. (1933) *How We Think: A Restatement of the Relation of Reflective Thinking to the Educative Process,* rev. edn. D.C. Heath, Boston.

DoH (Department of Health) (2001) *Consent – What You Have a Right to Expect: A Guide for Adults.* http://www.dh.gov.uk/en/Publichealth/Scientificdevelopmentgeneticsandbioethics/Consent/Consentgeneralinformation/index.htm

DoH (Department of Health) (2003) *The NHS Confidentiality Code of Practice.* Department of Health, London.

DoH (Department of Health) (2008a) Nursing quality to be measured for compassion of care. Speech by Alan Johnson, Health Secretary. www.dh.gov.uk

DoH (Department of Health) (2008b) *The NHS 60 Years On: High Quality Care for All*. Lord Darzi, Minister for Health. Department for Health, London.

DoH (Department of Health) (2009) *The NHS Constitution*. Department of Health, London.

Dollaghan, C. (2004) Evidence-based practice: Myths and realities. *The ASHA Leader*, April: 4–5, 12.

Fulford, K.W.M. (2004), *Ten Principles of Values-Based Medicine*. In Radden, J. (ed.) *The Philosophy of Psychiatry: A Companion*, pp. 205–34. Oxford University Press, New York.

Gibbs, G. (1988) *Learning by Doing: A Guide to Teaching and Learning Methods*. Oxford: Further Educational Unit, Oxford Polytechnic.

Gibbs, G. (1998) *Learning by Doing: A Guide to Teaching and Learning*. FEU, London.

Healthcare Policy and Strategy Directorate (2008). *Information Sharing between NHS Scotland and the Police*. www.sehd.scot.nhs.uk.

Johns, C. (1995) Framing learning through reflection within Carper's fundamental ways of knowing in nursing. *Journal of Advanced Nursing* **22**: 226–34.

Laming, Lord W.H. (2003) The Victoria Climbié Inquiry. Presented to Parliament by the Secretary of State for Health and the Secretary of State for the Home Department by Command of Her Majesty. HMSO, London.

Luquis, R. and Perez, M. (2003) Achieving cultural competence: the challenge for health educators. *American Journal of Health Education* **34**(3): 131–9.

Mahabeer, S. (2009) A descriptive study of the cultural competence of hemodialysis nurses. *Journal of the Canadian Association of Nephrology Nurses and Technicians* **19**(4): 30–3.

McCray, J. (2009) *Nursing and Multi-professional Practice*. Sage, London.

Muir Gray, J.A. (2001) *Evidence-based Healthcare*. Churchill Livingstone, Edinburgh (copyright Elsevier).

National Audit Office (2007) *Improving Quality and Safety Lessons for the New Primary Care Trusts: Progress in Implementing Clinical Governance in Primary Care*, Health Services Management Centre University of Birmingham.

National Centre for Social Research (2005) *British Social Attitudes: the 22nd Report – Two Terms of New Labour: The Public's Reaction*. NATCEN, London.

National Institute for Health and Clinical Excellence (2009) *Guidance for Health*. NICE London. http://www.nice.org.uk/guidance/index.jsp

NHS (2009a) *NHS Choices, Your Health, Your Choices*. http://www.nhs.uk/Pages/HomePage.aspx

NHS (2009b) *The History of Choice in the NHS*. http://www.nhs.uk/Tools/Pages/Patientchoice.aspx

NMC (Nursing and Midwifery Council) (2005) *NMC Guide for Students of Nursing and Midwifery*. NMC, London. www.nmc-uk.org.

NMC (Nursing and Midwifery Council) (2008) *The Code: Standards of conduct, performance and ethics for nurses and midwives*. NMS, London. www.nmc-uk.org

NMC (Nursing and Midwifery Council) (2009) *Record Keeping: Guidance for Nurses and Midwives*. NMC, London.

Office of Public Sector Information (2005) The Mental Capacity Act. OPSI, London. http://www.opsi.gov.uk/acts/acts2005

Office of the Public Guardian (2009) The Mental Capacity Act 2005. http://www.publicguardian.gov.uk/

Olavarria, M., Beaulac, J., Belanger, A., Young, M. and Aubry, T. (2009) Organisational cultural competence in community health and social service organisations: how to conduct a self-assessment. *Journal of Cultural Diversity* **16**(4): 140–50.

Polit, D.F., Beck, C. T. and Hungler, B. P. (2006) *Study Guide to Accompany Essentials of Nursing Research: Methods, Appraisal and Utilization*, 6th edn, Lippincott Williams and Wilkins, Philadelphia.

PHRU (Public Health Resources Unit) (2009) *Appraisal Tools*. PHRU, Oxford http://www.phru.nhs.uk/Pages/PHD/resources.htm

Ritchie, J.H., Dick, D. and Lingham, R. (1994) *The Report of the Inquiry into the Care and Treatment of Christopher Clunis*. HMSO, London.

Royal College of Nursing (2005) *Informed Consent in Health and Social Care Research*. RCN Guidance for Nurses. Available at www.rcn.org.uk

Sackett, D.L., Rosenberg, W.M.C., Gray, J.A.M., Haynes, R.B. and Richardson, W.S. (1996) Evidence based medicine: what it is and what it isn't. *British Medical Journal* **312**: 71–2.

Sackett, D.L., Straus, S.E., Richardson, W.S., Rosenberg, W. and Haynes, R.B. (2000) *Evidence-based Medicine: How to Practice and Teach EBM*, 2nd edn. Churchill Livingstone, Edinburgh and New York.

Scally, G. and Donaldson, L.J. (1998) Clinical governance and the drive for quality improvement in the new NHS in England. *British Medical Journal* **317**: 61–5.

Schön, D.A. (1983) *The Reflective Practitioner*. Basic Books, New York.

Seeleman, C., Suurmond, J. and Stronks, K. (2009) Cultural competence: A conceptual framework for teaching and learning. *Medical Education* **43**: 229–37.

Smith, Dame J. (2005) *The Shipman Inquiry*. Sixth and final report. HMSO, London.

Smyth, J. (1989) Developing and sustaining critical reflection in teacher education. *Journal of Teacher Education* **40**(2): 2–9.

Storey, J., Bate, P., Buchanan, D., Green, R., Salaman, G. and Winchester, N. (2008) *New Governance Arrangements in the NHS: Emergent Implications*, NHS-SDO funded project SDO/129. www.open.ac.uk

Sutherland, K. and Coyle, N. (2009) *Quality in Healthcare in England, Wales, Scotland, Northern Ireland: An Intra-UK Chart-book*. The Health Foundation, London.

Woodbridge, K., and Fulford, K.W.M. (2004) *Whose Values? A Workbook for Values-based Practice in Mental Health Care*. Sainsbury Centre for Mental Health, London.

4

Developing Skills for Reflective Practice

📖 Contents

☑ Learning outcomes

This chapter explores ways in which we can learn from our experiences and develop reflective skills that help us to make decisions about the best form of care to give to our patients. Reflective practice is one of the key ways that practitioners work as professionals – a hallmark of which is lifelong learning and development. For reflective practice to be used to its optimum effect, the skills need to be developed and learnt as part of the way nursing and midwifery is learnt. At the end of this chapter, you should be able to:

- Identify and discuss the key features of reflective practice
- Discuss the significance of reflective learning for professional practice
- Use reflective processes as ways of learning from your experiences
- Identify ways in which reflective learning has become part of your practice as a student practitioner
- Justify action taken as a result of reflection
- Identify learning opportunities in the practice environment
- Write reflectively in order to identify your learning and devise action plans
- Compile a portfolio utilising evidence and reflective writing to demonstrate the achievement of your objectives and learning outcomes.

What Is Reflective Practice?

It is probably true to say that the main way we learn throughout our lives is through learning from experiences. Most of the time we do not consciously think about our learning, we just file the experience away in our heads and probably subconsciously avoid or repeat actions and ways of doing things as a result. Sometimes though, these subconscious thoughts find their way into our conscious mind and we are aware of them. How many times have you caught yourself thinking 'I did that last time and it worked really well, so I'll try it again'. And, on the other hand, 'I tried that last time, and what a mess that turned out to be; so, let's try something different.'

These two outcomes are the essence of **reflective practice** – first of all that we learn to think consciously about our actions and evaluate them and repeat those that are successful and eliminate those that are not. Secondly, reflective practice is about taking some sort of action – it is not simply about thinking things over in some way. Of course we all use some form of reflection every day to ensure that we link our past experiences with what we are planning to do now, or in the future. Try Activity 4.1 to see how you already use reflection in your work.

Very little that we do is unrelated to things we have done in the past. We tend to momentarily recall, even if subconsciously, experiences we have had that are similar to the ones we are faced with in the present. We build up, over time, a reservoir of '**paradigm cases**' (Benner, 1984) or examples of each type of case and then draw on these to inform our current action. Hence, the name 'reflective practice'. Reflective practice is about how we practise as a result of our reflective activity. It is not reflection alone, as practice is about *doing* something as a result of the learning that has taken place during reflection. It can be summarised by using the ERA (experience-reflection-action) cycle described by Jasper (2003) in Figure 4.1.

Although this is a cycle, because action taken as a result of reflection will result in a different understanding and perspective being taken about something, it is important to see it as an eternal triangle. If one element of the triangle is removed, the concept itself ceases to exist. This is significant for the idea of reflective practice in that if reflection on an experience does not result in action being taken – or a change in the behaviour of the person reflecting – then clearly it is not reflective *practice* that is happening. You might be *practising reflection*, which is thinking about things that have happened to you, but this is not the same as *practising reflectively* which involves the conscious use of reflection to inform practice. Practice itself always involves some sort of action, a 'repeated exercise to improve a skill, action as opposed to theory' (*Collins English Dictionary*, 2001). This definition identifies the common feature of the word 'practice' in that it assumes growing competence of a skill through repetition; but practice as a professional involves

✳ Activity 4.1

Think yourself back to your last day in clinical practice and identify a task you undertook.
- What did you do?
- How did you do it?
- Why did you do it that way?
- Had you done this task before?
- If so, what knowledge and skill did you draw on from that time that you used to inform this time?
- If not, what related knowledge and skill did you draw on that helped you with this task?
- Did you do anything differently as a result of the development of your knowledge and skills?

reflective practice
professional practice guided by structured reflection on feelings, experience and empathy in order to make practice robust and enhance learning

paradigm cases
examples of patterns, particular perspectives that inform meaning and action

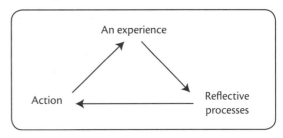

Figure 4.1 The ERA cycle

Source: Jasper (2003). With kind permission of Nelson Thornes.

much more than that. It also involves thoughtful consideration of alternatives for action, based on the best evidence and the knowledge and insight gained through experience. It is the conscious processes of reflective practice that turn the *practice as in repetition* to the *knowledgeable and discerning practice of the professional,* which involves practising to think reflectively as well as practising skills.

Much of the learning that a student practitioner does is within the practice environment, yet there are no formal strategies, as when you are learning in a classroom or learning from books or the internet, that ensure you revisit the knowledge or skill and 'embed' it as part of you. Classroom or book learning often involves repetition, or consideration of what you are learning, so that it is remembered.

But, of course, being a practitioner involves a great deal more than simply remembering knowledge – it is about transferring that knowledge into action – about the 'practising' of being a practitioner. The consequences therefore of not knowing or understanding what you are doing as a practitioner are far-reaching in terms of the harm that you might do to someone in your care. Reflective practice, and developing the skills of constantly practising reflectively, go in some ways to helping practitioners to avoid making mistakes and helps to ensure that actions taken can always be justified and explained against the practitioner's experience and evidence base. This is just one of the reasons why practitioners need to practice reflectively. Jasper (2003, p. 5) suggests others, as summarised in Figure 4.2.

In sum, however, these probably boil down to three main purposes of reflective practice:

1   Reflective practice is a learning activity.
2   Reflective practice contributes to improvements and developments in patient care.
3   Reflective practice contributes to the development of practice theory about nursing and midwifery and informs our knowledge base.

✴ Activity 4.2

Consider the different learning and teaching methods that you use as a student in university. Invariably, a lecture providing knowledge about a subject will be followed by seminar or group discussion work to consider the subject so that the key points are reinforced. How does this reinforcement happen with the other types of learning experiences you may have:
- reading books and journal articles
- practical work in a skills laboratory
- web-based learning
- educational visits
- practice placements.

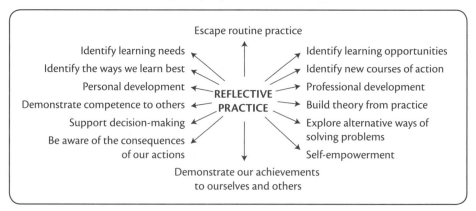

Figure 4.2 Reasons why professional practitioners need to practise reflectively
Source: Adapted from Jasper (2003).

The Reflective Practitioner

Professional practice is a complicated business. Nurses and midwives are registered with a professional body – the Nursing and Midwifery Council (NMC) – upon qualification, and from that time become accountable for their actions as practitioners. It is therefore important that they continue to develop the knowledge base for their practice, and that they expand the range of skills and experiences that enable them to develop beyond the basic level of competence and safe practice that qualification certifies.

However, it would be unrealistic to think that all practitioners continue to study in the formal way that involves the working towards qualifications or accredited learning that happens at the pre-registration stage. While many will inevitably return to formal learning opportunities to extend their qualifications, they also need to find ways of recognising and using the learning opportunities in their practice environment and to expand and develop their practice for the benefit of their clients. In fact Schön (1983) suggests that this is the primary way that all professionals work in action, as professional practice becomes a cycle of drawing on previous knowledge, considering its application for the problem at hand, and testing out new ideas and variations to find one that fits this new situation.

Schön (1983) identified two main types of reflection that professionals use in their everyday practice – reflection-in-action and reflection-on-action. A comparison of the characteristics of each of these is made in Table 4.1.

⬮ Link

Chapter 3 explores the responsibilities of being a registered practitioner and what it means to be professionally accountable.

Table 4.1 Characteristics of reflection-in-action and reflection-on-action

Reflection-in-action – the way that people think and theorise about practice while they are doing it	Reflection-on-action – conscious exploration of an event to discover more about it and learn from it
Perceived as automatic Seen as an unconscious activity Often called 'intuitive' practice Results from a combination of knowledge, skills and practice Difficult to articulate and explore	Retrospective – it occurs after the event has happened Conscious, deliberative activity It is a cognitive process involving analysis, interpretation and recombination of information It results in new perspectives being taken on the event It acknowledges the knowledge being used and results in knowledge deficits being identified Active process of transforming experience into knowledge Contributes to the development of practice theory

It is important to distinguish between these types of reflection because although both contribute to reflective practice, it is mainly reflection-on-action that is used as a learning strategy as a result of its conscious and deliberative nature.

Reflection-in-action

Reflection-in-action is more than simply 'thinking-while-doing'. According to Schön (1983), reflection-in-action has two components – thinking back about the action that is being taken, and thinking about the knowledge that is contributing

reflection-in-action
reflection on an event as it is being experienced

✴ Activity 4.3

Think back to your last day in practice and mentally run though the day. Can you remember:
- things that you did automatically, without having to think about them;
- occasions where you found yourself thinking through what you were doing and questioning whether you were doing the right things;
- asking yourself whether you could do anything differently;
- questioning, in your head, the knowledge you were drawing on;
- referring back to similar situations with which you had already dealt.

⚭ Link

Chapter 1 considers practice in more detail.

reflection-on-action

in-depth reflection on an event after it has finished

to that action. Schön (1983) describes the combination of these as 'knowing-in-action', but emphasises that for most of the time the practitioner uses this subconsciously. In other words, the practitioner is constantly reacting to the stimuli of the practical situation and scanning her knowledge and experience base for the 'paradigm cases' identified by Benner (1984), which she can compare to the present situation and then take action. Schön (1983) considered that thought and action were inseparable; they are two parts of the same process of reflection-in-action. This process usually happens so rapidly that it is unconscious – that is, the practitioner is not aware of doing it unless something happens to make them stop and think or challenge what they are doing. It is then that it becomes a learning activity. Of course, reflection-in-action depends entirely on the bank of experience that each person carries in their head. As a result, it is often seen as the characteristic way that advanced practitioners, or experts, practise, rather than the way that beginning practitioners function in the practice setting. But, anyone who has practical experience will begin to draw on their memory of paradigm cases once they have developed confidence in certain abilities and their knowledge base. Try Activity 4.3 for an illustration of this.

Probably the most important aspect of reflection-in-action for the student nurse or midwife is learning to recognise when you are doing it and to take note of what is happening. This is significant because it means that we are constantly aware of our practice, we are selecting from alternatives and challenging the ways in which practice occurs. This helps to guard against routinised practice that can be seen to have characterised nursing and midwifery in the past (Walsh and Ford, 1989).

It also enables you to note areas for your future development – whether this means extending your formal knowledge, discussing what happened with your mentor or considering, by yourself or with others, whether there are different ways in which that situation could be approached in the future.

Reflection-on-action

When you carry forward these examples for further work they become **reflection-on-action**, which takes place away from the arena of the experience and after the event itself. This allows you to put all your concentration into exploring the event that has happened from all perspectives and using it as a stimulus for your own learning. It is the development of strategies for reflection-on-action that will enable you to become a reflective practitioner, as well as helping you to make the most of the experiences you encounter in the practise setting. It is also these skills that, once embedded in the way you practise, will stay with you throughout your professional career, and enable you to be a 'life-long learner' in practice.

Skills for Beginning Reflective Practice

While to some extent being reflective is part of being human, Atkins and Murphy (1993) suggest that there are certain underlying skills needed for the development and use of reflective practice and for reflection to be successful as a strategy for learning. They define these as:

- self-awareness
- description
- critical analysis
- synthesis
- evaluation.

We will now discuss these five skills in more detail.

Self-awareness

Atkins (2004, p. 29) says that 'to be self-aware is to be conscious of one's character, including beliefs, values, qualities, strengths and limitations. It is about knowing oneself.' Self-awareness enables the practitioner to look at themselves, and the part they play in human interactions, honestly, and acknowledge the roles they played. The notion of honesty is probably the key to self-awareness, because if we are not able to stand back and own our actions, words and thoughts, it is unlikely that we will develop into reflective practitioners who are able to explore their role, their knowledge and understanding, and their actions in any given event. To some extent, self-awareness is linked with maturity (but not necessarily chronological age) and the ways in which we have been encouraged to take responsibility for our own actions in the past. It is also dependent on whether we have been encouraged to understand ourselves as an individual and recognise, for instance, what our fundamental beliefs and values are, what our beliefs and values about nursing are, and what our beliefs and values about ourselves are.

Description

The key to successful reflection is the ability to describe an experience – accurately identifying its key characteristics and without expressing a judgement – so that someone else can recognise and understand it. This may be verbally or in writing.

Good description takes a lot of practice, as it is tempting to stray away from an objective account into subjective observations or demonstrative language. It is also easy, until you have practised a great deal, to be side-tracked from the central features of the experience and end up a long way from where you started! Atkins (2004, p. 33) suggests that 'the account contains the following key elements: significant background factors (the context), the events as they unfolded in the situation, what you were thinking at the time, what you were feeling at the time, and the outcome of the situation.' Particularly difficult is recounting the personal emotive aspects of the event, without imposing some judgement at the same time.

The purpose of the description is to provide you with the substance to reflect on. This must come from your own experiences and arise from your own actions in practice if it is to be meaningful in helping you to learn from the experience. The description also needs to relate to your own actions, as opposed to assigning meaning to the actions of others.

> ☀ Activity 4.4
>
> Complete the following:
> - The three values I hold most strongly are...
> - I believe nursing/ midwifery to be...
> - The three attributes in other people that I value most are...
> - The three things I like about myself most are...
> - The three things I like most in others are...
> - My understanding of professional practice is...

Critical analysis

Critical analysis involves, first, being able to break an experience down into its component parts, and then to make judgements about the strengths and weaknesses of them. Being 'critical' does not mean finding fault with something. It involves considering, in an objective way, good parts of an experience, what went well for example, or what part you played in the experience that was effective; and then identifying those parts that could have been done better, or areas where you consider you need further development. This is where the attribute of self-awareness really comes into play, as it involves taking an honest, and sometimes critical, look at our part in an experience. Atkins (2004, pp. 36–7) suggests that being critically analytical involves:

- Identifying and illuminating existing knowledge of relevance to the situation
- Exploring feelings about the situation and the influence of these
- Identifying and challenging assumptions made
- Imagining and exploring alternative courses of action. (Adapted from Brookfield, 1987)

Identifying existing knowledge

The theoretical knowledge that we acquire in our pre-registration education, or even in post-qualifying courses, underpins the decisions that we take on a daily basis. Often, we are not aware of accessing that knowledge, but consider it as part and parcel of the way we practise. However, knowledge develops at a rapid rate, and there is always new evidence being published that needs to be taken into account when deciding on the most appropriate care for our patients.

Reflective practice often involves exploring the knowledge that we used when making decisions and taking action, thus it is important to be able to identify that knowledge and how we used it.

∞ Link

Chapter 3 explores the concept of evidence-based practice in clinical decision-making.

✹ Activity 4.5

Select one of the experiences you identified in Activity 4.3. Divide a piece of paper into four and head each section with the following: theoretical or scientific knowledge, ethical or moral knowledge, personal knowledge, and the 'art' of nursing. Think about the experience you have identified, considering the types of knowledge you used to inform that experience. Write these down under the headings.

Chart 4.1 Analysing an experience to identify the sources of knowledge that inform it

Description of the experience: Dawn was caring for Arthur, an 80-year-old man suffering from the end stages of bowel cancer. He and his wife had decided they wanted him to end his days in his own home. The care being provided was palliative, as Arthur was unconscious and surrounded by his family – his wife, two sons and daughters-in-law. Dawn was aware that Arthur would die soon, probably in the next hour. She had supported Arthur and his family as a visiting Macmillan nurse since his diagnosis and referral to the service via the hospice. She considered her role as having several aspects in terms of caring for the dying, unconscious patient and maintaining his dignity at the end of his life. However, her role also included caring for the family at this time, offering support with compassion and sensitivity.

Theoretical or scientific knowledge	Ethical or moral knowledge
The dying processes	Understanding the legal parameters of what professionals are able to do when helping people at the end of their lives
Bereavement theory	The principles of beneficence, non-maleficence, confidentiality and informed consent
Physical care of the dying patient	The NMC Code of Professional Conduct

Physical care of the unconscious patient	A cultural understanding of right and wrong
Personal knowledge	*The 'art' of nursing*
Being a person and understanding the importance of personal dignity to all people	Professional experience as a Macmillan nurse caring for other patients in similar circumstances
Being a daughter and watching her father die	Being with the patient and their family at this distressing time
Experience of caring for other dying patients	'Knowing', by experience, that the time of death was approaching and how to support the family at this time

Having completed Activity 4.5, depending on the experience you selected, you may find that you have a longer list in one box than another, and this will always happen, dependent upon the types of experience you explore. What this exercise shows us is that we inevitably have to draw on a range of sources of knowledge (Carper, 1978) to inform our practice, and rarely simply use one source of knowledge. This is illustrated in Chart 4.1.

Exploring feelings related to the situation

Feelings, and the emotional components of an experience are as important as the actions taken and the outcomes that result. Sometimes though, these are the most difficult to express to others, or even to own for oneself. Often, we choose to reflect on painful experiences, or those that have made us uncomfortable, and it is essential to explore these experiences for the roots of these feelings and why they are important to us. Conversely, we may reflect on good experiences that invoked positive emotions, particularly when something went very well or resulted in a positive outcome. Again, it is important to identify these emotions and seek out the source of these so that we can attempt to reinforce these activities and plan to be successful.

Identifying and challenging assumptions

Much of modern health-care practice is built upon the successes of the past – what worked or did not work in other people's experiences. As a result, it is easy for caring activities to become 'custom and practice' or part of the culture of a clinical area. How often have you asked a question about something only to be told 'it's the way we've always done it'. Being critical involves being willing to explore these 'taken- for-granted' ideas, practices and assumptions and maintaining an open mind about the ways in which things are decided and done. Sometimes this is not a comfortable process, as it involves challenging the status quo, and often challenging those in authority at the same time.

Imagining and exploring alternative courses of action

Again, key to this stage is the ability to retain an open mind and be willing to accept that there may be another way of doing something, even if it has 'always been done like that'. This involves being willing to think creatively and 'outside the box'.

Synthesis

Synthesis means recombining the individual elements of something, often in a different way and informed by the critical analysis that has gone on, in order to take a new perspective, or see new things as a result. This is combined with new sources of information and knowledge, such as in the approach of evidence-based practice. It involves professional creativity, and should result in the optimum care for each one of our patients as individuals.

Evaluation

★ **Activity 4.6**

Look back on the skills Atkins and Murphy (1993) identify as being prerequisites for reflective practice. How confident are you that you have these skills, and which ones do you feel require more development? Who can you get to help you to develop them?

Finally, a prerequisite for reflective practice is the ability to make a judgement about something, or to 'give it a value'. This is exactly what evaluation is – judging the value of something. Thus it means that a practitioner must be able to form their own opinions about the standards of care and whether care can be improved by changes to practice.

The idea of reflection suggests a solitary and independent activity, largely in the hands and under the control of the reflector themselves. However, within a professional capacity, and as a strategy for learning, the skills of reflection need as much support and facilitation if they are to be as successful as any other learning strategy. Hence, within your programme of study, it is likely that you will receive formal teaching regarding reflection within the university, as well as help in developing the skills, in the practice environment, from your mentors and supervisors. You will also have opportunities to practise reflection in group activities and in one-to-one supervision sessions with your mentor. As a result you will slowly develop these skills until they become an automatic part of the ways in which you also practise.

Choosing an Experience to Reflect on

Experiences that you reflect on in a formal way for the purpose of learning are often referred to as 'critical incidents'. This doesn't mean that they are great big dramatic events, or necessarily important to other people. What matters is that the incident or experience is important to you, and has meaning for you in some way. This may be because what happened was extraordinary or unusual and sticks in your mind for some reason. It may have been a really good experience that makes you feel happy, or confident, or you felt you did a good job. Other experiences that stand out are often those with less good outcomes, or as Atkins and Murphy (1993, p. 1189) suggest, arise from 'an awareness of uncomfortable feelings or thoughts. This stems from a realisation that, in a situation, the knowledge one was applying was not sufficient in itself to explain what was happening in that unique situation.'

It is worth remembering that for the majority of our time, for the majority of our lives, things go well. Indeed, if you think back over the past week, how many times can you remember when things went wrong? Yes, they might not have gone as you expected, but, how often does the way things work need to go exactly as you had imagined or planned for? Actually, there are usually many ways in which events might go, none of them necessarily being better than others as long as an acceptable outcome is achieved. This is the foundation for the notion of learning from your experiences – it is by using reflection that we learn to move away from fixed ways of thinking, to think creatively and find different ways of tackling problems, so moving practice forward.

Hence, it is important to view all types of experiences as opportunities for learning, and to embrace those events that caused us 'uncomfortable feelings or thoughts' simply as ways in which we can explore and develop our practice. These might well be the stimulus for expanding our knowledge base for practice, or for seeking help with areas of practice that we are having difficulty mastering. The key to responsible and accountable practice is for us to recognise the limits of our knowledge and competence in order to provide safe practice for our patients and clients. Hence, using examples of knowledge deficit, and developing the skills of reflective practice as a tool within professional practice, is vital in being a registered practitioner. Chart 4.2 lists some examples of experiences that can be used as 'critical incidents' as a basis for reflective practice.

> **✹ Activity 4.7**
>
> Think back over the past two shifts you worked in practice. What stands out in your mind? These events are probably just the sort of critical incidents that could be used as material for reflective learning.

Chart 4.2 Examples of 'critical incidents'

- The first time a particular skill is practised: such as feeding or bathing a patient, giving an injection, delivering your first baby
- The first time a new learning environment is experienced: for example a new ward placement; nursing in the home or general practice surgery; encountering patients and clients in hospital departments such as outpatients, clinics or for diagnostic tests
- Witnessing new events: for example a cardiac arrest; a chest drain being inserted; a baby being born by instrumental or operative delivery
- Events which have gone well for you: such as getting a good grade for an assignment; where you have made a difference to the outcome for a patient; where you have changed the course of something; the first time you carry out actions without direct supervision
- Events that you have found challenging: such as dealing with anxious, violent or aggressive patients; giving bad news to patients, or supporting them after others have done this; dealing with patients who you felt powerless to help; dealing with conflict with other members of staff
- Events that have made you feel uncomfortable: for example witnessing poor or dangerous care; events where you feel you could have acted differently; events that made you question your ambition to be a nurse or midwife; situations in which you felt you were unfairly treated
- Events that you cannot get out of your head for some reason: these events provide a rich source of material for reflection, because exploring them to uncover the reasons why they are sticking in your mind often provides a great deal of personal insight

Reflective Processes

Having ensured that you are familiar with the skills needed for reflective practice, we can now move on to exploring the processes that reflective practice involves. There are many models and frameworks suggested that provide a structured approach for reflective practice. These essentially build on Kolb's (1984) experiential learning cycle, a four-stage process starting with *observation* and going through the stages of *reflection* leading to *concept development/theorising*, and resulting in an *action*. Kolb's four stages, when applied to a practitioner's situation, can be extended into six stages, all of which are included within the majority of published frameworks, or those that you might be asked to use by your lecturers or supervisors. These stages are summarised in Chart 4.3.

You will notice from Chart 4.3 that you are asked, as you move through the stages, to try to think outside the ways that you normally think. At first this is challenging, and when doing this initially, it often helps to work with someone else who can ask you questions and draw you along avenues that you would not normally go down. As with any learning strategy, the amount you learn is often directly related to the amount of effort put in and the amount of commitment you give it. Learning by reflection is not necessarily easy, nor is it comfortable, as it involves us in reconsidering and exploring some of the fundamental ways in which we see and understand the world, and questioning those. It also asks us to consider our actions and relationships with others, and to look at the ways we interact with people, often asking ourselves whether what we did was appropriate or could have been done differently. Reflective learning is probably the only learning strategy that uses your own experiences as the raw material in this way, and the only strategy that actively engages you in exploring your own actions, feelings and consequences as part of the learning experience. This is why Atkins (2004) suggests that anyone engaging in reflection as learning needs to have self-awareness and a degree of insight and acceptance of responsibility for their own actions before starting out on that road.

Reflective learning has entered professional practice as a learning strategy because of the move of nursing and midwifery education into higher education. The ability to think critically is expected of any person who graduates from higher education, and has been recognised as one of the essential attributes of those engaged in independent professional practice. Using reflective processes to develop critical thinking abilities will help you to become a critical thinker. When starting out on reflective activity, it is often helpful to use a reflective framework, or model, that has been specifically designed to draw you through the stages of the reflective processes.

The following section gives a brief overview of a few of the frameworks available for use by students for reflection.

Using Models and Frameworks to Guide Reflective Activity

All frameworks for reflective activity are designed with differing underpinning beliefs and values, and with different purposes in mind. Hence, it is important to be able to select a suitable framework for the type of reflection you want to engage in, the purposes you are using it for, and the outcomes you want to achieve. As a student practitioner, it is likely that you have been given at least one framework to use within your programme. This will have been selected because it fits with the philosophy that underpins the programme and reflects other elements of the course itself, such as the practice assessments you undergo, or the teaching strategies that are fundamental to helping you to acquire the knowledge and skills you will need as a registered practitioner. This section, then, does not provide an 'off-the-shelf' package using one author's reflective framework; rather, it presents some criteria that you might use to select a framework for use.

As you will have deduced we use reflective strategies for many different reasons, but these can be grouped into three main purposes:

- As a learning strategy: to identify our knowledge base, or deficit
- To improve patient care
- To develop practice and practice theory.

Although each may arise from the other, in that if our knowledge about something improves then this will be translated into more evidence-based care and therefore develop practice, using one framework all the time will not necessarily enable us to achieve all these aims. These criteria then, as outcomes of your reflective activity, can be used as the criteria for selecting a framework to use.

As a student, learning is likely to be the primary purpose for reflection. This will also increase your knowledge base. Therefore it is useful to identify and use a framework that has its origins in particular educational beliefs and values. As professional practitioners, we are all adults and beyond the pedagogy associated with school learning, so we require a framework that respects us as independent learners, and recognises the individual nature of our experiences. Hence, we might look to frameworks for reflection that arise from the **andragogical** paradigm identified by Carl Rogers (1983); these frameworks value the self-direction of learners and tap into their own motivation and urgency to learn. This is reflected in Gibbs' (1988) reflective cycle, which focuses essentially on the experiences of the individual as central to learning and results in an action plan that relates to the person's own self-development.

Gibbs' 'reflective learning cycle' is probably the one most commonly used in health-care professional education at present, and is considered 'user-friendly' because it can be used at any stage of a practitioner's career, from student to advanced practitioner. It incorporates the six stages of the reflective process, but focuses initially on the emotions of the person who is the reflector, developing the understanding of the experience from this. This framework is useful, therefore, for a student who wants to identify their learning and knowledge as a result of experiences, but who also wants to develop an action plan arising from these. Chart 4.4 provides the stages of this framework.

Similar to Gibbs' model is a framework that arose from Atkins and Murphy's (1993) original work, which again uses the reflector's feelings as the vehicle for exploration of an event. The specific stages used in this framework are:

- Being aware of uncomfortable feelings or thoughts
- Describing the situation, including thoughts and feelings
- Analysing the feelings and knowledge relevant to the situation

andragogical
adult learning – recognises that adults' learning style is different from that of children – adults are predisposed to seeking knowledge as self-motivators and independent learners

co Link
Chapters 3 and 18 also explore reflection.

- Evaluating the relevance of the knowledge
- Identifying any new learning that has occurred
- Putting it into action.

⁕ Activity 4.8

Use Gibbs' framework to work through an experience you have had. You can either think this through, write it down, or use it verbally with another person.

It must be remembered that this work arose from a literature review of the concept of reflective practice at the time – a view that has developed and moved on since then. This is particularly so in relation to the stimulus for reflective activity, which is generally accepted as having moved on from 'being aware of uncomfortable feelings' to any critical incident that is complete enough in itself to be described in full. This moves the emphasis from discomfort as the only source of reflective activity, and has been responsible for the wider acceptance of the methods of reflection entering the mainstream learning and teaching strategies in nursing and midwifery as well as in other health-care professions.

Although all reflective frameworks will increase the understanding of the practitioner about their situation and result in learning, one framework that originally focused specifically on uncovering and understanding the knowledge being used in a particular situation is Johns' model of structured reflection. This model arose from one of the first nursing development units and has been developed and refined continuously since the early 1990s. The 13th version was published in 2000, and adapted in Johns' book *Guided Reflection: Advancing Practice* in 2002. This framework uses a series of questions and prompts to guide the reflector through re-experiencing the event. These questions relate to:

- identifying significant issues
- exploring feelings
- consequences of actions taken
- the role and feelings of others
- the underpinning knowledge used
- comparing the situation with previous ones
- current feelings about the experience
- the individual moving forward from the experience.

What has occurred in the development of this framework is first its apparent complexity, but also a subtle change in its focus towards outcomes for patients as well as for the practice of the individual nurse. Although Johns' framework appears more complicated than Gibbs', the complexity lies in the detailed way the reflector is drawn though the list of cues, rather than it being a difficult, or complex framework to grasp. What is required, however, is a paper copy of the cue questions on hand to act as that guide, whereas Gibbs' is easy to remember once you are familiar with it and it can be carried in your head for spontaneous verbal reflection.

Another framework, focusing not so much on learning but development, is that presented by Holm and Stephenson (1994) as a 'practitioner's framework'. While this has been published, it was originally devised by the practitioners, when they were students themselves, to guide their own practice. Again, and similar to Johns, it asks specific and focused questions as opposed to the more generalised ones used by Gibbs, and Atkins and Murphy. The questions ask about the role the person took in an incident; the actions taken; how the

Chart 4.3 Stages in reflective processes used in reflective practice

- *Stage one – Selecting an event to reflect on*
  Any experience that is complete enough in itself to be described as a separate entity can be used. This is often referred to as a critical incident. It is important to select this carefully, depending on what it is you want to learn from the experience, who is likely to be party to your reflections, and whether there may be consequences from it, especially in professional terms. Similarly, if you are discussing this with others, are you likely to need consent from any third party involved in the event

- *Stage two – Observing and describing the experience*
  This provides the raw material for your reflective activity by giving a full description of what happened, including the context of the experience. Different frameworks or models will ask you to structure this in a different way, depending on the type of outcome you want to achieve. One useful way of doing this is to answer the questions who, where, when, what, why and how? Writing an incident down may give you a different description to verbally describing it

- *Stage three – Analysing the experience*
  This involves breaking down the experience into component parts. Useful questions at this stage are the why and how? You will be forming conclusions about the experience at this stage, using evaluative skills, and may designate different parts as 'good' or 'bad'. At this stage, you may start to perceive the situation differently, and possibly see your role in it in a different light

- *Stage four – Interpreting the experience*
  Here you widen out your analysis to consider the experience in the light of other knowledge. At this stage, you may choose to focus on different aspects of the experience and concentrate on those that seem most important. You will start to get explanations at this stage, and may bring in theoretical knowledge or other wider experiences to consider this experience through

- *Stage five – Exploring alternatives*
  Having thoroughly explored the experience itself, you can now move on to consider whether other courses of action could have happened, which would have resulted in a different ending to the experience. Remember, the purpose of this activity is to learn from this experience; simply validating what you or someone else actually did is not necessarily going to help you learn anything. This stage may be uncomfortable as it asks you to step outside your normal frames of reference and take different viewpoints

- *Stage six – Framing action*
  This where you need to commit to some sort of action, for example you may resolve to go and talk about the experience with someone else, go to the library to increase your knowledge base, or perhaps change your practice in some way. At this stage, it is worth considering what you would do differently if the situation, or something similar, happened again. You may see this as an opportunity to engage in practice development activities in the area in which you are working

Source: Adapted from Jasper (2003).

Chart 4.4 A worked example using Gibbs' reflective framework

- Description – what happened?
- Feelings – what were you thinking and feeling?
- Evaluation – what was good and bad about the experience?
- Analysis – what sense can you make of the situation?
- Conclusion – what else could you have done?
- Action plan – what would you do if this situation arises again?

situation could have been improved for all concerned; what changes could be made; learning; new knowledge, broader issues such as ethical or social issues that have arisen.

This framework presents not only the main questions, but follow-up questions that invite the reflector to explore their experiences more fully and ask questions they perhaps would not have thought of themselves. While models and frameworks that look more complicated may initially be off-putting to students, they have the advantage of presenting an easy to follow structure that aids the reflector through the reflective processes in a particular way. This is a definite bonus for beginning reflectors, as it takes practice, and some courage, to ask oneself difficult questions, particularly if we don't like the idea of the answer!

One model that looks more simple than any of the others is the original work of Borton (1970). It is another developmental model, encouraging the reflector to consider the experience from whatever viewpoint, or focus, they want to take to achieve their own outcomes. It is structured through three question stems:

- *What…?* Questions that describe the situation such as: What happened? What did I do? What did others do? What did I feel?
- *So what…?* Questions that invite the reflector to look behind the experience and explore the knowledge and theory base and her personal understanding of the situation, resulting in a personal theory. These might be: So what evidence informed my decisions? So what was I trying to achieve? So what experiences have I had previously that contribute to my understanding of the situation?
- *Now what…?* Questions that encourage the reflector to plan active intervention based on the theory developed, such as: Now what am I going to do? Now what do I need to find out? Now what needs to change?

This is the only one of the frameworks that ask the reflector to commit to action, rather than it remaining hypothetical. It is extremely easy for reflectors to use at all stages in their development as reflective practitioners, provided they are confident enough to devise their own questions based on what they want to achieve. In many ways, though, these are its weaknesses as well, as it is dependent upon the reflector, or the person acting as the questioner, to ask the questions that will challenge the reflector sufficiently.

> ★ **Activity 4.9**
>
> Consider the frameworks presented here.
> Which of these appeals to you most? Why is this?

A note of caution has to be made here, in that it is always worth finding out more about the origins of a framework before using a shorthand version presented in this way. The original references for all these have been provided. In the case of Borton's framework however, which is significantly older than the rest, I'd like to signpost the reader to Rolfe et al.'s (2010) discussion and development of this model, which also incorporates some of the strategies of other frameworks presented here to make it more 'user-friendly' for the reflector.

Reflective Learning in the Practice Environment

Most of the opportunities for learning from practice will be found in the practice environment, and this practical experience will make up 50 per cent of your course. It is therefore extremely important for you to devise strategies that will make the most of the opportunities available and to gain the maximum knowledge and skill from your placements. It is worth taking some time to prepare for your placements so that you know what it is you need to get out of it and how you might do this.

Preparing for a placement

As already identified, all our experiences are built on what we already know. So, no matter what stage you are at in your course, you will have some experiences as the basic building blocks. So your first reflective activity when preparing for a new placement needs to be a review of your last placement, your practice assessment documents and your learning outcomes, to assess what it is you need to achieve in your new placement. It is likely that you will also have theoretical assignments to complete during your placement, so these need to be counted in with the learning outcomes from practice over the time period.

If you have completed Activity 4.10, you will be beginning to realise where you need to put the most effort in over the next few months, and the amount of work that needs to be done. Part of this work is to identify the learning experiences in the clinical environment that will help you to achieve your outcomes, and, if you are lucky, will provide the material for a theoretical assignment.

It is also worth reflecting on the sorts of opportunities that your next placement will offer so that you can maximise these in fulfilling your learning objectives. Find out as much about the placement area as you can before you arrive for your first shift. It may be worth making a preliminary visit and meeting your supervisor informally. Many areas provide information booklets about the type of work that goes on in the area, the types of patients received and the conditions treated. Similarly, midwifery areas differ in the services they offer to their clients – even if you are returning to a similar sort of area to one you have worked in before, the experience will offer a different philosophy of care, different customs and practices and different ways of doing things that you will need to adjust to.

> **✴ Activity 4.10**
>
> Make a list of what you need to achieve by the end of your next clinical placement. Review this list in terms of outcomes almost achieved, those that are part achieved, and those that are completely new to you.

Taking a positive-action approach to learning

You will have given yourself a head start in achieving your objectives if you have completed the tasks in the previous section. The next involves planning to use the opportunities you have identified to the full. This may involve keeping some sort of clinical log or diary to ensure that you record your activity, and then selecting from this as an *aide-memoire* when doing reflective activity that will help you learn from your experiences. Similarly, you can take an active part in organising your learning by ensuring that you know what is going on in the environment on a daily basis and are in the right place at the right time to experience activities. Finally, it is worth discussing with your supervisor, at an early stage in the placement, what it is you need to complete, and what you'd like to experience, as part of this time.

Using others to support your learning

Not only is there a wealth of learning opportunities in the clinical environment, there is also a large pool of different people who can contribute to your learning. In most clinical environments you will be working as part of an inter-professional team of health-care professionals, each of whom take a different approach and bring a different perspective to patient care. So, it is not just the nurses and midwives who will be able to support your learning, but also the allied health professionals, medical staff and supporting staff such as chaplains, social workers, clinical psychologists and others.

Primarily though, you will be working under the direction of your own supervisor, whose role it is to ensure that you have a range of learning experiences and opportunities to enable you to fulfil your learning needs. It is your supervisor's responsibility to help you to practise and develop reflective skills in relation to the clinical experiences you have with them in order to begin your own reflective practice. Therefore, it is important for you to use this person to maximum effect and take up any opportunities offered for reflective work. This may be through prearranged clinical supervision meetings, but it is more likely that these opportunities will arrive ad hoc during your shift, and it will take effort from both of you to ensure that you reflect informally whenever the opportunity arises.

Reflective dialogues are one of the main ways that you will be learning through other people. This may be through clinical supervision sessions, which are planned and structured in some way, or informal occurrences that happen opportunely when there is an event worthy of developing reflectively. It is not only qualified practitioners who will help you in this way; very often you learn as much by working reflectively with your student colleagues. In particular, colleagues are very useful for practising reflection using a reflective framework, as the more you do this, the more you will become comfortable with the technique and it will be part of the way you practise. Try to take the opportunity, when talking over your experiences, of suggesting that you talk through it in a structured way. Working in pairs, one can be the reflector, the other the facilitator. It is the latter's role to ensure that the reflector stays within the framework's structure when talking about their experience. After an agreed time period, swap roles, giving the other person the same amount of time to work through their experience. The facilitator has the responsibility of ensuring that the reflective cycle is completed – that is, that some sort of action is planned and that the other person is committed to taking that action.

Self-directed reflective learning in the clinical environment

There are various simple strategies that you can use to ensure that you make the most of what the clinical environment has to offer. A quick and simple way to use reflection daily is to get into the habit of reviewing the day and identifying what has happened to you and what you have learnt. Although this is a superficial activity, as with all reflective work, it is likely to lead to other things. For instance, if you use a technique called 'three-a-day' (outlined in Chart 4.5) you will give yourself plenty of material to reflect on, especially if you focus the 'three' on particular areas of knowledge or skills.

Another way to use reflection on a regular basis is to make the effort to write up or discuss, at least one critical incident each week using a reflective

Chart 4.5 Using the 'three-a-day' reflective technique

The three-a-day technique is simply a way of focusing your thoughts back over a particular time period. You can choose to focus on anything, but the trick is to identify the 'top' three of those. Several examples are given below, but for this to be of most use to you, it is worth getting into the habit of creating your own foci. These might arise from your knowledge or skills needs or your learning outcomes, for instance. Or you might need to give your confidence a bit of a boost, or perhaps, if you are doing well, to identify your weaknesses that could do with some work. Some examples are:

- Three things that went well today are …
- Three things that I enjoyed today are …
- Three things that I learnt today are …
- Three skills that I used today are …
- Three things that I am good at are …
- Three things that I find difficult are …
- Three drugs that I am familiar with are …
- Three people who I admire as role models are …
- Three people who I don't admire are …

This list is endless!

However, the key to this activity is not really the answers you gave, but what you then go on and do with these answers. For instance, look back to the last two sentences about people you may or may not admire. Having identified these people, you might like to think about why you admire them, or not; what it is about the way they conduct their practice that makes them a role model; what it is you can learn from them, or decide to avoid, from having observed them.

Getting into the habit of using this technique every day is a simple way of learning reflectively from practice. You may then decide to pick on one of these experiences as a focus for more formal reflective activity using a reflective framework. With practice, you can do this mentally, arriving at new perspectives or defining courses of action that you will take as a result of your experience.

---

framework. If you write these and keep them in your portfolio, this will not only provide you with regular practice of reflective learning techniques and develop your skills, it will also give you a dynamic record and evidence of your experiences and development in practice, and provide material for theoretical assignments.

Finally, always keep your eye on the future, both short and long term. Developing the habit of periodically reviewing your learning outcomes and your progress towards meeting them will ensure that you identify any deficits along the way and have time to plan to rectify them. As with the reflective frameworks that work through asking questions, try to develop the habit of continually questioning yourself.

> ✸ **Activity 4.11**
>
> Take a few minutes to review the opportunities and ideas presented in this section and jot down some examples for each one that you could use during your own placements.

Recording your Reflective Work

Most of the reflective work you do will be informal, within the workplace, either by yourself or with others, or by yourself away from the workplace. However, many university programmes now require formalised reflective activity to be demonstrated, either within written assignments or as components within a portfolio. Even if you are not required, as part of your course, to write reflectively, it is certainly worth considering doing this in a reflective journal or log, to enhance the value of the experiences you have in practice (Jasper, 2008) and as a self-directed learning strategy.

Written reflection is a different strategy to verbal or informal mental reflection and often results in different outcomes. This is partly because of the particular features of reflective writing as identified by Jasper (2003):

- We always write for a purpose – it is not random activity but is deliberate.
- Reflective writing takes place in the first person – it is impossible to put ourselves at the centre of our writing if we don't.
- Writing requires us to order our thoughts – whatever we use to do this, a structured framework or one devised by ourselves, all writing has some sort of order to it.
- Writing creates a permanent record that we can return to again and again and view differently each time.
- Writing helps to develop our creativity by enabling us to see connections between previously disparate items of information.
- Writing enhances our analytical ability by helping us to break things down.
- Writing reflectively helps us to be critical thinkers as we explore alternatives and weigh different ways of perceiving things.
- Writing can be used to develop new understanding and knowledge.

Writing reflectively does not need to take the same form all the time, although you may be required to use a specific format within your course.

Most common, in terms of reflective writing as a student, is likely to be the recording and analysis of critical incidents, and the use of reflective reviews at specific periods in your course.

Critical incident analysis

🔗 Link

Chapter 1 details the nursing process.

It is usual for students to be asked to use a framework to analyse a critical incident in a written format, to provide the practice of using a structure to analyse a problem. In many ways, this is no different to using, for instance, the nursing process to assess patient needs, diagnose nursing care, plan and implement a care strategy and evaluate it once delivered. The frameworks simply provide you with a way of structuring and ordering your writing in a certain way, while giving emphasis to particular elements of it. Any of the frameworks presented in this chapter can be used in this way. However, as you become more confident in your reflective activity, you may find that you want to adapt frameworks to suit the purpose of your reflection, or even to create your own in the way Holm and Stephenson (1994) did.

Reflective reviews

Reflective reviews differ from critical incident analysis in that they take a wider look at an experience, a series of experiences or over a period of time. For instance, you might be asked to evaluate your learning within a specific placement, or to review your progress towards a set of learning outcomes. The simplest way of doing this is to start off with the learning outcomes as a framework, and then construct a discussion showing how your experiences demonstrate your achievements. But, many people will want to develop more creative ways of doing this, by focusing on one particular patient's case history, for instance, and linking skill and knowledge developments and achievements to that. While there is no one way to write reflective reviews, it is important that the central feature of them is reflective learning and practice, thus they need to demonstrate how learning has been achieved through reflective processes. This will inevitably involve self-critique and evaluation, showing that you are working towards the self-assessment and evaluation of your own practice required of a registered practitioner.

Using Reflective Writing in Portfolios

In creating a permanent record through reflective writing you will be beginning to produce evidence that can be used within a portfolio to demonstrate your achievements. In many courses portfolios are used to collect evidence for practice assessment and to demonstrate your competence at each stage of your course. Sometimes portfolios will be used as module assessment, to create and reflect on evidence of specified learning outcomes and experiences that demonstrate the understanding of theory and its application to the student's practice. Finally, on completion of your course, you will need to keep an on-going professional portfolio to demonstrate your competence as a practitioner for the purposes of triennial registration with the NMC. A summary of the uses that may be made of portfolios is presented in Table 4.2.

Table 4.2 Uses of portfolios

As a student	As a practitioner
Public use	
• For coursework assessment	• To fulfil the NMC's PREP requirements for continuing professional development for triennial registration
• For assessment of your practice competences	• To demonstrate to others your accountability for your competence as a practitioner
• To collect evidence of your achievements	• As part of the annual employee appraisal process
• For use in applying for your first post as a qualified practitioner	• As part of the interview process for selection onto a course
	• As part of selection process for a new job
	• To keep together evidence of your ongoing development, for example records of attendance at conferences and study days, independent reading and so on
Private use	
• As a self-directed learning strategy	• As part of lifelong learning, using your experiences as the focus for development
• As a learning strategy to compile an ongoing record of your development	• To work through experiences in practice in order to learn from them
• To keep a record of your experiences	
• To work through your experiences reflectively as a learning strategy	

At the very minimum, a portfolio is a collection of artefacts that presents a picture of you as a practitioner. In your professional career it will be collected for a specific purpose and to demonstrate certain things – this may be while you are a student, where the parameters will be closely specified for you, or it may be for the NMC's purposes in verifying standards for post-registration education and practice (PREP).

However, you may decide to widen the contents and use of your portfolio and incorporate within it a reflective journal or log, or any of the reflective work that you do while you are on placement. It is important to remember that a portfolio is a private document and belongs to you. No-one can make you show it, in its entirety, to anyone else. Where it becomes a public document, open to the scrutiny of others, is where it forms part of a course of study, or may be requested by the NMC for audit purposes, and the only parts that you need to show, and can select from, are those specified in an agreement – such as the assessment criteria of your course, or the requirements of the NMC. Even so, you can select what is contained within your portfolio, and can remove parts of it if you want to, making sure that what remains and is open to scrutiny will do you no harm in a public arena. Many practitioners use reflective writing to explore events in practice that they find disturbing or maybe do not reflect on themselves in a particularly good light. It would be naive for those practitioners to leave these sorts of writings in their portfolios.

The purpose of the majority of portfolios is to demonstrate your achievements – whether this be against specified learning outcomes as a student, or to demonstrate accountable competent practice as a registered practitioner.

Using Personal Development Plans

Personal development plans (PDPs) are increasingly being used within higher education to enable students to plan and focus their learning activities. These are therefore ideal for incorporating within reflective practice, because they demand an element of forward planning and identification of both your learning needs and the achievements that need to result during your course of study. It is possible that these will even be the start of your reflective activity, as they often contain action plans to be completed, and review stages throughout your course to enable you to evaluate your progress towards your goals.

The range of PDPs available is vast, as they are usually designed to meet the needs of a specific institution or course, hence it is not appropriate to explore these in detail here, because if you are required to use them, you will be introduced to them as part of your programme. Similarly, many employers now require all their employees to have a PDP that is reviewed annually at performance review. These serve the purpose of helping the employee to consider their own future within the organisation, or their own career, and plan a strategy that will contribute to their personal and professional development.

Chapter Summary

This chapter has presented the basic elements of reflective practice as a requisite component of professional practice. Indeed, if these are acquired by every pre-registration student throughout their three years of studying for the professional register, it will contribute considerably to the standards of practice and quality of care experienced by our service users. Equally as important, developing the skills of reflective practice empowers the practitioner in making judgements and supporting their decision-making, resulting in the development of practice theory and a knowledge base that derives from practice experiences. These skills are just a beginning, however; following course completion, it is likely that the majority of the learning and development that you do will arise from practising as a reflective practitioner. So, not only are these skills important to ensure our patients' quality of care, they are significant for every individual practitioner in gaining the most out of their working lives.

? Test yourself!

1   What is reflective practice and what are its components?

2   What is the difference between reflection-in-action and reflection-on-action?

3   Why do professionals need to practise reflectively?

4   What are the six stages of the reflective processes?

5   How might models and frameworks of reflection help you to reflect?

6   What criteria would you use in choosing a model of reflection?

7   How can you maximise the learning opportunities in the clinical environment by using reflective techniques and practice?

8   How is writing reflectively different from reflecting in other ways?

Burns, C. and Schutz, S. (eds) (2004) *Reflective Practice in Nursing: The Growth of the Professional Practitioner*, Blackwell Publishing, Oxford.

Jasper, M.A. (2003) *Beginning Reflective Practice.* Nelson Thornes, Cheltenham.

Rolfe, G., Jasper, M., Freshwater, D. (2011) *Critical Reflection in Practice: Generating Knowledge for Care*, Palgrave Macmillan, Basingstoke.

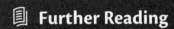 **Further Reading**

For live links to useful websites see: www.palgrave.com/nursinghealth/hogston

References

Atkins, S. (2004) Developing underlying skills in the move towards reflective practice. In Bulman, C. and Schutz, S. (eds) *Reflective Practice in Nursing.* Blackwell Publishing, Oxford.

Atkins, S. and Murphy, K. (1993) Reflection: a review of the literature. *Journal of Advanced Nursing* **18**: 1188–92.

Benner, P. (1984) *From Novice to Expert.* Addison-Wesley, Menlo Park, CA.

Borton T. (1970) *Reach, Touch, Teach.* McGraw-Hill, London.

Brookfield, S.D. (1987) *Developing Critical Thinkers:*

Challenging Adults to Explore Alternative Ways of Thinking and Acting. Open University Press, Milton Keynes.

Carper, B. (1978) Fundamental patterns of knowing in nursing. *Advances in Nursing Science* **1**: 15–23.

Gibbs, G. (1988) *Learning by Doing: A Guide to Teaching and Learning Methods.* Further Education Unit, Oxford Polytechnic, Oxford.

Holm, D. and Stephenson, S. (1994) Reflection – a student's perspective. In Palmer, A., Burns, S. and Bulman, C. (eds) *Reflective Practice in Nursing.* Blackwell Scientific, Oxford.

Jasper, M.A. (2003) *Beginning Reflective Practice.* Nelson Thornes, Cheltenham.

Jasper, M. (2008) Using reflective journals and diaries to enhance practice and learning. In Burns, C. and Schutz, S. (eds) *Reflective Practice in Nursing: The Growth of the Professional Practitioner.* Blackwell Publishing, Oxford.

Johns, C. (2002) *Guided Reflection: Advancing Practice.* Blackwell Publishing, Oxford.

Kolb, D. (1984) *Experiential Learning as the Science of Learning and Development.* Prentice Hall, Englewood Cliffs, NJ.

Rogers, C. (1983) *Freedom to Learn for the 80s.* Merrill, Columbus.

Rolfe G., Jasper M. and Freshwater D. (2010) *Critical Reflection in Practice: Generating Knowledge for Care,* 2nd edition, Palgrave Macmillan, Basingstoke.

Schön, D. (1983) *The Reflective Practitioner.* Temple Smith, London.

Walsh, M. and Ford, P. (1989) *Nursing Rituals: Research and Rational Actions.* Butterworth Heinemann, Oxford.

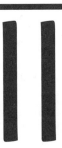

Nursing Interventions

5

Infection Control

📖 Contents

- Control of Infection
- Health-Care Associated Infections (HCAIs)
- Universal Infection Control Precautions

- Chapter Summary
- Test Yourself!
- Further Reading
- References

☑ Learning outcomes

This chapter describes the policies and procedures for the control of infection. It is intended that this chapter will provide practitioners with evidence-based knowledge to carry out procedures in a manner that will safeguard them and the patients in their care. By the end of the chapter, you should be able to:

- Demonstrate a basic knowledge of microbiology
- Define health-care associated infection (HCAI)
- Describe how microorganisms are spread
- Understand the need for universal precautions
- Discuss the management of clinical waste
- Describe the role of the infection control team.

Throughout the chapter you will be given an opportunity to undertake some exercises that will assist you in further developing your knowledge, skills and competence. Some of these activities may initially be practised in a skills laboratory under supervision, may also require you to access and read additional policies relevant to your health-care setting and suggested textbooks listed at the end of the chapter.

Control of Infection

The threat that infection poses to human health has become widely acknowledged as a result of the 'swine flu' pandemic caused by the influenza type A virus (H1N1) throughout the world (WHO, 2009) and the more resistant Methicillin-Resistant *Staphylococcus Aureus* epidemic (MRSA: also referred to as the superbug), and *Clostridium Difficile* (*C-Diff*) bacteria found in hospitals. Furthermore, the public have become more aware of health-care associated infections (HCAIs) such as MRSA as a likely complication and probable cause of death following hospitalisation. As a consequence, it has become necessary for organisations to develop strategies for preventing HCAIs. This chapter describes the policies and principles which nurses must follow to prevent HCAIs.

Health-Care Associated Infections (HCAIs)

Infection is a term used to describe the colonisation of the human body by pathogens such as bacteria, viruses, parasites, prions and fungi. A secondary infection denotes that an infection developed during or following the treatment of an existing primary infectious condition. A health-care associated infection (HCAI) is a term used to describe any infection acquired via the provision of health care.

The normal human skin is colonised with bacteria, with different parts of the body having varied numbers of bacterial counts. Bacteria found on hands are divided into two categories; the resident and the transient. The resident bacteria are attached to the deeper layers of the skin and more resistant to removal. The transient bacteria are often acquired by nurses through direct contact with patients or from surfaces that are contaminated, for example commodes. The transient bacteria are often associated with HCAIs and these transient micro-organisms can be removed by routine handwashing.

The prevalence of HCAIs in England in 2006 was 8 per cent, with the risk of acquiring an HCAI increasing with age, the elderly being at greatest risk. The length of stay in hospitals is also linked to the increased risk of acquiring an infection (National Audit Office, 2009). A host of additional factors may contribute to the development of HCAIs and these include:

- critically ill patients with weakened immunity
- increase in invasive procedures
- high turnover of patients
- poor compliance with good practice
- lack of cleanliness
- inappropriate use of antibiotics.

The development of modern-day health care, including complex invasive surgical interventions on critically ill patients with a greater susceptibility to infection, has increased the risk of acquiring an infection while in a health-care setting. The National Audit Office (2009) reported that the most common types of HCAIs included the following types of infection:

- Urinary tract: 20 per cent (80 per cent caused by indwelling catheters)

- Lower respiratory tract: 20 per cent (common in ventilated patients)
- Gastrointestinal: 22 per cent (70 per cent were associated with *C-Diff*)
- Surgical site: 14 per cent
- Blood stream: 7 per cent (associated with invasive procedures)
- Skin and soft tissue: 10 per cent (including pressure ulcers)
- Others such as bone, joint and the central nervous system: 7 per cent.

Many infectious diseases have the capacity to spread in nursing and residential care homes where large numbers of elderly people live in close proximity, have indwelling urinary catheters and wounds such as pressure ulcers. Many of these infections may be serious and in some cases may result in death.

Many of the common HCAIs such as MRSA originate from micro-organisms that people usually carry safely on their skin and cause infection only when they gain access to the blood stream. For an HCAI to occur there has to be a source or reservoir of organisms that can cause the infection and a means by which the germs are transmitted. The most likely means of transmission of infectious organisms is by direct contact or the percutaneous inoculation of infected material. Measures to control HCAI are twofold: if possible, the source of infection should be eliminated and, second, strategies should be implemented to break the chain of infection (Figure 5.1).

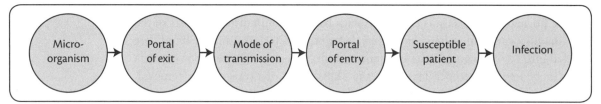

Figure 5.1 Chain of infection

The most effective and efficient way of breaking the chain of infection is to follow the standard precautions in daily practice. As many patients are unaware or unwilling to disclose any infection that may be present, the only way to ensure that the risk of transmission is reduced is by following standard precautions across all patients.

The Department of Health (DoH) has produced several major documents, such as *Winning Ways: Working Together to Reduce Healthcare Associated Infection in England* (2003), *Towards Cleaner Hospitals and Lower Rates of Infection: A Summary of Action* (2004), The Health Act 2006 (2006a), *Essential Steps to Safe, Clean Care: Reducing Healthcare-associated Infections* (2006b), *Infection Control: Guidance for Care Homes* (2006c), and it is beyond the scope of this chapter to discuss them all. However, following a critical review of the recommendations for good practices, the subsequent sections focus on essential core procedures and staff behaviour that are crucial in reducing HCAIs.

⊕ Link

Chapter 18 also discusses hospital-acquired infections.

Universal Infection Control Precautions

Hand hygiene and use of personal protective clothing

Good hand hygiene is the single most important activity for reducing the spread of HCAIs (Pratt et al., 2007, Bandolier, 2000, DoH, 2006b). Many infections spread by contact and hands are a major vehicle in the transmission of infection (Royal College of Nursing, 1992). Normal skin has a resident population of micro-organisms and additional transient organisms are picked up during contact in the delivery of nursing care, with species such as *klebsiella* surviving for up to two and a half hours (Casewell and Phillips, 1977). The aim of handwashing is to remove these micro-organisms or to reduce their numbers below that of an infective dose. Health-care workers should be trained in effective handwashing and hands should be washed following the procedures shown in Chart 5.1.

Chart 5.1 Indications for handwashing

• Before direct contact with patient	• Before serving meals
• When hands are visibly soiled or potentially contaminated	• After removing aprons and gloves
	• At the beginning and end of duty
• After handling contaminated items	• If in any doubt about the cleanliness of hands
• After handling body fluids	

Hands can be decontaminated by applying an alcohol-based hand rub or washing hands with soap and running water from a tap. An effective handwashing technique involves three stages: preparation, washing and rinsing, and drying. In the preparation phase, the hands are wet and an appropriate antimicrobial preparation applied. The solution must be applied to all the skin surfaces of the hands. The hands should be rubbed carefully for about 10–15 seconds ensuring that the tips of fingers, the thumb and the areas between the fingers, palm and back of hands have been attended to before rinsing thoroughly and drying using paper towels as shown in Figure 5.2.

Thorough rinsing under running water is an important part of the procedure. The final step is to dry the hands thoroughly using a paper towel for each hand – this not only prevents soreness, but also further reduces the number of transient bacteria that may still be present after handwashing.

When using alcohol hand rub, it is important to ensure that hands are free of dirt or organic matter otherwise handwashing using soap and water is recommended. The decontamination agent should come into contact with all surfaces of the hands and rubbed vigorously until all the alcohol has evaporated. Alcohol hand rub is significantly better than soap in reducing hand contamination (Gould, 1996; Girou et al., 2002). In 2004, hospitals were advised to introduce 'near patient' alcohol-based hand rubs – for example, attached beside beds and at entrances to wards – by April 2005 (National Patient Safety Agency, 2004). Archer et al. (2007) reported that poisoning from ingestion of alcohol hand rub has increased since the widespread introduction of their use in clinical areas and

✴ Activity 5.1

Identify the local and national guidelines concerning the control of infection in your place of work.

warn against the danger of toxicity especially among the young, the confused and those with alcohol dependency.

	Description
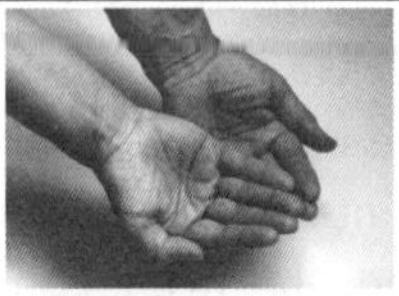	First wet your hands thoroughly then apply the soap.
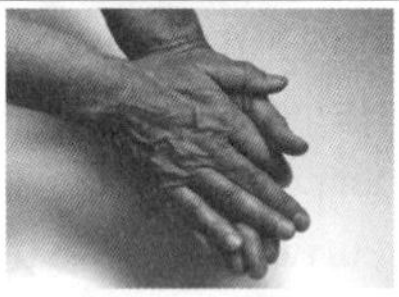	Rub your hands together (palm to palm) so that you achieve a visible lather that covers all surfaces.
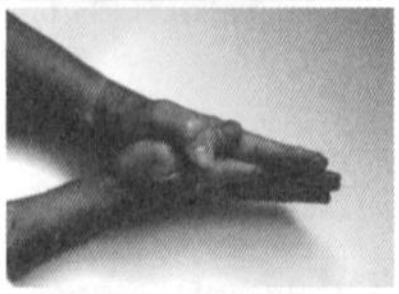	Rub the back of your left hand with the palm of your right. Then change over and rub the back of your right hand with your left palm.
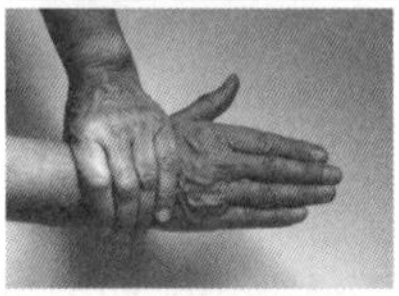	With your fingers interlinked rub your palms together.
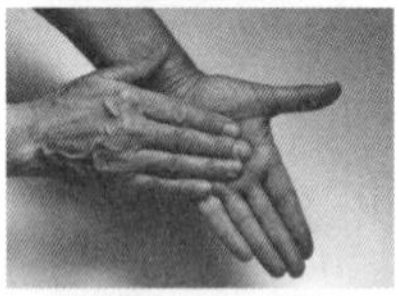	With your fingers interlaced, as close to the palm as you can, rub your fingers together.
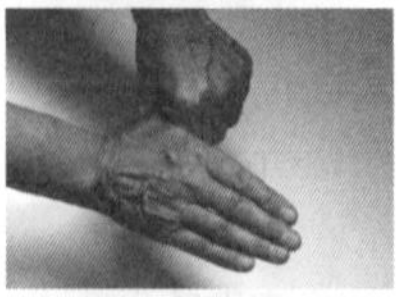	Interlock your fingers. Rub the backs of the fingers of your left hand in your right palm. Then do the same with the fingers of your right hand in your left palm.
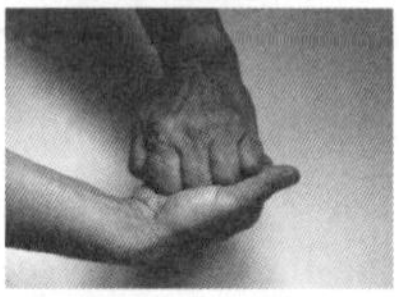	Clasp your right thumb in your left palm. Rotate your thumb. Then do the same with your left thumb in your right palm.
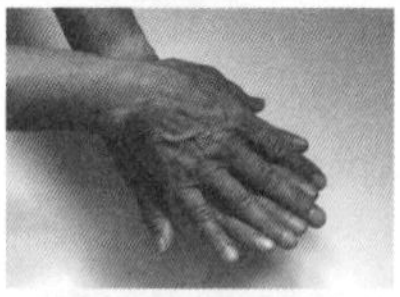 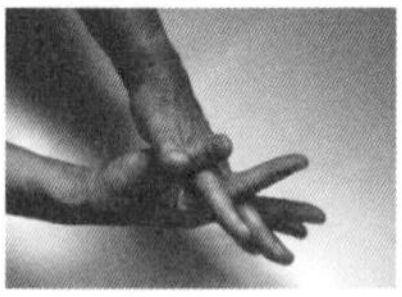	a) Rub the fingers of your left hand in a circular pattern in your right palm. Then repeat with the fingers of your right hand in your left palm. b) Using clasped index finger and thumb wash wrists.
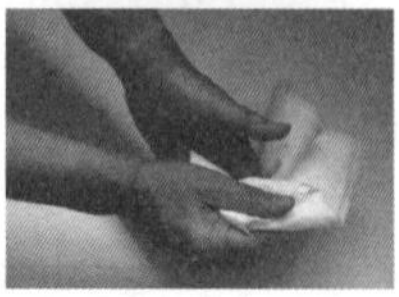	Rinse your hands thoroughly. Shake hands without splashing. Dry hands thoroughly using disposable paper towels.

Figure 5.2 Handwashing technique

The skin should be intact and any cuts or abrasions should be covered with waterproof dressings. Staff should also avoid contact with clinical waste and refrain from undertaking invasive procedures.

Use of protective wear

Staff should wear protective equipment depending on the risks to themselves and other patients. Gloves should be worn in the following situations:

- Contact with open wounds
- Contact with sterile sites
- Contact with mucous membranes
- Contact with body fluids
- When handling body secretions and excretions
- When managing contaminated equipments.

Gloves are not a substitute for effective hand hygiene. Gloves must be discarded after each activity in order to prevent the transmission of micro-organisms. For example, gloves worn to wash patients should not be used to clean the urinary catheter. After the removal of gloves hands should be washed with soap and water using the techniques described in Figure 5.2.

Plastic aprons must be worn as single-use items per patient when there is a risk of spillage of body fluids. Other protective clothing such as goggles, face masks and boots should be worn on the basis of an assessment of the risks of cross-infection.

Aseptic technique

All invasive clinical procedures should be carried out aseptically (Tremayne and Parboteeah, 2006). Gloves should be used as single-use items and sterile gloves must be used for **aseptic procedures**. Gloves should be applied immediately before a procedure and removed when the course of action is complete. Gloves must be changed in between patients and in some instances when undertaking different activities for the same patient, such as washing and aseptic dressing.

Proper handling of equipment

When equipment is being used for a group of patients, such as a communal bath and commodes, these must be cleaned and disinfected after each use and between patients. If it is not possible to clean and disinfect the equipment, then single-use or disposable equipment should be considered.

Safe handling and disposal of sharps

The use of sharp items such as needles, scissors, blades and scalpels is an everyday occurrence for health-care practitioners. It also increases their risk of injuries and the inoculation of germs. It is therefore essential that extreme care is taken in the safe use and disposal of sharps. The handling of sharps should be kept to a minimum. Needles and syringes must not be disassembled before disposal. Needles must not be resheathed and used sharps must be discarded into a sharps container conforming to British Safety (BS) standards. Staff should ensure that they have had training in the use of the equipment.

> ☀ Activity **5.2**
>
> Identify the different methods of hand decontamination used in different areas of practice, such as hospitals, health centres and patients' homes.

aseptic procedure
a procedure that is performed under sterile conditions to prevent contamination

Waste disposal

All waste must be handled and disposed of safely as it can potentially cause infection to another person coming into contact with it. The National Health Service (NHS) has a legal responsibility for the safe disposal of clinical and hazardous waste. Furthermore, all employers have a legal obligation under the Health and Safety at Work Act (1974) to ensure that all their employees are appropriately trained and proficient in procedures for working safely. All clinical areas should also have a written policy on waste disposal.

All waste is categorised into household waste and clinical waste. Household waste includes items such as paper, cardboard, flowers and those of a non-hazardous, non-contaminated nature. It is disposed of in an appropriate bag (please consult local policy for types/colour of bag to be used).

The legal definition of clinical waste is given in the Controlled Waste Regulations 1992 as:

> any waste which consists wholly or partly of human or animal tissue, blood or other bodily fluids, excretions, drugs or other pharmaceutical products, swabs or dressings, or syringes, needles or other sharp instruments, being waste which unless rendered safe may prove hazardous to any person coming into contact with it; and any other waste arising from medical, nursing, dental, veterinary, pharmaceutical or similar practice, investigation, treatment, care, teaching or research, or in the collection of blood for transfusion, being waste which may cause infection to any person coming in contact with it.
> (Environment Agency, 2004)

Clinical waste is categorised into five groups as shown in Table 5.1.

The following principles should be followed when handling waste:

• Bags should be filled no more than two-thirds full

✳ Activity 5.3

Identify how the following types of waste are dealt with in your hospital/community: used linen, soiled linen, infected linen, patients' personal clothing and duvets.

Table 5.1 Guidance for the recovery and disposal of hazardous and non-hazardous waste

Categories of waste		Method of disposal
Group A	Soiled dressings, swabs, and all other contaminated waste. Waste materials from cases of infectious diseases. All human tissues.	Waste placed in yellow clinical waste bag (in accordance with local policy).
Group B	Used syringes, needles, cartridges, broken glass, glass ampoules, cannulae and any other sharp instruments.	Yellow-coloured Sharps container which complies with BS 7320 and of a type approved by the infection control team.
Group C	Microbiological cultures and potentially infected waste from pathology departments, research laboratories and post-mortem rooms.	Yellow clinical waste bag placed in locked bins.
Group D	Pharmaceutical products that are unsuitable for use on safety grounds and chemical waste such as amalgam.	Yellow clinical waste bag. Cytotoxic waste should be disposed of in a designated cytotoxic waste container.
Group E	Used disposable items such as bed pans, urinals, incontinence pads, stoma bags and any items that do not fall into Group A.	Contents of disposable items can be disposed of via the toilets. If assessment indicates a risk, then follow instruction as for disposal of Group A waste.

Source: Environment Agency (2004). Reproduced under the Open Government Licence v1.0.

- Bags should not be compressed when closing
- Bags must be secured using a plastic tie or tying a knot at the top
- Avoid bodily contact with bags and handle them by the top end.

The following principles should be followed when handling sharps:

- Only fill container up to three-quarters full
- Use the handles provided to handle the containers
- On no account should attempts be made to open a sealed sharps container
- Place sharp items at the point of use
- Do not resheath needles and syringes before disposal.

Isolation of patient with HCAI

The isolation of patients with proven or suspected infection has been shown to reduce transmission of the germs and is one aspect of a hospital strategy for preventing HCAIs. Patients should ideally be placed in single rooms (DoH, 2005b). Single rooms must contain hand hygiene facilities and a wall-mounted antibacterial hand-cleaning gel dispenser. These rooms should also have full en suite facilities, including a toilet. In areas where there are shared toilet facilities, residents/patients with infectious diarrhoea must have sole use of a toilet, which must be thoroughly cleaned between each use. Advice should be sought from the Infection Control Team in hospitals or from the Public Health Laboratory for private nursing homes. If single rooms are not available, patients should be put in cohorts (having the same infection) and cared for by designated staff. Staff should follow strict hand hygiene and protective clothing procedures as outlined earlier and follow specific guidelines for the cleaning and decontamination of equipment, waste and linen disposal. There should be restricted movement of the patient and movement should only be allowed for clinical reasons.

Staff adherence to good infection control practices

It has been reported that despite aggressive educational initiatives, non-adherence of good infection control practices such as handwashing has remained low (Boyce and Pittet, 2002) due to a number of factors such as lack of time, lack of institutional support and lack of professional training. To improve adherence, it is important to understand why non-adherence occurs and to develop specific interventions that can help with the behaviour change. The provision of information to increase knowledge will not result in behaviour change (Delamater, 2006) unless managers understand that behaviour change is part of an interpersonal process requiring a staff-centred approach to management, a collaborative relationship, good communication and the provision of information at the earliest opportunity, when staff are ready to learn more about the new guidelines.

Several new initiatives have been developed by the DoH since 2004, such as the Cleanyourhands campaign (National Patient Safety Agency, 2004); *Saving Lives* (DoH, 2007), The Health Act (DoH, 2006a), to tackle HCAIs. Most of these are, however, policy documents that require hospitals to develop local strategies to deal with the causes of HCAIs and they are beyond the scope of this chapter.

✷ Activity 5.4

Discuss how an educational strategy can be developed in a care environment such as a nursing home or a hospital to educate staff on prevention and management of HCAIs.

✷ Activity 5.5

Discuss, with your mentor, how and when you would contact the infection control team in your placement environment, for example acute care, community care settings and nursing homes.

Chapter Summary

This chapter has focused on the practical aspects of reducing HCAIs in the day-to-day management of patients by following evidence-based guidelines. From the review of the literature, it is clear that staff should take personal responsibility for reducing HCAI by changing their behaviours and for organisations to have a strategic approach for managing the whole situation, with the formation of 'Infection Control Teams' to support and advise staff.

? Test yourself!

1 What does HCAI stand for?

2 What stages are involved in the 'chain of infection'?

3 What are the commonest sites for HCAIs?

4 Describe the classification for clinical waste.

Gould, D. and Brooker, C. (2008) *Infection Prevention and Control*. Palgrave Macmillan, Basingstoke.

Weston, D. (2008) *Infection Prevention and Control: Theory and Practice for Healthcare Professionals*, John Wiley & Sons, Chichester.

Smith, B. (2010) *Student Nurse Infection Control Survival Guide*. Pearson Education.

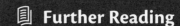

📖 Further Reading

For live links to useful websites see: www.palgrave.com/nursinghealth/hogston

References

Archer, J.R.H., Wood, D.M., Tizzard, Z., Jones, A.L. and Dargan, P.I. (2007) Alcohol hand rubs: hygiene and hazards. *British Medical Journal* **335**: 1154–5.

Bandolier (2000) Washing hands reduces hospital-acquired infection. http://www.medicine.ox.ac.uk/bandolier/band82/b82-2.html (accessed 25 June 2009).

Boyce, J.M. and Pittet, D. (2002) Guideline for hand hygiene in health-care settings: Recommendations of the Healthcare Infection Control Practices Advisory Committee and the HICPAC/SHEA/APIC/IDSA Hand Hygiene Task Force. *Morbidity and Mortality Weekly Report* **51**: 1–44. http://www.cdc.gov/mmwr/preview/mmwrhtml/rr5116a1.htm

Casewell, M. and Phillips, I. (1977) Hands as a route of transmission for Klebsiella species. *British Medical Journal* **2**: 1315–17.

Delamater, A. M. (2006) Improving patient adherence. *Clinical Diabetes* **24**(2): 71–7.

DoH (Department of Health) (2003). *Winning Ways: Working Together to Reduce Healthcare Associated Infection in England*. Report from the Chief Medical Officer. DoH, London. http://www.dh.gov.uk/assetRoot/04/06/46/89/04064689.pdf (accessed 28 June 2009).

DoH (Department of Health) (2004). *Towards Cleaner Hospitals and Lower Rates of Infection: A Summary of Action*. DoH, London. http://www.dh.gov.uk/assetRoot/04/08/58/61/04085861.pdf (accessed 28 June 2009).

DoH (Department of Health) (2005a) *Action on Health Care Associated Infection in England*. DoH, London.

DoH (Department of Health) (2005b) *Saving Lives: A Delivery Programme to Reduce Health Care Associated Infection (HCAI) Including MRSA*. DoH, London. http://www.dh.gov.uk/PolicyAndGuidance/HealthAndSocialCareTopics/HealthcareAcquiredInfection/ (accessed 28 June 2009).

DoH (Department of Health) (2006a) *The Health Act 2006, Chapter 28*. The Stationery Office, London.

DoH (Department of Health) (2006b) *Essential Steps to Safe, Clean Care: Reducing Health Care Associated Infection*. DoH, London. http://www.dh.gov.uk/en/Publicationsandstatistics/Publications/PublicationsPolicyAndGuidance/DH_4136212 (accessed 5 August 2010).

DoH (Department of Health) (2006c) *Infection Control: Guidance for care homes*. DoH, London.

DoH (Department of Health) (2007) *Saving Lives: Reducing Infection, Delivering Clean and Safe Care*.

Environment Agency (2004) Guidance for the recovery and disposal of hazardous and non hazardous waste. http://www.environment-agency.gov.uk/static/documents (accessed 26 June 2009).

Girou, E., Loyeau, S., Legrand, P., Oppein, F. and Brun-Buisson, C. (2002) Efficacy of handrubbing with alcohol based solution versus standard handwashing with antiseptic soap: randomised clinical trial. *British Medical Journal* **325**: 362–5.

Gould, D. (1996) Can ward-based learning improve infection control? *Nursing Times* **92**: 42–3.

National Audit Office (2009) *Reducing Health Care Associated Infections in Hospitals in England*. The Stationery Office, London.

National Patient Safety Agency (2004) *Patient Safety Alert: Clean Hands Help Saves Lives*. http://www.npsa.nhs.uk/cleanyourhands

Pratt, R.J., Pellowe, C.M. and Wilson, J.A. (2007) epic2: National evidence-based guidelines for preventing health care associated infections in the NHS hospitals in England. *Journal of Hospital Infection*, **65**, S1–S64. www.epic.tvu.ac.uk/pdf%20files/epic2/epic2-final.pdf

Royal College of Nursing (1992) Safety Representatives Conference Committee. *Introduction to Methicillin Resistant Staphylococcus Aureus*. RCN, London.

Tremayne, P. and Parboteeah, S. (2006) *Fundamental Aspects of Adult Nursing*, Quay Publishing, London.

WHO (World Health Organisation) (2009) Epidemic and pandemic alert response. http://www.who.int/csr/disease/swineflu/newsbriefs/h1n1_antiviral_resistance_20090708/en/index.html (accessed 24 June 2009).

SOMDUTH PARBOTEEAH

6

Administration of Medications

📖 Contents

- Introduction
- Patient Assessment
- Administration of Medications
- Chapter Summary
- Test Yourself!
- Further Reading
- References

☑ Learning outcomes

This chapter describes the procedures for the safe administration of medications. It provides a step-by-step guide for the preparation of the patient, the equipment and medications required, and the safe techniques for administering medications, which is evidence based. At the end of this chapter, you should be able to:

- Understand the legislation and professional code (for example, Nursing and Midwifery Council) governing the administration of medicines by health-care professionals
- Assess patients to ascertain suitability
- Prepare drugs to be administered
- Safely administer drugs to patients by a variety of routes
- Be involved in the storage and preparation of drugs
- Demonstrate ability to calculate drug dosages
- Understand how drugs work.

Throughout the chapter you will be asked to undertake exercises that will assist you in developing your knowledge, skills and competence. Some of the skills, such as giving an intramuscular injection, may initially be practised in a skills laboratory under supervision prior to undertaking such procedures in the clinical areas. In this chapter, the term 'health-care professional' is used to refer to a person who is qualified to administer medications, such as a registered nurse.

Introduction

The administration of medicines is an important aspect of the professional practice of health-care practitioners. The health-care practitioner is responsible for assessing, planning, implementing and evaluating drug therapies as well as educating patients about their drug regimens. It is more that a mechanistic task, requiring thought and the exercise of professional judgement (NMC, 2008). To be effective, the practitioner must have an understanding of the fundamental principles of drug action, the purposes of drug use and the actions necessary to bring about beneficial outcomes. The student is advised to consult textbooks listed in the further reading section at the end of this chapter for more comprehensive information on drug actions and pharmacokinetics. The administration of medications via the intravenous and the epidural routes using electronic devices, for example pumps, are not described in this section as they require further post-qualifying training.

In the UK, the range of substances intended for medicinal use must conform to standards specified in the *British Pharmacopoeia* or the *British Pharmaceutical Codex* and must satisfy the relevant government legislation listed in Chart 6.1. Some of the earlier Acts have been superseded by the current legislation. Failure to comply with legal requirements and errors may result in disciplinary action by the relevant professional bodies, employers and criminal prosecution.

Chart 6.1 Statutes controlling substances intended for medicinal use

• The Misuse of Drugs Act 1971	• The Medicines Act 1968, 1983
• The Poisons Act 1972	• The Prescription by Nurses Act 1992

Patient Assessment

A thorough patient assessment is an essential component in the process of drug administration. A detailed assessment guideline should include:

- Medications that the patient is currently taking
- Frequency and dosage of all medications
- Any home remedies being taken
- Other complementary therapies being used
- Allergies to any drugs
- Height, weight, blood pressure, temperature and respiration, as some drug dosages, for example dopamine infusion, are calculated on body mass, and side effects can affect blood pressure
- General fitness and health, as such information can influence decisions about the routes and methods of drug administration; for example, an emaciated patient may not be able to tolerate deep intramuscular injections
- Diet; for example, if foods such as cheese, yogurt, broad beans, marmite, red wine and beer are administered to a patient who is receiving monoamine oxidase inhibitors (MAOIs), dangerous side effects may ensue.

✸ Activity 6.1

In your practice, carry out a patient assessment using the above guidelines and discuss your findings with your mentor.

Prescriptions

Prescriptions have traditionally been written on paper prescription charts. With an increase in computers, prescriptions are now available in electronic form in hospitals or the community (ePrescribing) and this is likely to expand. Health-care practitioners should ensure that a prescription has been written prior to the administration of medicines.

Regardless of the modality used all prescriptions should include information necessary for the safe administration of the drug and should include:

- The name of the patient, date of birth, address and hospital ID
- The date that the prescription was issued and the signature of the prescriber
- The medication
- Form, dosage and strength
- The route for administering the drug
- The time of administration
- Any specific information, for example, that it is to be taken with meals.

For hand-written prescriptions the following criteria should be adhered to in order to prevent drug errors:

generic drugs
drugs that are made up of the same ingredients as the brandname drug but are not protected by patent or exclusive rights of the innovator company

controlled drugs
those drugs, such as morphine, subject to the prescription requirements of the Misuse of Drug Regulations 1985

1 The prescription must be legible, and the approved or **generic drug** name should be used.

2 Details of the patient's name and address, the dose required and the frequency and route of administration must be clearly stated. For certain drugs (for example, antibiotics), the proposed duration of therapy should be stated.

3 **Controlled drugs**, that is, drugs that are subject to the prescription requirements of the Misuse of the Drug Regulations 2001, should be clearly monitored.

4 A prescription should not be altered once it has been written and should be written out in full again if a change in dose or frequency is indicated.

5 When a prescription is to be cancelled, it should be crossed out and signed and dated by the doctor.

6 In emergencies, telephone orders for the administration of medicines can be accepted by a first-level registered health-care practitioner (providing there is local agreement) if the doctor is unable to attend the ward. The prescription must then be written and signed by the health-care practitioner, stating that it is a verbal prescription. The doctor's name should be recorded on the prescription sheet and the doctor should sign the prescription as soon as possible. No telephone orders should be repeated.

ePrescribing systems have reduced some of the errors associated with prescriptions. However, ePrescribing systems have introduced new problems of their own and health-care practitioners should therefore be vigilant and adhere to the 'five Rs' of drug administration (see below).

Administration of Medications

When administering medications, the health-care practitioner's first task is to check the prescription for completeness; then he or she can prepare to administer the drug. In preparing medications, it is important to ensure cleanliness of the hands, a clean surface and sterility of all the materials used. All the components must be assembled in a well-lit room and medicines prepared in a safe area away from distraction, following guidelines for the Control of Substances Hazardous to Health (COSHH). A general guide to ensure patients' safety in the administration of medications is to check the 'five Rs':

✴ Activity 6.2

In your practice examine the prescription chart of a patient for its legibility, accuracy and completeness as outlined above.

1 The right medication
2 The right amount
3 The right time
4 The right patient
5 The right route.

Right medication

After checking the prescription, the health-care practitioner selects the right medication, carefully checking the labels on the containers. The practitioner administering the drug 'must know the therapeutic uses of the medicine to be administered' (NMC, 2008, p. 4). Medications from a container that is unlabelled, defaced or illegible must never be used. The health-care practitioner should read any instructions pertaining to the medication and check the expiry date. Health-care practitioners must never administer a drug prepared by someone else because the health-care practitioner administering the drug will still be held accountable for any errors made by others during preparation. Medications must never be decanted from one container to another. The health-care practitioner should be familiar with essential information about the drug including its action, contraindications and side effects, and current reference books, such as the *British National Formulary* (BNF), should be available at all times.

Controlled drugs should be administered according to relevant legislation and local protocols. A secondary signatory is recommended for the administration of controlled drugs in a hospital environment. A student health-care practitioner/midwife can be a 'second signatory' (NMC, 2008, p. 5) and must also ensure that he / she witnesses the whole process of drug administration.

Right amount

To prepare the right amount of medication, the health-care practitioner must be familiar with the different measurement systems (such as milligram, millilitre) and common abbreviations used (Table 6.1). Many of the terms are derived from latin such as guttae for drops.

When preparing liquid medications for oral administration, it is important to shake all suspensions and emulsions to ensure a proper distribution of the drug. A calibrated medicine pot or syringe may be used to draw up the right amount of medication. If the medication is poured from the container, the medicine pot

Table 6.1 Common abbreviations used in prescriptions

Abbreviation	Latin	Meaning
a.c.	ante cibum	before meals
b.i.d.	bis in die	twice daily
caps	capsula	capsule
elix		elixir
gtt(s)	gutta(e)	drops
IM		intramuscular
IV		intravenous
mcg		microgram
mL		millilitre
nebul	nebula	a spray
p.c.	post cibum	after meals
p.o.	per os	by mouth
p.r.n.	pro re nata	as needed
SC		subcutaneous
SL		sublingual
STAT	statim	immediately
supp	suppositorium	suppository
t.i.d.	ter in die	three times a day
t.r.		tincture
q.i.d.	quarter in die	four times a day
q.d.	quaque die	daily
q.h.	quaque hora	every hour

meniscus
the curved surface of a column of fluid

★ Activity **6.3**

You have reviewed the common abbreviations used when prescribing drugs. Scrutinise at least six prescription charts and see if you understand the abbreviations used.

should be placed on a flat surface. To check for accuracy, the pot should be raised to eye level and the measurement read at the lowest point of the **meniscus**.

Some medications, for example eye drops, are measured with a dropper. The dropper must be held vertically, and the bulb should be slowly squeezed and released until the required dosage is reached.

The administration of injections depends on the drugs prescribed. Some injectables, for example pethidine, are available in liquid form, and the required amount can easily be drawn up. Administering the correct amount also depends on the strength of the drug. For example, heparin is available in 5,000, 10,000 or 25,000 units/ml, so the amount injected will vary. Other injectables, such as penicillin, are produced in 'powder form' and require dilution before they can be administered. Where fluid is added, the solution displacement value must be taken into account. This can be found in the literature accompanying the vial and is usually 0.02 ml. If this value is not checked, it can result in erroneous doses being administered. When drugs are supplied at strengths different from the dosages that have been prescribed, the health-care practitioner must determine the quantity of drug that is to be administered. Special formulae are available, but it is also essential for the health-care practitioner to have a basic knowledge of arithmetic. A student who is experiencing difficulty should consult one of the many drug calculation workbooks now available (see reading list at end of chapter), seek help from lecturers and clinical practice mentors.

Right time

In order to achieve maximum therapeutic effectiveness, the doctor will specify the number of times within a 24-hour period the drug is to be given. It is important to adhere to this regimen as closely as possible in order to maintain a relatively constant blood plasma level of the drug; this is also referred to as the therapeutic window (Figure 6.1). The minimum effective concentration (MEC) is the lowest concentration of the drug that will produce the desired effect and the minimum toxic concentration (MTC) is the lowest concentration of the drug in the blood that will cause an adverse response. The peak is the highest concentration and the trough is the lowest concentration of drug measured in the blood. The trough should not fall below the MEC level and should be reached just before the next dose of drug is due.

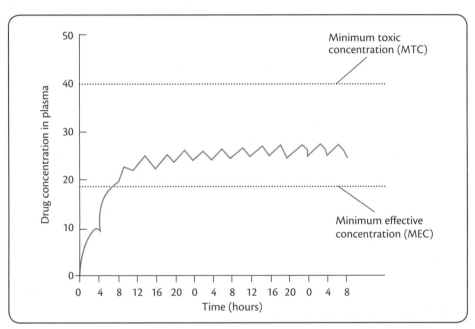

Figure 6.1 Plasma level versus time plot of a drug administered at four-hourly intervals in order to keep the plasma concentration of the drug in an effective but not toxic range

Right patient

The NMC (2008, p. 4) suggests that practitioners 'must be certain of the identity of the patient to whom the medicine is to be administered'. The following principles should be employed as a matter of routine regardless of the number of patients involved:

- In acute care settings, check the wrist identity bracelet against the details on the drug chart.

✳ Activity 6.4

Undertake a survey of your patients to find out whether they receive their medications on time. Discuss your findings with your mentor or lecturer and the effects a delay will have on the treatment programme.

✳ Activity 6.5

Consider the importance of administering medicines via the prescribed route with your mentor, tutor or peeers. What information is given to the patients in anticipation of the procedure?

- If the patient is not confused, ask him to state his name but never prompt or say 'Are you Mr/Mrs …?'
- If the patient questions the dosage, appearance or method of administration, always double-check the prescription and medication.
- Never leave medicines for a patient who is not available during the drug round.
- Never administer medications if you cannot confirm the identity of the patient.

> **! Specific points on children's medications**
>
> - If the child is too young, ask the parents to confirm the child's identity.
> - Children and parents have a right to know about the treatments and they should always be addressed by name.

Right route

The doctor must specify the route by which the medication is to be administered. If there are any discrepancies, the doctor should be consulted. If the health-care practitioner is concerned about the safety of administering any drugs via a particular route, the doctor should be asked to prepare and administer the drug.

Drugs may be administered via different routes (Chart 6.2) and the choice of route depends on factors such as the rate of absorption, onset of action, chemical nature of the drug, duration of action, control of dose, the first pass effect (drugs absorbed from the gastrointestinal tract pass through the liver where a fraction of the drug may be eliminated before it reaches the rest of the body), the patient's general condition and side effects.

Health-care practitioners are not responsible for the administration of drugs by all of these routes but may have to assist doctors, for example with intrathecal administration.

Chart 6.2 Routes of drug administration

- Oral – given by mouth
- Sublingual – under the tongue
- Injections: intramuscular, subcutaneous, intradermal – into soft tissues
- Rectal – inserting drug into the rectum
- Vaginal – inserting drug into the vagina
- Topical – placing on the skin or mucous membranes
- Inhalation – via the respiratory tract
- Optic – into the eye
- Aural – into the ear
- Nasal – into the nose
- Intra-articular – into the cavity of a joint*
- Intrathecal – into the spinal fluid*
- Intravenous – into a vein*
- Intracardiac – into the heart*

* Students should not be involved in the checking or the administration of medications via these routes. Students should also adhere to local policies.

Oral medications

The **oral route** is the most frequently used route for drug administration. Oral medications in liquid (for example, elixir), or solid (for example, tablet or capsule) form, have a high degree of stability and provide accurate dosage. The gastrointestinal tract may, however, alter the gut pH, gastric motility as well as the rate of absorption. Some patients are sometimes prescribed modified release preparations and these tablets are coated with materials that delay release of the drug until after they leave the stomach. These tablets should never be crushed or chewed as they may lead to specific drug complications.

oral route
via the mouth

Guidelines for oral drug administration

1   Wash your hands and wear gloves (as necessary).
2   Check the prescription for completeness of date, time, drug to be given, dosage, route, frequency and duration of therapy. The health-care practitioner must know the therapeutic uses of the drug, its normal dosage, side effects, contraindications and specific precautions. Check that the drug has not already been given and is due.
3   Check that the patient is not allergic to the medication.
4   Select and check the required medication for contamination and expiry date. Liquids should be checked for discolouration and precipitation.
5   Prepare the dosage as prescribed. Do not crush enteric-coated, sublingual or sustained-action tablets. Empty the required dose into a medicine pot. To prevent contamination, avoid touching the preparation. If dispensing liquid, the bottle should be held with the label towards the palm of the hand to prevent spillage obscuring the name of the drug.
6   Check the labels on containers again.
7   Take the medication and the prescription chart to the patient. Check the patient's identity (as described earlier) and the drug to be given.
8   Position the patient as upright as possible to aid swallowing, and instruct the patient accordingly. A glass of water or juice (50 ml or more) should be given to facilitate swallowing. The health-care practitioner must ensure that the patient has swallowed the medication. Infants and young children should be supported firmly to avoid spilling the medication.
9   Make the patient comfortable and ask the patient/client to stay upright for a few minutes.
10   Immediately complete all the necessary records.
11   Clear all the equipment.

There is a growing interest in **enteral** feeding as a means of delivering medication, particularly to **dysphagic** patients. Medications may also be given via feeding tubes if other routes are not available. The choice and size of tubes depend on the aims of the treatment and the condition of the patient. However, the type of tube, tube location in the gastrointestinal tract, site of drug action and absorption and the effects of food on drug absorption must be evaluated. The procedure for administering the drug via this route is described below. Liquid

enteral
within the gastrointestinal tract

dysphagic
painful or difficult swallowing

🔗 **Link**

Chapter 7 contains a section on enteral feeding via a nasogastric tube.

medications will flow easily down the tube by gravity; tablets and other solid medications should be avoided and alternative drugs used.

Guidelines for administering drugs via nasogastric tube

1 Wash hands and use gloves as necessary. Turn off pump to stop continuous feeding. Explain the procedure to the patient and gain his/her cooperation. Maintain privacy of the patient. If possible, elevate the patient's head 30–45 degrees to avoid aspiration during and following administration of medication.

2 Check the placement of the nasogastric tube by aspirating a small quantity of gastric contents and measuring for pH, using pH indicator strips/paper (Tremayne and Parboteeah, 2006, NPSA, 2005).

3 Remove plunger from 60 ml syringe and connect to tubing. For adults put 30 ml of water in syringe barrel and flush tubing using gravity flow (20ml for children (Pickering, 2003).

4 Prepare the medication (follow guidelines for preparing drugs as outlined above) and pour in barrel of syringe. Hold the barrel of the syringe about 15 cm (6 inches) higher than the patient's nose and allow the fluid to flow into the stomach by gravity as shown in Figure 6.2.

5 Between medications – flush the tube with 5 ml of water or prescribed amounts of fluids. After medications have been given, flush tubing with 15–30 ml of water. Clamp tubing and detach syringe if no feeding is in progress.

6 If the patient is on continuous feeding, the feeding is recommenced as prescribed.

Staff should avoid crushing tablets or opening capsules in order to administer the drug via the nasogastric tube as this process is in breach of the Medicines Act 1968 (Griffith, 2003) and the manufacturer will assume no responsibility for any harm to the patient. When a medicine is prescribed to be administered in an 'unlicensed' form, a percentage of liability will still lie with the person administering the drug. The drug must be prescribed in milligrams and not ml as several strengths may be available.

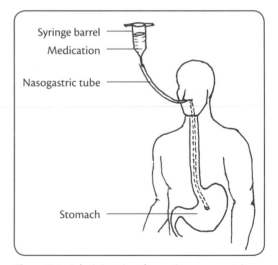

Figure 6.2 Administering drugs via a nasogastric tube

The medication should not be added to a 'feed'. Instead, the continuous feeding should be interrupted and resumed after administration of the drug. The tube should be flushed with water prior to and after the administration of the drug.

> **! Specific points on children's medications**
>
> - Flush the nasogastric tube with 20 ml water.

The administration of medications via enteral feeding tubes may present a number of problems which the health-care practitioner must be aware of and all preparations must be reviewed to eliminate the problems. Enteral feed coming into contact with the medication may precipitate. The drug may also bind to the inner lining of the enteral feeding tube thus reducing the amount of drug available for pharmacokinetic effects. The point at which the drug is delivered in the gastrointestinal tract may also affect the **bioavailability** of medications.

Although the newer feeding tubes share the capacity for medication delivery, their use for the administration of drugs may induce intolerance and/or result in less than optimal drug absorption. Reasons for this include:

- Crushing oral tablets or opening capsules for the purposes of enteral administration may alter bioavailability, resulting in unpredictable serum concentrations or tube occlusion.
- Drugs may bind to the enteral feeding tube, reducing drug absorption.

Policy where/when tablets can be crushed

In exceptional circumstances where the patient is unable to swallow and no alternative medicines are available, medical and dental practitioners can author-ise the use of unlicensed medicines. For example, the NMC indicates that 'A registrant may administer an unlicensed medicinal product with the patient's informed consent against a patient-specific direction but NOT against a patient group direction (NMC, Standard 22, Section 7). In such cases the pharmacist should endorse the drug chart where medications can be crushed prior to admin-istration and an entry is made in the patients' notes. Hospitals should have local guidelines for such practices and should be used in conjunction with the Control of Substances Hazardous to Health (COSHH) guidelines for wards (HSE, 2002).

Parenteral medications

The term '**parenteral**' refers to the act of administering medications by a route other than the alimentary tract. The term is most commonly used to indicate the injection routes such as intramuscular, subcutaneous and intravenous. Less common ways by which medications are administered include intrathecally (into the spinal fluid), intra-articularly (into a joint cavity such as a knee joint), intra-cardiac (directly into the heart) and intra-arterially (into an artery), these more specialized procedures being performed by doctors. Drugs given parenterally are absorbed more readily into the blood achieving a high plasma level very quickly for rapid treatment. The possible disadvantages include the introduction of microorganisms (discussed in Chapter 5), injury to tissues, nerves, veins and arteries.

✹ Activity 6.6

Under direct supervision, assist qualified staff to administer oral drugs to clients/patients.

bioavailability
the level at which medications become available for use by the body after its administration

parenteral route
a route other than via the alimentary canal

∞ Link

Chapter 5 discusses microorganisms.

✹ Activity 6.7

Identify the different gauge needles that are used for intradermal, subcutaneous, intravenous and intramuscular injections, and for drawing up medications.

Injections

Giving an injection is a procedure routinely undertaken by health-care practitioners and health-care professionals. The practitioner must have a good knowledge and understanding of human anatomy in order to identify safe areas for injecting. The practitioner must also develop safe injection technique so that injections become a less painful and less traumatic experience for the patient. An injection is defined as a procedure that introduces a substance into the body by piercing the skin, especially by means of a hypodermic needle.

There are many different syringes and needles, suiting many different procedures (Table 6.2). A range of syringes are available which can hold volumes of 0.1 to 5 ml for injections. Most hospitals use plastic disposable syringes; however, glass syringes may be required for patient who are allergic to latex or for some types of drugs such as paraldehyde.

Needle selection should be based on the route for the injection (intramuscular, subcutaneous, and intradermal), the size of the individual (obese or thin person), the volume to be administered and the viscosity of the injectate. A fine gauge needle can be used for clear fluids. The selection of the right length needle for an intramuscular injection is important as medications deposited in the subcutaneous tissues can cause more pain and be less effective (Lenz, 1983).

Table 6.2 Selection of needles for different types of injection

Type of injection	Suggested needle gauge		Size of syringe
	Adult	Child	
Intradermal	26 G × ⅜″	26 G × ⅜″	1 ml calibrated in
	(0.45 × 10 mm)	(0.45 × 10 mm)	0.1 ml divisions
Subcutaneous	25/26 G × ⅝″	26 G × ⅝″	1 ml calibrated in
	(0.45 × 16 mm)	(0.45 × 16 mm)	0.1 ml divisions
Intramuscular	21 G × 1½″	23 G × 1¼″	5 ml calibrated in
	(0.6 × 30 mm)	(0.8 × 40 mm)	0.2 ml divisions

cytotoxic

any substance that is toxic to cells

Gloves should be worn to prevent cross-infection or if the drug is likely to cause skin sensitisation with frequent use. For example, dermatitis can be caused by frequent contact with drugs such as penicillin, streptomycin and chlorpromazine. When cytotoxic drugs are given, vinyl gloves should be worn; goggles and a mask may also be necessary.

Skin cleansing prior to administration of an intradermal, subcutaneous or intramuscular injection

A review of the literature by the Scottish Center for Infection and Environmental Health (SCIEH) (2005) reported that there is little evidence at this time to support the need for skin disinfection prior to intradermal, subcutaneous and intramuscular injections. The skin should be clean prior to the administration of an injection. If the skin is visibly soiled, it should be cleaned with soap and water. If the local policy requires disinfection, the injection site should be cleaned with a pre-medicated 70 per cent alcohol swab. The site should be cleaned for 30 seconds and allowed to dry for a further 30 seconds to ensure bacteria are rendered inactive.

✹ Activity 6.8

Describe the policy for the safe disposal of used needles, syringes, vials and glass ampoules (refer to Chapter 5 for guidelines on safe disposal of sharps). Find out what actions should be taken in the event of an accidental needle injury.

Preparation of medications

Drawing medication from a single-dose ampoule

- Check the ampoule for cracks, cloudiness and precipitation.
- Gently tap the upper area of the ampoule to release any medication trapped at the top of the ampoule.
- Cover the neck of the ampoule or use an 'ampoule breaker' when snapping it open.
- Insert the needle into the ampoule and withdraw the required amount. Avoid contaminating the medication.
- Change the needle and dispose of it as per hospital/clinical setting policy.
- Tap the barrel to dislodge any air bubbles towards the needle and expel the air.

Drawing medication from a multi-dose vial solution

- Remove the metal cover from the vial and inspect the medication as above.
- Clean the rubber cap with antiseptic solution and let it dry.
- Withdraw the prescribed amount of solution. Two methods can be used to draw the solution:

  Method 1. Insert a 19 G needle into the cap to vent the vial. Insert the assembled needle and syringe, and draw up the required amount.

  Method 2. Assemble the needle and syringe. Fill the syringe with the same volume of air as the medication that will be withdrawn. Insert the needle through the rubber stopper, holding the vial at an oblique angle, and inject the air into the vial. Keep the needle in the solution, invert the vial and allow the medication to enter the syringe. The volume can be adjusted by using the plunger, and the needle is removed when the required amount has been drawn up.

- Change the needle as it may have become blunted/damaged.
- Tap the barrel to dislodge any air bubbles towards the needle and expel the air.

It is preferable to use single-dose vials rather than multi-dose vials whenever possible as these multi-dose vials remain prone to bacterial contamination (Simon et al., 1993).

Reconstituting a powdered medication

- Clean the rubber cap with an antiseptic and allow it to dry.
- Check for the displacement value of the drug (see below).
- Add the required amount of diluents carefully down the wall of the vial, and allow an equal amount of air to escape into the syringe.
- Remove the needle and syringe.
- Shake the vial to dissolve the powder.
- The reconstituted solution can now be withdrawn as described for removing solutions from a multi-dose vial.

Displacement values when reconstituting powdered medication

When dry powder medications are reconstituted, the powder displaces a certain volume of fluid know as the displacement volume of the drug. Hence, the total volume in a reconstituted vial should be equal to the sum of the displacement value of the drug and the volume of diluents added. If displacement values are not considered, dosage errors will occur when a portion of the solution is used, especially in paediatric patients. For example, you have been asked to prepare a drug in the concentration of 20 mg/ml to produce 5 ml of the solution. The drug is available in powder form with a displacement value of 0.15 ml/100mg. The volume of diluents that should be added is 4.85 ml to make 5 ml of the solution with a concentration of 20 mg/ml. If 5 ml of diluents is added, then the concentration will be 19.4 mg/ml and not 20 mg/ml. Displacement values for drugs can be found in drug data sheets.

Intramuscular injections

intramuscular route
into a muscle

The **intramuscular route** is used to administer medications that are irritating or painful. Skeletal muscles are well perfused with blood and have fewer pain receptors, so pain is minimal causing less discomfort (Newton et al., 1992). Up to 5 ml of injectate may be given into the large muscles (1–2 ml into the deltoid muscle, for example).

Guidelines for intramuscular injection

To give an intramuscular injection:

1   Collect and check all the equipment to ensure sterility. If the outer packaging is damaged, replace the pack.
2   Wash your hands.
3   Prepare the needle(s) and syringe on a tray. Check for any defects.
4   Check the patient's prescription(s) for completeness.
5   Select the drug and verify it against the prescription.
6   Prepare the drug using gloves if necessary.
7   Identify the patient and explain the procedure. Patients report high levels of distress during painful procedures and interventions should be deployed to reduce distress. MacLaren and Cohen (2005) compared two distraction strategies and found that children in the passive condition (watching a movie) were more distracted and less distressed compared to children in the interactive condition (playing with a toy).
8   Select injection site and position patient for easy access to the injection site, comfort and privacy. In obese patients, select an appropriate site to ensure the injection in given into the muscles and not the subcutaneous fat. Infants and children should be held firmly so that they do not move as this could cause injuries during the procedure.
9   Clean the site with antiseptic and allow the alcohol to evaporate (as per local policy).
10   Holding the needle at 90 degrees (Figure 6.3), quickly insert the needle into the muscle. Leave a third of the needle shaft exposed. If the needle breaks from the hub, it can then be removed safely.

11   Pull back the plunger for 5–10 seconds. If blood appears, withdraw the needle and repeat the procedure with a sterile needle in a different place. Explain to the patient what is happening.

12   If no blood appears, depress the plunger and inject the drug slowly.

13   Quickly withdraw the needle and apply gentle pressure over the puncture site.

14   Position the patient comfortably.

15   Dispose of the needle and syringe as per hospital/clinical setting policy.

16   Complete all the necessary records.

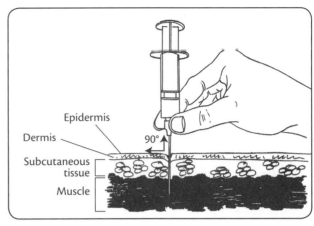

Figure 6.3 Intramuscular injection

Sites for intramuscular injection

Five possible sites for intramuscular injections are currently advocated for giving an intramuscular injection: the deltoid, the dorsogluteal, the ventrogluteal, vastus lateralis and the rectus femoris (Tortora and Derrickson, 2008). Each of these sites will be described in detail next. When choosing a site, it is important to identify the anatomical landmarks in order to avoid injuring nerves, striking bones or puncturing blood vessels. The site must also be inspected for its suitability, for example:

* Is there sufficient muscle mass?
* Does the area to be injected have a good blood supply?
* Is there any skin damage?

* Is there evidence of fibrosis or infection?
* Is there too much subcutaneous fat?

✴ Activity 6.9

Using a mannikin or a picture of the body, identify the sites for intramuscular injections. Discuss the advantages and disadvantages of using the different sites in your current area of practice. Investigate current evidence and recommendations and reflect on your current practice.

The deltoid muscle in the upper arm

The deltoid is used for small quantities of injectate, 1 ml or less (Covington and Trattler, 1997) of clear non-irritating medication, for example vaccines. The volumes of injectate that can be tolerated by this muscle group appear to be based on its smaller muscle mass rather than research studies. The muscle is located in the lateral aspect of the upper arm. The injection site (Figure 6.4) is located 4–5 cm below the acromion process and above the deltoid groove in adults, and approximately 2 cm below the acromion process in older children.

The dorsogluteal site in the buttocks

The dorsogluteal site has a larger muscle mass and can tolerate volumes of up to 5 ml. If the dorsogluteal site (Figure 6.5) is chosen for the intramuscular injection, the health-care practitioner must have a full understanding of the anatomy of the site and surrounding anatomical structures, be able to accurately identify anatomic landmarks and site boundaries, and administer the injection with meticulous technique, as

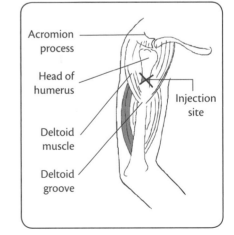

Figure 6.4 Deltoid injection site

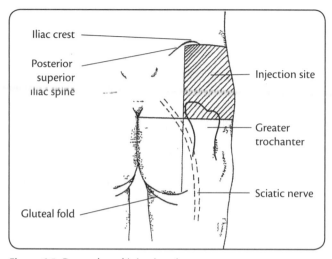

Figure 6.5 Dorsogluteal injection site

the sciatic nerve and the superior gluteal artery run close to this site. The injection site is identified by palpating the anatomical landmarks of the posterior superior iliac spine and the greater trochanter (at the head of the femur). A line is drawn between these two points and safe injection sites are in the area above and lateral to this line. The area below this line should be avoided to prevent damage to the sciatic nerve.

Chan et al. (2006) and Burbridge (2007) have demonstrated that the majority of assumed intramuscular injections were actually injected in the subcutaneous tissue in the dorsogluteal site. Nisbet (2006) and Zaybak et al. (2007) have shown that standard needles do not reach the gluteal muscles and therefore an alternative site should be chosen to optimise the effectiveness of the medication.

The patient should be asked to lie prone with the toes pointing inwards to relax the buttocks. This site should not be used in infants or children who have not been walking for at least 1 year since this muscle is not developed.

Practitioners should at all times consider the cultural diversity of their patients and maintain their dignity especially when injecting in the dorsogluteal site and adhere to any specific cultural needs.

The ventrogluteal site in the hip area

There is wide agreement in the literature that the ventrogluteal site is preferable to the dorsogluteal site for intramuscular injections as it is free of major nerves and blood vessels (Beecroft and Redick, 1990; Covington and Trattler, 1997; Rodger

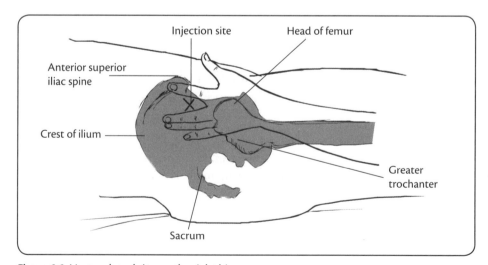

Figure 6.6 Ventrogluteal site on the right hip area

and King, 2000). The injection is given in the gluteus medius and gluteus maximus muscles. The patient is placed on his/her side or can be allowed to stay in the supine or prone position. To find the injection site on the right hip (the most convenient site for right-handed practitioners) palpate the greater trochanter, the iliac crest and the anterior superior iliac spine. Place the palm of the left hand on the greater trochanter and the left index finger towards the anterior superior iliac spine (Figure 6.6). Move the middle finger away from the index finger to form a V between the fingers. The injection is given into the centre of the V. This is the preferred site for infants and children who have not been walking for a year (Beecroft and Redick, 1990; Whalley and Wong, 1995) because the pelvis is concave below the iliac crest and contains a relatively large muscle mass.

The vastus lateralis in the thigh

This muscle is situated in the lateral thigh and can be used for both adults and children. The volume of fluid that can be given in this site is from 1–5 ml (Covington and Tattler, 1997; Rodger and King, 2000). This site (Figure 6.7) is preferable because there are no major blood vessels or nerves in the area. The patient is asked to lie in the supine position with the thigh well exposed, pointing the toe inwards to give a better exposure of the lateral aspects of the thigh. The injection site can be located by dividing the thigh horizontally and vertically into thirds by

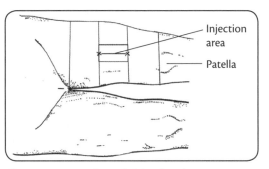

Figure 6.7 Vastus lateralis injection site

placing one hand's breadth below the greater trochanter at the top of the thigh and one hand's breadth from the knee. The thigh is then measured vertically, this time by placing one hand's breadth along the middle of the inner side of the thigh and one hand's breadth on the outer side of the thigh, thus creating a rectangle in the middle where it is safe to inject. This strip is between 2 and 4 cm long in children and about 7 cm long in adults. The needle is directed into the tissues at a right angle.

The rectus femoris site

This muscle is found in the middle third of the anterior thigh (Figure 6.8). It is easily accessed for self-administration (Springhouse Corporation 1993). Workman (1999) suggests that in adults 5 ml and in children 1–3 ml can be injected in the rectus femoris. In children and very thin adults, this muscle may need to be bunched up in a handful to provide sufficient muscle depth. Newton et al. (1992) suggest that the uptake of medications from this region is slower than from the arm but faster than from the buttock, thereby facilitating better drug serum concentrations. Berger and Williams (1992) caution that injections in this area may cause considerable discomfort.

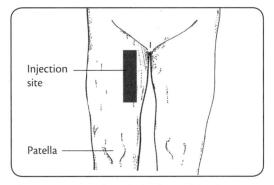

Figure 6.8 Rectus femoris site for IM injection

> ## ! Specific points on children's injections
>
> Injections can cause substantial distress to children and many view injections as the most traumatic experience of being in a hospital (Cordoni and Cordoni, 2001; Cummings et al., 1996). An important factor in helping children cope with the procedure is to enable them to have some control of the situation, such as indicating their preferences with respect to time and events, positive reinforcements or even some form of rewards.
>
> - Sites for intramuscular injection in infants and children who have not been walking for one year
>   1 Ventrogluteal (Figure 6.6)
>   2 Vastus lateralis in the middle third of femur (Figure 6.7)
> - Sites for intramuscular injection in older children who have been walking for more than 1 year
>   1 Vastus lateralis (Figure 6.7)
>   2 Dorsogluteal site in the gluteus medius muscle (Figure 6.5)
>   3 Deltoid muscle for older children (Figure 6.4)

Z-track intramuscular injection

This technique for intramuscular injection has been primarily reserved for use with medications such as iron preparations that are known to be particularly irritating and can permanently stain the subcutaneous tissue. During this procedure, there is lateral displacement of the cutaneous tissue prior to injection, and the tension is released immediately after injection. When utilising the Z-track technique, the health-care practitioner grasps the muscle and pulls it laterally about 2.5 cm until it is taut, holding the tissue in this position. The needle is inserted at a 90 degree angle. After ensuring the position of the needle, the medication is injected. Following withdrawal of the needle, the skin is immediately released.

Complications of intramuscular injections

The health-care practitioner should be aware of the possible complications of injections and make every effort to prevent them.

Infection

The introduction of infection via a needle may lead to local (abscesses) or systemic (septicaemia) complications. It is important to maintain strict asepsis during all invasive procedures. All equipment should be sterile, and good hand washing is essential.

Muscle myopathy

Intramuscular injections, by their very nature, cause injury to tissues. Needle myopathy damage can be prevented by good injection technique using the optimum-sized needles. Focal myopathy can be caused by the injectates and by using injectorates of neutral pH.

Wrong route

Injectates may accidentally be given into a vein or an artery, resulting in a rapid physiological response. Depending on the drug used, severe complications and even death may occur. The syringe should be aspirated before the drug is injected. If blood appears in the barrel of the syringe, the needle is withdrawn and an alternative site used. The patient should be informed of the reasons for this. Drugs injected in an artery may cause thrombosis with disruption of the blood supply.

Nerve damage

Nerve damage (to the sciatic nerve) in the dorsogluteal region should be avoided. The health-care practitioner should identify the landmarks, as shown in Figure 6.5 and select a safe area for injection. Sciatic nerve injury can result from erroneous injection, causing client discomfort, morbidity and lasting disability (Small, 2004).

Subcutaneous injections in adults

A **subcutaneous** injection is administered as a bolus dose into the subcutaneous layer of the skin, below the dermis and above the muscles. The subcutaneous layer is rich in capillaries and absorption of the medication occurs via slow diffusion into the capillaries. This route is suitable for drug administration when the medication cannot be taken by mouth or it will be destroyed. Therefore, it is ideal for drugs such as insulin and heparin, and up to 1–2 ml can be injected.

subcutaneous route
under the skin

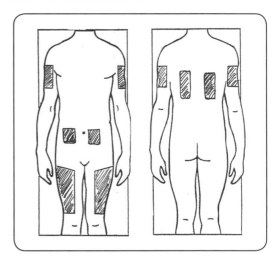

Figure 6.9 Subcutaneous injection site

In adults, the sites for administering subcutaneous injections include the lateral aspects of the upper arm, the abdomen on either side of the umbilicus, the middle and outer area of the thigh and the back (Figure 6.9).

Guidelines for administering a subcutaneous injection

1 Explain the procedure to the patient and gain his co-operation.
2 Select the site and assist the patient into position to maintain his comfort and dignity.
3 Expose the injection site; in a viable injection site the health-care practitioner should be able to pinch at least 2.5 cm of subcutaneous tissue. Check the rotation chart if one is in use.
4 Wash your hands thoroughly to prevent infection.
5 Prepare medication.
6 Ensure site is clean and safe for injecting medication.
7 Grasp the skin firmly between the thumb and forefinger, as shown in Figure 6.10.
8 Maintain the fold and insert the needle almost to its full length at an angle of 90 degrees.
9 Inject the medication.
10 Remove the needle and release the skin fold.

11   Do not recap the used needle.

12   Safely dispose of the syringe and needle.

13   Wash your hands.

14   Complete all the relevant records.

Subcutaneous injections in babies and children

The subcutaneous route is commonly used in babies and children to administer a range of medications. The sites for the administration of subcutaneous injections include the abdomen, the thighs and the upper arms (Cocoman and Barron, 2008). The abdominal site is the preferred site when faster absorption is required and is less affected by muscle activity. The front of the thigh is the preferred site for slower absorption, for example, longer acting insulins.

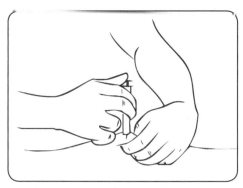

Figure 6.10 Current recommended method for injecting insulin at right angles with the skin pinched

Choosing the needle length

The depth of insertion of the needle determines whether the drug is deposited in the subcutaneous layer or in the muscles. It is therefore vital that the correct length needle is used. Zuckerman (2000), Tubiana-Rufi et al. (1999) and Wales (1997) support the use of 5, 6 or 8 mm long needles as children need different needle length based on the amount of subcutaneous fat that they have. It is therefore imperative that an individualised assessment is carried out in order to determine the amount of subcutaneous tissue present and to select the most appropriate needle length. (If a 5mm mini-pen needle is used to inject insulin, the needle can be inserted at a 90 degree angle without having to pinch the skin (Becton Dickinson, 2009).)

Administration of vaccine

The Department of Health (2006) recommends that injectable vaccines should be given by intramuscular injection. The preferred sites are the deltoid area of the upper arm (Figure 6.4) and the anterolateral aspects of the thigh, the target muscle being the vastus lateralis. The exact site of injection is the middle third portion between the greater trochanter and the lateral femoral condyle of the anterolateral thigh. The anterolateral site is the preferred site for infants under 1 year old as it provides a large muscle mass for the injection. Cook and Murtagh (2005) reported that the World Health Organisation (1984) recommended technique for intramuscular thigh vaccination in infants and toddlers using a 25 gauge 16 mm long needle inserted at a 90 degree angle to the long axis of the femur with the skin compressed between the index finger and the thumb had fewer side adverse reactions compared to the Australian technique of using a 23 gauge 25 mm long needle inserted at the junction of the upper and middle third of the vastus lateralis at a 45–60 degree angle to the skin pointing to the knee, and the United States technique of a 23 gauge 25 mm long needle inserted into the upper lateral quadrant at a 45 degree angle to the long axis of the femur and posteriorly at 45 degrees. Hence it is vital for practitioners to review their local policies for administering vaccines.

Intradermal injections

Intradermal administration is frequently used for diagnostic purposes, the injectate being placed within the layers of the skin just below the epidermis (Figure 6.11). Small amounts of medication, usually between 0.1 and 0.5 ml are administered because of the small tissue spaces. The site most often used is the central forearm, but other areas, such as the back and the chest, are acceptable.

intradermal
within the layers of the skin

Guidelines for giving an intradermal injection

1   Wash your hands. Check the prescription for completeness as described earlier. Prepare the equipment (a 1 ml syringe with a 26 G × 16 mm needle).
2   Explain the procedure to the patient and gain his cooperation.
3   Select the site and assist the patient into position to maintain his comfort and dignity. Select a site with minimal, or preferably no hair and skin blemishes.

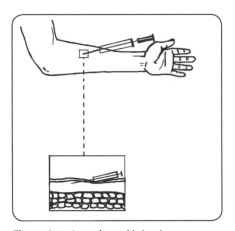

Figure 6.11 Intradermal injection

4   Clean the area with antiseptic solution. Avoid using iodine solutions as the residual stain may interfere with interpreting the results of the skin test. If the skin is oily, cleanse the area with acetone to remove any fat deposits. Allow the skin to dry.
5   Support the patient's arm and stretch the skin taut.
6   Place the bevel of the needle almost flat against the patient's skin and insert the needle with the bevel side up at an angle of 10–15 degrees (Figure 6.11). The needle should be about 3 mm below the skin surface. The medication is slowly injected while watching for a wheal to develop which verifies that the medication has entered the dermis (McConnell, 2000).
7   Once the wheal appears, withdraw the needle and circle the injection site with an appropriate marking pen.
8   The area should never be massaged as it may interfere with the test results.
9   If the test is carried out to determine sensitivity, follow the text instructions to determine, for example, signs of local reaction.
10 Dispose of the equipment as per hospital policy.

11   Wash your hands.

12   Complete all the relevant records.

When testing for allergies, it is essential that resuscitation equipment and expertise is available in case the patient develops a hypersensitive reaction (anaphylactic shock).

Topical medications

topical
applied to the skin or mucous membranes

inunction
rubbing a drug mixed with a fatty base into the skin; also the name given to the mixture

Topical administration refers to the application of medications to the skin or mucous membranes to achieve local or systemic effects. The medication may be incorporated into a base such as an oil, lotion or cream, which is rubbed into the skin (**inunction**), the area being cleaned with soap and water before application. The inunction can be applied with the fingers and hands, or using cotton wool balls or gauze swabs. If there is a risk of infection or application is to the mucous membranes, gloves should be worn.

Guidelines for the topical administration of drugs

1   Wash your hands. Check the prescription as discussed above before administering the drug.

2   Explain the procedure to the patient, who is positioned to expose the area, and carry out any assessments. Observe for any changes. The patient's privacy and dignity should be maintained.

3   Apply gloves as necessary.

4   Prepare the equipment, and follow aseptic guidelines if there is risk of infection. Remove solid or semisolid medications with a sterile spatula.

5   Apply the medication to the site.

6   Inform the patient if the preparation is likely to cause skin staining or soiling of clothing.

7   Dispose of used items according to local policy.

8   Complete the appropriate records.

Transdermal drug administration

transdermal route
application directly on to the skin, the substance applied then being absorbed via the skin

Transdermal drug administration represents a viable way of administering a number of drugs such as fentanyl and morphine, and an effective means of delivering drugs that currently require intramuscular, intravenous, or subcutaneous injections or have poor oral availability. Current transdermal drug delivery (TDD) relies mostly upon occlusive patches and there are more than 35 TDD products (Thomas and Finnin, 2004) approved for use in the USA for the treatment of a wide range of conditions such as hypertension, pain, angina and female menopause.

The advantages of using this route includes sustained delivery of drugs to provide a steady plasma profile, avoidance of first-pass metabolism effect for drugs with poor bioavailability, convenient and friendly option with flexibility for dosage adjustment according to needs, and the ability for self-administration by the patient. TD patches should not be applied on broken skin.

Guidelines for application of a transdermal patch

1   Wash your hands.
2   Check the prescription.
3   Explain the procedure to the patient, who is positioned to expose the area and carry out any assessments.
4   Apply gloves as necessary.
5   Remove previously applied patch from the patient's skin and wipe any residual medication from the skin.
6   Open package and remove new patch.
7   Follow manufacturer's instruction and expose the adhesive surface.
8   Apply the patch to a dry, hairless area of skin.
9   Write the date, time and initials on the patch.
10 Dispose of any waste and wash hands.
11 Complete the necessary documentation.

The side effect of using TDD includes toxicity, inflammation and skin irritation. To prevent skin complications, the site should be rotated and recorded on a rotation chart. The practitioner must also monitor the patient to ascertain the effectiveness of the therapy or lack of it and must be able to recognise signs of toxicity. The patient should be advised to keep the patch away from external sources of heat such as a heating pad. Some patches may be worn while bathing or showering and the health-care practitioner should check the manufacturer's advice. If a patch falls off, the health-care practitioner should follow recommended guidelines or discuss the issue with the doctor.

> **⚖ Link**
>
> Chapter 9 discusses methods of delivering drugs by inhalations

Eye medication

Eye medications are available in two forms: eye ointments and eye drops. The administration of eye drops and eye ointment will initially be the responsibility of the health-care practitioner, but he or she may also be involved in instructing the patient as well as other members of the family to administer the medication. It is important that the correct eye is treated. The prescription must be carefully checked and any abbreviations verified. The patient should be informed if her vision is going to be affected after the procedure. Although the eye is not sterile, it is important to use aseptic techniques when performing eye treatment. If infection is present in both eyes, the least affected eye is treated first to prevent cross-contamination.

Guidelines for administering eye drops and eye ointments

1   Explain the procedure to the patient, emphasising that her nose may feel as if it is 'running' because the punctum of the eye drains into the nasal space. The patient may also get a taste of the drug at the back of her throat.
2   Ideally, the patient should be lying flat with her head tilted backwards to allow easy access to the eyes. The health-care practitioner should stand behind the patient's head as it is easier to administer the drug from that position.

3   Prepare all the necessary equipment. Warm the eye drops and ointments to room temperature.

4   Wash your hands, and put on gloves if necessary.

5   Check the eye and perform eye toilet as necessary.

6   Gently pull down the lower lid to form a pouch, as shown in Figure 6.12. Gently drop the required number of drops into the pouch. Ask the patient to close the eye gently for about 2 minutes. The patient should avoid blinking, as this activity may squeeze the medications out of the eye, or squeezing the eye lids closed as this may forces the drops out of the eye onto the cheek. If two different types of eye drops are being administered, a five-minute interval should be allowed between drops thus allowing the first drug to be adsorbed.

7   For eye ointment, start from the angle near the nose (the inner canthus) and work towards the ear, gently squeezing the tube along the inner edge of the lower lid. Avoid touching the eye with the sharp nozzle. An eye pad may be applied if requested. Separate tubes/bottles should always be used for the left and right eyes.

8   The patient should be advised not to rub or squeeze the eye. Leave the patient comfortable.

9   Remove any gloves used. Wash your hands.

10   Complete all the necessary documentation.

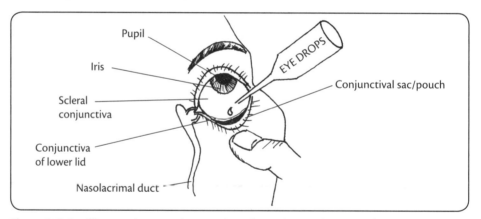

Figure 6.12 Instilling eye drops or ointment into the conjunctival sac/pouch

> **! Specific points on children's medications**
>
> - The health-care practitioner should get extra help so that the head can be held still during eye and ear treatments, to prevent the child rubbing his eyes or ears, and to provide comfort and reassurance.

Ear medications

Eardrops may be instilled to treat infection, soften ear wax, reduce discomfort and inflammation. *Instillation of eardrops is contraindicated if the patient has a perforated eardrum.* However, in some individual cases, medications may be prescribed which should be administered with caution while maintaining strict asepsis.

Guidelines for administering ear drops

1   Wash your hands and put on gloves if necessary.
2   Prepare all the necessary equipment and check the prescription that the medication is due. Each patient should have their own dropper.
3   Warm the medication to room temperature as cold drops may cause pain and dizziness.
4   Ask the patient to lie on the side with the ear to be treated facing upwards.
5   Examine the patient's ear canal and clean the outer canal if necessary using normal saline.
6   In children below 3 years of age, straighten the auditory canal by gently pulling the pinna downwards and backwards as in Figure 6.13a. In adults and children over 3 years old pull the pinna upwards and backwards as shown in Figure 6.13b (Craven and Hirnle, 2008).
7   Allow the prescribed number of drops to fall on the side of the ear canal and allow the drops to flow in until they disappear.
8   Advise the patient to remain in that position for 5 minutes.
9   When the patient is allowed to sit up, cleanse the external ear of any spillages or leakages, and make the patient comfortable.
10   Remove gloves and wash your hands.
11   Complete all the relevant records.

If both ears are to be treated, wait for 15 minutes between instillations.

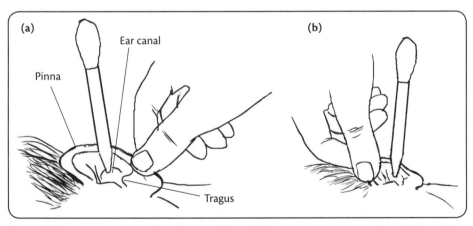

Figure 6.13 Administration of ear drops in (a) a child less than three years old and (b) a child who is over three years old and adults

Nasal medications

The intranasal route offers an alternative means of administering medications when traditional routes are not available or desirable. The drug may be used to achieve a local or a systemic effect and a number of drugs (midazolam, ephedrine) are available for use via this route. Nasal medications may be administered as nasal drops or sprays. Nasal drops may flood the sinuses or dribble down the throat and be ingested. This may induce an unpleasant taste in the mouth and the patient should be given a drink of juice to eliminate this taste. The patient should be advised to expectorate any drug going down the throat rather than swallow it. The patient should be able to breathe through each nostril as a blocked nostril will prevent the medication from reaching its intended target and will be wasted. The timing of these drugs is important, and they should be administered 20 minutes before meals so that the nasal passages will be clear during feeding.

Guidelines for administration of nasal medication

1   Wash your hands and put on gloves and masks if necessary.
2   Prepare all the necessary equipment, and check the prescription for completeness.
3   Explain the procedure to the patient as his cooperation is vital.
4   Support the patient to clear his nasal passages.
5   For a nasal spray using a pump bottle: keep the head in an upright position slightly tilted forward. Close the nostril that is not being treated by gently pressing on the side of the nostril. Whilst keeping the container upright, gently insert the spray tip about 0.5 cm into the nostril. Squeeze the container as instructed and instruct the patient to take a deep breath through the nose and breathe out by the mouth. After removing the nozzle out of the nostril, ask the patient to tip the head back for several seconds to aid absorption of the drug. Clear any excess drainage and ask the patient to avoid blowing their nose for 15 minutes. Repeat with the other nostril if required.
6   For nasal drops, it is better if the patient is lying down or holding their head back. Insert the dropper approximately 0.5 cm into the nostril and instil the required amount of medication. The patient should maintain this position for about 2 minutes to avoid the medication spilling out of the nostril. The tip of the dropper should not become contaminated and each patient should have their own dropper. Young children may be held on the lap with the neck extended.
7   After the procedure, make the patient comfortable and wash hands.
8   Complete all the relevant documentation.

Administering medications via a nebuliser

The respiratory tract, which includes the nasal mucosa, hypopharynx, and large and small airway structures, provides a large mucosal surface area for drug absorption. This route of administration is useful for treatment of pulmonary conditions. The commonest indication for nebulised therapy is the emergency treatment of acute asthma and exacerbations of chronic obstructive pulmonary disease. A number of drugs are now available for administration via a nebuliser for their action in the respiratory system; bronchodilators, corticosteroids and anticholinergics. Administering a drug via a nebuliser produces a mist enabling the drug to be inhaled directly into the lungs (Porter-Jones, 2000; Currie and Douglas, 2007; Jevon, 2007).

Before starting the procedure, it is important to ensure that the equipment is in good working order and if a cylinder of gas is used, that there is sufficient gas to complete the treatment and that Health and Safety regulations are met.

Guidelines for administration of medication via a nebuliser

1   The health-care practitioner should prepare all the equipment, compressed air, mouthpiece or mask, nebuliser system and tubing, and ensure that they are all safe to use and meet the COSHH standards. Patients with chronic obstructive pulmonary disease (COPD) should have their nebulisers driven by air and those with asthma by oxygen (BMA/RPSGB, 2009).

2   The patient should be sat in a comfortable upright position to maximise lung expansion.

3   The patient should be informed if the equipment is likely to generate any noise (air compressor) in order to allay anxiety.

4   The patient must be encouraged to adopt a normal pattern of breathing when receiving the nebuliser.

5   Prepare the medication as instructed.

6   Unscrew the nebuliser and pour the contents of the drug/solution into the nebuliser chamber.

7   Screw the nebuliser back together, attach the mouthpiece or mask to the nebuliser and connect the tubing to the nebuliser and attach to either the air compressor or cylinder.

8   If using an air cylinder, turn the flow rate to 6–8 litres per minute which produces particles of less than 5 microns in diameter and small enough to be deposited in the lungs. Once the mist begins to appear at the mouthpiece ask the patient to insert the mouthpiece into their mouth or to put the mask on and breathe normally. If the patient is well enough to hold each breath for 2–3 seconds then they should be instructed to do so as this will allow the medication to settle in the airways.

9   The treatment is complete when there is no further mist being produced and the nebuliser makes a sputtering noise. The gas supply is switched off and the nebuliser equipment is disposed of or cleaned according to hospital policy.

10   Observe for any side effects.

11   Record peak flow to monitor the effectiveness of nebulised medication.

12   Make patient comfortable at the end of the procedure.

13   Complete all documentation.

Rectal medications

The human rectum is the slightly dilated part of the colon measuring about 13 cm long and represents a body cavity in which drugs can be introduced and retained so that absorption of the drug can take place. The rectum's wall is thin and has a rich blood supply allowing the drug to be readily absorbed with acceptable therapeutic efficacy (Karunajeewa et al., 2007). However, the absorption of drugs from the rectum can be variable as absorption may be limited due to the small surface area of mucosa that the medication is in contact with and the presence of faeces in the rectum. The **rectal route** is used as an alternative route of drug administration during convulsion, nausea and vomiting, the uncooperative patient, nil by mouth peri-operatively and the unconscious patient.

rectal route
via the rectum

The action of the drug can be local (for example, lubricant suppositories) or systemic (for example, aminophylline). These medications are in the form of a suppository, cream or solution. It is vitally important to gain the patient's consent. Young patients are sensitive about this procedure. Vyvyan and Hanafiah (1995) found that patients preferred to discuss this beforehand and there was greater acceptability among males compared to female patients (Bhagat et al., 2003).

Application of creams or suppository

1 Wash your hands.
2 Prepare all the equipment, and check the prescription for completeness.
3 Explain the procedure to the patient and provide privacy.
4 Put gloves on.
5 Position the patient on his left side and only expose the buttocks. Gently lifting the upper buttocks will expose the rectal opening.
6 External creams can be applied directly using gloved finger or gauze. Internal rectal medicine such as enemas should be administered with greater care. The tip of the applicator should be lubricated with a water soluble lubricant and inserted for the required length (as per manufacturer's recommendations). The medication is squeezed into the rectum slowly. To insert a suppository, the lubricated (water-soluble lubricant) tapered end of the suppository should be placed at the anus and gently pushed into the rectum past the anal sphincter. Clean away any excess lubricant.
7 Make the patient comfortable and instruct the patient accordingly. Drugs used for systemic effects should be retained and prevented from being expelled. If the medication has been administered to relieve constipation, appropriate toileting arrangements should be in place.
8 Children and infants may be held or cuddled to distract them.
9 Dispose of all equipment, and wash your hands.
10 Complete all the relevant records.

> **! Specific points on children's medications**
>
> - When giving a suppository to an infant or toddler, he can lie on his back with his legs flexed. The suppository is inserted using the index finger for children over 3 years. In children of 3 years or less, the little finger may be used.

∞ Link

Chapter 8 also discusses administration of suppositories.

Vaginal medications

The vagina has been shown to be an alternative route for the administration of drugs for women. The vagina is a thin walled tube approximately 8–10 cm long and extends from the cervix to the exterior (Marieb, 2004). Drugs are absorbed through the vaginal wall owing to its highly permeable structure and abundant blood supply which also contributes to an effective systemic distribution of the drugs.

Several drugs have proven to be suitable and effective for vaginal administration (Neves et al., 2008). For example, hormonal contraception has become more widely used in recent years. A number of preparations achieve serum levels sufficient to have systemic effects allowing the administration of lower doses with steady drug levels and less frequent administration (Alexander et al., 2004). Medications intended for administration via the **vaginal route** are available in many forms – pessaries, creams, medicated douches and vaginal rings. Societal taboo against speaking about the vagina can create discomfort for both patient and health-care professional and the possibility of administering drugs via this route should be discussed in a sensitive manner.

vaginal route
into the vagina

Application of vaginal creams

The patient should be encouraged to empty her bladder as she is expected to remain lying down for 20 minutes after insertion of the medication.

1   Wash your hands.
2   Prepare all the equipment, and check the prescription for completeness.
3   Explain the procedure to the patient and provide privacy. Select the appropriate position, either supine with the knees drawn up and legs parted, or left lateral with the knees drawn up.
4   Wash your hands and put on gloves.
5   Lubricate the pessary or applicator.
6   Insert the pessary along the posterior vaginal wall and into the top of the vagina. If using an applicator, insert the barrel of the applicator into the vagina as far as it will go. Squeeze the tube to insert the drug while holding the applicator steady. Withdraw the applicator, and make the patient comfortable.
7   Provide the patient with sanitary towels and advise her to remain in position for 20 minutes.
8   Discard the equipment or clean it for reuse.
9   Remove gloves and wash your hands.
10 Complete all the relevant documentation.

Medication adherence

Adherence can be defined 'as the extent to which patients follow the instruction they were given for prescribed treatments' (Haynes et al., 2009, p. 1). In this context, the term 'adherence' is used to be non-judgemental, a statement of fact rather than of blame of the patient, prescriber or treatment.

> ✱ Activity **6.10**
>
> Discuss with your mentor, tutor or lecturer the benefits of administering drugs rectally. What are the ethical and cultural issues when administering drugs via the rectal and vaginal routes?
>
> Identify which drugs are routinely given via these routes.

There are many reasons that exist for non-adherence and these have been categorised into (a) intentional – when the patient decides not to follow the treatment recommendations, and (b) unintentional – when the patient is prevented from doing so by barriers that are beyond their control (NICE, 2009). NICE advises that non-adherence should not be seen as a patient's problem but as a limitation in the delivery of health which requires a multi-factorial approach to its management.

Patients known to be at risk of non-adherence should be managed as follows:

- The adoption of a 'no blame' approach that encourages the patient to voice any concerns about taking the medications (NICE, 2009).
- A patient-centred approach that encourages adherence, taking into account the patient's needs and preferences, including the involvement of the family and the patient's rights.
- Review of each medication to ensure that it is still required.
- Identification of barriers to adherence.

General principles when administering medications to children

It is essential to provide safe and effective drug therapy to children. Because of anatomical and physiological differences, the drug's pharmacokinetic properties – absorption, distribution, metabolism and excretion – may be affected. For more details of drug pharmacokinetics in children and infants, you should consult the latest recommendation from the BNF.

General guidelines for giving medications to children

1 It is important to establish a trusting relationship with the child and to identify any preferences. Always be honest regarding painful injections or distasteful medications. Remain calm.

2 Adequate time should be allowed prior to and after the administration of drugs to comfort the child. It may take longer than expected to explain to the child and to give any instructions that they must follow to enhance the effectiveness of therapy.

3 The health-care practitioner should be kind but firm when approaching the child.

4 Organise help to control and support children. Do not interrupt what the child is doing; make medicine-taking a part of it.

5 Identify the child correctly, checking with the parents. If possible, organise drug administration when the parents are present.

6 Explain the procedure to the child and parents. Parents may provide information on how the child likes to take her medication. Offer a choice, for example taking it from the parent or health-care practitioner.

7 Avoid mixing medications in milk or essential foods or the child may avoid those foods and develop malnutrition or dehydration.

8 If possible, allow children to participate, for example choosing the juice to be drunk with the medicine.

9   Reward children for taking their medications, but avoid punishing children who are uncooperative.
10 Do not anticipate difficulty: the child quickly picks up your anxiety.
11 Never make a promise you cannot keep.

! Specific guidelines when giving injections to children

- The aseptic and safe-checking procedures should be followed as discussed.
- Prepare the equipment, and check the prescription for completeness.
- Explain the procedure to the child in a manner consistent with the child's age and understanding. Audiovisual aids such as booklets or dolls may be used to get the message across. Parents should be informed and involved in supporting the child.
- Appropriate restraint, for example a blanket, may be required.
- Select the injection site (see above).
- The procedure should be undertaken quickly and gently.
- Support is provided as necessary by the health-care practitioner and/or parents.

Giving medications to clients with learning disabilities

Clients with learning disabilities may have varying degrees of mental and physical disabilities, and it may be as difficult for the health-care practitioner to explain and for the patient to understand. Following the 'five Rs' of drug administration should secure the client's safety. The client may also suffer from physical deformities, which may require adapting methods and in some cases changing the form of the drug and the route of administration. With difficult situations, the practitioner should consult the pharmacist who may be able to help with special preparations. Liquid preparations are safer than tablets or capsules.

Giving medications to patients with mental illness

The Mental Capacity Act 2005 sets out in law the principle that people should be presumed to have capacity to make their own decisions and that decisions made on behalf of those who lack capacity should be made on the individual's best interests. The side effects of some medications used to treat mental health

Chart 6.3 Side effects of anti-psychotic drugs

- Unusual body movements
- Feeling drowsy and sedated
- Heart arrhythmia
- Weight gain (Clozapine, olanzapine)
- Diabetes
- Excess salivation
- Stroke
- Dizziness
- Blurred vision
- Hormonal changes: increased levels of prolactin causing osteoporosis,
- reduced libido, impotence

Link

Chapters 3 and 13 also discuss the Mental Capacity Act.

problems may cause physical symptoms (Mentality, 2003) and it is very important that regular reviews are in place to monitor for side effects. Side effects of anti-psychotic drugs are listed in Chart 6.3.

Mentality (2004) recommends that patients are closely monitored to assess the impact of medication on physical illness.

Medication errors

A medication error is defined as any preventable event that may cause or lead to inappropriate medication use or patient harm while the medication administration is in the control of the professional practitioner (Hicks et al., 2008). The UK National Patient Safety Agency Report (2007) highlighted that medical errors cause a large number of deaths each year and that the error can occur at any stage of the medication use: prescribing, dispensing and administration.

To prevent medication errors, the health-care practitioner should adhere to the 'five R' principles: right medication, right amount, right time, right patient and the right route as discussed earlier in this chapter.

Any incidents involving medication errors should be reported immediately to the health-care practitioner in charge and the doctor. The patient should be monitored for any side effects. A senior member of staff should inform the patient of what has happened and what actions are being taken. Preventative measures may be taken to control the effects of the drugs. The incident is usually investigated, and if the health-care practitioner has been found to be negligent, disciplinary action may be taken by the employing authority and the NMC. The patient can also take legal action against the health-care practitioner or the employer.

Chapter Summary

This chapter has described some of the key aspects of safe practice in the administration of medicines. Every activity that the health-care practitioner undertakes carries considerable risk to the patient as well as to the health-care practitioner. By applying the principles described in this chapter, the health-care practitioner can ensure that procedures are carried out safely, that patients are not harmed and that their care is optimised.

? Test yourself!

1   Name the five Rs in relation to drug administration.
2   Which five sites can be used for injections?
3   What side effects can arise from using anti-psychotic drugs?

Greenstein, B. (2004) *Trounce's Clinical Pharmacology for Nurses*. 17th edn. Churchill Livingstone, Edinburgh.

Shihab, P. (2009) *Numeracy in Nursing and Healthcare: Calculations and Practice*. Pearson Education, Harlow.

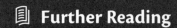

Further Reading

For live links to useful websites see: www.palgrave.com/nursinghealth/hogston

References

Alexander, N.J., Baker, E., Kaptein, M., Karck, U., Miller, L. and Zampaglione, E. (2004) Why consider vaginal drug administration? *Fertility and Sterility* **82**(1): 1–12.

Becton Dickinson (2009) How to inject insulin. http://www.bddiabetes.com

Beecroft, P.C. and Redick, S.A. (1990) Intramuscular injection practices of paediatric nurses: site selection. *Nurse Educator* **15**(4): 23–8.

Berger, K.J. and Williams, M.S. (1992) *Fundamentals of Nursing: Collaborating for Optimal Health*. Appleton and Lange, Stamford, CT.

Bhagat, H., Malhotra, K., Tyagi.C., Gangwar, N. and Pal, N. (2003) Evaluation of preoperative rectal Diclofenac for perioperative analgesia in ENT surgery. *Indian Journal of Anaesthesia* **47**(6): 463–6.

BMA (British Medical Association)/RPSGB (Royal Pharmaceutical Society of Great Britain) (2009) *British National Formulary 57*. BMA/RPSGB, London. www.bnf.org/bnf

Burbridge, B.E. (2007) Computed tomographic measurement of gluteal subcutaneous fat thickness in reference to failure of gluteal intramuscular injections. *Canadian Association Radiology Journal* **58**(2): 72–5.

Chan, V.O., Colville, J., Persaud, T., Buckley, O. and Torreggiani, W.C. (2006) Intramuscular injections into the buttocks: are they truly intramuscular? *European Journal of Radiology* **58**(3): 480–4.

Cocoman, A. and Barron, C. (2008) Administering subcutaneous injections to children: what does the evidence say? *Journal of Children and Young People's Nursing* **2**(2): 84–9.

Cook, I.F. and Murtagh, J. (2005) The WHO technique for intramuscular thigh vaccination in infants and toddlers had fewer adverse reactions than 2 other techniques. *Medical Journal of Australia* **183**: 60–3.

Cordoni, A. and Cordoni, L.E. (2001) Eutectic mixture of local anesthetics reduces pain during catheter insertion in paediatric patients. *Clinical Journal of Pain* **17**: 115–18.

Covington, T.P. and Trattler, M.R. (1997) Bull's eye! Finding the right target for IM injections. *Nursing* **27**: 62–3.

Craven, R.F. and Hirnle, C.J. (2008) *Fundamentals of Nursing: Human Health and Function*. 6th edn. Lippincott Williams & Wilkins, Philadelphia.

Cummings, E.A., Reid, C.J., Finley, G.A., McGrath, P.J. and Ritchie, J.A. (1996) Prevalence and source of pain in paediatric inpatients. *Pain* **68**: 25–31.

Currie, G. and Douglas, J. (2007) Oxygen and inhalers. In Currie, G. (ed.) *ABC of COPD*. Blackwell, Oxford.

DoH (Department of Health) (2006) *Immunisation against Infectious Diseases*. The Stationery Office, London.

Griffith, R. (2003) Covert administration of medicines. *The Pharmaceutical Journal* **271**(7258): 90–1.

Haynes, R.B., McDonald, H.P. and Garg, A.X. (2009) Helping patients follow prescribed treatment. *Journal of the American Medical Association* **228**(22): 2880–3.

Hicks, R.W., Becker, S.C. and Jackson, D.G. (2008) Understanding medication errors: Discussion of a case involving a urinary catheter implicated in a wrong route error. *Urologic Nursing* **28**(6): 454–9.

HSE (Health and Safety Executive) (2002) *COSHH Guidelines*. http://www.hse.gov.uk/pubns/indg136.pdf

Jevon, P. (2007) Respiratory procedures: use of a nebuliser. *Nursing Times* **103**(34): 24.

Karunajeewa, H.A., Manning, L., Mueller, I., Ilett, K.F. and Davies, T.M.E. (2007) Rectal administration of artemisinin derivatives for the treatment of malaria. *Journal of American Medical Association* **297** (21): 2381–90.

Lenz, C.L. (1983) Make your needle selection right to the point. *Nursing* **13**: 50–1.

MacLaren, J. and Cohen, L. (2005) A comparison of distraction strategies for venipuncture distress in children. *Journal of Pediatric Psychology* **30**(5): 387–96.

Marieb, E.N. (2004) *Human Anatomy and Physiology*. 6th edn. Pearson/Benjamin Cummings. San Francisco.

McConnell, E.S. (2000) Administering an intradermal injection. *Nursing* **30**(3): 17.

Mentality (2003) Not all in the mind – the physical health of mental health users. Radical

Mentalities Briefing Paper 2. Mentality, London.

Mentality (2004) Healthy body and mind: promoting healthy living for people who experience mental distress. Mentality, London.

National Coordinating Council for Medication Error Reporting and Prevention (2009) What is a medication error. http://nccmerp.org/aboutmederrors.html (accessed on 14 September 2009).

Neves, J.D., Santos, B., Teixeira, B., Dias, G., Cunha, T. and Brochado, J. (2008) Vaginal drug administration in the hospital setting. *American Journal of Health-System Pharmacy* **65**: 254–9.

Newton, M., Newton, D.W. and Fudin, J. (1992) Reviewing the three big injection routes. *Nursing* **22**: 34–42.

NICE (National Institute for Health and Clinical Excellence) (2009) *Medicine adherence: involving patients in decisions about prescribed medicines and supporting adherence CG76.* National Collaborating Centre for Primary Care/Royal College of Physicians. http://guidance.nice.org.uk/CG76/NiceGuidance/doc/English

Nisbet, A.C. (2006) Intramuscular gluteal injections in the increasingly obese population: retrospective study. *British Medical Journal* **332**(7542): 637–8.

NMC (Nursing and Midwifery Council) (2008) *Standards for Medicine Management.* NMC, London.

NPSA (National Patient Safety Agency) (2005) *Advice to the NHS on Reducing Harm Caused by the Misplacement of Nasogastric Feeding Tubes.* NPSA, London. http://www.npsa.nhs.uk/nrls/alerts-and-directives/alerts/nasogastric-feeding-tubes/

NPSA (National Patient Safety Agency) (2007). *Safety in Doses: Medication Safety Incident in the NHS: The Fourth Report from the Patient Safety Observatory.* NPSA, London.

Pickering, K. (2003) The administration of drugs via the enteral feeding tubes. *Nursing Times* **99**(46): 46–9.

Porter-Jones, G. (2000) Nebulisers – 1: Preparation. *Nursing Times* **96**(36): 45–6.

Pringle, B., Hilley, L., Gelfand, K., Dahlquist, L. M., Switkin, M., Diver, T., Sulc, W. and Allen, E. (2001) Decreasing child distress during needle sticks and maintaining treatment gains over time. *Journal of Clinical Psychology in Medical Settings* **8**(2): 119–30.

Rodger, M. and King, L. (2000) Drawing up and administering intramuscular injections: a review of the literature. *Journal of Advanced Nursing* **13**: 574–82.

Royal College of Paediatrics and Child Health (2002) *Position Statement on Injection Techniques.* RCPCH, London.

Scottish Centre Infection and Environmental Health (2005) *Review of Skin Injections.* SCIEH.

Simon, P.A., Chen, R.T., Elliot, J.A. and Schwartz, B. (1993) Outbreak of pyogenic abscesses after diphtheria and tetanus toxoids and pertussis vaccination. *Pediatric Infectious Disease* **12**: 368–71.

Small, S.P. (2004) Preventing sciatic nerve injury from intramuscular injections: literature review. *Journal of Advanced Nursing* **47**(3): 287–96.

Springhouse Corporation (1993) *Medication Administration and IV Therapy Manual.* 2nd edn. Springhouse Corporation, Philadelphia, PA.

Thomas, B.J. and Finnin, B.C. (2004) The transdermal revolution. *Drug Discovery Today* **9**(6): 697–703.

Tremayne, P. and Parboteeah, S. (2006) *Fundamental Aspects of Adult Nursing Procedures.* Quay Publishing, London.

Tortora, G. and Derrickson, B. (2008) *Principles of Anatomy and Physiology,* 12th edn. Wiley, Hoboken, NJ.

Tubiana-Rufi, N., Belarbi, N., Pasquier-Fadiasvsky, L., Polak, K., Kakou, B. and Leridon, L. (1999) Short needle (8 mm) reduce the risk of intramuscular injections in children with type 1 diabetes. *Diabetes Care* **22**(10): 1621–5.

UK National Patient Safety Agency Report (2007) *Reducing the Harms Caused by Misplaced Nasogastric Feeding Tubes: Patient Safety Alert 05.* NPSA, London.

Vyvyan, H.A. and Hanafiah, Z. (1995) Patients' attitudes to rectal drug administration. *Anaesthesia* **50**(11): 983–4.

Wales, J. (1997) Insulin strategies. Cited in: Court, S. and Lamb, B. (eds) (2001) *Childhood and Adolescent Diabetes.* John Wiley & Sons, Chichester.

Whalley, L.F. and Wong, D.L. (1995) *Nursing Care of Infants and Children,* 4th edn. Mosby, London.

Workman, B. (1999) Safe injection techniques *Nursing Standard* **13**: 47–53.

World Health Organisation (1984) Immunisation in practice (a guide for health workers who give vaccines). When and how to give vaccines. EPI/PHW/84/3 Revision 1. World Health Organisation, Geneva, Switzerland.

Zaybak, A., Günes, U.Y., Tamsel, S., Khorshid, L. and Eser, I. (2007) Does obesity prevent the needle from reaching muscles in intramuscular injections? *Journal of Advanced Nursing* **58**(6): 552–6.

Zuckerman, J.N. (2000) The importance of injecting vaccine into muscle. *British Medical Journal* **321**: 137–8.

SUE M. GREEN

Chapter

Eating and Drinking

7

📖 Contents

- The Role of the RN and the MDT in Nutritional Care
- Diet, Foods and Nutrients
- Public Health Nutrition
- Clients' Nutritional Needs
- Nutritional Support

- Ethical Issues
- Chapter Summary
- Test Yourself!
- Further Reading
- References

☑ Learning outcomes

The purpose of this chapter is to introduce you to basic nutritional concepts and the role of the Registered Nurse (RN) in enabling clients to consume a diet which is optimal to their health in all settings. At the end of the chapter, you should be able to:

- Outline the role of the RN and the multidisciplinary team (MDT) in nutritional care
- Define the terms diet, foods and nutrients
- Identify the main macronutrients in the diet and discuss their role in the body and name the two main types of micronutrient giving examples of each type and their role in the body
- Discuss the importance of oral fluid intake
- Outline the difference between the concept of public health nutrition and clients' nutritional needs
- Discuss political, social and economic influences on dietary choice and the influence of appetite on food intake
- Identify methods of screening and assessing nutritional status
- Describe the condition of malnutrition
- Outline the way in which food intake can be promoted for clients with different dietary requirements.

The Role of the RN and the MDT in Nutritional Care

Eating and drinking is an activity that is fundamental to a body's survival. Eating and drinking provides the body with fluid and nutrients that enables cells to function. Without appropriate nutrients and fluids in appropriate quantities the health of cells and consequently the body is threatened. The role of the registered nurse (RN) in ensuring a client receives appropriate nutrients and fluids for their needs in the right quantities and at the right times is a fundamental part of nursing care. The nutritional care of a client can range from providing information on healthy eating to ensuring complex nutritional support regimes, for example parenteral nutrition, are given appropriately as prescribed. The importance of the RN in ensuring appropriate nutritional care is emphasised by incorporation of an essential skill category 'Nutrition and Fluid Management' within the Essential Skills Clusters (NMC, 2007) for pre-registration nursing programmes. This chapter focuses on nutrition and briefly considers fluid intake.

The Essential Skills Cluster (NMC, 2007) relating to nutrition outlines that clients can trust a newly qualified RN to:

- Provide assistance with selecting a diet through which they will receive adequate nutritional and fluid intake.
- Assess and monitor nutritional status and formulate an effective care plan.
- Provide an environment conducive to eating and drinking.
- Ensure that those unable to take food by mouth receive adequate nutrition.

These activities are likely to be outlined in your assessment of practice portfolio but in order to achieve competency in the skill an underpinning knowledge and understanding of nutritional concepts relating to client care is required.

There are a number of other important publications which guide the way in which RNs should give nutritional care in the UK. The clinical guidelines produced by the National Institute for Health and Clinical Excellence (NICE) concerning the management of nutrition support and obesity (NICE, 2006a, 2006b) are essential reading for this chapter. In addition the publication *Essence of Care* (DoH, 2010) should also be consulted. This document aims to enable practitioners to identify best practice and improve care and one of the eight areas covered is 'food and nutrition'.

It is also important to consider nutritional care by the RN from a European perspective. The Council of Europe and other European organisations have produced several documents on nutrition that can be related to nursing practice. These include guidelines on food and nutritional care in hospitals (Council of Europe, 2003) and recommendations for initiatives for tackling malnutrition (European Nutrition for Health Alliance, 2007) and obesity (Commission of the European Communities, 2007).

Basic nutritional care of clients can be provided by the RN but beyond this other members of the multidisciplinary team must be involved. Most often this involves referring the client to the dietitian and doctor; however, it may also involve referring the client to the pharmacist, speech and language therapist, occupational therapist or RN nutrition specialist. Some practice areas have a Nutrition Support Team. This is a team of health-care professionals (usually including an RN, doctor, dietitian, pharmacist and sometimes laboratory scientists) with expertise in nutritional care. Nutrition Support Teams have a range of responsibilities concerning advanced nutritional care, education, and standards of clinical practice in nutritional support.

The Nutrition RN Specialist (NNS) is an RN with expertise in nutritional care. The role of the NNS varies according to the practice area but generally involves the management of advanced nutritional support, training, the development of clinical guidelines and audit.

★ Activity **7.1**

Access the British Dietetic Association website (BDA, 2010) to learn about the dietitian's role: http://www.bda.uk.com/

Diet, Foods and Nutrients

The diet consists of what we eat and drink over the course of a period of time. Some clients may not be able to eat and drink and may be given nutrients and fluid via a tube into their gastrointestinal tract (for example, gastrostomy and naso-gastric nutrition) or, more rarely, directly into their venous system (parenteral nutrition).

Foods that we eat, when considered altogether, constitute the diet. Some clients' diet consists of only a few foods whereas others may consist of a wide variety of foods, sometimes termed a 'varied diet'. There are many different types of food and the reason why a person chooses to eat particular foods depends on many factors, such as cost, culture and individual taste preference.

Foods themselves are composed of different types of nutrients and other substances which add to the characteristics of the food but are not nutrients in that they do not provide any nutritive value (for example caffeine). Nutrients are substances which are required by the body to enable it to function. They form the structure of the body, provide energy for the cells or form part of the metabolic processes that enable cells to live. Nutrients can be categorised into macronutrients and micronutrients. Macronutrients are the nutrients required in large amounts: protein, fat and carbohydrate. Micronutrients are nutrients required in only small amounts and comprise of vitamins and minerals.

Macronutrients

Macronutrients provide energy for the body to function. In nutrition energy is measured in joules, kilojoules (1 kJ = 1,000 joules) and megajoules (1 MJ = 1,000 kJ or 1,000,000 joules). Kilocalories (kcal) are older units of measurement which are still commonly used, the lay term for which tends to be 'calories'. For people whose body weight lies within the 'normal' range, energy (or kilocalorie) intake should be enough to maintain a reasonably constant body weight when an adequate amount of exercise is taken. If we eat more energy than our body needs we gain weight and if we eat less we lose weight. Energy requirements vary according to age, gender, and level of physical activity. For example, people with well-developed muscles have a faster metabolism than sedentary people and older people tend to have a slower metabolism than younger people. A physically active person with lots of metabolically active muscle requires more energy than a relatively sedentary one with a higher percentage of body fat.

Carbohydrate

Carbohydrates are classified according to their structure. The smallest unit of a carbohydrate is a monosaccharide. Carbohydrate is absorbed as monosaccharides for use by the body. The monosaccharides are also known as 'simple sugars' and include glucose and fructose. Glucose is a very important nutrient for the body as body cells usually produce the energy they need to carry out activities from glucose. Oligosaccharides consist of a small number of monosaccharides linked together and include sucrose (table sugar), lactose (milk sugar) and maltose. Polysaccharides, sometimes termed complex carbohydrates, consist of many monosaccharides linked together and include starch and non-starch polysaccharides ('fibre'). Starch is digested by enzymes in the gastrointestinal tract so it can be absorbed as monsaccharides. Non-starch polysaccharides ('fibre') cannot be digested by enzymes produced by the salivary glands and small intestine and so pass through the body and form the bulk of faeces.

> ✳ **Activity 7.2**
>
> Review the metabolic pathway that produces energy from glucose in human cells in your anatomy and physiology text book.

Carbohydrate is used by the body for energy with each gram yielding about 17 kjoules (4 kcals). A limited amount of carbohydrate can be stored in the body in the form of glycogen. The process of forming glycogen from glucose is termed glycogenesis and the breakdown of glycogen to glucose when carbohydrate is needed by the body is termed glycogenolysis. A healthy adult's diet should obtain at least 50 per cent of food energy from carbohydrate, mainly in the form of starch (BNF, 2009). Foods rich in carbohydrate include bread, rice, breakfast cereals, pasta, potatoes, yams, bananas, corn and oats. Other sources of carbohydrate include cakes, biscuits and pastry, but these also tend to have high levels of fat.

Protein

The smallest unit of a protein is an amino acid. Protein is absorbed as amino acids in the gastrointestinal tract. There are 20 or so different amino acids required by the human body, which are classified into:

- *Essential* – those which cannot be synthesised by the body
- *Non-essential* – those which can be synthesised by the body.

> 🔗 **Link**
>
> Chapter 11 describes factors needed for wound healing.

Protein is essential for the formation of cells and forms components of many of the metabolic processes that take place within the body. An adequate protein intake is essential for growth, body defence mechanisms and repair of damage to the body. Protein can be used by the body for energy with each gram yielding about 17 kjoules (4 kcals); this process is termed gluconeogenesis. In a healthy adult individual approximately 10 to 20 per cent of total energy should derive from protein which is about 0.75 grams per kg of body weight (Pavlovic et al., 2007). There is some evidence that excessive dietary protein may contribute to demineralisation of bone and may have some effect on renal function (AHA, 2009).

Rich sources of protein include meat, fish, eggs, pulses (peas, beans and lentils), nuts, tofu, soya and textured vegetable protein. It is possible to get all the essential amino acids from vegetable sources, providing that the right amount, combination and range of protein-containing foods are consumed.

Fat

Triglycerides are the main fat used by the body and the main components of these are fatty acids and glycerol. Fatty acids can be, in chemical terms, saturated or unsaturated. Saturated fatty acids have only single bonds between the carbon atoms that make up the molecule, whereas in unsaturated fatty acids there may be one (monounsaturated) or more (polyunsaturated) double bonds between carbon atoms. In general, fats that contain mainly saturated fatty acids are solid at room temperature, whereas those which contain mainly unsaturated fatty acids are liquid at room temperature (though they usually solidify when chilled).

Saturated fatty acids are mainly of animal origin and a high intake is associated with an increased risk of cardiovascular disease (Denny, 2008). Certain cancers, such as breast cancer, have also been linked to a high intake of saturated fats (Cancer Research UK, 2008).

The two main types of polyunsaturated fats are omega-3 (linoleic acid) and omega-6 (alpha-linolenic acid). These are sometimes termed essential fatty acids as they need to be consumed in the diet.

Trans fatty acids are fatty acids that have been altered in the manufacturing process in order to make them suitable for use in some food products, for example biscuits. They are metabolised in the body in the same way as saturated fatty acids.

It is important to understand the different types of fat and the effect that they can have on the body because of their influence on blood cholesterol level. Cholesterol is obtained from the diet (contained, for example, in eggs, offal and shellfish) and made by the liver. Cholesterol is transported in the plasma by carrier proteins called lipoproteins. Low density lipoprotein (LDL) cholesterol is associated with atherosclerosis and high density lipoprotein (HDL) cholesterol is associated with reduced risk of the formation of atherosclerosis. Both the total amount of fat and the relative amounts of saturated and unsaturated fat affect the concentration of the two lipoproteins in the plasma. A high intake of total fat, especially saturated fat, is associated with a high LDL cholesterol level whereas a relatively low intake of fat, with a high proportion in the form of unsaturated fat, is associated with a lower LDL cholesterol level. Triglycerides are also transported in the blood and a high level is associated with the development of atherosclerosis.

One gram of fat provides 38 kJ (9 kcal) of energy. It is, therefore, the most energy-dense nutrient.

For adults and older children, it is recommended that no more than 35 per cent of food energy should come from fat (BNF, 2004).

This can be subdivided into:

- no more than 10 per cent of total energy from saturated fatty acids, for example butter
- no more that 2 per cent from *trans*-fatty acids, in for example biscuits and pastry (as hydrogenated vegetable oil or fat).

A restricted dietary fat intake is not recommended for those below the age of five years.

Fat is used by the body as an energy source, to provide an insulating and protective layer and to form parts of cells (for example cell membranes) and hormones.

Fat is found in many foods, for example meat, nuts, cereals and some vegetables and fruit (e.g. avocado). It is also one of the ingredients for food products (for example biscuits, cakes and pastry) and many foods are cooked in fat (for example potatoes). Foods rich in monounsaturated fat include olive and rapeseed oil. The principal source of the polyunsaturated omega-3 fatty acids is fish oil, and people living in the UK are advised to eat two portions of fish a week, one of which should be oily (FSA, 2009). However, there are recommendations for the maximum amount of oily fish that should be consumed in a week because of pollutants contained in the fish (FSA, 2009). Females who might one day have a baby and those pregnant or breastfeeding should not eat more than two portions a week. Other people should not eat more than four portions of oily fish a week. Vegetarians and vegans do not eat fish and should be directed to the information sheets provided by the Vegetarian Society (2009). Omega-6 sources include corn, sunflower, rapeseed and soya bean oils.

Consumption of dietary fat also supplies vitamins A, D, E and K as these are fat soluble and so found in fatty or oily foods.

Alcohol

Alcohol is not usually classified as a nutrient but its contribution to the diet needs to be considered because metabolism of alcohol provides energy for the body. Each gram of alcohol yields 7 kcals (29 kJ). Alcoholic drinks are enjoyed in moderate quantities by many people. Some alcoholic drinks (for example red wine) contain antioxidants which can protect against some diseases when drunk in moderate amounts (Streppel et al., 2009). Alcoholic drinks can enhance the enjoyment of a meal, promote appetite, and are often used to celebrate life events. Problems arise when alcohol is taken in excess or in 'binges'. As alcohol provides the body with energy, people who drink large amounts habitually may reduce the amount of food they eat which can lead to a deficiency in intake of nutrients, or weight gain may be promoted if the diet remains the same. The liver is the organ that is largely responsible for metabolising alcohol. Habitually drinking large amounts of alcohol damages the liver and can lead to liver disease. 'Binge' drinking causes many health problems even if the individual is not considered to be alcohol dependent. Alcohol's psychogenic effects can lead to risk taking behaviour and misjudgement in social and other situations. Large amounts taken at one time cannot be metabolised by the liver quickly enough to prevent build-up of levels in the blood which causes neurological changes, dehydration as fluid balance mechanisms are disturbed and can result in loss of consciousness and death.

Current guidelines suggest women can drink up to 2–3 units per day and men up to 3–4 units per day without significant risk to health (FSA, 2009). One unit equates to half a pint of standard strength beer, lager or cider or a pub measure of spirit.

Non-starch polysaccharide

Non-starch polysaccharide (NSP) is the scientific term for 'roughage' and 'fibre'. NSP may not be classified as a nutrient as it provides no nutrients and minimal energy for the body. However, it is very important in terms of maintaining gastrointestinal health. NSP is found in plant cells and cannot be digested by the digestive enzymes produced by the human gastrointestinal tract. NSP aids the passage of food through the bowel and enables elimination of waste products. Sources of NSP include fruit and vegetables, whole grains, wholemeal bread, cereals, beans and pulses. There is no NSP in animal food sources such as milk, meat, cheese and eggs. It is recommended healthy adults consume 18 g a day, with the range being 12 to 24 g per day. Ensuring a good intake dietary intake of NSP requires the consumption of fruit and vegetables (whole and unpeeled where possible) and whole grain (rather than refined versions) products such as wholemeal bread, brown rice and wholemeal pasta. A minimum of five different fruits and vegetables a day is recommended for most people (FSA, 2009). There are two sorts of NSP: soluble and insoluble.

> **∞ Link**
> Chapter 8 discusses the effects of diet on faecal elimination.

Soluble NSP forms a gel-like matrix in the gastrointestinal tract and helps to maintain a steady blood glucose level by slowing the absorption of glucose across the intestinal wall. Soluble NSP may help to decrease a blood cholesterol level by preventing bile acids and cholesterol in the intestine from being reabsorbed. Rich sources are pulses, oats, barley, rye, beans and lentils, but it is also found in fruits and vegetables.

Insoluble NSP passes through the digestive system and giving bulk to the food in the digestive system and therefore aiding passage of waste products. Large amounts of insoluble NSP can reduce the absorption of some micronutrients. It is found in wheat-based breakfast cereals, bread, rice, maize, pasta, fruits and vegetables.

> **✴ Activity 7.3**
> Think about your 'fibre' (non starch polysaccharide) intake over the past seven days. Do you eat enough fibre?

Micronutrients

Micronutrients is the general term used to describe vitamins and minerals. Micronutrients are required in small amounts and either play a role in the various metabolic processes that take place in the body or are structural materials. The vitamins include A, B complex, C, D, E, K and folate. Vitamins are water soluble or fat soluble. A regular intake of water soluble vitamins is required because excess intake is excreted in the urine rather than being stored in the body. The minerals include calcium, phosphorous, magnesium, sodium, potassium, chloride, iron, zinc, copper, selenium, iodine and several others. For a description of each micronutrient and its function please refer to a text book on human nutrition.

Thiamine (B_1), vitamin C and vitamin D (cholecalciferol), calcium and iron, will be briefly considered in this chapter as these are relatively common micronutrient deficiencies in the United Kingdom (UK). It is important to recognise that micronutrients are required in adequate amounts for optimal physiological functioning; however, excessive amounts can also be dangerous to health. Ingesting amounts in excess of that recommended by the Department of Health or 'mega' doses is not advised unless they have been prescribed by a medical doctor.

Thiamine (B1)

Thiamine is a water soluble vitamin which has a role in many metabolic pathways in the body, including the pathway which produces energy. Deficiency is caused by poor diet and increased use within the body. People at risk of thiamine deficiency in the UK are the alcohol dependent. The metabolism of alcohol requires thiamine which is why those who drink excessive amounts are at particular risk. Deficiency in the alcohol dependent can cause Wernicke-Korsakoff syndrome which includes Wernicke's encephalopathy and Korsakoff's psychosis. Deficiency can also cause a disease called beriberi which can cause neurological changes and heart failure. Thiamine is found in many foods and rich sources include unrefined cereal grains, fortified flour and some breakfast cereals.

Vitamin C

Vitamin C is a water soluble vitamin which has a range of functions in the body. It is important for collagen formation and is an antioxidant. Deficiency is generally caused by poor diet. Those at risk of vitamin C deficiency include older adults, alcohol dependent individuals and smokers. The features of vitamin C deficiency include lassitude, gum changes, bruising and petechial haemorrhages, anaemia, poor wound healing and joint changes. Fresh vegetables and fruit, particularly spinach, tomatoes, broccoli, strawberries and citrus fruits are good sources of vitamin C.

Vitamin D (cholecalciferol)

rickets
a condition in children where vitamin D deficiency results in poor bone development and softening and bending of long bones

osteomalacia
a condition in which adults experience bone softening due to vitamin D deficiency or deficiency of calcium and phosphate or excessive absorption from the bones

Vitamin D is a fat soluble vitamin that controls calcium and phosphate levels in the blood. It is required for absorption of calcium and phosphate in the small intestine, mobilisation of these minerals from the bones, and reabsorption in the kidneys. Deficiency is associated with inadequate exposure to sunlight and those particularly at risk are children and women of Asian origin, people who always cover their skin when outside, older adults and the house-bound. Deficiency may also be caused by poor dietary intake and malabsorption. Deficiency causes disruption of calcium homeostasis and bone mineralisation and can result in **rickets** in children and **osteomalacia** in adults. The major source of vitamin D is exposure to sunlight but it is also found in dietary form in fatty fish, liver, milk, eggs and fortified food such as margarine, breakfast cereals. It is recommended that pregnant or breastfeeding women take supplements containing 10 mcg of vitamin D a day (FSA, 2009).

Calcium

Calcium is a mineral that has many roles with the body. It is a structural component of the body essential for cell membranes and organelles and bone mineralisation. It is also important in nerve function and muscle contraction. Deficiency is associated with fat malabsorption, poor dietary intake and the consumption of large amounts of phytates. The effects of deficiency are widespread and include stunted growth and bone malformation in children and skeletal and tooth changes in adults. Rich sources of calcium include milk, cheese, small fish (sardines), some green leafy vegetables, soybean products, fortified wheat flour and breakfast cereals and some nuts.

Iron

Iron deficiency is the most common nutritional disorder in the world (WHO, 2009). Iron is an essential nutrient for the formation of red blood cells. Those at risk of iron deficiency include infants, toddlers, adolescents, menstruating women and older adults. The causes of iron deficiency are insufficient dietary iron and blood loss. Features of iron deficiency are pallor, glossitis, angular stomatitis, lowered immunity, spoon shaped nails, fatigue, giddiness and impaired cognitive function. Rich dietary sources include liver, meat, beans, nuts, dried fruit, fish, enriched cereals, soybean flour and dark leafy green vegetables. There are dietary factors that influence uptake of iron from the gastrointestinal tract. These include the form of iron ingested (vegetable or meat origin), the presence of vitamin C and the presence of phytates.

Nutritional requirements

The optimal intake of a particular nutrient varies according to a body size, gender, activity level, state of health and age. The Department of Health has published recommendations of nutrient intake for sections of the population (DoH, 1991), termed Dietary Reference Values. These are not recommendations for intake by individuals but are estimates for healthy populations. They can be used to consider the adequacy of an individual's diet but should not be used as a prescription for intake. A person who eats a diet that follows healthy eating guidelines should be able to obtain all their nutrient requirements. Individuals who have a medical condition that affects absorption and utilisation of nutrients or those with a poor dietary intake may be prescribed vitamin and/or mineral supplements to ensure they obtain their daily requirements. In addition it is recommended that some groups within the population take additional supplements of some nutrients, for example women who wish to become pregnant or are in the first 12 weeks of pregnancy are advised to take folic acid tablets to supplements their dietary intake. Please refer to the Food Standards Agency website for further information (FSA, 2009).

> **Link**
>
> Chapter 7 outlines the functions for gastrointestinal and renal systems related to elimination

Fluid

Water is the main constituent of the body, comprising more than half of adult body weight. Water is gained from food but, with the exception of exclusively breast or bottle fed babies, fluid also needs to be drunk to ensure sufficient is obtained. Adults need to drink six to eight glasses of water or other fluids each day (FSA, 2009). This requirement may increase, for example, in hot weather, if physical activity is taken which causes sweating or if a person has diarrhoea. A low fluid intake can lead to health problems, such as a reduction in urine flow increasing the risk of urine infection, and constipation. However, people with conditions affecting their heart or renal system may be advised by their doctor to drink less each day. Older people may feel less thirsty when dehydrated than younger people and some medical conditions may make it difficult for a person to recognise that they are dehydrated, for example people with dementia. It is therefore important that the RN monitors fluid intake and encourages fluid intake if required.

In the acutely ill person fluid intake may be reduced or in excess of the body's requirements. In order to ensure fluid homeostasis is maintained careful monitoring of fluid intake and output, clinical condition and levels of electrolytes and other indicators of fluid status are undertaken. An infusion of fluids may be required or drugs which promote diuresis may be given.

> **✴ Activity 7.4**
>
> Write definitions of the following terms: homeostasis, electrolytes, diuresis.

Public Health Nutrition

> **∞ Link**
>
> Chapter 18 discusses the role of health-care professionals and nutrition.

Public health nutrition can be defined as the 'promotion of good health through primary preventions of nutrition-related illness in the population' (Margetts, 2004, p. 1). RNs are generally involved in giving one-to-one advice and support to clients; however, part of the role of some RNs does involve public health nutrition. For example, school RNs work to promote healthy eating in school children.

Clients' Nutritional Needs

> **∞ Link**
>
> Chapter 1 discusses assessment and care planning.

RNs are most frequently required to give nutritional care to individuals. Nutritional care is a process which commences with screening and assessment of nutritional status. Following this care can be planned and implemented according to need. The final stage of the process is evaluation to ensure the plan of care is appropriate for the client. Before undertaking nutritional screening and assessment it is important to have an understanding of factors which influence the nutritional intake of an individual and the concept of malnutrition.

Political, economic and social factors influencing food intake

There are many reasons why people eat the type of diet that they do and it is important to understand what can influence people's behaviour in terms of dietary intake. Political, economic and social factors shape what food is eaten as they influence the types and amount of food available. Some people are, for political, economic or social factors unable to access sufficient food or foods that constitute a healthy diet. Political factors influence the food that is available to a population. If the political climate results in inadequate food distribution or poor availability of a varied diet, individuals are unable to obtain the food and consequently diet that they require. Economic factors affect both the supply of food to individuals and the ability of the individuals to purchase the foods. Some people cannot afford to access or buy a range of foods that enable them to follow healthy eating guidelines. For example, people who have no access to supermarkets due to a lack of transport may have to rely on local shops which often contain a limited range of foods. People who live in temporary accommodation or who are homeless are unable to store and prepare food easily so have to rely on prepared food. Finally, cultural factors influence the type of diet eaten and it is vitally important that the RN asks any individual that they are caring for what type of diet they prefer to eat and if there are any foods they should not be offered. It is very distressing for a person to be offered food that is not acceptable to them on religious grounds. All care settings should offer an appropriate menu for individuals from different religions.

Children are particularly vulnerable to the effect of poor dietary intake and recently efforts have been made to address social and economic factors which may influence dietary intake of children by the provision of foods that promote a healthy diet. For example, the School, Fruit and Vegetable Scheme (part of the 5 A DAY programme) aims to increase fruit and vegetable consumption of all 4- to 6-year-old children in LEA-maintained infant, primary and special schools. According to this scheme these children are entitled to a free piece of fruit or vegetable each school day. Examples of other government initiatives aimed at increasing the quality of nutritional intake can be viewed on the Department of Health website (DoH, 2009). It is also important that RNs are aware of the Food Standards Agency, which is an independent government department set up in 2000 to protect the public's health and consumer interests in relation to food. The website for this agency contains up-to-date information on diet and health issues and is easily accessible to both clients and those caring for them (FSA, 2009).

Appetite and its influence on food intake

In this chapter appetite can be defined as a desire for food which is usually associated with hunger. Hunger is a sensation that is caused by a variety of signals being received by the central nervous system. These signals are both nervous and hormonal and caused by factors such as lack of food in the stomach and small intestine and nutrient levels in the blood. Hunger leads to a desire to eat which generally results in the acquisition of food and the act of eating. Sometimes people will exert volitional control over their desire and refrain from eating. This may be because they find the food on offer unacceptable or they may be consciously restricting their intake in order to maintain or lose weight. Once we experience a desire to eat, and choose to follow that desire, there are many factors which influence what and how much we eat. These include internal factors, such as low mood or nausea, and external factors. External factors can include foods that are available for us to eat, the circumstance that we are eating in and

✸ Activity 7.5

When you are in placement identify a client who is underweight and discuss with your mentor the reasons why he/she is underweight.

who we are eating with. People tend to eat more if they are feeling comfortable and are offered a wide variety of palatable foods in a pleasant environment with friends. It is useful to remember this when encouraging a person to eat in a health-care setting. Eating a meal in a busy acute hospital ward when unwell often does not promote food intake. Appetite can be affected by disease process. Anorexia (a loss of appetite) is common in many conditions, for example some cancers and gastrointestinal diseases. Anorexia can also be caused by treatments and medication.

Malnutrition

Malnutrition can refer to both under and over nutrition. This section will consider obesity which is a form of over nutrition and protein-energy malnutrition which is a form of under nutrition. These two types of malnutrition are common in the UK and RNs are frequently involved in the care of people with obesity and protein-energy malnutrition.

Protein-energy malnutrition

Protein-energy malnutrition is a condition that is caused by a lack of protein and energy (or 'calorie') intake resulting in loss of body fat and muscle. It is common in people who have a medical condition that affects intake, digestion and loss of nutrients from the body. In children it is subdivided into two conditions called Kwashiorkor and marasmus and students who are studying paediatric nursing should read further on these conditions. Protein-energy malnutrition leads to muscle weakness, poor wound healing and lower immunity and, therefore, can prolong recovery from illness and surgery (Gibney et al., 2005). Management of the person with protein-energy malnutrition involves referral to the dietitian and doctor and the provision of high energy, high protein foods. However, it is dangerous for a person to receive too many nutrients when first treated for malnutrition. This is because the body adapts to an intake of low levels of nutrients and does not cope well with a sudden influx of energy or nutrients (termed **refeeding syndrome**). For this reason it is essential that the doctor and dietitian inform the plan of care.

Obesity

Obesity is a major public health issue in the UK and most other countries in the world. In the past 30 years or so there has been a rise in the number of individuals who are obese each year. Obesity is defined as a body mass index of 30 kg/m^2 or more. Obesity is related to the development of some medical conditions such as Type II diabetes mellitus, sleep apnoea and coronary heart disease (ASO, 2009). The treatment of obesity should be individualised and include assessment and goal setting. The initial aim of obesity management is to stabilise weight and prevent further weight gain. Following this a moderate weight loss can be attempted followed by further weight loss and weight maintenance. If diet, activity and behavioural change are unsuccessful in isolation drug therapy or surgery may be offered. The RN's role in preventing and reducing obesity is to

refeeding syndrome in starvation, levels of electrolytes, particularly phosphate, in the cells are low. When a person who has been starved is given food containing carbohydrate, insulin release is stimulated leading to electrolytes in the extracellular fluid moving into the cells, which can result in abnormally low levels outside the cells. This results in metabolic changes in the body causing serious illness (Mehanna et al., 2008)

be competent to give advice to clients on how to adhere to a 'healthy diet' and increase levels of physical activity. If the client is unsuccessful in their efforts to stabilise or lose weight then more intensive support may be required and the client should be referred to the doctor or dietitian or another appropriate health-care professional. The Department of Health has published a number of resources for health-care professionals relating to obesity including a care pathway (DoH, 2009). Prevention is, of course, better than cure and currently there are lots of national and local initiatives to try to address the significant public health problem of obesity in this and other countries.

Screening and assessing nutritional status

The aim of screening and assessing nutritional status is to identify those with, or at risk of, malnutrition and highlight potential causes. If an individual is screened and considered to be at risk of, or to have malnutrition, then a more detailed assessment should be undertaken. This will usually be undertaken by the dietitian but may be undertaken by another health-care professional, for example a speech and language therapist will be asked to see the client if a swallow deficit is suspected. Screening and assessment enables identification of nutritional needs, planning of nutritional interventions and setting of nutritional goals. Following this, interventions can be implemented which should be regularly evaluated and modified.

There are five principal methods of screening or assessing for nutritional status; assessment of dietary history and intake, clinical examination, functional tests, biochemical tests and anthropometric measures. Factors other than nutritional status can affect functional and biochemical tests of nutritional status and, therefore, analysis is not straightforward. For example, a low haemoglobin can result from poor iron intake but can also be due to other factors such as blood loss. These ways of assessing nutritional status are not considered here.

Dietary history and intake

Recording a client's past or current dietary and fluid intake gives an indication of the type of diet they are eating and fluids they are drinking. Dietary intake can be recorded on a food chart and fluid intake on a fluid chart following each meal or snack in a residential care setting. This is a useful way of assessing whether a client is ingesting sufficient food and fluids. Clients can also record their own intake over a period of days and this can be used to give advice on how the diet can be changed. Asking a client what they have eaten and drunk recently can enable the RN to assess the adequacy of recent intake or identify foods or drinks that may be contributing to a current health problem. If there are issues of concern the client should be referred to the dietitian as the dietitian is able to carry out a more reliable and detailed assessment. The client's ability to access food and fluid normally, in terms of shopping, storing, cooking or cutting up food, must also be considered. General lifestyle questions will include an assessment of activity levels, how much time they spend out of doors, whether they smoke and what their level of alcohol consumption is. Clients must also be asked about the type

★ Activity 7.6

Explore what initiatives are in place in your local area that aim to help people prevent or address obesity in the local population.

of diet they prefer to eat as it is the RN's responsibility to ensure that they are provided with a diet appropriate to meet their cultural needs.

Clinical assessment

Observation of clients will include a clinical assessment to see whether they appear well nourished, and will include looking at the fit of their clothes, the condition of their skin, mouth, eyes, hair and nails, how they move and how alert or apathetic they appear. These can all give an indication of nutritional status but can be difficult to interrupt so if any issues are identified the client should be referred to the doctor, dietitian or specialist RN.

Anthropometric measures

Anthropometry refers to the measurement of the human body. Simple anthropometric measures can be used by RNs to screen and assess nutritional status. It is important to weigh clients on admission to care to provide a baseline measure, and at regular intervals subsequently to identify any losses or gains. If possible, the person should be weighed on the same scales at the same time each day, in similar clothes after voiding.

Percentage weight can be used to assess weight loss or gain and is calculated using the equation:

$$\% \text{ weight loss/gain} = \frac{\text{usual weight} - \text{current weight (kg)} \times 100}{\text{usual weight (kg)}}$$

A loss of 10 per cent in the previous three months is suggestive of malnutrition. It must be remembered though that weight changes for other reasons too, such as dehydration or oedema.

body mass index (BMI)
a figure derived from a person's height and weight, which indicates whether his or her weight is within a range that is considered to promote health best

Weight in relation to height is a more accurate way of assessing the degree to which a person is under or overweight. Body mass index (BMI) is commonly used for this reason. This can be calculated by dividing body weight in kilograms (kg) by the height in metres squared (m²). If height cannot be measured it can be estimated in other ways, for example, by the use of ulna length (BAPEN, 2006a). A BMI of less than 18.5 suggests a person is underweight, a BMI of 18.5 to 24.9 is considered normal. A BMI of 25.0 to 29.9 suggests a person is overweight and a BMI of 30 or more suggests a person is obese (IOTF, 2003). The use of BMI with very old people may not be appropriate (BDA, 2003).

Measuring waist circumference is increasingly being carried out to screen for cardiovascular risk in primary care. Men with a waist circumference of greater that 102 cm and women with a waist circumference of greater than 88 cm are at increased risk of cardiovascular disease and should consider losing weight (Lean, 2000).

Anthropometric measures that assess fat levels or muscle mass of the body are sometimes used, such as skinfold measures to estimate body fat and mid-arm muscle circumference to estimate skeletal muscle mass.

As with all equipment it is important that weighing machines are cleaned and checked for accuracy according to Trust guidelines.

To try to identify those with malnutrition and at risk of malnutrition on admission to care many nutritional screening and assessment tools have been developed (Green and Watson, 2005). Most have a series of questions to be answered, these being scored to identify the client's level of risk of malnutrition. A national valid and reliable tool (the 'MUST' tool) has been developed for use recently by the British Association of Parenteral and Enteral nutrition (BAPEN, 2006b). It is for use in all clinical areas.

As highlighted by NICE (2006b) recently it is important that clients are screened for malnutrition on admission to care. Only then can an appropriate plan of care be made. The plan of care may require referral to another member of the multidisciplinary team, for example the dietitian or doctor, for nutritional needs to be assessed fully and met. Or it may require the RN to assist the client to meet their nutritional needs. The plan of care must be evaluated to ensure that it is effective. This can be done by returning to the process of screening and assessing. For example, if a person is provided with modified cutlery by the occupational therapist as a result of a problem being identified with handling normal cutlery on assessment, then the ability of the client to consume adequate amounts of food with the modified cutlery needs to be assessed to ensure the intervention has been successful.

> **✷ Activity 7.7**
>
> Identify how clients are screened for malnutrition in your current or next practice placement.

Casebox 7.1

Lin Chang is a 65-year-old lady who has been admitted to the trauma orthopaedic ward where you are undertaking your placement. She has sustained a fractured neck of femur. On admission you identify her as being at risk of malnutrition and estimate her BMI is 17.5. How may her nutritional status influence her recovery from her injury?

Factors to consider

Her BMI indicates that she is underweight and therefore malnourished. This may influence her ability to recover from the surgery.

Her poor nutritional status may:
- delay her wound healing
- compromise her immune system leading to increased risk of infection
- cause her to feel lethargic and low in mood
- reduce her muscle strength resulting in poorer mobility and increased risk of chest infection
- increase her risk of pressure ulcers as she has little fat protecting her bony prominences and lower levels of circulating nutrients.

Casebox 7.2

Elijah Gray is an 18-year-old man who lives at home with his family and is currently studying for A levels at college. He has made an appointment to visit the practice nurse in the Health Centre where you are undertaking a community placement because he wants to lose weight. His BMI is calculated as 32 and he reveals that he smokes 10 cigarettes a day. What health promotion activities should the practice nurse undertake?

Factors to consider

- The first health promotion activity that should be undertaken is to enable him to give up smoking.
- Following this, health promotion activities related to promoting the consumption of a healthy diet and increasing physical activity should be undertaken.

It is important to assess his current physical activity level and type of diet consumed before giving any advice. His BMI may classify him as obese whereas he may be very physically active and have a high muscle mass and low fat mass. He should still be advised to eat a 'healthy diet' but may not need to increase his physical activity level or reduce the amount of food he eats.

Promoting dietary intake

Following screening and assessment the type of intervention that best meets the client's needs should be identified. The doctor and dietitian, and in some cases pharmacist, will inform the plan of nutritional care made in order to meet the nutritional needs of the critically ill client. Generally the acutely unwell client should be advised to follow a dietary intake that they find acceptable. If appetite is poor this may comprise of energy dense foods so that sufficient nutrients to meet their needs can be obtained. The doctor and dietitian will inform the plan of nutritional care for the acutely ill client who is malnourished, requires a therapeutic diet or has a condition that affects nutrient intake, absorption or utilisation.

For the non-acutely ill, normal weight, overweight and obese client the RN should promote a 'healthy diet'. The UK's guidelines for a healthy diet are represented in the health promotion tool 'The plate model' (FSA, 2009) shown in Figure 7.1. This shows the five major food groups and the proportion each should contribute to the dietary intake. This model outlines that the diet should consist of 33 per cent vegetables and fruit, 33 per cent complex carbohydrate, 12 per cent protein containing foods, 15 per cent dairy products or similar foods and 8 per cent fat and sugar containing foods. Additionally it is recommended

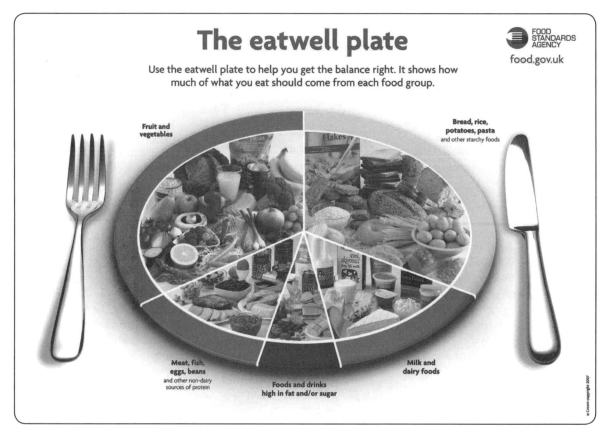

Figure 7.1 The eatwell plate model

Source: Food Standards Agency (food.gov.uk). Reproduced under the Open Government Licence v1.0.

each individual should eat 5 or more portions of a variety of fruit and vegetables a day (DoH, 2007). Chart 7.1 identifies tips for eating well produced by the Food Standards Agency (2009). This type of diet is not suitable for those under five years of age. Clients who are undernourished require a more energy dense diet in order to obtain sufficient nutrients to meet their needs and therefore adherence to healthy eating guidelines may not be appropriate.

Chart 7.1 Tips for eating well

1	Base your meals on starchy foods	6	Get active and try to be a healthy weight
2	Eat lots of fruit and veg	7	Drink plenty of water
3	Eat more fish	8	Don't skip breakfast
4	Cut down on saturated fat and sugar		
5	Try to eat less salt – no more than 6g a day		

Source: FSA (2009). Reproduced under the Open Government Licence v1.0.

Functional foods

Foods termed 'functional foods' now appear on food shelves for purchase by the general public. A functional food is defined as a food which has health-promoting benefits and/or disease promoting properties in addition to usual nutritional value (Barasi, 2003). Examples of functional foods include omega-enriched eggs and sterol-enriched margarine.

> **✸ Activity 7.8**
>
> Next time you go food shopping identify a functional food in the supermarket and find out its mode of action.

Casebox 7.3

Ra Shah is 21 years old and has Down's syndrome and moderate learning disabilities. He is moving into a new home and on admission his BMI is noted to be 26. How should his main carer be advised to ensure his nutritional needs are met?

Factors to consider

- Ra needs to avoid increasing his BMI as he is just within the overweight category.
- His carer should enable him to eat a 'healthy diet' and increase his physical activity level.

- Ra should be involved in food shopping and meal preparation to enable him to make healthy dietary choices on a day-to-day basis.
- Ra's weight should be recorded at regular intervals to assess weight loss or gain.

Meal-time in institutional care settings

The RN is responsible for ensuring that the environment that the client is in is conducive to eating. Clients should be offered toilet facilities and facilities to wash their hands prior to the serving of meals. It is important that mealtime activities take precedence over other activities when food is served. This enables the client to focus on and enjoy their meal and not be subject to numerous disturbances. Recently the concept of protected mealtimes has been emphasised by several national bodies (NPSA, 2008). This concept involves the planning of clinical activities to avoid unnecessary interruptions at mealtimes. The RN is responsible for ensuring each client in the clinical area receives appropriate food in appropriate quantities for their needs at mealtimes and that food is available in-between meals if required. The RN is also responsible for ensuring food intake of clients is documented where appropriate and appropriate action taken if food intake is inadequate. Relatives and carers may bring in favourite foods provided hospital policy is adhered to.

Assisting a client to eat and drink

Clients or patients require assistance to eat if they are unable to eat adequately without assistance. Assistance to eat and drink can range from prompting the client during a meal to actually transferring food to the client's mouth. The type of assistance required should be identified at the screening and assessment stage and documented in the client's plan of care. The first stage in assisting the client to eat is to prepare them and their environment for a meal. Clients should receive analgesia or anti-emetics prior to the meal if these are required. The next stage is to ensure that toileting and handwashing facilities are available and the environment is appropriate. In addition it should be ensured that the client's dentures are in place. In some clinical areas it is possible to take clients into a dining room for meals, although a person who needs assistance to eat may prefer not to sit with other clients. Clients eating at the bedside should have their bed-tables cleared of objects such as urinals and wiped clean prior to the meal being presented. The client should sit as upright as possible to facilitate swallowing.

The next stage in assisting clients to eat is serving appropriate food in an appropriate manner. Staff should wear an apron as per hospital policy. Hot foods should be served hot and cold foods cold to enhance their palatability. It is important food looks appealing when presented to the client. The tray should be arranged so the client can reach and access everything. Condiments should be offered to flavour food. Appropriate cutlery should be provided and food cut up as required. A drink should also be available. Clients should be offered protection for their clothes. When serving a food or a meal to a person who is partially sighted or blind ensure that the food is described verbally so the person knows what to expect. The 'clock face' can be used to describe where different foods are sited on a plate.

If the client is unable to eat and drink themselves the following procedure should be followed:

- Check the client's dietary needs
- Introduce yourself to the client, explain the procedure and obtain consent to assist the client
- Set up the area appropriately and position correctly
- Ensure the client's mouth is clean and dentures in place if appropriate
- Wash your hands and put on an appropriate apron
- Prepare any equipment needed
- Sit or stand at the same eye level as the client
- Check the food and drink is not too hot prior to offering
- Feed small amounts of the meal each mouthful
- Ensure each mouthful is swallowed
- After a pause offer the next mouthful
- Offer a drink periodically

- When the client has finished eating offer a mouthwash or check their mouth for retained food
- Clear any unswallowed food in the mouth with a drink, swab or toothbrush
- The client should stay sitting up right for about 30 minutes to reduce the chance of **reflux**
- Communicate verbally with the client during the procedure but allow them to focus on eating rather than answering questions
- Document how much the client has eaten

If the client's voice sounds wet or gurgly, shows signs of choking or there is food pocketing in mouth no more food or drink should be offered and the RN in charge informed.

Oral fluid intake

In the care setting drinks should be readily available to clients taking into account their preferences. Fluid intake should consist of different drinks and water. Coffee and some teas contain caffeine which has a stimulating effect and so moderate amounts should be drunk. Drinks high in sugar and carbonated drinks should be avoided between meals as they can promote tooth damage and add to the energy intake of the diet. If it is suspected a client is dehydrated or overhydrated the RN in charge or doctor should be informed. The client's fluid status will need to be assessed in order to decide on an appropriate course of action. It may be that the client requires an intravenous or subcutaneous fluid infusion or a change in the type of medication they are taking.

Promoting dietary intake

Where possible, clients should be encouraged to fulfil their nutritional needs by eating appropriate foods rather than relying on supplements or fluids. Clients who are not malnourished should be encouraged to follow healthy eating guidelines. Not all clients, however, can eat the full range of foods and fluids represented in the plate model. Clients with a food allergy will be required to avoid the food or drink that causes the allergy. Clients with particular medical conditions are also required to avoid some foods and drinks. For example, people with coeliac disease avoid gluten containing foods and people with phenylketonuria avoid phenylalanine containing foods and drinks. The types of diets that people are required to follow as a result of a medical condition tend to be termed 'therapeutic diets' and should always be prescribed by a Registered Dietitian. Clients who have dysphagia are often required to consume foods and fluids that have had their texture modified, for example meat which has been puréed and fluids that have been thickened. The purpose of modifying the texture of a diet is to ensure that food can be swallowed safely. Foods that are lumpy in texture, dry or require chewing are more difficult to swallow. Clients who are malnourished should be encouraged to eat foods high in energy and nutrients to enable them to correct any nutrient deficits. Although, as discussed above, dietary intake should be introduced gradually and with medical and dietetic supervision to avoid refeeding syndrome.

reflux
a backward flow of food and fluid up the gastrointestinal tract

✳ Activity 7.9

If you care for a client who requires assistance to eat in your current or next placement, under the supervision of your mentor assist them to eat and then discuss with your mentor how you facilitated their dietary intake.

✳ Activity 7.10

Identify a client who is prescribed a therapeutic diet and research why they have been prescribed the diet and the types of foods they can and cannot eat.

Rosa Perez has just been admitted to the nursing home where you are undertaking your first placement. She is 82 years of age, has dementia and following nutritional screening has been identified as at risk of malnutrition. What do you think should be included in her plan of care to try to address her nutritional needs?

Factors to consider

- She should be referred to the dietician if this facility is available and the speech and language therapist if any difficulties with swallowing are noted.

- Her dietary preferences should be ascertained and used to inform her care plan.

- Her relatives and friends should be encouraged to bring in her favourite food and drinks (if in accordance with the clinical area's policy).

- She should be encouraged to eat several small meals rather than one or two large meals each day.

- She should receive snacks between meals and before bedtime.

- She may find it easier to eat finger foods rather than use a knife, fork or spoon.

- If she has a poor appetite she should be encourage to eat energy dense foods (for example foods that are high in kilocalories) rather than

foods that have fewer calories. An example would be the consumption of full fat milk rather than skimmed milk.

- She should be prompted to eat and complete her meal if she appears distracted. Eating with others may prompt her to eat more.

- She may benefit from dietary supplements if her dietary intake is poor.

- Her plan of care should be evaluated weekly.

Nutritional Support

When a client is unable to eat sufficient normal foods to meet their nutritional needs the decision may be taken to provide some form of nutritional support. Generally, the decision to give nutritional support is made with the doctor and dietitian, although other members of the multidisciplinary team are involved with the advanced forms of nutritional support. If the gastrointestinal tract is functioning nutritional support should be given orally, however, if the client is unable to swallow adequately or is unable to consume sufficient orally to meet their needs nutritional support can be given via a tube. The tube may pass into the stomach or small intestine (enteral nutrition by tube) or directly into the venous system (parenteral nutrition). Oral dietary supplements can be given to clients able to swallow adequately. Oral dietary supplements take the form of milk, fruit or vegetable flavoured energy and nutrient dense drinks, puddings or soups. Vitamin or mineral supplements may be prescribed if there is evidence of a specific nutrient deficiency or if the diet is considered to be limited and, therefore, lacking in micronutrients.

nasogastric tube
a wide bore nasogastric tube can be used for aspiration of stomach content

The most common types of tube used for enteral feeding are **nasogastric tubes** and gastrostomies. Nasogastric tubes for delivering enteral nutrition are fine-bore polyurethane or PVC tubes which pass through the nose and terminate in the stomach. The smallest possible tube is used to reduce discomfort and minimise the risk of nasal mucosal ulceration. RNs are required to be able to pass nasogastric tubes and care for clients with enteral feeding tubes in situ where appropriate for branch. However, doctors or specialist RNs are responsible for the insertion of nasogastric tubes in clients with maxillo-facial disorders or surgery, laryngectomy, and disorders of the oesophagus due to the risk of perforation. Nasojejunal and nasoduodenal tubes may also be used but these tend to be used in specialist areas only and RNs should not pass these types of tubes unless it is specified that it is part of their specialist role. Please refer to Dougherty and Lister (2008) and the policy and guidelines for your clinical area for information on the procedure of passing and removing a nasogastric tube. It is essential to check that the tip of the nasogastric tube is in the stomach before feeding begins. This should be done by aspiration of the tube for acid residual or x-ray (see NPSA, 2005). The tube should be flushed with 30 to 50 mls of water before and after each feed and before and after drug administration. Sterile water should be used to flush tubes in acute health-care settings and all tubes which terminate in the jejunum (Skipper et al., 2003). In the community setting, cooled, freshly boiled water or sterile water from a newly opened container should be used if the individual is immunosuppressed (NICE, 2003). Fifty millilitre bladder tip syringes or enteral syringes should be used as these are considered incompatible with intravenous systems. Warm water should be used to dislodge blocks in the tube. Fluids or air should never be forced into the tube though as the tube may split. The nasogastric tube and giving sets used to infuse feed should be replaced according to local clinical guidelines. The type and rate of feed given should be prescribed by the dietitian or in some specialist units may be prescribed by the doctor. The client's head and shoulders should be elevated by at least 30 degrees when the feed is in progress and for one hour after it has stopped unless contraindicated. Critically ill clients may not absorb feeding solution in the stomach so the residual volume in the stomach should be aspirated and measured periodically in order to determine whether the feed is being digested and absorbed. Algorithms detailing what should be done according to how much is absorbed are usually available in units where this is carried out.

> **⊂⊃ Link**
>
> Chapter 6 discusses the use of nasogastric tubes in relation to the administration of medicines

Complications of nasogastric tubes include displacement, naso-pharyngeal irritation, occlusion of the tube, biochemical disturbances and infection. Malpositioning of the tube in the trachea or bronchus may cause the accidental intrapulmonary administration of feed and it is important to check the tube position according to national and local guidelines. NICE (2006a) guidelines identify that monitoring protocols which integrate a variety of observations and measurements are required in order to ensure nutritional support is given safely and in appropriate amounts. Local guidelines should identify the monitoring that is required for clients receiving NG feeding. If these are not available NICE guidelines (NICE, 2006a) should be consulted.

Enterostomies

enterostomy
the formation of an external opening into the small gastrointestinal tract

For clients who need enteral feeding for a long period (usually more than four weeks), a tube can be inserted directly into the gastrointestinal tract across the abdominal wall. Usually tubes are inserted into the stomach (gastrostomy) (Figure 7.2) but in some specialist areas they may be inserted into the jejunum (jejunostomy). This procedure can be carried out in endoscopy, radiology

Reginald Allen has been admitted to the care of community psychiatric nurse as he has recently been diagnosed with depression. Reginald is 58 years of age, lives at home alone and does not feel able to go out shopping for food currently. How could you ensure that he is enabled to meet him nutritional needs?

Factors to consider

- Screening and assessment of nutritional status should be undertaken.
- If he is not undernourished he should be encouraged to follow a 'healthy diet'.
- He could undertake his food shopping on the internet if

he does not want to leave the house or he could use a company that provides meals to people at home. Alternatively he may have a friend or relative willing to go shopping for him.
- He should be encouraged to leave home to shop when he feels able to do so.

ascites
excess fluid in the peritoneal cavity

or the operating theatre. Contraindications to the insertion of gastrostomy feeding tubes include **ascites**, blood clotting abnormalities and gastric malignancy. Instructions as to when feeding can be started – usually on same day the tube has been inserted – should be issued by the person who inserted the tube. As with tubes via the nose enterosotomy tubes should be flushed with the same frequency and in the same way as nasogastric tubes. The gastrostomy site must be observed daily for signs of gastric acid leakage and infection. Before it

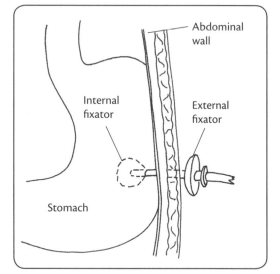

Figure 7.2 Gastrostomy feeding tube with internal and external retention discs

is healed the gastrostomy site should be cleaned ascetically with normal saline but once it is healed it should be cleaned daily with soap and water. A dressing is not generally required unless there is discharge. It may be advised that the gastrostomy tube is pushed in by 1 cm and rotated daily once the tract is healed to avoid tissue adhering to the tube. Local guidelines should be consulted on this issue as practice does vary according to policy and the type of tube used. Complications of gastrostomy feeding tube insertion include: peritonitis (inflammation of the peritoneal cavity), pulmonary aspiration of the feed, peristomal (around the hole) infection and migration of the tube. As with nasogastric feeding local guidelines should identify the monitoring that clients require when receiving this form of nutritional support.

Clients who receive their nutritional needs via tube may be unable to keep their mouth clean and moist without assistance. It is important, therefore, that the client is assisted to clean his mouth regularly and use lip salve as required. The client's mouth should be inspected daily for signs of infection and for observation of general condition.

Medication may be given via feeding tubes. The pharmacist should advise on the appropriate preparation and administration. For further information see the BAPEN website (BAPEN, 2006b).

The RN must be aware of the psychosocial impact of enteral feeding by tube. Clients who cannot eat are often unable to join in with the social aspects of eating and drinking. Some clients may eat and drink small amounts and this should be encouraged if they can.

Drug-nutrient interactions

Food intake, absorption and metabolism can be influenced by some drugs and some nutrients may influence drug absorption and metabolism. This is an important issue for RNs to be aware of because of their role in the administration of medications. A good example of a drug-nutrient interaction is the interaction of the antiepileptic drug phenytoin with enteral feed. Phenytoin needs to be administered when the client's stomach is empty to ensure optional absorption of the drug. The pharmacist can provide advice on this issue. Older adults are particularly at risk as they are often prescribed more than one drug and experience more than one disease (Mallet et al., 2007).

> ✳ Activity **7.11**
>
> In your current or next practice placement identify one commonly used drug which can interact with food eaten by the client.

Ethical Issues

A chapter on nutrition is not complete without some consideration of ethical issues surrounding the provision of food and fluids to client. Clients may make the decision not to eat and drink to meet their nutritional needs and may decline administration of nutrition via a tube when the health-care team considers this is in their best interests. Foods and fluid cannot be given to a client without their consent unless they are being treated against their will in accordance with the mental health legislation of the country in which they are hospitalised. In addition the decision to administer nutrition via tube involves ethical consideration as well as consideration of the nutritional aspects of the support as some clients may not benefit from the nutritional support. This is a complex area and has been reviewed by Körner et al. (2006).

Chapter Summary

This chapter has reviewed the basic concepts of nutritional science and considered the nutritional care of clients. The chapter has highlighted that the process of nutritional care involves screening and assessing nutritional status, planning and implementing nutritional interventions and evaluating care given. Nutritional care is a basic nursing skill but close working with other members of the multidisciplinary team is a requirement in order to meet clients' nutritional needs.

? Test yourself!

1   List the five sections that make up the 'plate model'.

2   What influence do saturated fatty acids have on blood cholesterol level?

3   What foods are rich in iron?

4   If your BMI was in the range of 25.0–29.9 what would you be classed as?

5   What is refeeding syndrome?

Dougherty, L. and Lister, S. (2008) *The Royal Marsden Hospital Manual of Clinical Nursing Procedures*. Wiley-Blackwell, Oxford.
Best, C. (2008) *Nutrition: A Handbook for Nurses*. John Wiley and Sons, Chichester.

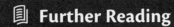

📖 Further Reading

For live links to useful websites see:
www.palgrave.com/nursinghealth/hogston

References

AHA (American Heart Association) (2009) *High Protein Diets*. http://www.americanheart.org/presenter.jhtml?identifier=11234 (accessed 20 July 2009).

ASO (Association for the Study of Obesity) (2009) http://www.aso.org.uk/ (accessed 20 July 2009).

BAPEN (British Association for Parenteral and Enteral Nutrition) (2006a) *Malnutrition Universal Screening Tool (the MUST)*. BAPEN, Redditch. http://www.bapen.org.uk/must_tool.html (accessed 20 July 2009).

BAPEN (British Association for Parenteral and Enteral Nutrition) (2006b) *Drug Administration via Enteral Feeding Tubes*. BAPEN, Redditch. http://www.bapen.org.uk/res_drugs.html (accessed 28 July 2009).

Barasi, M.E. (2003) *Human Nutrition: A Health Perspective*. Arnold, London.

BDA (British Dietetic Association) (2003) Effective Practice Bulletin issue 32: Challenging the use of Body Mass Index (BMI) to assess undernutrition in older people. *Dietetics Today* **38**(3): 15–19.

BDA (British Dietetic Association) (2010) *The British Dietetic Association*, http://www.bda.uk.com/ (accessed 16 August 2010).

BNF (British Nutrition Foundation) (2004) *Energy and Nutrients*. http://www.nutrition.org.uk/home.asp?siteId=43&sectionId=320&parentSection=299&which=1 (accessed 20 July 2009).

BNF (British Nutrition Foundation) (2009) *Carbohydrate*, http://www.nutrition.org.uk/nutritionscience/nutrients/carbohydrate (accessed 16 August 2010).

Cancer Research UK (2008) *Lifestyle and Cancer*, http://info.cancerresearchuk.org/cancerstats/causes/lifestyle/diet/#fat (accessed 20 July 2009).

Commission of the European Communities (2007) *A Strategy for Europe on Nutrition, Overweight and Obesity Related Health Issues*, http://www.eufic.org/page/en/fftid/European-Commission-seeks-action/ (accessed 20 July 2009).

Council of Europe (2003) *Resolution ResAP (2003)3 on Food and Nutritional Care in Hospitals*, http://www.bapen.org.uk/pdfs/coe_adoption.pdf (accessed 20 July 2009).

Denny, A. (2008) An overview of the role of diet during the ageing process. *British Journal of Community Nursing* **13**(2): 59–67.

DoH (Department of Health) (1991) *Dietary Reference Values for Food Energy and Nutrients for the United Kingdom*, Report of the Panel on Dietary Reference Values of the Committee on Medical Aspects of Food Policy. HMSO, London.

DoH (Department of Health) (2003) *The Essence of Care: Patient-focused Benchmarks for Clinical Governance*. HMSO, London.

DoH (Department of Health) (2007) *5 a Day General Information*, http://www.dh.gov.uk/en/Publichealth/Healthimprovement/FiveADay/FiveADaygeneralinformation/DH_4001494 (accessed 28 July 2009).

DoH (Department of Health) (2009) *Welcome to the Department of Health*, http://www.dh.gov.uk/en/index.htm (accessed 20 July 2009).

Dougherty, L. and Lister, S. (eds) (2008) *The Royal Marsden Hospital Manual of Clinical Nursing Procedures*, 7th edn. Wiley-Blackwell, Oxford.

European Nutrition for Health Alliance (2007) *From Malnutrition to Wellnutrition: Policy to Practice*, www.european-nutrition.org/files/pdf_pdf_38.pdf (accessed 20 July 2009).

FSA (Food Standards Agency) (2009) *Latest News*, http://www.food.gov.uk/aboutus/contactus/ (accessed 20 July 2009).

Gibney, M.J., Elia, M., Ljungqvist, O. and Dowsett, J. (2005) *Clinical Nutrition*. Blackwell Science, Oxford.

Green, S.M. and Watson, R. (2005) Nutritional screening and assessment tools for use by RNs: literature review. *Journal of Advanced Nursing* **50**(1): 69–83.

IOTF (International Obesity Taskforce) (2003) *About Obesity*. https://www.iotf.org (accessed 2 July 2009).

Körner, U., Bondolfi, A., Bühler, E., MacFie, J., Meguid, M.M., Messing, B., Oehmichen, F., Valentini, L. and Allison, S.P. (2006) Ethical and legal aspects of enteral nutrition. *Clinical Nutrition* **35**: 196–202.

Lean, M.E.J. (2000) Pathophysiology of obesity. *Proceedings of the Nutrition Society* **59**: 331–6.

Mallet, L., Spinewine, A. and Huang, A. (2007) The challenge of managing drug interactions in elderly people, *Lancet* **370**(9582): 185–91.

Margetts, B. (2004) An overview of public health nutrition. In Gibney, M.J., Margetts, B.M., Kearney, J.M. and Arab. L. (eds) *Public Health Nutrition*. Blackwell Science, Oxford.

Mehanna, H.M., Moledina, J., and Travis, J. (2008) Refeeding syndrome: what it is, and how to prevent and treat it. *British Medical Journal* **336**: 1495–8.

NPSA (National Patient Safety Agency) (2005) *Advice to the NHS on Reducing Harm Caused by the Misplacement of Nasogastric Feeding Tubes.* NPSA, London.

NPSA (National Patient Safety Agency) (2008) *Protected Mealtimes.* http://www.npsa.nhs.uk/nrls/improvingpatientsafety/cleaning-and-nutrition/nutrition/protected-mealtimes/ (accessed 20 July 2009).

NICE (National Institute for Health and Clinical Excellence) (2003) *Prevention of Healthcare-associated Infections in Primary and Community Care.* NICE, London.

NICE (National Institute for Health and Clinical Excellence) (2006a) *Nutrition Support in Adults.* http://www.nice.org.uk/page.aspx?o=cg032#summary (accessed 20 July 2009).

NICE (National Institute for Health and Clinical Excellence) (2006b) *Obesity: The Prevention, Identification, Assessment and Management of Overweight and Obesity in Adults and Children.* http://www.nice.org.uk/guidance/index.jsp?action=byID&o=11000 (accessed 20 July 2009).

NMC (Nursing and Midwifery Council) (2007) *Essential Skills Clusters*, Circular 07/2007 Annexe 2. NMC, London.

Pavlovic, M., Prentice, A., Thorsdottir, I., Wolfram, G. and Branca, F. (2007) Challenges in harmonizing energy and nutrient recommendations in Europe. *Annals of Nutrition and Metabolism* **51**: 108–14.

Skipper, L., Cuffling, J. and Pratelli, N. (2003) *Enteral Feeding Infection Control Guidelines.* Infection Control Nurses Association, Bathgate.

Streppel, M.T., Ocké, M.C., Boshuizen, H.C., Kok, R.J. and Kromhout, D. (2009) Long-term wine consumption is related to cardiovascular mortality and life expectancy independently of moderate alcohol intake: the Zutphen study. *Journal of Epidemiology and Community Health* **63**: 534–40.

Vegetarian Society (2009) Information sheet. http://www.vegsoc.org/info/omega3.html (accessed 20 July 2009).

WHO (World Health Organisation) (2009) *Micronutrient Deficiencies.* http://www.who.int/nutrition/topics/ida/en/index.html (accessed 28 July 2009).

Chapter

BARBARA A. MARJORAM

8 Elimination

📖 Contents

☑ Learning outcomes

The purpose of this chapter is to explore the urinary and faecal elements of elimination, explaining the normal and abnormal processes and influences on it. At the end of the chapter, you should be able to:

- Explain the development of elimination that an individual experiences throughout the life span
- Identify specimens that may be collected and common abnormalities that may be found
- Understand the causes of constipation and diarrhoea, and the nursing care of clients experiencing these
- Outline the types of urinary and faecal incontinence and the possible treatments and interventions available
- Introduce the different types of stoma and the specific care that clients with them require.

The chapter provides an opportunity for you to undertake activities that will assist you in your understanding of some aspects of client care. It also includes case study scenarios to illustrate points made in the text.

Faecal Elimination

> Elimination of excess water and wastes is a basic need for all forms of life.
> (Lewis and Timby, 1993)

Successful elimination in humans depends on the individual having an intact and fully functioning gastrointestinal tract, urinary tract and nervous system.

The lower gastrointestinal tract (Figure 8.1) includes the small and large intestines. The small intestine (duodenum, jejunum and ileum) is approximately 610 cm (20 feet) long and 2.5 cm (1 inch) in diameter in an adult. The partially digested food (chyme) leaving the stomach is moved along the small intestine by **peristalsis**. The large intestine (caecum, colon, rectum and anus) is approximately 152 cm (5 feet) long and 6 cm (2.5 inches) in diameter. The faeces – the waste material of digestion that is passed out of the body via the anus or any other opening (stoma) designed for this purpose following surgery (see below) – are moved along the length of the large intestine in response to food entering the stomach. This **gastrocolic reflex**, which propels the faeces by mass peristalsis and is associated with eating, usually occurs three or four times a day, during or immediately after a meal.

The defaecation reflex is initiated by the response to faeces entering the rectum. This reflex encourages the internal anal sphincter to relax, the need to defaecate being conveyed to the brain and interpreted by the individual as an awareness of the requirement to eliminate faeces. The 'normal' defaecation pattern varies from one individual to another, some defaecating three times a day, others only once a week.

peristalisis
the coordinated serial contraction of smooth muscle propelling food through the digestive tract

gastrocolic reflex
a mass peristaltic movement of the large intestine occurring shortly after food enters the stomach

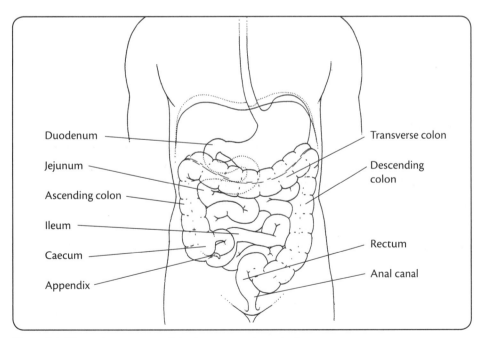

Duodenum

Jejunum

Ascending colon

Ileum

Caecum

Appendix

Transverse colon

Descending colon

Rectum

Anal canal

Figure 8.1 The main structure of the lower gastrointestinal tract

Development of faecal elimination

Infant

At birth, the muscles of the infant's intestines are poorly developed and control by the nervous system is immature. The intestines contain some simple digestive enzymes but are unable to break down complex carbohydrates or proteins, so the infant can, therefore, digest only simple foods (Cox et al., 1993).

The infant's first bowel movement usually occurs within the first 24 hours of birth and comprises **meconium**, which contains salts, amniotic fluid, mucus, bile and epithelial cells. It is greenish-black to light brown in colour, almost odourless and of a tarry consistency. With the introduction of milk feeding, the characteristics of the infant's faeces change. The infant who is breastfed will have a stool that is bright yellow, soft and semiliquid, whereas the bottle-fed infant's stool will be light yellow to brown in colour and more formed (Berman et al., 2008). During the first four weeks of life, the infant will have up to four to eight soft bowel movements per day. This number gradually decreases so that, by the fourth week, the number of bowel movements is two to four per day. By four months of age, the infant has gradually developed a predictable pattern of faecal elimination.

Toddler to preschool

The nervous and gastrointestinal systems gradually mature and are, by the age of 2–3 years, ready to control the function of faecal elimination. The infant develops patterns of defaecation so the parents can identify when their child will have success on the potty. Eating stimulates peristaltic activity and defaecation (see above), and this can be used as a sign to take the child to the toilet. As elimination is a natural process, it is important that the child does not feel that it is a dirty or unnatural procedure.

The child, even though toilet trained, can still have 'accidents', often when the urge to defaecate is allowed to progress inappropriately. If the child becomes so engrossed in what he is doing, he may ignore the need for defaecation and become constipated.

School-aged child

During the school years, the gastrointestinal system attains adult functional maturity. Individuals with learning disabilities may not reach the indicated maturation milestones because of their disability or lack of perception.

Adolescent

Adolescence is important as the developing bowel habits will take them through their adult life. Adolescents often find it difficult to talk about any elimination problem as they develop sexually.

Adult

There may be an increasing incidence of intestinal disorders (colonic and rectal carcinoma, and other gastrointestinal conditions such as **irritable bowel syndrome** and **Crohn's disease**) in adulthood. These can be caused by a decrease in

---

meconium

the thick, sticky material that accumulates in the intestines of the foetus and forms the newborn's first stools

✳ Activity 8.1

Make a list of all the words you have heard or read that describe bowel habit. You may like to discuss this list with your colleagues. This will help you to understand some of the 'language' your clients may use.

irritable bowel syndrome

abnormally increased motility of the bowel, often associated with emotional stress

Crohn's disease

a chronic, often patchy, inflammatory bowel disease of unknown origin, usually affecting the ileum

the excretion of digestive enzymes (pepsin, ptyalin and pancreatic enzymes) and gastric acid. Elimination patterns are affected by changing lifestyle, for example marriage, having children and changes in employment, which may precipitate stress and anxiety. As the ageing process progresses the large intestines gradually lose their tone resulting in an increase prevalence of constipation (Berman et al., 2008).

Ageing adult

The elimination process may be affected by the slowing of peristalsis and decrease in muscle tone of the intestines causes increased fluid re-absorption and therefore constipation (Berman et al., 2008). Severe constipation, causing faecal impaction, can result in urinary retention and also faecal and urinary incontinence. It may also be affected by changing dietary intake caused by a reduced production of saliva, fewer taste buds and the loss of natural teeth, which are replaced by dentures, caps, crowns and bridges as well as reduced levels of mobility. There are increasing numbers of individuals with learning disabilities living into old age resulting in 59 per cent of them who live 50–65+ years experiencing continence and excretory health problems (Walker and Walker, 1998; Bland et al., 2003). Some older adults who consistently use laxatives, to treat their constipation, find that continued use often requires them to increase the dose to encourage defaecation (see section on constipation).

> ✷ **Activity 8.2**
>
> For further information on physiology and factors affecting defecation, read Kozier et al. (2008, pp. 378–415).

Specimen collection

Faecal specimens

Faecal **specimens** may be analysed to detect abnormal characteristics or contents, for example blood, parasites, parasite eggs and pathogens (see Chart 8.1).

> **specimens**
> samples of tissue, body fluids, secretions or excretions

Chart 8.1 Reasons we collect specimens

Specimens are collected:
- To identify the nature of any disease or for diagnosis
- To assess the effect of treatment
- To confirm or eliminate a specific site of the body as a focus of infection or colonisation
- To determine whether a client who has had an infection is still harbouring the pathogen responsible for it. Clients who have Salmonella food poisoning may, for example, still harbour the bacteria in their stools even though their signs and symptoms have disappeared

It is essential that the faecal specimen is not contaminated, so the client is asked to void urine separately into a toilet, bedpan or urinal; urine can interfere with the examination of the faeces, for example destroying some parasites. The client is then asked to pass the faeces into a bedpan. The nurse transfers approximately 15 g (3 teaspoons) of the faeces into the specimen collection container. Care should be taken not to contaminate the outside of the specimen container with the faeces (containers usually have a built-in spatula to assist with this).

Assessment of normal bowel habit

✹ Activity 8.3

For further information on faecal collection, read Dougherty and Lister (2008, p. 785).

Each individual develops their own bowel habit that is 'normal' to them but this can change throughout the lifespan (see start of this chapter). It is, therefore, essential that a note of the normal bowel habits of clients is included in the admission procedure and recorded. In order to assess the type and consistency of faeces eliminated the Adult Bristol Stool Form Scale (Figure 8.2) and Children's Bristol Stool Form Scales (Figure 8.3) could be used, therefore ensuring accurate and consistent observations are maintained.

Altered faecal elimination

Constipation

Constipation refers to the abnormally difficult or infrequent passage of hard faeces and is caused by a decreased motility of the intestines. Some elderly individuals find it difficult to pass soft, bulky faeces. The longer the faeces remain in the intestine, the more water is absorbed from them, which makes them become harder and dryer.

✹ Activity 8.4

List all the factors that you think may predispose the individual to constipation.

Lembo and Camilleri (2003) identify that, in the Western world, constipation affects up to 27 per cent of the population. Many individuals wrongly regard themselves as being constipated if they do not defaecate every day. Some individuals who are constipated have episodes of diarrhoea that can be the result of the hard faeces irritating the colon (often termed constipation with overflow).

Causes of constipation

Causes of constipation include the following:

Hirschsprung's disease
congenital abnormality that causes megacolon

megacolon
very dilated colon – often congenital but can also occur in infancy or childhood

diverticular disease
a condition in which pouch-like extensions develop through the muscular layer of the colon, affecting the passage of faeces

paraplegia
paralysis or sensory loss of the lower limbs, usually including the bladder and rectum

hypokalaemia
low potassium levels in the blood

- *Drugs:* tranquillisers, analgesics (especially those containing codiene), opiates (e.g. morphine), diuretics (leading to excess water and potassium loss), anti-Parksonian drugs, anticholinergics (e.g. oxybutynin), iron supplements, antidepressants (e.g. amitriptyline) and antacids containing aluminium, as these reduce the motility of the intestines.
- *Laxatives:* the abuse of laxatives or frequent enemas. The normal reflexes then diminish, causing the abuser to need more laxative to provide a result and thus become dependent on laxatives.
- *Pregnancy:* limits the space for the faeces to pass through the intestine. Peristalsis slows because progesterone causes an excessive absorption of water from the faeces.
- *Disease:* obstruction from outside or within the intestine, for example from an abdominal or intestinal tumour, adhesions, **Hirschsprung's disease, megacolon**, interfering with the passage of faeces. Other causes include irritable bowel syndrome, **diverticular disease** and neurological deficiencies such as **paraplegia**, multiple sclerosis, Parkinson's disease, endocrine disorders for example hypothyroidism, **hypokalaemia** (causing electrolyte imbalance).
- *Pain:* for example, from an anal fissure (a longitudinal ulcer in the anal canal) or external haemorrhoids (varicose veins in the anal canal,

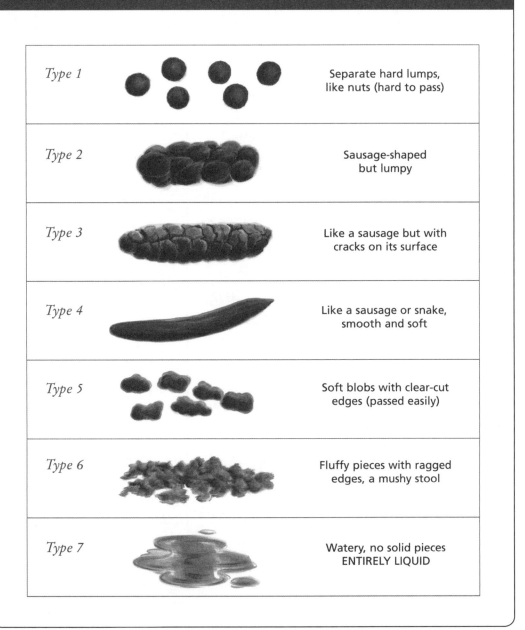

THE BRISTOL STOOL FORM SCALE

Type 1		Separate hard lumps, like nuts (hard to pass)
Type 2		Sausage-shaped but lumpy
Type 3		Like a sausage but with cracks on its surface
Type 4		Like a sausage or snake, smooth and soft
Type 5		Soft blobs with clear-cut edges (passed easily)
Type 6		Fluffy pieces with ragged edges, a mushy stool
Type 7		Watery, no solid pieces ENTIRELY LIQUID

Figure 8.2 Adult Bristol stool chart

Source: Reproduced by kind permission of Dr K. W. Heaton, Reader in Medicine at the University of Bristol.
©2000 Norgine Pharmaceuticals Ltd. Manufacturers of Movicol®

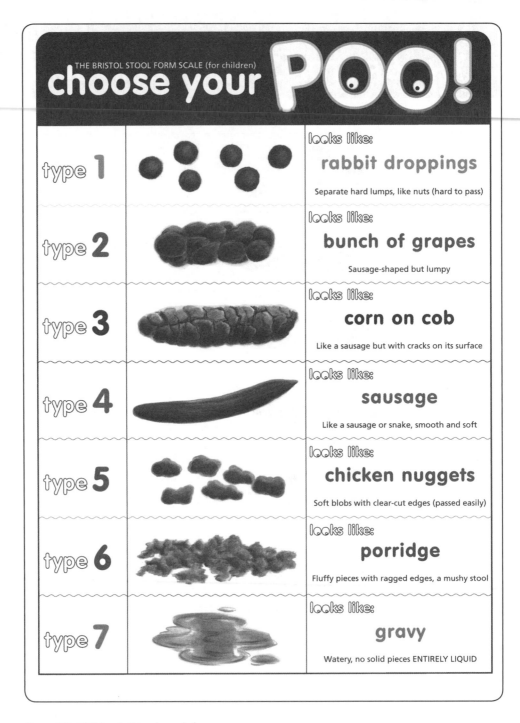

Figure 8.3 Children's Bristol stool chart

Source: Concept by Professor D.C.A. Candy and Emma Davey based on the Bristol Stool Form Scale produced by Dr K.W. Heaton, Reader in Medicine at the University of Bristol. ©2005 Norgine Pharmaceuticals Limited. Manufacturers of Movicol® Paediatric Plain

colloquially known as piles) resulting in a reluctance to defeacate due to the discomfort.

- *Psychiatric/psychological reasons:* depression, leading to reduction in gastro-intestinal motility as well as a lack of interest in the surroundings and diet, chronic psychoses and anorexia nervosa, which can cause an imbalanced or inappropriate dietary intake and therefore a low fibre and fluid intake. Those with any form of cognitive impairment, for example dementia, may be unaware of their nutrition, hydration and elimination needs.
- *Diet:* food low in fibre – resulting in low levels of waste products which then results in lack of stimulation of gastro-colic reflex or an inadequate food intake.
- *Lack of fluid:* either an insufficient intake of fluid or, rarely, an excessive loss of fluid through vomiting and/or sweating.
- *Immobility:* any disease that predisposes to immobility or any enforced immobility from bedrest reducing the motility of the gastrointestinal tract, as a result of decreased activity levels in the ageing adult.
- *Ignoring the call to defaecate:* this allows more fluid to be absorbed from the faeces, thus making them harder and more difficult to eliminate.
- *Psychological factors:* unfavourable lavatory conditions, poor hygiene, lack of privacy or having to use commodes and bedpans, which may result in the client delaying the defaecation process.

There are increasing numbers of individuals with learning disabilities who live to old age and with this comes the normal ageing factors. Added to this, individuals with Down's syndrome experience an increased risk of hypothyroidism, an Alzhiemer's type disease which can result in an increasing risk of constipation (Evenhuis et al., 2000, Holland et al., 1998, Hutchinson, 1999).

Casebox 8.1

Tracey, aged 32, uses the mental health services for depression and takes her antidepressants as prescribed. She has found it difficult to hold down a job and is at present unemployed, living on benefit payments in her bedsit.

What is the probable impact of depression on Tracey's elimination status?
Identify the associated symptoms and signs that Tracey may experience as a result of her elimination problem.

- A lack of interest in her surroundings and diet, as well as her medication, may cause Tracey to become constipated.
- The symptoms and signs that Tracey may experience are highlighted later in the chapter.

Casebox 8.2

Molly, aged 5, was upset by her father's drinking and her parents' subsequent divorce. She has become chronically constipated.

Define constipation.
How would you relieve Molly's constipation? (See also Chapter 7.)

- Constipation refers to the abnormally difficult or infrequent passage of hard faeces and is caused by the decreased motility of the intestines.
- To relieve Molly's constipation, first assess her diet and fluid intake, and advise accordingly.

Try to assess whether she is depressed because of the divorce, with a view to referring her for counselling if necessary.

- Monitor using the Children's Bristol Stool Chart (Figure 8.3)

Care of client with constipation

With his or her help, a history must be taken of the patient's normal elimination pattern. If a diagnosis of constipation is made, an assessment can be undertaken to aid the planning of the client's care.

It is the nurse's responsibility to promote an understanding of the measures available to overcome constipation. The client needs to be educated in the signs and symptoms that are associated with constipation, for example:

- Altered bowel habit, with a lower than usual frequency
- Straining on defaecation
- Abdominal and/or back pain
- Changing shape of the faeces
- Hard, formed faeces
- A palpable abdominal mass
- Halitosis (bad breath)
- Headache (owing to possible dehydration and the build-up of toxins)
- Impaired appetite
- An increased frequency of **micturition** because of increased pressure on the bladder from an increased mass in the large intestines.
- Clients may require advice on:
  - *Dietary intake:* increasing the proportion of fibre
  - *Fluid intake:* increasing fluids and avoiding excess alcohol as this acts as a diuretic. The client should be advised to drink 30–35ml/kg per day (unless other medical conditions restrict this)
  - *Mobility:* doing more exercise, if other medical conditions allow, to aid in increasing the motility of the gastrointestinal tract.

micturition
the voiding of urine

Although laxatives should be avoided, they may be used only as a short-term measure as prolonged use can lead to dependency, which may result in faecal impaction at a future date.

Other measures to treat constipation include the use of enemas and suppositories. Suppositories are bullet shaped and are designed to melt once they have been inserted into the rectum. Some suppositories soften the faeces and some lubricate the anal canal, whereas others use chemicals to stimulate peristalsis. Other types of suppository that the nurse may use do not promote elimination but are treatments for other conditions, for example infections and pain; these include antibiotic and analgesic preparations. Enemas are solutions that are instilled into the large intestine, the most common being a type of cleansing solution used to empty the lower intestinal tract of faeces.

To insert or introduce a suppository or enema, the client is asked to lie on his left side with his knees bent and drawn up gently towards his abdomen (Figure 8.4). The left side is the preferred side for lying on as the bowel will be angled downward, which will aid the retention of the suppository or enema and help to prevent trauma to the rectum. The suppository or enema is gently introduced into the rectum and the client is asked to retain it for approximately 15 minutes

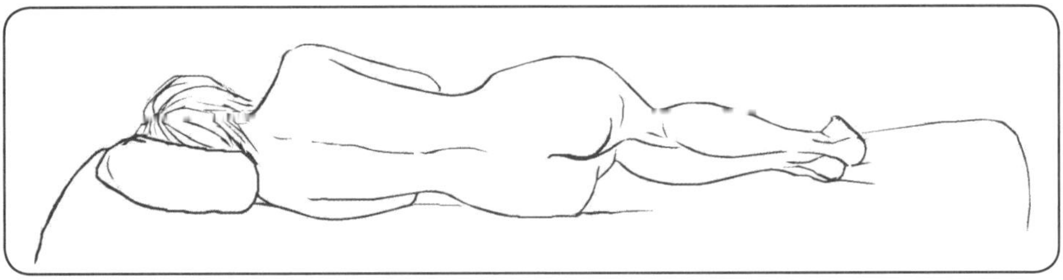

Figure 8.4 Left lateral position

to allow the chemicals to stimulate defaecation. Clients often feel that they wish to defaecate as soon as the suppository or enema has been introduced into the rectum because of stimulation caused by the insertion: the anus and rectum react to the stretching of the muscle by sending the information to the brain that the rectum is full.

For some clients, for example those who are paraplegic/quadriplegic or grossly constipated, the only method of faecal elimination available to them is manual evacuation.

The client is required to lie on the left side, and the nurse will remove the impacted faeces by hooking them out of the rectum using a gloved finger or two fingers to break them up. This should be used only in exceptional circumstances and not as a routine alternative to other methods of aiding faecal elimination.

> **✷ Activity 8.5**
>
> Calculate your fluid intake over 24 hours and compare it with the recommendation of 30–35 ml/kg per day.

Casebox 8.3

Mrs Abasolo is 89 and has been living in a residential care home for three years. She used to walk in the garden each day but now finds it difficult, requiring a helping hand for safety. Mrs Abasolo spends most of her day sitting in either the lounge or her bedroom. Her gums are very sore as her dentures are not fitting properly, so she will only eat 'sloppy' food.

Why does Mrs Abasolo have a potential risk of suffering from constipation (see Chapter 7)? What drugs can treat constipation but when abused can cause it?

- There is a risk of constipation because of immobility, ignoring the call to defaecate, possible depression, leading to a lack of interest in her surroundings and diet, a lack of fibre and, because

of her immobiliy, drinking only the amount of fluid on offer, which may not be sufficient.

- Laxatives can both treat and predispose to constipation.

Casebox 8.4

Mark, aged 50 years, has learning disabilities and multiple physical disabilities. He has just moved to a group home in the community. He suffers from chronic constipation as a result of long-term care in an institution where he had a poor diet (lacking in fruit and vegetables), restricted access to fluids and little exercise. Previous care to relieve his constipation included enemas and laxatives.

Mark's new GP has advised the discontinuation of the enemas and laxatives in order to treat his constipation.

What changes to Mark's lifestyle would you consider to improve his elimination problems (see also Chapter 7)?

- Mark needs to increase his mobility. His diet should be assessed and relevant advice

given, emphasising an increase in the amount of fruit and vegetables. Fluid intake should also be assessed, the target being an intake of 30–35 ml/kg per day. Discourage Mark from ignoring the call to defaecate, and gradually reduce his enemas and laxatives.

- Assess using the Adult Bristol Stool Chart (Figure 8.2)

✷ Activity 8.6

For further information on manual evacuation read Dougherty and Lister (2008, pp. 342–4).

✷ Activity 8.7

List all the factors that you think may predispose an individual to diarrhoea.

Do not employ the procedure without specific instruction as there is an associated danger of perforation of the lower gastrointestinal tract.

The Essence of Care Benchmark identifies that 'all bladder and bowel care is given within an environment that is conducive to the patients individual needs' (NHS Modernisation Agency, 2003, p. 3).

Diarrhoea

Diarrhoea results when movements of the intestine occur too rapidly for water to be absorbed. Faeces are therefore produced in large amounts and may range from being 'loose' to being entirely liquid. If the diarrhoea is severe, large amounts of fluid, consisting of ingested fluids and digestive juices together with sodium and potassium, are lost in the faeces; this can rapidly result in dehydration and electrolyte imbalance.

Causes of diarrhoea

Causes of diarrhoea include:

- *Lack of hygiene:* for example, poor hygiene when preparing food after elimination, handling contaminated items, causing the contamination of ingested food.
- *Drugs:* laxatives resulting from laxative abuse, iron, antibiotics.
- *Infected food: Staphylococcus pyogenes, Salmonella, Escherichia coli* and *Campylobacter*.
- *Stress:* excitement, stress, anger and/or anxiety, causing an increased rate of peristalsis so that the faecal material moves faster through the intestines and less water is absorbed.
- *Diet:* excessive fibre-rich foods, and allergy to some foodstuffs, causing irritation of the intestine. Enteral feeding via a nasogastric tube.
- *Disease:* diseases such as chronic pancreatitis, **ulcerative colitis**, Crohn's disease, diverticular disease and irritable bowel syndrome can result in swings between diarrhoea and constipation. Malabsorption syndrome can cause fatty diarrhoea (**steatorrhoea**). Side effects of some treatments, for example radiotherapy.

ulcerative colitis
a chronic inflammatory disease of the large bowel

steatorrhoea
fatty diarrhoea

Care of the patient with diarrhoea

It is essential that fluid balance is maintained as the client can quickly become dehydrated. The nurse must therefore assess the client for signs of dehydration (tachycardia and decreased skin turgor), and the client's input and output of fluid must be accurately recorded. Oral fluid should be high in added potassium and sodium, for example commercially prepared drinks such as Dioralyte or flat cola with a pinch of salt. In severe cases, an intravenous infusion may be required. Clients should also be encouraged to eat foods high in carbohydrates, for example rice, pasta and soon (NHS Direct, 2005). Some herbal teas, for example rosehip, orange and rhubarb, should be avoided as they exacerbate diarrhoea (Newell et al., 1996).

A careful and thorough history must be taken from the client to ascertain the possible cause of the diarrhoea. All clients suffering from diarrhoea must be treated as potentially infectious until proved otherwise by laboratory examination of the faeces.

Skin care of the perianal region must be maintained as faecal matter is made up of 60 per cent bacteria which can destroy the skin's cellular defence; this can lead to skin breakdown and infection. This can also result in the bacteria tracking up the urethra and causing a urinary tract infection (Whitman, 1991). Barrier creams may be applied to the area once it has been thoroughly but gently cleaned and dried.

Faecal incontinence

Faecal incontinence is the inability to control faecal and gaseous discharge through the anal sphincter (Berman et al., 2008) and is very distressing for the individual as it is difficult to disguise expelled faeces and/or flatus. Bliss et al. (2005, p. 36) suggest that the incidence of faecal incontinence, in the total population, is 2 per cent. However, they also suggest that the prevalence increases with age and is as high as 4–17 per cent in individuals in the elderly population, with an even bigger increase for those in care of the elderly homes being 20–54 per cent. It is essential that a complete history is taken from the client as it may identify possible causes of the incontinence. These include:

- Disease or injury: permanent or progressive conditions such as spinal cord damage, cerebrovascular accident (stroke) or multiple sclerosis: 50 per cent of patients with multiple sclerosis and 61 per cent of those with spinal injuries suffer from faecal incontinence (Kamm, 1998)
- Impacted faeces with overflow (spurious diarrhoea)
- Temporary loss of control caused by diarrhoea
- Caffeine abuse – as this acts by stimulating colonic motor activity giving a laxative effect
- Pudendal nerve damage after childbirth
- Infection
- Ulcerative colitis or Crohn's disease, which can lead to faecal urge incontinence
- Stress incontinence caused by chronic straining, trauma or a congenital defect, or arising post-partum
- Congenital malformation, for example anal atresia
- Rectal prolapse, rectal intussusception
- Iatrogenic injury (trauma/injury to anal sphincter)
- Mega rectum (rectum grossly dilated – Horton, 2004)
- Anxiety
- Individuals with severe cognitive impairment (NICE, 2007)
- Frail older individuals (NICE, 2007)
- Individuals with learning disabilities (NICE, 2007)

✳ Activity 8.8

Try the following exercise to assess skin turgor. Pinch the supraclavicular skin (above the collar bone). If a person is dehydrated, the skin fold will remain. In normal hydration, the skin will return to its normal position almost immediately. Older skin reacts more slowly than younger.

✳ Activity 8.9

Identify the impact of diarrhoea on an individual's lifestyle.

- Drugs – some tranquilisers or hyponotics (e.g. benzodiazepines, tricyclic antidepressants that reduce alertness), drugs that can predispose to loose stools (e.g. laxatives, metformin, antibiotics) and drugs that can alter sphincter tone (e.g. nitrates, calcium channel antagonists)

Management of faecal incontinence

Feacal incontinence is a very distressing problem and can be socially isolating for all who experience it, therefore it is important to give psychological support to your client. NICE (2007) have identified that incontinence in adults, urinary and faecal, costs the NHS an estimate of £500 million per year; this accounts for approximately 2 per cent of the UK's total annual health-care budget. NICE (2007) have identfied that up to 10 per cent of adults are affected by faecal incontinence, with 0.5–1 per cent of adults experiencing regular episodes that affect their quality of life.

The management will depend on the cause but will include:

- Administering suppositories or an enema every 2–3 days if the condition has been caused by faecal impaction, and then instigating a regimen to prevent recurrence
- Advice on changing the diet to one that is well balanced and high in fibre with an increased fluid intake (if other medical conditions allow)
- The treatment of any diarrhoea
- Controlling and trying to eliminate laxative intake if the condition has been caused by laxative abuse
- Advising clients to attend to their elimination needs after a meal to take advantage of the body's normal gastrocolic reflex
- The use of incontinence aids, such as pads, pants and bed protection
- Pelvic floor exercises (see below). For severe cases of stress incontinence, surgery is indicated, for example post-anal repair or repair after **rectoplexy** for rectal prolapse
- Surgery – sphincter repair, **colostomy** or feacal diversion
- When caring for clients with learning disabilities, a behavioural programme that involves prompt sitting on the toilet and other measures such as increased fluid intake and the use of fibre supplements or bulking agents to help normal bowel function (Smith et al., 1994).

rectoplexy
the fixation of the rectum by suturing to surrounding tissue

colostomy
an opening of the colon on to the abdominal wall

Stoma care

The word 'stoma' is derived from Greek meaning mouth or opening. A stoma is formed following surgical intervention for a disease process, its full name being determined by its site. A stoma for elimination purposes is therefore an opening on to the surface of the abdomen through which faecal elimination from either the small or large intestine (or urinary elimination; see below) takes place.

The formation of either a temporary or permanent stoma may be the result of elective surgery or an emergency procedure.

Colostomy

A colostomy is an opening from the colon, which may be temporary or permanent and is indicated for the treatment of the following conditions·

- Malignancy of the colon or rectum; Black (2000) reporting that colorectal cancer is the second most common malignancy in the Western world
- Diverticular disease
- Inflammatory disease of the intestine (for example Crohn's disease or ulcerative colitis)
- Faecal incontinence (in severe cases)
- Hirschprung's disease
- Bowel **ischaemia**
- Trauma to the large intestine
- The relief of acute intestinal obstruction or perforation
- The protection of a distal **anastomosis**, the stoma being formed in a position higher in the gastrointestinal tract than the join between the two ends of intestine that remain after a section of bowel has been removed.

ischaemia
poor blood supply

anastomosis
the joining of two hollow structures

A permanent colostomy is required when the distal segment of the large intestine has been removed, for example when the rectum has been excised because of cancer. The stoma is created by bringing the proximal end of the colon out through an opening on to the anterior wall of the abdomen.

A temporary colostomy is usually necessary to divert the flow of faeces away from the distal part of the large intestine. The surgical technique permits the stoma to be closed once the condition requiring the surgery has been resolved.

The faecal material eliminated from a colostomy depends on the site of the stoma (Chart 8.2).

Chart 8.2 Faecal consistency

- Ileostomy: fluid faeces (of a porridge-like consistency), normally 500–800 ml every 24 hours
- Transverse colostomy: unformed faeces, semiliquid
- Descending colostomy: more formed faeces, near to the normal output for that patient

Ileostomy

An ileostomy is an opening into the ileum on to the abdominal wall and can be indicated for the treatment of inflammatory disease of the intestine, for example Crohn's disease or ulcerative colitis, or as a temporary measure to rest the large intestine after major large bowel surgery. An ileostomy can be a permanent stoma when the colon has been removed (panproctocolectomy) or temporary to allow the disease process to resolve. A temporary stoma can be closed by anastomosis at a later date and the intestine returned to normal functioning.

The faecal material eliminated through an ileostomy (Chart 8.2) is liquid in consistency, containing digestive enzymes that can cause **excoriation** and erosion of the skin if it is not well protected.

excoriation
injury to the skin caused by trauma such as scratching, rubbing or chemicals, for example the combination of urine and/or faeces and air

Management of a client with a stoma

Preoperative care

The client will require a rigorous preoperative assessment, particularly if presenting with a history of chronic disease, weight loss or anorexia. Such clients may be debilitated, so malnutrition and electrolyte imbalances must be corrected to ensure optimum recovery to facilitate wound healing (Berman et al., 2008). Clients also require psychological preparation to prepare them for the change in body image, to reduce anxiety and for reassurance that they can return to their previous place in society.

The stoma nurse should ensure that the client is offered counselling prior to surgery. She or he, or the consultant if no stoma nurse is available, should mark appropriate sites for the stoma so that the surgery does not interfere postoperatively with normal activities of living (Chart 8.3). The client should be shown and allowed to discuss the appliances available (Figure 8.5).

> **✳ Activity 8.10**
>
> For further information on colostomy and ileostomy, read Dougherty and Lister (2008, pp. 362–76).

Chart 8.3 Sites to be avoided to facilitate the easy management of a stoma

• Old scars	• The umbilicus	• Skin folds
• Bony prominences	• The pubic area	

Postoperative care

Up to 20 per cent of clients who have a stoma experience significant psychological problems postoperatively (White, 1998; Black, 2000) and will therefore require a great deal of support, especially in the initial days, weeks and months after its formation. The elimination process of the body has changed, as has

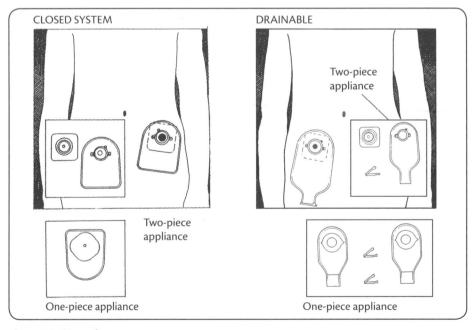

Figure 8.5 Stoma bags

body image. Clients therefore have to be helped to adapt to the changes: preoperative counselling may help them to make a full recovery, returning home to a 'normal' life. Patients may initially demonstrate evidence of withdrawal and depression. Overcoming this is an important part of nursing care; if nurses can show that they accept the clients, this will give their clients confidence.

The formation of the stoma concerns not only clients, but also their partners, one reason being that the change in body image may cause their partners psychological difficulties because of an inability to accept it. Clients who have an ileostomy or colostomy may experience sexual dysfunction (impotence in males and **dyspareunia** in females), but even if they suffer no problems, clients may not be able to return to their normal activities, including sexual activity, for two or three months after the operation. This may be because of the trauma and oedema at the site of the surgery, or sometimes because of nerve damage.

Within our multicultural society, care must be provided that is appropriate to the health practices, values and beliefs of the client. As an example, clients who practise the Muslim religion of Islam are required to pray five times a day, before which they are required to perform a washing ritual called *al-wadhu* to signify the body's cleanliness inside and out. The client will need to apply a clean stoma appliance at each prayer time, so a two-piece appliance may be most suitable (Black, 2000).

dyspareunia
the occurrence of pain in the labial, vaginal or pelvic region during or after sexual intercourse

> **∞ Link**
>
> Chapter 15 mentions the impact of stoma surgery on body image.

Care specific to the stoma

Postoperatively, the stoma must be checked regularly – its colour and size, whether it is retracting or prolapsing (Chart 8.4) and its function – to ensure its viability. The stoma may initially discharge some **haemoserous** fluid, and this will be followed, once bowel sounds return, by the passage of some **flatus**, mucus and fluid. Once solid food has been reintroduced, the stoma will discharge faecal matter that is often very liquid at first but gradually becomes fluid or semisolid, depending on the stoma site, over the following few days or weeks. The client will be unable to control the passage of flatus, which can cause them embarrassment.

haemoserous fluid
serous fluid containing a small amount of blood

flatus
gas in the gastro-intestinal tract, which is often expelled through a body orifice, especially the anus

Chart 8.4 Appearance of a normal stoma

- Pinkish red (the colour resembling that of the inside of the mouth)
- Initially postoperatively, the stoma is oedematous

The client will require dietary advice as some gas-forming foods (for example onions, fizzy drinks, cabbage, baked beans and spicy food) may produce excess flatus and pain. The client is therefore advised to try out foods gradually in order to identify which ones cause problems. Clients who have an ileostomy should be advised to increase their fluid intake as their faeces will contain large amounts of water that would previously have been absorbed by the large intestine.

It is important that clients are shown how to care for their own stoma and that, prior to discharge, they are proficient in its management, for example in changing stoma bags, cleaning the stoma and disposing of equipment and soiled stoma bags.

Urinary Elimination

The normal anatomy of the urinary system is shown in Figure 8.6.

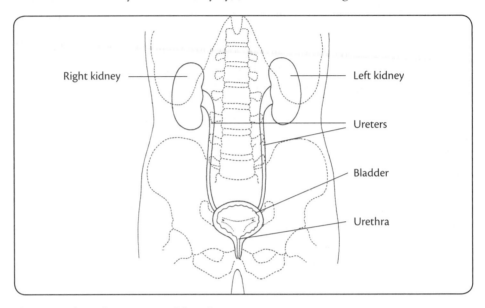

Figure 8.6 The main structures of the urinary system

Development of urinary elimination

Infant

At birth, both nervous system control and renal function are immature, so there is an inability to concentrate the urine and urinary elimination is involuntary. Urinary output is affected by fluid intake, the amount of activity and the environmental temperature. If the infant is more active or the temperature is raised, more fluid will be excreted through the skin and more water vapour via exhaled air. During the first year urine output increases to 250–500 ml a day (Berman et al., 2008).

Toddler to preschool

The bladder increases in size with the growth of the child and is now able to hold more urine. By two years of age, the kidneys are maturing and can conserve water and concentrate urine almost as well as those of the adult. The nervous system is mature enough for the toddler to control bladder functioning and, as Martini (2002) suggests, toilet training is not physiologically possible until this time.

Day-time bladder control is attained first, followed by night-time control. Even when toilet training has been achieved, however, there may be times of regression and 'accidents'.

School-aged child

The urinary system has now reached maturity. Between the ages of 5 and 10 the kidneys double in size. For some children there may also be issues related to **enuresis** at this age which can be very distressing for the child. Non-judgemental, non-blame and positive approaches should be utilised to ensure that the child is not psychologically affected by these incidences.

Adolescent and young adult

There are no noticeable changes in urinary elimination during this time.

Adult

There is a decrease in renal function with ageing as the result of a gradual decrease in the number of nephrons. Bladder tone gradually diminishes, and urinary elimination is therefore more frequent as the ability to store urine prior to voiding decreases. In a healthy adult, the decrease in renal function is so gradual that the effects are minimal until later in the ageing process (Cox et al., 1993).

Ageing adult

The nephrons continue to decrease in number so renal function gradually lessens. This, combined with **arteriosclerosis**, decreases the glomerular filtration rate, thus decreasing the concentrating ability of the kidneys. Waste products are still processed effectively by the kidneys, but this takes longer than before (Berman et al., 2008).

The loss of smooth muscle elasticity affects the bladder and reduces its capacity. Inhibited bladder contraction can result in frequency and a premature urge to urinate. In the older male, the enlargement of the prostate gland can lead to **urethritis**, especially if there is urinary stasis, which may result in a urinary tract infection (UTI). This leads to dribbling of urine, difficulty in commencing urination, a poor stream, incomplete emptying of the bladder and increased frequency. Slack et al. (2008) identify that 25 per cent of males with enlarged prostates will develop bladder symptoms related to outflow obstruction. These changes can cause nocturia (the need to urinate at night) and therefore disturbed sleep. The decrease in oestrogen level in females can predispose to urinary urgency and urinary frequency (Berman et al., 2008).

Factors affecting urinary elimination include:

- Lack of privacy
- Fluid intake, for example alcohol and caffeine related drinks which increase urinary output (cola, coffee, tea)
- Weather – hot weather increases sweating so decreases fluid output via urinary elimination, unless client adjusts fluid intake to account for this
- Medication, for example diuretics, alpha-blockers
- Disease, for example diabetes melitus, kidney failure, enlarged prostate
- Developmental stage of client
- Obesity may be a contributory factor for urge and stress incontinence.

enuresis
an involuntary discharge of urine after the age by which bladder control should have been established. In children, a voluntary control of urination is usually established by the age of 5 years. Nocturnal enuresis is, however, present in about 10 per cent of otherwise healthy children at age 5 years, and 1 per cent at age 15 years

ateriosclerosis
thickening of the walls of the arterioles with a subsequent loss of elasticity and contractability

urethritis
inflammation of the urethra

✹ Activity 8.11

List the types of urine specimen you have been asked to collect and why.

Specimen collection

Urine specimens commonly collected are:

- Urine test for *routine screening*, for example on admission or as an outpatient screening procedure

diurnal

occurring over a 24-hour period

- *Early morning urine* (EMU): because of **diurnal** variation, the first voided urine of the day is usually the most concentrated and is the preferred specimen when testing for substances present in a low concentration, for example hormones in a pregnancy test
- *24 hour urine collection*: used to assess the amount of a substance that is lost in the urine. Depending on the substance to be measured, a preservative may be required in the collection bottle, as in the creatinine clearance test (an increased amount of creatinine being found in the urine in the advanced stages of renal disease)
- *Midstream specimen of urine* (MSU), the object of collection being to obtain a specimen of urine uncontaminated by bacteria that may be present on the:
  - skin
  - external genital tract
  - perianal region
  - distal third of the urethra.

Infected urine and urinary stasis can lead to crystallisation of the urine; both this and foreign bodies can cause urinary tract stones. There are several other factors that predispose to urinary stone formation and they are: dehydration, immobility, disease processes, for example gout and hyperparathyroidism, and the most common is **idiopathic** (Burkitt et al. 1990).

idiopathic

of unknown or spontaneous origin

Principles of collecting an MSU

Any bacteria present in the urethra are washed away in the first portion of urine voided, which is not collected. An avoidance of contamination by other bacteria is achieved by thorough cleansing and a good clean technique.

Catheter specimen of urine

A catheter specimen of urine (CSU) is taken using an aseptic technique. The specimen portal is cleaned using an injection/alcohol swab and allowed to dry. A sterile needle (21G × 1½ inches) (however some catheter tubing has needleless sampling ports) is inserted into the sampling port, and a specimen of approximately 10–20ml of urine is withdrawn into the syringe, the needle then being removed. The specimen should then be transferred to a sterile container, ensuring that the container is not contaminated. It is important that specimens are taken only from the sampling port that has been designed for this procedure as using any other site may cause the catheter, catheter bag or tube to leak. Urine taken from the catheter bag is too old and possibly too contaminated for an accurate test result.

Urine specimens should, if possible, be taken before antibiotics are commenced as any treatment may affect the result.

✶ Activity 8.12

List the observations that may be made on a specimen of urine without using a test.

✶ Activity 8.13

For exact details on how to test urine during routine screening, read the guidelines that are enclosed with all containers of urine test strips; these will be stocked in your clinical area.

Urine testing for screening

It is important to remember that urine is a body fluid, so all precautions (as identified in a care setting's control of infection procedure book) must be taken for the nurse's safety.

All clients being admitted to hospital should have a urine test. This is one of the few times that urine is screened, and it can highlight any previously undiagnosed medical conditions, for example diabetes mellitus. It will also give baseline information on the client and may precipitate further investigations. The urine must be observed for its colour and odour before being tested with a reagent stick. Normal urine is pale and straw coloured, but the urine may be darker because of a loss of extra fluid through perspiration during hot weather, or from a limited fluid intake. Normal urine, when fresh, has little smell, but if left it may develop an odour of ammonia. Infected urine may be foul-smelling immediately after voiding and become worse on standing. The normal 'straw' colour may alter because of substances present in the urine (Figure 8.7).

> ✸ Activity **8.14**
>
> For further information on urine specimens, read Dougherty and Lister (2008, pp. 390–1).

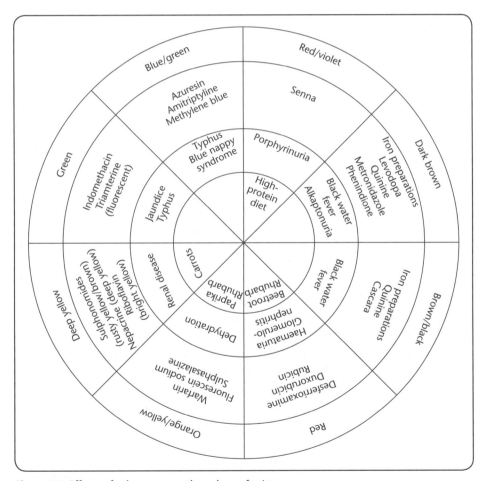

Figure 8.7 Effects of substances on the colour of urine
Source: Adapted from Ford (1992).

Fluids containing alcohol increase the urinary output by inhibiting the production of antidiuretic hormone (Berman et al., 2008). Likewise fluids that contain caffeine (for example tea, coffee, cola drinks) have a diuretic property so increasing urine production.

Casebox 8.5

Mrs MacDonnell, aged 72, has visited her GP complaining that her urine has been red.

What urinary test will the GP perform, and what do you expect the result to be?
What foods could Mrs MacDonnell have been eating that would turn her urine red?

• A routine urine test and an MSU will be taken. These findings may be positive for haematuria, or negative if the problem is diet related. Even though Mrs MacDonnell is aged 72, vaginal bleeding (which could be disease related) should not be ruled out.

• Beetroot or rhubarb could have this effect on her urine.

Altered urinary elimination

Incontinence

Incontinence can be either permanent or temporary. It can be defined as the involuntary loss of urine and/or faeces at an inappropriate time or in an inappropriate place. This is a 'silent problem', many individuals being thought not to seek medical help because of embarrassment. It is identified that 5–7 per cent of 15 to 44-year-olds, 8–15 per cent of 45 to 64-year-olds and 10–20 per cent of over 65-year-olds experience incontinence, 20 per cent of women aged over 40 years being affected by urinary incontinence with 23 per cent of males aged 40–79 years experiencing dribbling and 14.5 per cent wet clothing (Hunskaar et al., 2004; Thakar and Stanton, 2000). Earnshaw and Bates (2001) identified that up to three million individuals experience urinary incontinence, in the UK, and that many of these have learning disabilities. Lennox et al. (2003) identified that 47 per cent of individuals with learning disabilities experience urinary incontinence but Bland et al. (2003) suggest 59 per cent. As well as causing clients considerable distress and discomfort, urinary and faecal incontinence costs the NHS approximately £500 million per year (NICE, 2007). Clients experiencing dementia may have normal bladder function but may 'void inappropriately' due to cognitive impairment and mobility problems, resulting in their inability to recognise the need to urinate or find a toilet.

Incontinence is not a disease but a symptom of an underlying disorder that can be mental, physical, social or environmental and affects both sexes at all ages. It may be primary, as in childhood enuresis or learning disability, or secondary to another cause such as multiple sclerosis, prostatic enlargement, obesity or constipation. It can also result from a combination of these; that is, the cause can be multifactorial. As Hunskaar et al. (2004) have identified, urinary incontinence affects the psychosocial, social, economic and physical well-being of individuals and their families. Urinary incontinence has an impact on feelings of sexuality, in its broadest sense, including sexual relationships, appearance, intimacy and caring (Roe, 1999). In a study of Pakistani women's perception of urinary incontinence Wilkinson (2001) identified feelings of being unclean and sinful. Wells and Wagg (2007) identified that Bangladeshi women viewed any bladder weakness as a personal problem and a loss of self-control rather than a medical problem requiring professional help. For practising members of the Muslim religion urinary incontinence has implications on religious obligations – their daily ritual of ablutions and prayer. They also felt more embarrassment when talking to males about incontinence issues. Eustice (2007) suggest that clients with dementia, confusion or disorientation may experience episodes of incontinence due to an inability to locate the toilet.

When assessing clients, their oral fluid intake should be reviewed as some herbal teas, for example elderberry, strawberry, rose, wild blackberry and nettle, act as diuretics (Newell et al., 1996).

There are four main types of urinary incontinence:

- Stress incontinence
- Urge incontinence
- Reflex incontinence
- Overflow incontinence.

NICE (2006) suggest that assessment of the client should be multidisciplinary, involving doctors, nurses, occupational therapists and physiotherapists.

The female and male urethras are shown in Figures 8.8 and 8.9 respectively (see also Chart 8.5).

Chart 8.5 The female urethra

- The urethra is embedded in the anterior wall of the vagina
- It runs downwards and forwards behind the symphysis pubis and opens at the external urethral orifice, which lies just in front of the opening of the vagina
- Its diameter is approximately 0.7 mm
- It is approximately 4 cm long
- The urethra is 'slit-shaped' rather than cylindrical
- If there is a weakness of the pelvic floor muscles and the urethra becomes more vertical, it is easier for urine to leak out (incontinence)

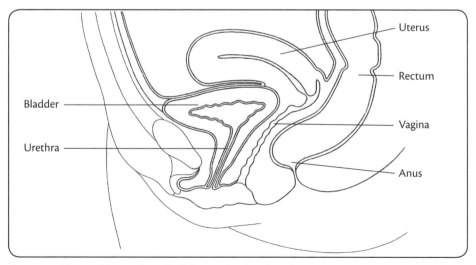

Figure 8.8 The position and angle of the urethra in a female

Source: Haslam (1997) Reproduced with kind permission of *Nursing Times*.

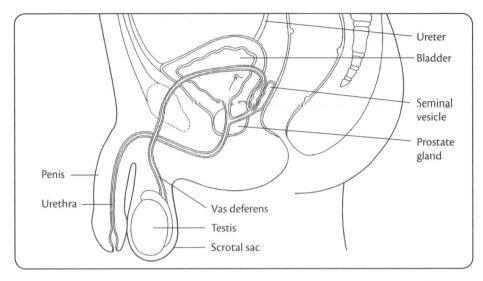

Figure 8.9 The position of the urethra in a male

Stress incontinence

This type of incontinence is more common in females than males and it is both a neuromuscular and anatomical condition. The main cause is sphincter deficiency – pelvic floor dysfunction, pudential/pelvic nerve damage, injury or degenerative changes as a result of hormonal deficiency, or age-related atrophy of the tissues (Bardsley, 2004). A small amount of urine is leaked on physical exertion, coughing, sneezing or laughing. This results from an incompetent urethral sphincter, which is caused by a weakness of the supporting pelvic floor muscles. Predisposing factors include childbirth, hormonal changes owing to the menopause, vaginal prolapse, obesity, inactivity and constipation; in men, stress incontinence can occur after prostatectomy.

Treatment includes pelvic floor exercises, weighted vaginal cones, electrical therapy that stimulates the nerves, causing the muscles to contract, periurethral bulking injections, pharmacological therapy, special tampons, vaginal pessary and, in the case of postmenopausal women, oestrogen hormone replacement therapy (Bardsley, 2004). Surgical intervention may include **vaginal repair** or insertion of sub-urethral tape which is inserted between the urethra and vagina, therefore lifting the middle part of the vagina.

Urge incontinence

Urge incontinence is the commonest type of incontinence in the older adult and causes the loss of a variable amount of urine which is caused by **detrusor muscle** instability (an unstable bladder), neuropathic conditions and outflow obstruction. The individual often complains that they have little or no warning of a need to micturate and is often incontinent on the way to the toilet. Causes include urinary tract infection, bladder stones, an enlarged prostate gland, a urethral stricture, faecal impaction, Alzheimer's disease, cerebrovascular accident, spinal cord lesions and Parkinson's disease. Residual volumes of urine, left in

★ Activity 8.15

List the causes of stress incontinence.

vaginal repair
following prolapse of the vagina and uterus, surgical repair is performed to return the structures to their normal position

detrusor muscle
the external longitudinal layer of the muscular coat of the bladder

the bladder after micturition, may occur causing urinary stasis and a subsequent UTI.

Treatment rarely involves surgery but does include bladder retraining exercises, **antimuscarinic** drug therapy and relaxation exercises.

There is a high level of mixed stress and urge incontinence, especially in the elderly.

Reflex incontinence

This type of incontinence manifests itself as the individual's failure to recognise the need to micturate and is usually caused by damage of the peripheral nerves to the bladder or of the spinal cord. The bladder fills and empties on a reflex cycle, and the condition may be combined with incomplete voiding and a high residual urinary volume.

Treatment may involve surgery, for example urinary diversion or urostomy (see below). In addition, catheterisation (indwelling urethral, suprapubic or intermittent self-catheterisation) and other techniques, such as the Valsalva or Credé manoeuvre (Chart 8.6), may be used.

Chart 8.6 Valsalva and Credé manoeuvres

Valsalva manoeuvre
The client is asked to inhale and then attempt to forcibly exhale, with the glottis (vocal cords), nose and mouth closed. This causes the diaphragm to flatten, thus increasing the intra-abdominal pressure. Unless the urethral sphincter is in complete spasm, the increased pressure forces urine to be voided. Clients with cardiac problems should not attempt this

Credé manoeuvre
The client is asked to apply pressure over the symphysis pubis. The pressure may be enough to produce spasm of the bladder or cause voiding of the urine

Overflow incontinence

Overflow incontinence occurs in men more frequently than females and is caused by urinary retention with overflow caused by:

- *An obstruction* from an enlarged prostate, prostatic cancer, urethral stricture, pelvic floor prolapse or faecal impaction; treatment includes prostatectomy, urethrotomy and the clearance of any faecal impaction.
- *A hypotonic bladder* (ineffective contraction of the bladder when voiding urine) caused by neuropathy (as in diabetes) or anticholinergic medication (such as imipramine); treatment includes intermittent self-catheterisation, drug therapy (for example carbachol) to enhance detrusor contractility and a review of drug regimens to ensure that other medication is not the cause of the hypotonia.
- *Detrusor–sphincter dyssynergia* (uncoordinated muscle activity) caused by neuropathic conditions, for example paraplegia and multiple sclerosis; treatment includes intermittent self-catheterisation and **biofeedback** to teach coordination.

An indwelling catheter should be used only as a last resort for clients with voiding difficulties.

antimuscarinic
opposing the action of muscarine or agents that mimic it, for example atropine and scopolamine

biofeedback
a training programme designed to develop one's ability to control autonomic (involuntary) nervous system

Cystitis

Cystitis is inflammation of the bladder usually occurring secondary to an ascending UTI. It is more common in sexually active females because of the close proximity of the urethra and the vagina. In the acute stage, clients complain of frequent and painful micturition; in the chronic stage, it is secondary to a lesion that may have pyuria as its only symptom. Antibiotics are used to treat the infection, and the client should be encouraged to drink 30–35mls per kilogram body weight of fluid per day (if the medical condition allows) to dilute the urine and decrease the pain on micturition.

Pelvic floor exercises

Pelvic floor exercises (Chart 8.7) are primarily intended to increase the strength of the levator ani muscles. In women, pelvic floor exercises involve the contraction and relaxation of the muscles that surround the vagina and anus, thus improving their tone. This helps to restore the normal anatomical relationships of the surrounding structures as well as the function of the urethral sphincter.

Chart 8.7 Pelvic floor exercises

The client needs to sit, stand or lie in a comfortable position and tighten the pelvic floor for approximately 10 seconds – there should be feeling of tightening the anus but not the buttocks, abdomen or legs. This should be repeated 10 times. Clients need to imagine that they are stopping a flow of urine. For females learning this exercise, a finger can be inserted into the vagina and 'squeezed'. Clients should progress so that, when passing urine, they can stop and start mid-flow; this should be carried out once a week to check the progress of the exercise regimen. Pelvic floor exercises should be performed at least twice daily

✷ Activity 8.16

If you do not already practise pelvic floor exercises regularly, you should start now by following the instructions in Chart 8.7.

In males, pelvic floor exercises should be taught before prostatectomy so that they can help to stop post-micturition dribbling following prostatectomy by improving urethral sphincter function.

NICE (2006) suggest that daily muscle training pelvic floor exercises, over a period of three months, is effective for stress and mixed urinary incontinence.

Urinary catheterisation

A urinary catheter is designed to remove fluid from or instil fluid into the bladder. Urinary catheterisation is a common procedure, between 16 and 25 per cent of hospital clients (Patel and Arya, 2001; Saint et al., 2000; Weinstein et al., 1999) and 4 per cent of clients in the community (Getliffe, 1995) being catheterised at any one time.

Indications for catheterisation are:

cytotoxic

toxic to cells; the term is usually applied to drugs used in the treatment of cancer

- Pre- and postoperatively to empty the bladder before or after abdominal, rectal or pelvic surgery
- The acute or chronic retention of urine
- To introduce drugs, for example antibiotics and **cytotoxic** drugs
- To irrigate the bladder in order to remove sediment and/or blood clots

- Trauma, for example any trauma to the pelvis or lower urinary tract (as any oedema resulting from the trauma may cause obstruction), in order to monitor for blood, and following burns to monitor urinary output
- The accurate measurement of urinary output
- Diagnostic investigations of bladder function
- Incontinence, when all other methods have failed.

Catheters

The nurse should assess the client prior to catheterisation and identify the reason for undertaking the procedure, the length of time the catheter is to remain in situ and the sex of the client. This will help to determine the type of catheter required. The size of catheter will depend upon whether clear urine or haematuria is to be drained (Chart 8.8). Catheters designed for women are shorter than those designed for men because the adult urethra is approximately 4 cm long in a woman and 20–23 cm in a man.

Chart 8.8 Catheter size

• Adult clients with clear urine:	10–16 Fr (Ch)
• Adult clients with haematuria:	18–30 Fr (Ch)
• Paediatric:	6–8 Fr (Ch)

(larger sizes may be required dependent on size of child and reason of catheterisation)
1 Fr (Ch) is equivalent to 0.3 mm, catheters being measured across their external diameter

Length
• Standard length:	40–44 cm
• Female length:	23–26 cm
• Paediatric length:	30 cm

In the majority of cases, a retaining balloon 5 ml in volume will be sufficient. The catheter will require 10 ml of sterile water for its insertion: 5 ml to fill the balloon and 5 ml to fill the balloon's inlet tubing. A balloon size of 30 ml volume should be discouraged, its main use being for clients following urological surgery, in particular prostatic surgery.

Common types of catheter
- *Teflon:* the latex is teflon coated to reduce urethral irritation; such catheters can be used for clients requiring short- or medium-term, up to one month, catheterisation.
- *Silicone:* these catheters are very soft, are less irritating and cause less crystal formation than the latex variety. They should be used for clients who require catheterising for more than two weeks, the catheters having a life span of approximately three months.
- *Hydrogel:* these catheters absorb water to produce a slippery surface and therefore decrease friction to the urethra. They are more resistant to encrustation and adherent bacteria, and have a life span of up to 14 weeks.
- *Conformable catheter:* these are designed to conform to the shape of the female urethra (slit-shaped) and allow partial filling of the bladder. They are approximately 3 cm longer than conventional female catheters.

Types of catheterisation

There are three types of catheterisation with the most common and probably the best known is indwelling catheterisation, the other two being intermittent self-catheterisation and suprapubic catheterisation.

Indwelling catheters

The insertion of a urethral catheter requires an aseptic technique, and it is preferable for the client to have a shower or bath prior to catheterisation to ensure good hygiene. The balloon size, the type of material and the size of the catheter used will depend on the reason for catheterisation.

It is important that meatal and perineal hygiene is maintained to reduce the risk of encrustation around the catheter and **meatus**. Perineal and meatal hygiene should be performed twice daily and the nurse or client must ensure that the area is thoroughly dried afterwards. Mild soap and water are sufficient to clean the meatal and perineal areas.

The type of urinary drainage bag will be determined by whether the client is mobile (for example clients able to continue normal mobility activities or clients in wheelchairs) or has limited mobility (for example after surgery or with a medical condition reducing mobility). Clients who are normally mobile may benefit from wearing a leg bag during the day, changing to a full-size drainage bag at night. Clients with limited mobility will normally wear a full-size bag until the catheter has been removed or 'normal' mobility restored.

To empty a urinary drainage bag, the nurse must wash their hands prior to and after carrying out the procedure, as well as wear gloves during the procedure. The outlet tap of the catheter system should be opened and the urine allowed to drain into a single-use receptacle, the outlet tap being closed after emptying. The urinary drainage bag must hang below the level of the bladder to ensure that urine does not seep back into the bladder; the bag can be supported by attaching it either to the side of the bed or to a stand specially designed for this purpose. If a leg bag is worn, it must be secured to the client's leg without causing traction to the catheter and therefore trauma to the urethra and bladder neck. The tap of the urinary drainage bag must not touch the floor as this will result in contamination and a possible UTI (Figure 8.10).

The adult client should be encouraged to drink 2–3 litres per day (unless other medical conditions restrict this) in order to reduce the risk of UTI, constipation (as this may cause pressure on the bladder and urethra) and the irritant effect of concentrated urine on the bladder. Constipation should also be avoided as it can contribute towards leakage

meatus
a passage or opening

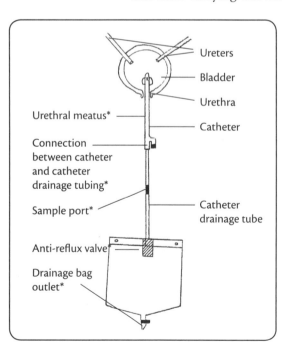

Figure 8.10 Points at which pathogens can enter a closed urinary drainage system (*)

around the catheter. Pomfret (2000) identified a number of risk factors or serious complications associated with urinary catheterisation including urethral perforation, trauma, stricture formation, urinary tract infection, encrustation and bladder calculi and possible carcinoma of the bladder. Urinary tract infections are the most common complaint for individuals with indwelling catheters (Simpson, 2001) and the incidence increases the longer the catheter is in situ (Curran, 2001). This is particularly increased when individuals have other infections, the catheter is being used to measure urinary output or individuals have existing chronic conditions, for example diabetes or malnutrition. Also females are at greater risk than males (Maki and Tambyah, 2001). The principles of care of the patient with a urinary catheter are shown in Chart 8.9. Roadhouse and Wellstead (2004) identify that the most common hospital-acquired infection is associated with catheter related infections, accounting for 35–40 per cent of all hospital infections.

> **⚭ Link**
>
> Chapter 15 explores issues of body image.

Chart 8.9 Principles of care for the client with a urinary catheter in situ

- Meatal hygiene – to minimise encrustation
- Fluid intake – adequate intake to reduce the risk of concentrated urine irritating the bladder and to lessen the risk of constipation
- Catheter selection – the appropriate size of catheter and balloon, in a material appropriate to the time proposed in situ, and of a length appropriate to gender; a shorter length for women can, for example, prevent accidental trauma from traction
- Catheter drainage bag – positioned lower than the level of the client's bladder and with effective support
- Catheter drainage bag tubing – ensuring that this is not kinked
- Catheter bag drainage outlet – must not touch the floor as this can cause contamination, leading to UTI
- Having a catheter in situ affects body image and sexual activity in the long term, therefore psychological support and understanding for the client and partner are essential

Intermittent self-catheterisation

Intermittent self-catheterisation is the periodic drainage of urine from the bladder. A catheter is inserted into the bladder via the urethra by the nurse, client or carer, and the bladder is emptied; the catheter is then removed until the next time voiding needs to take place. This method of emptying the bladder is particularly useful for clients who have difficulties in passing urine and/or have a post void residual greater than 100 ml – for example clients with neurological problems and those who suffer from urinary incontinence – thus allowing them to gain control of their bladder. Prior to instruction, clients and/or carers should be assessed in terms of whether they are suitable to undertake this procedure (Chart 8.10).

Chart 8.10 Criteria for clients undertaking intermittent self-catheterisation

Clients should:
- Be incontinent of urine (overflow incontinence)
- Have good manual dexterity and mobility
- Have the mental ability to learn and understand
- Show good motivation
- Possess an intact urethra

The catheter's length will be determined by the client's gender. For a man, the catheter should be 38 cm long, and for a woman 20 cm as the female urethra is shorter than the male.

The actual principles and procedure of intermittent self-catheterisation are the same as for the insertion of an indwelling catheter, but this is a 'clean' procedure rather than an aseptic one. Catheters may be used more than once and may be self-lubricating. Urinary tract infections are lower in incidence in this group than in clients with indwelling catheters.

Suprapubic bladder drainage

A self-retaining catheter is inserted through a suprapubic incision or puncture into the bladder (Figure 8.11). This is a temporary measure to divert the flow of urine from the urethra when the urethral route is impassable or impossible because of, for example:

- Trauma
- Stricture
- Prostatic obstruction
- Pelvic fractures
- Gynaecological operations: vaginal hysterectomy and vaginal repair.

Drainage can be maintained for several months.

✷ Activity 8.17

For further information on urinary catheterisation, refer to Dougherty and Lister (2008, pp. 378–93) or Berman et al. (2008, pp. 1303–11).

✷ Activity 8.18

For further information on suprapubic catheterisation, read Doughertyand Lister (2008, p. 383) or Berman et al. (2008, pp. 1313–15).

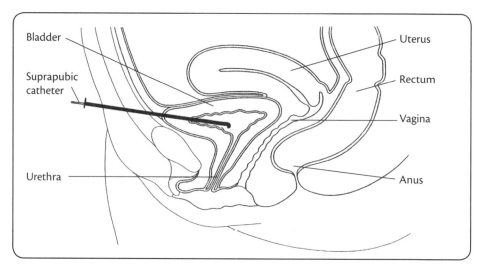

Figure 8.11 A suprapubic catheter in situ

Bond and Harris (2005) suggest that, for suprapubic catheterisation, the catheter used should be no smaller than 16 CH with a 10 ml baloon as this ensures that the tract between the bladder and skin is maintained.

Urostomy

A **urostomy** is performed when the bladder is being removed or is diseased (Chart 8.11). It is an opening from the ureters into a resected section of (usually) ileum, approximately 15 cm in length, which then channels the urine through a stoma that has been formed on the abdominal wall (known as an ileal conduit) and is fashioned into a spout to aid drainage.

urostomy
an opening in the abdominal wall to allow the diversion of urine

Chart 8.11 Indications for urostomy formation

- Malignant disease of the bladder
- Malignant disease of the pelvis
- Trauma
- Neurological damage
- Congenital disorders
- Intractable incontinence

Urine that is eliminated through a urostomy can excoriate the surrounding skin if it is not well protected. The urine will constantly 'dribble' from the stoma into a urostomy drainage bag (Figure 8.12). The management of a urostomy is the same as for stoma care.

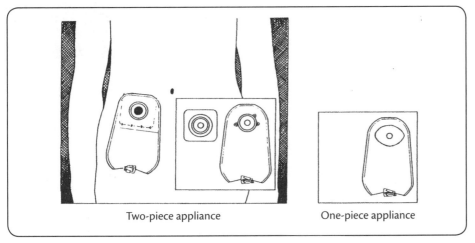

Two-piece appliance   One-piece appliance

Figure 8.12 Urostomy bags

Chapter Summary

This chapter has explored both the urinary and faecal elements of elimination. It explains the normal anatomy and physiology and then identifies the abnormal processes of and influences on elimination. It explores possible treatments, the advice available and nursing care for the conditions identified.

? Test yourself!

1   What information do you need to obtain when making an assessment of your client's elimination needs?

2   List and explain the factors that may cause a client to become constipated.

3   Identify four types of incontinence.

4   What is the difference between an ileostomy, a colostomy and a urostomy?

5   Identify the psychological factors that affect both urinary and faecal elimination.

6   How much fluid should a healthy individual weighing 65 kg drink in a day?

Benson, D. (2003) The importance of a thorough continence assessment. *Nursing Times* **99**(29): 53.

Brooker, C. and Waugh, A. (eds) (2007) *Foundations of Nursing Practice – Fundamentals of Holistic Care.* Mosby Elsevier, Philadelphia.

Fultz, N.H. and Herzog, A. (2001) Self-reported social and emotional impact of urinary incontinence. *Journal of the American Geriatrics Society* **49**: 892–9

Getliffe, K. (2003) How to manage encrustation and blockage of Foley catheters. *Nursing Times* **99**(29): 59.

Marieb, E.N. (2009) *Essentials of Human Anatomy and Physiology*, 9th edn, Pearson Education, San Francisco.

Marieb, E.N. and Hoehn, K. (2010) *Human Anatomy and Physiology*, 8th edn. Pearson Education, San Francisco.

Marklew, A. (2004) Urinary catheter care in the intensive care unit, *Nursing in Critical Care* **9**(1): 21–7.

Peate, I. (2003) Nursing role in the management of constipation: use of laxatives. *British Journal of Nursing* **12**(19): 1130–6.

Further Reading

For live links to useful websites see: www.palgrave.com/nursinghealth/hogston

References

Bardsley, A. (2004) Key trends in the management and treatment of stress urinary incontinence. *Professional Nurse* **19**(10): 30–2.

Berman, A., Snyder, S., Kozier, B. and Erb, G. (2008) *Fundamentals of Nursing: Concepts, Process and Practice*, International 8th edn. Pearson Education, New Jersey.

Black, P. (2000) Practical stoma care. *Nursing Standard* **14**(41): 47–53.

Bland, R., Hutchinson, N., Oakes, P. and Yates, C. (2003) Double jeopardy? Needs and services for older people who have learning disabilities. *Journal of Learning Disabilities* **7**(4): 323–44.

Bliss, D.Z., Fisher, L. and Savik, K. (2005) Managing fecal incontinence: Self-care practices for older adults. *Journal of Gerontological Nursing* **31**(7): 35–44.

Bond, P. and Harris, C. (2005) Best practice in urinary catheterisation and catheter care. *Nursing Times* **101**(8): 54–8.

Burkitt, H., Quick, C. and Gatt, D. (1990) *Essential Surgery: Problems, Diagnosis and Management.* Churchill Livingstone, Edinburgh.

Cox, H.C., Hinz, M.D., Lubno, M.A. and Newfield, S.A. (1993) *Clinical Applications of Nursing Diagnosis: Adult, Child, Mental Health, Gerontic and Home Health Considerations*, 2nd edn. F.A. Davis, Philadelphia.

Curran, E. (2001) Reducing the risk of health-acquired infections. *Nursing Standard* **16**: 45–52.

Dougherty, L. and Lister, S. (eds) (2008) *The Royal Marsden Hospital Manual of Clinical Nursing Procedures*, 7th edn. Wiley-Blackwell, Oxford.

Earnshaw, K. and Bates, A. (2001) Continuing professional development: continence. *Learning Disability Practice* **4**(2): 33–9.

Eustice, S. (2007) Frail elderly. In Getliffe, K. and Dolman, P (eds) *Promoting Continence*, 3rd edn. Balliere Tindell, London.

Evenhuis, H., Henderson, C.M., Beange, H., Lennox, N. and Chicione, B. (2000) *Healthy Aging: Adults with Intellectual Disabilities: Physical Health Issues.* World Health Organisation, Geneva.

Ford, A. (1992) Feeling off-colour. *Nursing Times* **88**(5): 64–8.

Getliffe, K. (1995) Long-term catheter use in the community. *Nursing Standard* **9**(31): 25–7.

Haslam, J. (1997) Floor plan. *Nursing Times* **93**(15): 67–70.

Holland, A.J., Hon, J., Huppert, F.A., Stevens, F. and Watson, P. (1998) Population based study of the prevalence and presentation of dementia in adults with Down's syndrome. *British Journal of Psychiatry* **172**: 493–8.

Horton, N. (2004) *Behavioural and biofeedback therapy for evacuation disorders.* In Newton, C. and Chelvanayagam, S. (eds) *Bowel Continence Nursing.* Beaconsfield Publishers, Beaconsfield.

Hunskaar, S., Lose, G., Sykes, D. and Voss, S. (2004) The prevalence of urinary incontinence in woman in four European Countries. *British Journal of Urology International* **93**(3): 324–30.

Hutchinson, N.J. (1999) Associated Down's syndrome and Alzheimer's disease: Review of the literature. *Journal of Learning Disabilities for Nursing, Health and Developmental Disabilities* **15**: 329–36.

Kamm, M.A. (1998) Faecal incontinence. *British Medical Journal* **316**: 528–32.

Kozier, B., Erb, G., Berman, A., Snyder, S., Lakr, R. and Harvey, S. (2008) *Fundamentals of Nursing: Concepts, Process and Practice*, Pearson Education, Essex.

Lembo, A. and Camilleri, M. (2003) Chronic constipation. *The New England Journal of Medicine* **349**(14): 1360–8.

Lennox, T., Nadkarni, J., Moffat, P. and Robertson, C. (2003) Access to services and meeting the needs of people with learning disabilities. *Journal of Intellectual Disabilities* **7**: 34–50.

Lewis, L.W. and Timby, B.K. (1993) *Fundamental Skills and Concepts in Patient Care.* Chapman & Hall, London.

Maki, D.G. and Tambyah, P.A. (2001) Engineering out the risk of infection with urinary catheters. *Emerging Infectious Disease* **7**: 342–7.

Martini, F.H. (2002) *Fundamentals of Anatomy and Physiology*, Prentice Hall, Englewood Cliffs, NJ.

Newell, C.A. Anderson, L.A. and Phillipson, J.D. (1996) *Herbal Medicines: A Guide for Healthcare Professions.* Pharmaceutical Press, London.

NHS Direct (2005) *Health Encycolpaedia.* www.nhs.direct.nhs.uk/en.aspx?ArticleID=131 (accessed 1 June 2009).

NHS Modernisation Agency (2003) *Benchmarks for Continence and Bladder and Bowel Care.* http://www.dh.gov.uk/en/Publicationsandstatistics/Publications/PublicationsPolicyAndGuidance/DH_4005475 (accessed 1 June 2009).

NICE (National Institute for Health and Clinical Excellence) (2006) *Urinary Incontinence: The Management of Urinary Incontinence in Women.* NICE, London.

NICE (National Institute for Health and Clinical Excellence) (2007) *Faecal Incontinence: The Management of Faecal Incontinence in Adults.* NICE, London.

Patel, H.R.H. and Arya, M. (2001) The urinary catheter: 'a-voiding catastrophe'. *Hospital Medicine* **62**(3): 148–9.

Pomfret, I.J. (2000) Multidisciplinary continence care. *Nursing Times* **99**(19): 59.

Roadhouse, A.J. and Wellstead, A. (2004) The prevention of indwelling catheter related urinary infections – the outcome of a performance improvement project. *British Journal of Infection Control* **5**(5): 22–3.

Roe, B. (1999) Incontinence and sexuality: findings from a qualitative perspective. *Journal of Advanced Nursing* **30**(3): 573–9.

Saint, S., Wiese, J., Amory, J.K., Bernstein, M.L., Patel, U.D., Zemencuk, J.K., Bernstein, S.J., Lipsky, J. A. and Hofer, T.P. (2000) Are physicians aware of which of their patients have indwelling urinary catheters? *The American Journal of Medicine* **109**(6): 476–80.

Simpson, L. (2001) Indwelling urethral catheters. *Nursing Standard* **15**(46): 47–53.

Slack, A., Jackson, S. and Wein, A.J. (2008) *Fast Facts: Bladder Disorders.* Health Press, Oxford.

Smith, L.J., Franchetti, B., McCoull, K., Pattison, D. and Pickstock, J. (1994) A behavioural approach to retraining bowel function after long-standing constipation and faecal impact in people with learning disabilities. *Developmental Medicine and Child Psychology* **34**: 41–9.

Thakar, R. and Stanton, S. (2000) Management of urinary incontinence in women. *British Medical Journal* **321**: 1326–31.

Walker, C. and Walker, A. (1998) *Uncertain Futures: People with Learning Difficulties and their Aging Family Carers.* Pavilion, Joseph Rowntree Foundation, London.

Weinstein, J.W., Mazon, D., Pantelick, E., Reagan-Cirincione, P., Dembry, L.M. and Hierholzwe, W.J. Jr (1999) A decade of prevalence surveys in a tertiary-care center: trends in nosocomial infection rates, device utilization, and patient acuity. *Infection Control Hospital Epidemiology* **20**: 543–8.

Wells, M. and Wagg, A. (2007) Integrated continence services in the female Bangladeshi population. *British Journal of Nursing* **16**: 516–19.

White, C. (1998) Psychological management of stoma related concerns. *Nursing Standard* **12**(36): 35–8.

Whitman, D. (1991) Intra-abdominal infections. pathophysiology and treatment. Hoechst, Frankfurt, Germany. Cited in Le Lievre, S. (2002) An overview of skin care and faecal incontinence. *Nursing Times* **98**(41).

Wilkinson, K. (2001) Pakistani women's perceptions and experiences of incontinence. *Nursing Standard* **16**(5): 30–2.

JAN DEAN, PAMELA DIGGENS AND ROB HAYWOOD

Chapter

9

Respiration

📖 Contents

- Respiratory Physiology
- Respiratory Assessment
- Nursing Interventions

- Test Yourself!
- Further Reading
- References

☑ Learning outcomes

The purpose of this chapter is to examine factors associated with respiratory function. It will explore the nurse's role in relation to the assessment of, and implementation of care with, clients who experience difficulties with respiration. At the end of the chapter, you should be able to:

- Outline normal respiratory processes
- Assess, interpret and monitor a client's respiratory signs
- Rationalise common deviations from normal values
- Identify techniques for supporting respiratory function
- Assist clients in maintaining effective respiratory function.

Respiratory Physiology

The purpose of respiration

The purpose of respiration is to ensure that a constant supply of oxygen is available to all the cells in the body and that carbon dioxide, a waste product of cellular metabolism, is excreted. This is achieved by the respiratory and circulatory systems working closely together, but for clarity this chapter will focus on the respiratory system in isolation.

Many specialist texts are available which describe in detail the anatomy and physiology of the respiratory system and as this chapter will only provide an overview of physiology and pathophysiology, a more detailed text should be consulted when required.

The mechanisms required to achieve a continuous supply of oxygen in the cells are:

- Ventilation (or breathing)
- Gaseous exchange in the lungs (sometimes termed external respiration)
- Transportation of gases around the body
- Gaseous exchange in the tissues (sometimes termed internal respiration)

An interruption in, or abnormality of any of these processes may result in an inadequate amount of oxygen reaching the tissues (hypoxia), and/or an accumulation of carbon dioxide in the body (hypercapnia) resulting in changes in pH levels (respiratory **acidosis** or **alkalosis**) which will rapidly have serious implications for the body. It is only possible to survive for 4 or 5 minutes if no oxygen reaches the brain.

Respiratory structures

The respiratory structures include the mouth and nasal cavity, pharynx, larynx and the trachea, which divides into right and left main bronchi, one in each lung (Figure 9.1). Within each lung, the main bronchi branch repeatedly into smaller bronchioles forming the 'bronchial tree'. The airways terminate in the alveoli (or air sacs) where gaseous exchange takes place.

Each lung is surrounded by two pleural membranes – the visceral pleura which cover the lung and the parietal pleura which line the thoracic cavity. There is a potential space between the two pleural membranes, and they glide over each other as the chest moves; pleural fluid is produced between the layers which act as a lubricant. Pleural fluid also causes the two layers of membrane to adhere to each other by surface tension, helping to create a slight negative pressure which holds the lungs to the chest wall enabling the lungs to expand and inflate during inspiration.

Respiratory structures are adapted to protect the airway and keep it patent (open) at all times as ventilation must be a continuous process. The epiglottis is a leaf-shaped flap of cartilage in the larynx which can 'close off' the trachea during swallowing to prevent food and fluid entering the trachea. If anything

acidosis
depletion of body's alkali reserve; abnormally low pH of the blood, as a result of an increase of acid in the blood, or loss of alkali from the blood.

alkalosis
the alkalinity of the body increases, resulting from either excess alkali or reduction of acid in the body

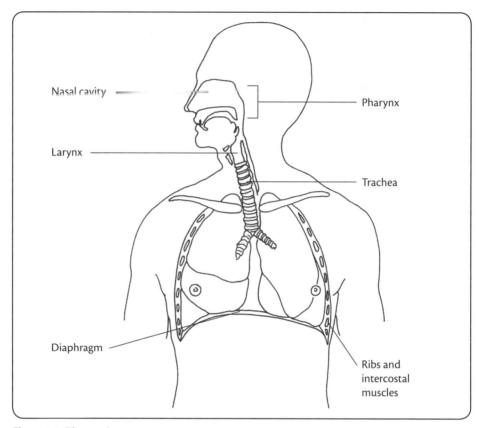

Figure 9.1 The respiratory system

other than air enters the trachea, the cough reflex is initiated in an attempt to expel it. The trachea is surrounded by C-shaped bands of cartilage which prevent its collapse during ventilation. However, the upper airways may become obstructed during deep unconsciousness; when the muscles of the tongue and in the pharynx are fully relaxed, they may block the airway. Careful positioning of unconscious patients can avoid this.

Babies and small children are not miniature adults in terms of respiratory anatomy and physiology, and this must be taken into account during assessment, when supporting their respiration and during cardio-pulmonary resuscitation.

Ventilation

Ventilation is the process by which air is drawn into the lungs as a result of pressure changes brought about by an alteration in the shape of the chest. During inspiration the respiratory muscles – the diaphragm and the intercostal muscles – contract, causing the ribcage to move up and outwards and the diaphragm (which is dome shaped) to flatten. The resultant increase in thoracic capacity causes a decrease in the pressure inside the lungs and air will flow in, provided that the airways are patent. This is because gases will always flow from an area of high pressure, to an area of low pressure, until the pressure is equalised.

Expiration is a passive process; when inspiration ends the natural elasticity of the lung tissue and relaxation of the respiratory muscles, will enable air to flow out of the lungs without active effort.

Other muscle groups – the accessory muscles of respiration in the neck, back and abdomen – may be recruited to assist in both inspiration and expiration, but this does not occur in normal ventilation.

The respiratory rate (ventilatory rate) is the number of inspirations and expirations recorded in one minute. Normal rates vary according to the age of the patient, with babies and young children breathing more quickly than adults: the respiratory rate of a baby under 1 year is 30–40 breaths per minute (bpm), between 1 and 2 years 25–35 bpm, and between 2 and 12 years 20–30 bpm. Children over 12 years of age would be expected to have a respiratory rate similar to an adult (Weiteska et al., 2005).

It is important to note that newborn babies may breathe very erratically with periods of bradypnoea (slow breathing) and tachypnoea (fast breathing) interspersed with occasional periods of apnoea. This is due to the immaturity of the respiratory regulatory centres in the brain.

The control of ventilation is mostly involuntary (unconscious), but voluntary override is possible to allow for particular ventilatory needs, such as singing, swimming, coughing or speaking. Such control of ventilation is temporary – involuntary control will be resumed after a period of time. It is important to remember that as voluntary control of ventilation is possible, patients may consciously alter their ventilatory pattern if they are aware that they are being observed. Thus a more accurate assessment of ventilatory rate and depth will be obtained if the patient is not aware that the nurse is observing them.

As well as voluntary control, ventilation can be affected by drugs such as opiates, sedatives and alcohol which depress ventilation, and can cause breathing to stop (apnoea) if administered in sufficient quantity.

Involuntary ventilation is controlled by a variety of complex mechanisms, which constantly 'fine tune' ventilatory effort to ensure that adequate oxygenation and removal of carbon dioxide is achieved. These mechanisms include:

- **Chemoreceptors** (chemical control)
- Stretch and irritant receptors (mechanical control).

Chemical control of ventilation

Chemoreceptors are specialised cells in the walls of the aorta and carotid arteries which monitor changes in the amount of oxygen and carbon dioxide in the arterial blood. A rise in the level of carbon dioxide detected by these receptors will stimulate ventilation to ensure that the excess carbon dioxide is excreted. A reduction in the amount of oxygen detected will have the same effect – ventilation will be stimulated. A decrease in the arterial pH level (acidosis), which is often associated with high levels of carbon dioxide, but may be due to other metabolic disorders, will also result in an increase in ventilation.

Signals from the chemoreceptors are transmitted to the respiratory control centres in the brain via the cranial nerves in the peripheral nervous system.

> ⌾ Link
>
> Chapters 8 and 14 further discuss effects of alcohol.

chemoreceptors
nerve endings or groups of cells that are stimulated by chemicals

The respiratory control centres in the brain are situated in the medulla and the pons (the brain stem) and consist of inspiratory and expiratory neurones. Stimulation of the inspiratory neurones will result in inspiration, and centres in the pons inhibit or stimulate the inspiratory neurone to 'fine tune' the ventilatory rhythm.

Mechanical control of ventilation

Stretch receptors within the airways and pleural membranes respond as the lung expands by inhibiting ventilation to prevent over inflation. Impulses are transmitted from the receptors to the respiratory control centres via the peripheral nervous system and inspiration will cease.

Irritants such as dust will stimulate receptors in the airways when inhaled into the respiratory system and initiate coughing and sneezing, which are protective reflexes designed to expel pollutants from the respiratory tract.

Ventilation may fail resulting in potentially life-threatening hypoxia for a variety of reasons. The airway may be partially or fully obstructed, the patient may be in a low oxygen environment, respiratory muscles may be paralysed by disease or drugs, or ventilatory effort may be inadequate following injury or surgery to the chest or abdomen. In these situations rapid assessment and intervention is crucial.

Gaseous exchange in the lungs (external respiration)

The air which enters the respiratory tract on inspiration is composed of 20.9 per cent oxygen, 78.6 per cent nitrogen and small amounts of carbon dioxide and water vapour. On reaching the alveoli, oxygen will diffuse into the blood from the alveolar air space, because the partial pressure of the oxygen is higher in the air than in the blood. Diffusion will occur in an attempt to equalise the pressure. The diffusion of oxygen can occur rapidly as the thin, moist alveolar membrane provides a huge surface area, with a closely related blood supply (pulmonary capillaries), which is ideal for gaseous exchange. Any change in these conditions, for example, excess fluid in the alveoli, thickening of the alveolar wall, loss of blood supply to the pulmonary capillaries, will reduce the efficiency of gaseous exchange and may result in an inadequate transfer of oxygen into the blood.

At the same time as oxygen is diffusing into the blood from the alveoli, carbon dioxide will diffuse out of the blood and into the alveolar airsacs, as the **partial pressure** of carbon dioxide in the blood, is greater than in the air. Therefore, as oxygen enters the blood stream, the main waste product of respiration, carbon dioxide, diffuses out of the blood and can be eliminated from the body by exhalation.

partial pressure
the pressure of a gas in a mixture of gases, related to its concentration

Transportation of gases around the body

The respiratory and circulatory systems are interdependent and must both function efficiently to ensure that oxygen, once in the arterial blood reaches the cells, and that carbon dioxide is transported from the cells via the venous system for excretion in the lungs. An inadequate circulation, for any reason, for example

∞ Link

Chapter 10 discusses hypotension in more depth.

hypotension (low blood pressure) or cardiac failure, will result in a lack of available oxygen in the cells, as although ventilation and gaseous exchange may be adequate, the oxygen cannot reach the cells that need it. As the pump in the circulatory system – the heart – is dependent upon a constant oxygen supply to function, it can be clearly seen that the two systems are reliant upon each other.

Transportation of oxygen

Most of the oxygen which diffuses into the blood in the alveoli combines with the haemoglobin (in the erythrocytes). A small amount (as little as 1 per cent) is dissolved in the plasma. Haemoglobin is a specialised protein, composed of iron and globin, and one molecule of haemoglobin can reversibly combine with four molecules of oxygen. Once four oxygen molecules are attached to the haemoglobin molecule – it is described as fully saturated. Pulse oximeters are now commonly used in clinical practice to measure the percentage of saturated haemoglobin in arterial blood, and so provide useful information about the patient's lung capacity for gaseous exchange. As not all haemoglobin molecules will always have 4 molecules of oxygen attached to them, the normal range for oxygen saturation is 97–99 per cent. Desaturated haemoglobin has a bluish colour, and this can be observed in the tissues as cyanosis.

Any reduction in the quantity of erythrocytes (red blood cells) in the circulation will reduce the body's ability to transport oxygen around the body and thus can result in **hypoxia** in the cells. This could be caused by anaemia, or haemorrhage.

hypoxia diminished amount of oxygen in the tissues

When blood reaches the tissues, the oxygen molecules are 'unloaded' from the haemoglobin and become available to the cells. The rate at which oxygen combines with, and is unloaded from, haemoglobin is affected by a variety of conditions. These can include the partial pressure of oxygen and carbon dioxide, blood pH and temperature, for example a rise in temperature, or reduction in pH, will facilitate the release of oxygen, therefore increasing availability to more metabolically active cells.

Transportation of carbon dioxide

Carbon dioxide is transported via three mechanisms, dissolved in blood plasma, attached to haemoglobin molecules and as hydrogen ions in the blood, the latter being the most significant, as the hydrogen ions affect the pH of the blood. Abnormally high levels of carbon dioxide in the blood, which can result from ventilatory failure, will result in acidosis which impacts negatively on all the metabolic processes in the body.

Gaseous exchange in the tissues (internal respiration)

Gaseous exchange in the tissues is the opposite of gaseous exchange in the lungs. On reaching the tissues, oxygen is 'unloaded' from the haemoglobin molecules and diffuses from the blood into the tissues, as the partial pressure of oxygen is higher in the blood than in the tissues. Carbon dioxide will diffuse from the tissues into the blood and will be transported back to the lungs for excretion.

Once oxygen enters the cells, it combines with glucose to produce adenosine triphosphate (ATP), the source of energy for all cellular activity. This process can be inhibited by cellular poisons, such as cyanide, again resulting in hypoxia.

Respiratory Assessment

Assessment is an essential element of the nursing process that enables a variety of information to be gathered about the patient. This can contribute to, or confirm diagnosis of a patient's condition, monitor current treatment or intervention and in healthy individuals serve as a baseline of information. The use of a structured approach when assessing, in both emergency and non-emergency situations, may assist in preventing any aspects from being omitted.

Although there are many approaches that can be used for assessing a patient's respiratory system, this chapter will follow a 'Look, Listen and Feel' approach. This approach can be used in conjunction with the Airway, Breathing, Circulation, Disability and Exposure (ABCDE) approach which is recommended in emergency situations (Smith, 2003). This will ensure that appropriate aspects of assessment are given priority where required and that both subjective and objective information is obtained from a variety of elements; patient history, physical assessment and investigations that may aid diagnosis.

Patient history

In non-emergency situations it is recognised that taking the patient's history may be extremely useful as it can contribute towards 80 per cent or more to the diagnosis (Epstein et al., 2008). It is, however, important to remember that subjective information obtained from the history depends upon each interviewer's ability and skill in communication techniques when gathering this information. Consequently, if questions are not asked or phrased correctly it may result in the omission of relevant information. With more experience greater time may be taken on questioning some of these components compared to others depending on the information required.

There are various components of the history including:

- presenting complaint
- past medical or surgical history
- medication (which should include prescription, non-prescription and recreational)
- social
- occupation
- environmental exposure to hazards
- travel – particularly abroad
- allergies
- familial
- smoking.

When discussing patients' smoking history it is important to establish if they have ever smoked, as conditions such as chronic obstructive pulmonary disease (COPD) are related to smoking but the symptoms may not be evident until years later.

Accessing any prior documentation or previous medical notes may be useful but it should be remembered that any previous or pre-existing condition may not necessarily be the cause of their current problem. It may also be useful to ascertain from each patient how their presenting complaint varies from their condition normally.

Physical assessment

This will involve using a variety of skills and techniques to gather objective information about the patient that can be seen, felt or heard. To enable a more thorough assessment it is useful to have patients positioned upright whenever possible so that access to both posterior (back), anterior (front) and lateral (sides) areas of the chest can be obtained (Moore, 2007). This position may not be possible for some patients and appropriate adjustments will have to be made when undertaking their assessment.

An initial, general assessment begins as you approach the patient. Some information can be assessed very quickly, for example their colour, effort of breathing and body position. On asking patients how they feel you can assess severity of breathlessness or difficulty breathing as this is evident by them not being able to reply back or only able to manage single words. In comparison, patients not experiencing severe distress will be able to speak in sentences.

Physical assessment – 'Look'

Looking at the patient, assess their colour, body position, effort of breathing and any shortness of breath (SOB). Gathering additional information may take more time as it will require direct access to the patient's thoracic cage and involve greater observation skills. Assessing the thoracic cage includes the lateral, anterior and posterior chest. Whenever possible compare the right side of the chest with the left as there are various conditions that may affect only one side.

Respiratory rate

It is important to observe and record the patient's respiratory rate. Looking at the chest movements for one minute, count the number of respirations. A patient's respiratory rate within the normal values is termed eupnoea. Numerous conditions can result in altered breathing rates termed **bradypnoea**, **tachypnoea** and **apnoea**.

It is important to acknowledge that a change in respiratory rate can often be an early indicator that a patient's condition is deteriorating and therefore it is essential that their respiratory rate is not omitted when taking other vital signs.

Respiratory rhythm

Normal breathing has a regular, evenly paced pattern consisting of an expiratory and inspiratory phase. Changes from the normal pattern of respirations may include:

- dyspnoea
- orthopnoea
- Cheyne-Stokes respiration
- Biot's respiration
- Kussmaul's respiration.

bradypnoea
slow breathing as a result of depression of the respiratory centre. It is normal during sleep but in ill health may indicate over sedation or the presence of a cerebral lesion

tachypnoea
an increase in the respiratory rate caused by the body's demand for extra oxygen, or by anxiety. It can be seen in shock, anaemia, cardiac and respiratory failure. It is a normal physiological response to exercise

apnoea
cessation of breathing which is usually abnormal and constitutes a medical emergency. However, short periods of apnoea can be observed in infants and small children due to the immaturity of respiratory control mechanisms

nasal flaring
the nostrils flare to decrease resistance to air entry

recession
the inward movement of the chest during inspiration due to extreme respiratory effort

Dyspnoea is difficult, laboured breathing, present when the airways are obstructed and is frequently accompanied by sweating or pallor. Asthma and COPD are conditions that may cause dyspnoea.

Orthopnoea is the ability to breathe without difficulty only when sitting upright. It may be as a result of heart failure with pulmonary oedema, or occur in an infant or small child when abdominal pressure is exerted on the diaphragm.

Cheyne-Stokes respirations are recognized by breathing cycles of gradually decreasing rate and depth, followed by cycles of increasing rate and depth. This alternating pattern is repeated at intervals of between 45 seconds and 3 minutes and frequently indicates impending death. There may be periods of apnoea during the cycles.

Biot's and Kussmaul's respiration are patterns of rapid, deep breathing often associated with metabolic acidosis, as the body tries to excrete excess amounts of carbon dioxide in the blood in an effort to neutralize the acidosis.

Respiratory depth and effort

Respiratory depth is assessed by observing the degree of movement in the chest wall. Depth of breathing can provide information on adequacy of ventilation. Hyperpnoea is shallow, rapid breathing, usually in an attempt to avoid pain originating from the thorax or abdomen. Deep, laboured breathing may occur when patients are struggling to breath, for example as in asthma and COPD. They may also have increased effort, this indicates that patients are utilising more energy to breathe and that breathing is now referred to as an active process rather than passive. This in turn involves use of accessory muscles, mentioned earlier. In severe respiratory distress, **nasal flaring** and chest wall **recession** may be observed.

In some patients assessing the rate, depth and pattern by observation alone can be very difficult and for this reason it can be useful to place a hand on their chest. Whenever possible, allow patients to rest before counting their respiratory rate as factors including exercise, temperature and smoking can increase the rate from their resting state. Patients with pre-existing or underlying conditions such as COPD, may have an altered 'normal' range due to their condition and in these cases this needs to be taken into account when assessing rate, rhythm and depth.

Colour

In healthy individuals the skin is warm, well perfused and the oral mucosa, lips, tongue and nail beds are pink in colour. There are, however, a variety of conditions that result in these having the physical appearance of a bluish colour, termed cyanosis. There are two types of cyanosis, peripheral and central, both caused by a variety of conditions. Peripheral cyanosis occurs when there is sufficient oxygenation but a problem with normal circulation. This can occur in a cold environment or due to an arterial obstruction, hypovolaemia or hypotension.

Central cyanosis indicates that circulating blood is lacking in sufficient oxygen due to a circulatory or ventilatory problem. This is evident by a bluish tinge affecting patients' lips, tongue and oral mucosa. Common conditions that may cause this include pneumonia, pulmonary oedema, COPD and severe asthma.

Thoracic shape

Look at the shape of the chest to assess for any skeletal structure abnormalities. Skeletal deformities may cause an inequality or inability of the lungs to fully expand and this may impact on cardiac function as well as respiratory function if severe. Unequal chest expansion may also be due to conditions such as pneumothorax, pneumonia and pleural effusions.

Normally the transverse diameter (width across the back) is twice the distance compared to the anterior-posterior diameter (front to back) so the normal ratio is two to one. Conditions such as COPD cause the normal chest shape and hence ratio to be altered resulting in a barrel-shaped chest.

Conscious level

Observe the patient's level of consciousness. If they are hypoxic and/or **hypercapnic** their level of consciousness may be altered and they may appear agitated, drowsy, confused or behave inappropriately.

Physical assessment – 'listen'

Usually breathing is a quiet, passive process and therefore normal respiration is soundless. It may be very obvious when patients are breathing if they are making any abnormal noises which may indicate either partial or complete obstruction. There are various noises that patients may make but some main ones are:

- stridor
- wheeze
- snoring
- cough.

Stridor, when heard, sounds very harsh and occurs on inspiration due to extreme difficulty breathing in. This sound if heard indicates an emergency situation and senior assistance should be sought immediately as there could be an obstruction to the patient's airway such as an object stuck in their airway.

Wheeze occurs when the airways are narrowed resulting in the airway being compressed. Wheezing may be audible on expiration and/or inspiration and may be audible with or without the aid of a stethoscope. Asthma, COPD and secretions in the airway are a few conditions that can cause wheeze.

Snoring occurs on inspiration through the nose, usually during sleep. It is indicative of partial obstruction of the upper airway and can be caused by various conditions such as inflammation of the nasal mucosa, tongue relaxing into the airway, enlarged tonsils or adenoids. In severe cases short cessations in respiration may occur known as sleep apnoea. This may require the patient to undergo further investigations to confirm diagnosis.

Cough is part of a response group that defends the bronchi, trachea and lungs against irritation from a foreign body or excessive secretions. It is a sudden, violent expulsion of air from the lungs which may contain a mix of mucus, cell debris, pus and microorganisms. Observe patients' tissues or sputum pots as this will provide information about any sputum expectorated (coughed up). In particular, try to assess its colour, consistency and quantity (Kennedy, 2007). Sputum can be described as **mucoid**, **mucopurulent**, **purulent**, **tenacious** and/or

---

hypercapnic respiratory failure
failure of the respiratory system resulting in greater than normal amounts of carbon dioxide in the blood (hypercapnia). This type of respiratory failure can occur in some patients with COPD

mucoid
has the appearance of raw egg and occurs in chronic bronchitis

mucopurulent
thick sticky, green/yellow in colour indicating infection

purulent
slimy and green/yellow in colour indicative of infection

tenacious
sputum which is sticky and difficult to expel; often associated with asthma or dehydration

frothy
bubbly white sputum which may be tinged with pink if blood is present and can indicate pulmonary oedema

To help you identify some respiratory sounds, use a stethoscope to listen to the chest of a patient or colleague, preferably one with a cough or an infection.

Is there any difficulty differentiating between inspiratory and expiratory noises? Can you hear the heartbeat as well?

frothy. Sputum can also be blood-stained indicating haemorrhage from the lungs (haemoptysis). Fresh blood from the lungs will be red but stale blood coughed up is rusty brown in colour.

Whenever possible, it can also be useful to observe patients when they are coughing to assess for any difficulty expectorating as this may potentially affect their ability to clear their airways.

Physical assessment – 'feel'

This involves touching the patient's chest to determine information about any pain, abnormalities, skin texture and temperature. When palpating a patient's chest it can aid the assessment if both hands are placed symmetrically to enable each side and same location to be compared.

Pain

Patients may experience pain, tenderness or discomfort which may be increased or become more evident on palpation. Patients may experience pain in the thoracic region for a variety of reasons, some of which may not originate from respiratory disorders.

Abnormalities and deformities

Lung expansion can be palpated by placing the hands, fingers spread apart and palms down symmetrically on both sides of the posterior chest so that the spine is in the middle of both hands. This position may be difficult to access particularly in those patients experiencing respiratory distress and in these situations the anterior chest can be assessed. On inspiration a patient's thoracic cage will move upwards and outwards and this movement can be felt by the hands. As expiration occurs the hands will feel this movement as it causes the hands to move nearer together, back to their start position. Although this technique assesses by feeling for equal expansion of both sides, it is also good practice to observe the hand movement whilst undertaking this part of the assessment. As mentioned earlier there are various reasons that can cause unequal chest expansion.

When a patient speaks vibrations, called fremitus, are transmitted throughout the bronchial tree. By placing the bony parts of the palms onto the patient's chest these vibrations can be felt more easily enabling any difference between each side and location to be identified. Vibrations should normally be felt equally, but decrease as the palm position moves down the chest. Fremitus may be decreased by conditions such as pleural effusion, pneumothorax, COPD and asthma which prevent or reduce the transmission of sound. Also, conditions including pneumonia and pulmonary oedema transmit sound better through a solid substance resulting in increased vibrations being felt.

Temperature and texture

A lot can be determined by feeling the temperature and texture of patient's skin. It is recognised that using the back of the hand to assess skin temperature is more useful than the palm. Hot and sweaty skin may be caused by conditions including infection, hot environment or problems with the hypothalamus and its regulatory centre. Whereas cold, clammy skin may indicate that perfusion is inadequate as in, shock.

Age considerations

There are a few variations that need to be taken into consideration when assessing patients across the age spectrum, in particular babies, infants, young children and older adults. Often in the younger age range there are more developmental considerations that need to be taken into account. Babies are predominantly obligatory nose breathers and use their abdominal muscles during respiration compared to the older child and adult. As previously mentioned their respiratory rates and rhythms are also altered. Their respiratory depth is assessed by observing the degree of movement in the abdominal wall in children under the age of seven years and in the chest wall in older children and adults (Hazinski, 1999).

As adults age there may be reduced lung function as elastic fibres are less compliant and therefore stretch less; this means that chest expansion may be reduced. In those patients that have structural chest deformities these may become more severe or pronounced due to the ageing process and hence may cause more restriction on lung function as they get older compared to when they were younger. Hence the older adult may start to develop problems related to their respiratory system later in life.

> **✷ Activity 9.3**
>
> Ask a physiotherapist to show you how they intervene with a patient who experiences difficulties in expectorating.
>
> Interventions may include postural drainage, percussion and vibration as well as breathing exercises.

Documentation

Once the assessment process is completed all findings must be carefully recorded. As with any aspect of nursing care it is a requirement that thorough and accurate documentation is maintained (NMC, 2008). Where this information is documented may vary in each clinical area, so ensure that the correct forms are being used to record information appropriately. Documentation recorded by student nurses must be countersigned by the supervising registered nurse. Findings must also be reported to senior nursing and medical staff with the appropriate degree of urgency.

Investigations

There are a variety of investigations that can be undertaken to confirm diagnosis or to provide information regarding effectiveness of any treatment or any changes in patients' condition. Those most commonly associated with the respiratory system are peak expiratory flow rate, pulse oximetry, arterial blood gas analysis (ABG) and chest X-ray. Only the former two will be addressed as they are non-invasive and easy to undertake both in clinical and non-clinical environments.

Peak expiratory flow rate (PEFR)

This may be referred to more frequently as 'peak flow' and will require the patient to take a deep breath and then blow/puff out as hard and fast as possible into a peak flow meter placed in their mouth (see Figure 9.2).

As the name suggests it provides information about the patient's ability to breathe out quickly. Conditions such as asthma and COPD mean that patients have difficulty breathing out as air becomes trapped within the alveoli. It is particularly useful to complete PEFR pre (before) and post (after) any treatment or medication, particularly bronchodilator medication to determine its effectiveness. Some patients find this very difficult to accomplish and this may affect their technique and therefore the measurement obtained may be inaccurate. Patients in any respiratory distress will be unable to perform this procedure until their condition has stabilised.

Pulse oximetry

pulse oximetry
a photodiagnostic method of monitoring arterial blood oxygen saturation (SaO$_2$)

Pulse oximetry is an easy, non-invasive method which can be performed anywhere and provides information about the percentage of haemoglobin that is saturated with oxygen (Higgins, 2005). It is often described as the fifth vital sign.

The pulse oximeter has a probe which consists of a light emitting diode (sensor) that transmits both red and infrared light waves which are received by a light sensitive photodiode (detector). Placing the probe onto a patient's fingertip enables these light waves to be transmitted through the skin and hence the peripheral vascular bed. As saturated and desaturated haemoglobin are a different colour, the oximeter can then detect the percentage of saturated haemoglobin in the blood. Other body sites that can be used include; toe, ear lobe and bridge of nose, although these may require different probes to be used.

The probe can either be placed on the patient's finger constantly to provide continuous information or when a reading is required. It is important to ensure that if continuous monitoring is required that the probe needs to change position to prevent the risk of pressure damage to the skin (Higgins, 2005).

The oxygen saturation, as recorded by pulse oximetry, can supply important information about the lungs' capacity for gaseous exchange, but it cannot measure ventilation or carbon dioxide levels in the blood and so must be regarded as part of the respiratory assessment strategy, and not relied upon alone.

There are various factors that can cause the pulse oximeter to obtain inaccurate information. These include patients who have severe anaemia, poor vascular perfusion, are wearing nail varnish, shivering, and have carbon monoxide poisoning which causes false high results.

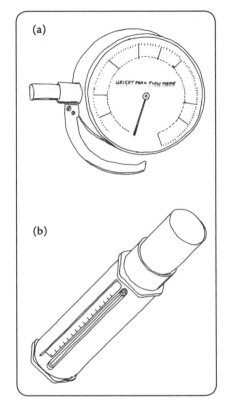

Figure 9.2 Peak flow meters

Nursing Interventions

Airway maintenance

The mechanism of breathing consists of two phases, inspiration and expiration. For breathing to occur, a **patent airway** is required at all times. If a patient is unable to maintain their own airway, interventions to maintain airway patency are essential.

Airway is a generic term for those parts of the respiratory system through which atmospheric air containing oxygen flows. If any part of the airway is obstructed the flow of air and oxygen is impeded and hypoxia can result. If not managed appropriately, this can lead to tissue injury, damage to vital organs, cardiac **dysrhythmias** and ultimately death.

Undergraduate medical and nursing training incorporates primary assessment of 'ABCDE' utilising a 'Look – Listen – Feel' approach to substantiate all clinical data to make an informed opinion about the patient. It is nurses in particular who are in a pivotal position to observe, monitor and intervene to ensure airway maintenance (Smith and Poplett, 2002).

Nursing interventions related to airway maintenance are:

- patient positioning
- simple airway manoeuvres
- use of airway adjuncts
- oro-pharyngeal suctioning
- administration of supplemental oxygen
- administration of drugs by inhalation.

Observing and questioning the patient will generate useful initial information with regard to their airway and respiratory status; if the patient is alert and orientated this instantly indicates that the airway is patent and cerebral perfusion is adequate.

Positioning

The most common cause of airway obstruction in the hospitalised patient is pharyngeal obstruction by the tongue due to an altered level of consciousness. The altered level of consciousness may be caused by an elective procedure which is managed by health-care practitioners (for example administration of **general anaesthetic** or other pharmacological agents including intravenous **sedation** and **opiate** analgesia).

The airway can be opened using a 'head tilt – chin lift' technique to move the tongue away from the oropharyngeal space (Figure 9.3). It must be remembered that this position must be continually held to achieve this outcome. As a busy health-care practitioner, holding this position indefinitely may well be impossible and the use of airway adjuncts and/or nursing the patient on their side will be necessary.

Appropriate positioning of the patient is fundamental to assist with airway patency and maximise 'vital capacity'. Vital capacity is the total amount of

patent airway
an airway that is opened and unblocked

dysrhythmias
irregular heart/cardiac rhythm

general anaesthetic
absence of sensation and consciousness as induced by anaesthetic drugs given by inhalation or intravenously

sedation
a state of quiet, calmness or sleep induced by a sedative or hypnotic drug

opiate
a powerful analgesic which can cause respiratory depression

tidal volume
the amount inhaled and exhaled during normal breathing

inspiratory reserve volume
the maximum amount of air that can be inhaled

expiratory reserve volume
the maximum amount of air that can be exhaled

orthopnoeic position
a body position that enables a patient to breath effectively. This is often sitting up, or bent forward with the arms supported on a table or chair arms

airway adjunct
a medical device utilised to maintain airway patency

laryngospasm
involuntary muscular contractions of the larynx which may obstruct the airway

exchangeable air and represents the sum of **tidal**, **inspiratory reserve** and **expiratory reserve volumes**.

Oxygenation is reduced in a patient in the supine position, the **orthopnoeic position** is the best position to maximise deep breathing and vital capacity, if the patient is conscious.

Deep breathing exercises should be encouraged as they assist airway clearance, improve respiratory muscle function and gaseous exchange.

Patients who are unable to maintain their own airway may benefit from the insertion of an **airway adjunct** to maintain patency.

Oropharyngeal airways

Oropharyngeal airways (still sometimes known clinically as Guedel airways, see Figure 9.4) can be used in the unconscious patient to maintain airway patency. It should be noted that if one of these adjuncts is inserted, the patient has to be in a completely unconscious state to tolerate the device. As the patient's level of consciousness increases the device will stimulate the gag reflex, which may initiate choking, **laryngospasm**, retching and/or vomiting resulting in an increased risk of aspiration of any stomach content into the lungs.

Oropharyngeal airways come in different sizes (colour coded) and are constructed from hard, curved, rigid plastic. The device has a reinforced and fully integrated bite block segment and the mouth piece rests between the patient's incisors. The bite block ensures that the patient cannot occlude the airway by biting on it. An approximate size assessment can be made by measuring the vertical distance between the angle of the mandible and centre of the incisors, which is roughly the length of airway required. The airway is inserted concave side uppermost (upside down) and rotated 180 degrees at the point where the hard palate meets the soft palate in the roof of the mouth. The device 'holds and maintains' the tongue within the curved segment and prevents migration into the oropharyngeal space.

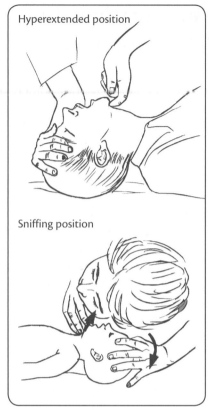

Figure 9.3 Airway opening manoeuvre

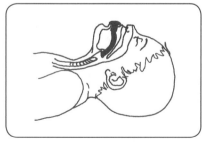

Figure 9.4 Guedel's (oropharyngeal) airway

Naso-pharyngeal airways

Another airway adjunct available to assist with airway patency is the naso-pharyngeal airway. This may be utilised in the patient who is in either a conscious or unconscious state. A contraindication for the use of this airway adjunct is in the patient with known nasal polyps or suspected base of skull fracture. Caution is also warranted in patients with coagulation disorders.

Some nasal airways require the insertion of a safety pin into the outer rim of the flange, to prevent the airway migrating into the nostrils. Other nasal airways have larger flanges which will ensure that this cannot occur. It is essential to ascertain whether or not a safety pin is required, and ensure that one is used if necessary.

Lubrication of the external component of the tube is necessary prior to insertion. Ideally, the tube is inserted into the right nostril, because when the tube is in position the bevel lies outermost within the oropharyngeal space, maximising airway patency. If the left nostril is used and the patient has any degree of angioedema (soft tissue swelling) of the oropharyngeal space, the tube may be partially occluded. If there is any obstruction or difficulty during the insertion procedure, the tube must not be forced. This could cause trauma to the nostrils and result in **epistaxis** which could compromise the airway further.

epistaxis
bleeding from the nose

Oropharyngeal suctioning

Oropharyngeal suctioning may be required to maintain the patency of the airway, by the removal of secretions or debris in the mouth (blood, vomit) to prevent obstruction and the aspiration of such material into the lungs. Appropriate infection control measures must be observed when undertaking suctioning.

If airway patency cannot be maintained using these methods then escalation to advanced airway/respiratory management will be required, necessitating intervention by senior nursing or medical staff.

Supplemental oxygen

The administration of **supplemental oxygen** should now be based on guidelines produced by the British Thoracic Society. This document outlines specific measures to ensure safe and effective administration of oxygen (British Thoracic Society, 2008).

The guideline suggests that supplemental oxygen should be administered to hypoxic patients to achieve normal or near normal oxygen saturations for all acutely ill patients, apart from those at risk of hypercapnic respiratory failure (Type 2 respiratory failure) or those receiving terminal palliative care. Hypercapnic respiratory failure can be worsened by high concentrations of oxygen, and any patient with a history of this type of failure, or who may be at risk – notably some patients with COPD – should be given oxygen in controlled amounts and under close observation.

Recommended target oxygen saturations are:

supplemental oxygen
the addition of a flow of oxygen via an oxygen device to remedy oxygen deficiency within the body

- 94–98 per cent for most acutely ill patients
- 88–92 per cent for those at risk of hypercapnic respiratory failure (type 2 respiratory failure).

Oxygen is one of the most widely used drugs in a variety of clinical settings and specialities. The principle highlighted by the guidelines is that oxygen should be treated in the same way as other prescribed medications – only to be administered to patients who have a clinical need. Oxygen saturations (SaO_2) must be measured by pulse oximetry to determine the effects of oxygen administration, and it should be administered to treat hypoxia (oxygen saturation below 94 per cent) and not breathlessness. Oxygen does not have any effect on the sensation of breathlessness in the non-hypoxic patient.

In an emergency situation, oxygen is administered to patients immediately without a formal prescription. The lack of a prescription should never preclude oxygen being given when needed in an emergency situation.

Oxygen delivery systems

This section outlines the main types of oxygen delivery systems available in clinical practice for the delivery of oxygen therapy.

Nasal cannulae

These are one of the most common devices for oxygen delivery. Nasal cannulae consist of two soft prongs attached to the oxygen supply tubing. The prongs are positioned in the patient's nostrils and the tubing is looped around the patient's ears and the 'toggle' adjusted to promote a secure and comfortable fit. Oxygen then flows from the cannulae into the patient's nasopharynx which acts as an anatomic reservoir. The actual concentration of the oxygen received by the patient will vary dependent upon the flow rate administered and the patient's breathing pattern.

The device is lightweight and well tolerated by patients; the patient is also able to eat, drink and speak with the device in situ. Nasal cannulae are contraindicated in any patient with nasal obstruction, but they can benefit 'mouth breathers'.

Oxygen can be delivered at up to six litres per minute in adults. Flow rates of 4 litres or less do not need to be humidified. Nasal cannulae are available in different sizes (from adult to paediatric).

As nasal cannulae can deliver low to medium concentration of oxygen, they are suitable for a wide variety of patients including some patients with COPD. They are not appropriate for the administration of high concentrations of oxygen.

Simple face masks

These devices are sometimes known as 'MC' or medium concentration masks and they offer another common clinical alternative for the delivery of low flow oxygen therapy. Face masks are indicated if higher concentrations of oxygen are required which cannot be met by nasal cannulae or when nostrils cannot be used. Face masks are available in different sizes (from adult to paediatric). Some masks have nose clips to improve comfort and fit and some have ear loops for simple fitting when the patient's head cannot be raised (for example cervical spine injury).

The flow meter (which ranges from 1–15 litres per minute) is set to give the prescribed oxygen concentration. The mask is then fitted over the patient's nose and mouth and the elastic tightened to give a secure and comfortable fit. If the mask has a nose clip, it is pinched to optimise overall fit and comfort. Aspiration of vomit is also more likely when a face mask is in place, as the mask may prevent vomit from being quickly expelled from the mouth.

If utilising facemasks for oxygen delivery, flow rate must be 5 litres and above to wash carbon dioxide out of the mask and prevent re-breathing and excessive respiratory work (British Thoracic Society, 2008).

Simple face masks can deliver between 40 and 60 per cent, but because the actual concentration delivered cannot be precisely controlled, such masks are not suitable for patients at risk of hypercapnic respiratory failure.

High concentration reservoir masks

High concentration reservoir masks (also known as non-rebreathing masks) are used to deliver oxygen in higher concentrations, mainly in high risk or critically ill patients. With these devices, as the patient breathes from the mask a non-return valve is opened so the breath is taken from the reservoir bag. Minimal room air is therefore inhaled and on exhalation air escapes from the mask through exhalation valves. This device delivers up to 80 per cent oxygen with flows between 10 and 15 litres of oxygen per minute.

The design and fit of the mask and the patient's breathing pattern will affect the amount of room air entrained and actual oxygen concentration delivered. Flow rate is initially set at 15 litres and the oxygen reservoir inflated by occluding the one-way valve in the mask with a finger and directing the oxygen flow into the reservoir. Once inflated the mask is securely and comfortably placed onto the patient. Oxygen flow rate must be adjusted (between 10 and 15 litres) to allow the reservoir bag to deflate by approximately one-third on each inspiration, but not empty completely. The minimal flow rate for this is 10 litres per minute.

When administering supplemental oxygen via nasal cannulae, simple face mask or high concentration reservoir masks, it is important to remember that although the oxygen flow rate can be set and recorded, the actual delivered oxygen concentration (**FiO2**) can vary and will depend on the following variables:

FiO$_2$
fraction of inspired oxygen, expressed as a percentage, for example 28 per cent

- tidal volume – the amount of air inhaled and exhaled during normal breathing
- peak inspired flow rate – the greatest rate of airflow that can be achieved during inspiration with the lungs deflated
- mask fit – how closely the mask is fitted onto the patient's face to minimise air leakage
- oral or nasal breathing pattern
- breathing rate.

Venturi masks

Venturi masks are used to deliver an accurate concentration of oxygen to the patient regardless of the oxygen flow rate. The oxygen concentration remains constant because of the **Venturi principle**: the flow of oxygen into the mask is diluted by room air which is entrained into the system via the colour-coded valve on the mask. Higher flow rates of oxygen will suck in more room air, so the concentration of oxygen remains the same. The Venturi mask system has several colour-coded valves which deliver varying concentrations of oxygen, and the manufacturer's instructions should be consulted to ascertain the correct flow rate required to deliver the prescribed percentage of oxygen.

Venturi principle
a principle of physics related to the flow of gases under pressure. This effect is a factor in the design of respiratory therapy equipment for mixing medical gases

Venturi masks are available to deliver 24, 28, 35, 40 and 60 per cent oxygen. They are suitable for any patient who requires a known concentration of oxygen, but the 24 per cent and 28 per cent masks are particularly suited to patients known to be at risk of carbon dioxide retention.

Humidification

Humidification is not required for the delivery of low flow oxygen or for the short-term use of high flow oxygen. Humidification is recommended for patients who require high flow oxygen delivery systems for more than 24 hours or for the patient who reports upper airway discomfort due to dryness (British Thoracic Society, 2008).

The administration of drugs by inhalation

⬭ Link

Chapter 6 discusses administration of drugs via inhalation.

A common intervention to support respiratory function is the administration of drugs. Drugs affecting the respiratory system can be administered orally or intravenously, as with other body systems; however, it is also possible to administer drugs by inhalation directly into the respiratory tract. The advantage of this route is that local effects can be achieved rapidly, whilst some of the side-effects which arise from oral administration can be avoided, as smaller doses can be administered which will still be effective (*British National Formulary*, 2007).

Inhaled drugs are administered via:

- inhalers
- nebulisers.

Inhalers

Inhalers are commonly used in the treatment of asthma and COPD. A wide variety of inhalers are available for prescription and they fall into three categories:

1 Metered-dose inhalers (MDIs) which use pressurised propellants to deliver the drug into the lungs when triggered manually by the patient. This involves a high degree of coordination between the patient's breathing in to inhale the drug, and dexterity in triggering the device at the correct moment .This is not achievable for babies and young children, and can be very difficult for the elderly and those with learning disabilities.

2 Breath-activated inhalers are triggered by the patient inhaling and so coordination is not required. Such devices may therefore be a more appropriate choice for some patients.

3 Dry powder inhalers, which are also activated by inhalation.

'Spacers' or holding chambers are plastic devices which are used in conjunction with MDIs to remove the need for coordination between triggering the MDI and inhalation. They are very effective in the administration of medication, significantly increasing the amount of drug delivered into the lungs; indeed evidence suggests that used correctly, a MDI in conjunction with a 'spacer' device is as effective as nebulisation in the treatment of acute bronchospasm (Cates et al., 2006). Spacers also reduce the incidence of oral thrush (oral candidiasis) which can be a side-effect of inhaled corticosteroid drugs, used to control asthma.

It is very important to ensure that patients can correctly use the device(s) prescribed for them, as poor technique can greatly reduce the amount of drug actually delivered into the airways, which can be as low as 7–20 per cent of the original dose administered (Price et al., 2004). Whenever caring for patients with respiratory disease, an assessment of inhaler technique is crucial, even when patients have been using their delivery system for some time, perhaps many years, as psycho-motor skills can deteriorate.

Nurses involved in such assessment should familiarise themselves with the manufacturer's instructions for the particular device, discuss these with the patient, and then observe the patient's technique on several occasions to ensure correct use. If the patient is unable to follow the instructions correctly, education should be provided or another device prescribed that is more appropriate.

Nebulisers

A nebuliser converts a solution of a drug into an aerosol for inhalation. They are used to deliver higher doses of a drug than can be administered with inhalers, particularly in emergency situations. They are usually driven by gas which can be either air or oxygen. For most patients (particularly those who are already suffering hypoxia or are dependent on additional oxygen), nebulised drugs should be administered via oxygen – indeed it could be very dangerous not to do so, as the time taken to deliver the required amount of drug solution may cause dangerous hypoxia if air is used. In a small number of patients with chronic lung disease (for example COPD, cystic fibrosis) changes to the respiratory control mechanisms in the brain can result in an inability to tolerate high levels of oxygen, and in these patients, nebulised drugs should be administered on air. It is suggested that controlled levels of oxygen (low levels) can be administered to such patients via nasal cannula, whilst they are receiving their nebulised medication. This will ensure that a constant oxygen supply is delivered (British Thoracic Society, 2008).

As with all drugs, only a registered nurse can administer inhalers, nebulisers or oxygen. Student nurses may participate in the administration of these drugs for education purposes, under the direct supervision of the registered nurse (NMC, 2007). In addition, local hospital trust's drug administration policies must be adhered to at all times.

Psychological care

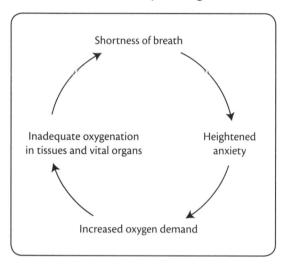

Figure 9.5 The vicious cycle of breathlessness and increased oxygen demands

All patients with respiratory problems will be anxious. Dyspnoea is a very distressing symptom and patients who feel that they cannot breathe properly for any reason will be very frightened indeed. Fear and anxiety may result in rapid, shallow, panicky ventilation which is inefficient in terms of oxygenating the body. As physiological stress responses increase the metabolic rate and therefore increase oxygen demand, a vicious cycle can develop (Cutler and Murch, 2003) (Figure 9.5).

Nurses should endeavour to interrupt this cycle, to reduce patient anxiety and enable more effective respiration to occur. Clearly this is not an easy task, but the development of a close, therapeutic relationship with the patient is important. A calm and knowledgeable approach, coupled with good communication skills is essential, and other strategies may prove helpful:

- Cognitive interventions, such as providing appropriate levels of information, to ensure that the patient understands what is happening.
- Behavioural interventions, such as controlled breathing and relaxation techniques.
- Sensory interventions, such as appropriate touch, and music.
- Pharmacological interventions, such as anxiolytic drugs are occasionally used, but this must be with extreme caution, as respiratory depression may be caused.

Some interventions will be more effective in some patients than others and it must be appreciated that it is not appropriate to try to teach deep breathing and relaxation techniques to an acutely dyspnoeic patient. Some patients with chronic lung disease, however, are very familiar with such strategies and can be encouraged to use them when necessary. For many patients the nurse can provide a reassuring presence, just 'being there' and encouraging the patient to breathe as slowly and deeply as they can, can be very helpful and has the advantage of ensuring that the patient is under constant observation.

Every nurse has a professional responsibility to ensure that they are prepared to interpret, and act upon, the findings of clinical assessment in a timely and appropriate manner. All nurses must be able to initiate and evaluate interventions commensurate with their level of training and scope of clinical practice, and be able to communicate appropriately the need for assistance from other specialist practitioners within the multidisciplinary team.

? Test yourself!

1   What is the normal respiratory rate for a 2-year-old child?

2   What are Cheyne-Stokes respirations?

3   Describe four types of sputum and their causes.

4   What is the target oxygen saturation range for adults with no history of lung disease?

British Thoracic Society (2008) The executive summary of the guideline for emergency oxygen use in adult patients. *Thorax* (October) **63**(6). www.brit-thoracic.org.uk/emergencyoxygen

Jarvis, C. (2004) *Physical Examination and Health Assessment*, 4th edn. Saunders, Philadelphia.

Marieb, E. and Hoehn, K. (2010) *Human Anatomy and Physiology*, 8th edn. Pearson Benjamin Cummings, San Francisco.

 Further Reading

For live links to useful websites see: www.palgrave.com/nursinghealth/hogston

---

References

British National Formulary 54 September. (2007) BMJ Publishing Group Ltd, London.

British Thoracic Society (2008) The executive summary of the guideline for emergency oxygen use in adult patients. *Thorax* (October) **63**(6). www.brit-thoracic.org.uk/emergencyoxygen

Cates, C.J., Crilly, J.A. and Rowe, B.H. (2006) Holding chambers (spacers) versus nebulisers for beta-agonist treatment of acute asthma. *Cochrane Database of Systematic Reviews*. Issue 2 Art. No. CD000052.

Cutler, L. and Murch, P. (2003) The respiratory system. In Bassett, C. (ed.) *Essentials of Nursing Care*. Whurr Publishers, London.

Epstein, O., Perkin, G., Cookson, J., Watt, I., Rakhit, R., Robins, A. and Hornett, G. (eds) (2008) *Clinical Examination*, 4th edn. Mosby, Edinburgh.

Hazinski, M. (1999) *Manual of Nursing Care in the Critically Ill*. Mosby, St Louis.

Higgins, D. (2005) Pulse oximetry. *Nursing Times* **101**(6): 34.

Kennedy, S. (2007) Detecting changes in the respiratory status of ward patients. *Nursing Standard* **21**(49): 42–6.

Moore, T. (2007) Respiratory assessment in adults. *Nursing Standard* **21**(49): 48–56.

NMC (Nursing and Midwifery Council) (2007) *Standards for Medicines Management*. NMC, London. www.nmc-uk.org

NMC (Nursing and Midwifery Council) (2008) *The NMC Code of Professional Conduct: Standards for Conduct, Performance and Ethics*. NMC, London. www.nmc-uk.org

Price, D., Foster, J., Scullion, J. and Freeman, D. (2004) *In Clinical Practice Series: Asthma and COPD*. Churchill Livingstone, London.

Smith, G. (2003) *ALERT; Acute Life Threatening Events: Recognition and Treatment*. University of Portsmouth, Portsmouth.

Smith, G. and Poplett, N. (2002) Knowledge of aspects of acute care in trainee doctors. *Post Graduate Medical Journal* **78**: 335–8.

Weiteska, S., Mackaway-Jones, K. and Phillips, B. (2005) *Advanced Paediatric Life Support: The Practical Approach*, 4th edn. BMJ Publishing Ltd, London.

10

Circulation

📖 Contents

- Introduction
- Common Disease Processes Affecting the Circulatory System
- Circulatory Assessment
- Nursing Interventions
- Chapter Summary
- Test Yourself!
- References

Learning outcomes

The purpose of this chapter is to examine factors associated with cardiac function. It will explore the nurse's role in relation to assessing and implementing care with clients who experience difficulties with maintaining circulation. At the end of the chapter, you should be able to:

- Monitor and interpret a client's cardiac vital signs
- Rationalise common deviations from normal values
- Identify techniques for maintaining cardiac function
- Assist clients in maintaining effective cardiac function
- Recognise the signs of cardiac arrest
- Describe the appropriate response and initial management of a collapsed client.

Introduction

The purpose of the circulatory system is to provide an adequate blood flow to vital organs such as the heart and brain. An adequate circulation ensures the delivery of oxygen and nutrients to the body tissues, the removal of carbon dioxide and waste products and the dissipation of heat from active organs to ensure temperature regulation. Effective circulation is achieved via two separate circuits, the systemic and pulmonary circulations, both of which originate and terminate within the heart. In order to better understand the physiological and anatomical principles of circulation and the cardiovascular system, your lecturers may recommend specialist texts on the subject, for example Marieb and Hoehn (2010).

This chapter will specifically focus upon the common disease processes which affect the circulatory system and detail the circulatory nursing assessments and interventions which are utilised when caring for patients.

Common Disease Processes Affecting the Circulatory System

As described above, an adequate circulation of blood is necessary to ensure **homeostasis**. Any disturbance in the circulatory system can therefore have a profound physiological impact.

Vascular disease (including coronary heart disease (CHD), stroke and kidney disease) is the biggest killer in the UK, leading to 200,000 deaths a year and is responsible for a fifth of all hospital admissions (DoH, 2007). Risk factors for the development of vascular disease include tobacco use, high cholesterol levels, hypertension, diabetes, familial risk factors and lack of physical exercise. In relation to the heart, **atherosclerosis** leads to the narrowing of coronary arteries, and the resultant decreased oxygen supply to the myocardium leads to **ischaemia**, which the patient may experience as angina. Further narrowing of the coronary arteries (normally due to a blood clot (**thrombus**) forming within the atherosclerotic artery) can lead to acute coronary syndromes, such as unstable angina and myocardial **infarction**, as well as sudden cardiac death (Resuscitation Council UK, 2006).

Changes in the heart rhythm can also decrease the efffectiveness of the heart as a pump, and **atrial fibrillation** (AF) in particular becomes more prevalent with age with 0.5 per cent of the population aged 50–59 having this condition, compared with 8.8 per cent of the 80–89 year age group (Swanton, 2003). AF can lead to a decreased cardiac output and is also a major cause of strokes as the ineffective pumping action of the heart can lead to the accumulation of clots within the left atrium of the heart, which can then be dispersed as arterial **emboli** (NICE, 2006).

Atherosclerosis is also a major contributing factor to the development of systemic arterial problems. Severe peripheral vascular disease may lead to leg ischaemia and subsequent gangrene which may neccesitate amputation, while atherosclerosis of the arteries, which supply the brain with oxygen, can lead to

homeostasis
the state of relative stability or equilibrium of the body

atherosclerosis
a build up of fats and white blood cells within the lumen of an artery. This narrows the lumen, and makes the vessel less elastic

ischaemia
insufficient blood supply to the tissues. May result in infarction

infarction
the death of tissues (necrosis) due to the lack of an oxygenated blood supply

thrombus (pl. thrombi)
a clot of blood formed in the heart or blood vessels

atrial fibrillation
an irregular and ineffective heart rhythm

embolus (pl. emboli)
an object that travels from one part of the body to another part within the blood stream, and then lodges in a blood vessel to either partially or completely block it. An embolus is most commonly a blood clot, but it can also be comprised of fat, air, bacteria, amniotic fluid or a foreign body

brain ischaemia and infarction. Abdominal aortic aneurysms (AAAs) are another significant systemic vascular problem which predominantly affect men aged over 65 years. A third of AAAs will suddenly rupture, leading to rapid cardiovascular collapse, and subsequent death unless emergency surgery is performed. Even with surgical intervention many patients, however, will still die due to profound cardiovascular instability, and factors such as co-morbidity and multi-organ failure; and the overall mortality rate for AAAs is 65–85 per cent (DoH, 2008a).

The main pathological condition affecting the pulmonary circulation is pulmonary embolus (PE). PEs have been identified as a common phenomena, which left untreated are associated with high morbidity and mortality and are thought to account for over 25,000 deaths in the UK each year (House of Commons Health Committee, 2005). Goldhaber (1997) identifies that the majority of PEs result from thrombi which have their origins in either the pelvic veins or the deep veins of the leg (deep vein thrombosis (DVT)). These DVTs are the result of a combination of factors, including sluggish blood flow, compression of a vein, hypercoagulopathy, or local injury (Camm and Bunce, 2005). Risk factors for the development of DVTs include surgery (especially orthopaedic and abdominal), decreased mobility, including hospitalisation, malignancy, pregnancy and long-distance sedentary travel (British Thoracic Society, 2003). When these thrombi dislodge, the subsequent emboli then follow the venous system through to the right side of the heart and then into the pulmonary arterial system. This can lead to chest pain and shortness of breath, while a massive PE can lead to collapse and death.

Any significant cardiovascular dysfunction can result in circulatory shock, whereby tissue perfusion with oxygen and nutrients is inadequate for the body's metabolic requirements. Some of the more common causes of shock are listed in Chart 10.1. Some of the early signs of shock can include an increasing pulse and respiratory rate, a narrowing pulse presssure (the difference between the systolic and diastolic blood pressures), and the increasing restlessness of the patient, while a drop in blood pressure is most often associated with more profound shock and decompensation (American College of Surgeons Committee on Trauma, 2008). The early identification of shock is therefore vital and the nurse needs to be vigilant for any deterioration in the clinical condition of the patient. It is vitally important that when the circulatory system and other vital signs are assessed, that the findings are both promptly interpreted and acted upon. Many

Chart 10.1 The common causes of shock

• Hypovolaemic	for example	Haemorrhage, Gastroenteritis, Burns
• Cardiogenic	for example	Heart failure, Arrhythmias
• Distributive	for example	Sepsis, Anaphylaxis
• Obstructive	for example	Tension pneumothorax, Cardiac tamponade, Pulmonary embolus
• Dissociative	for example	Anaemia, Carbon monoxide poisoning

Source: *Advanced Paediatric Life Support: The Practical Approach*. 4th Edition. Advanced Life Support Group (2005). Reproduced with permission.

hospitals now use early warning scores (EWS), and NICE (2007) have proposed that such strategies are necessary to ensure that nursing staff are empowered to alert specialist teams when the condition of patients deteriorates. Consider the patient in Casebox 10.1, and determine what course of action would be most appropriate in this case.

Mabel Thompson, a 55-year-old lady, has returned to the day surgery unit from the operating theatre following surgical removal of varicose veins in her right leg. Her initial blood pressure on return to the ward was 114/65, heart rate was 86, and respiratory rate was 16. Her pain score was 2 out of 10.

One hour later one of the health-care assistants on the ward reports that the vital signs are as follows:

- BP = 88/62
- HR = 118
- RR = 28

Mabel is restless and agitated. What should the nurse do now?

- The nurse needs to call for additional help, and should assess the patient in more detail. One system of assessment is the primary survey (Airway Breathing Circulation Disability Exposure – Resuscitation Council (UK) 2006).

On exposing the patient's wound site (as part of the circulatory assessment), the primary survey reveals that both the dressings and the bed linen are soaked with blood. What should the nurse do now?

- The nurse has noted a significant post-operative bleed, which has led to hypovolaemic shock. The nurse needs to apply pressure to the wound site, elevate the leg and ensure that any prescribed fluid and oxygen are administered. The patient has a high Early Warning Score, and thus the nurse should initiate a call to the surgical team who performed the operation; and in some hospitals a Medical Emergency Team can also be summoned – they will be able to assist with stabilising the patient's condition prior to a transfer back to theatres.

Circulatory Assessment

Due to the prevalence of conditions such as those detailed in the section above, it is essential that a thorough physical assessment of cardiovascular function should be undertaken as an integral part of the nursing process. This assessment should include an examination of heart rate, blood pressure, peripheral perfusion and fluid balance. In the context of chest pain, an electrocardiogram (ECG) and pain assessment should also be undertaken.

Heart rate

The heart rate is most commonly assessed by calculating the pulse rate. As the left ventricle of the heart contracts, blood is forced from the left ventricle into the aorta. This creates an arterial pressure change, which in turn leads to a wave of distension which can be felt in the arterial wall. This is known as the **pulse** (Chart 10.2).

The pulse rate is the number of beats in a 60-second period. It is calculated most accurately by counting the number of beats felt within a full period of 60 seconds or, at a minimum, over a 30-second period, then doubling the result. Accuracy is particularly important and is most difficult in patients who have a fast or irregular heart rate. Normal heart rates for children and adults are shown in Table 10.1.

✴ Activity 10.1

Count your resting pulse and respiratory rate. Run up a flight of about 10 stairs five times. Count your pulse and respiratory rate now and again after 2 minutes. Chart these readings and note the correlation between the respiratory and pulse rates.

Consider what physiological changes have occurred. There is usually a 1:4 or 1:5 differential between the respiratory and pulse rates.

pulse
the wave of distension felt in an artery as the heart contracts

Chart 10.2 Hints for pulse measurement

The pulse is detected by placing two fingers over an artery close to a bony or firm surface. The most common site used for pulse rate detection in adults and children over the age of one years is the radial pulse because it is one of most easily detected and accessible sites. This can be felt on the anterior aspect of the wrist (Figure 10.1). The arm should be supported and relaxed, and the palm rotated uppermost. The pulse should be felt with the index and middle fingers over the groove along the thumb side of the wrist. Toddlers may need distracting to ensure accurate counting of the pulse. Further sites available for pulse rate palpation are shown in Figure 10.2. In infants (children under one year of age) the most reliable method used for calculating the heart rate is to measure the apical rate by placing a stethoscope over the chest at the apex of the heart (Glasper et al., 2007). When assessing a person's pulse, three factors should be observed: its rate, rhythm and strength.

tachycardia
a heart rate which is faster than 100 beats per minute in an adult

A heart rate faster than the normal values shown in Table 10.1 is known as a **tachycardia**. In adults this is considered to occur when the heart rate is over 100 beats per minute. Causes of an increased heart rate include exercise, stress, fear, excitement, pyrexia (fever), blood or fluid loss, certain drugs and heart conditions (for example **atrial fibrillation** and cardiac failure).

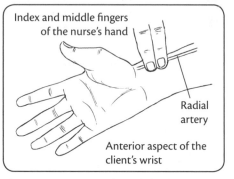

Figure 10.1 Locating the radial pulse

A heart rate slower than the normal values shown in Table 10.1 is known

bradycardia
a heart rate which is slower than 60 beats per minute in an adult

digoxin
a drug that slows, steadies and strengthens the heart beat, and is used for arrhythmias such as atrial fibrillation

beta-blockers
drugs that slow the heart rate and reduce the blood pressure

as a **bradycardia**. In adults this is considered to occur when the heart rate is less than 60 beats per minute. Causes of a slow heart rate include hypothermia, certain drugs (for example **digoxin** and **beta-blockers**), activation of the parasympathetic nervous system (for example during sleep or rest), certain heart conditions (such as heart block, which results from a disorder of the conduction system) and raised intracranial pressure following a brain haemorrhage. A slow heart rate may also be a normal finding in fit athletic individuals.

Table 10.1 Normal heart rates for children and adults

Age (years)	Heart rate (beats per minute)
<1	110–160
1–2	100–150
2–5	95–140
5–12	80–120
12–Adult	60–100

Source: *Advanced Paediatric Life Support: The Practical Approach.* 4th Edition. Advanced Life Support Group (2005). Reproduced with permission.

✳ Activity 10.2

Identify three drugs that can increase the heart rate. Look up how they do this in a pharmacology reference book.

Now carry out Activity 10.2. Did you consider:
- *Atropine:* increases the heart rate by inhibiting the parasympathetic nervous system. It can be used in asystolic cardiac arrests; with patients who are unwell with bradycardias; and pre-operatively to limit the effects of the vagal nerve.
- *Thyroxine:* replacement therapy for clients with an underactive thyroid gland. When taken in excess this drug will increase the metabolic rate and heart rate.

- *Adrenaline* (epinephrine): its actions resemble those of the sympathetic nervous system, thereby increasing heart rate and strength of contraction. It also causes peripheral vasoconstriction, which allows more blood to be diverted to the central organs, such as the heart and brain (Resuscitation Council (UK), 2006). It is for this reason that adrenaline is one of the key drugs used in cardiac arrest.

The accurate recording and reporting of an abnormally fast or slow heart rate is essential. It will often indicate a sudden change in a person's condition that needs to be further assessed and possibly treated. Furthermore, extreme bradycardia and tachycardia result in inadequate filling of the coronary arteries, which can lead to myocardial ischaemia and infarction. In addition, a lack of oxygenated blood to the brain (hypoxia) initially leads to confusion and disorientation, and can ultimately lead to brain damage.

The strength or volume of the pulse is important because it can provide an indication of the person's cardiac function, cardiac output and probable blood pressure. Table 10.2 outlines the relationship between palpable pulse sites and systolic blood pressure. A pulse that is weak and difficult to feel is often described as 'thready'. A thready pulse will usually be rapid and may be obliterated by pressure on the artery, suggesting that the patient is dehydrated, bleeding or exhausted. In such cases, it may be necessary to feel the carotid or femoral pulse. A very strong and bounding pulse may be the result of infection, stress, anaemia or exercise. A pulse which quickly disappears or 'collapses' may indicate a Corrigan's or waterhammer pulse, which is a feature of aortic valve regurgitation (Swanton, 2003). The first half of the pulse is normal or full but, after reaching its peak, the wave suddenly recedes under the finger.

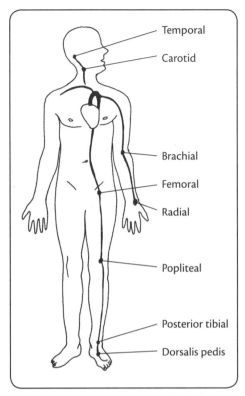

Figure 10.2 Common sites in the body for pulse palpation

Table 10.2 The correlation between palpable pulses and systolic blood pressure

Palpable pulse site	Systolic blood pressure
Radial	>80 mmHg
Femoral	>70 mmHg
Carotid	>60 mmHg

Source: Greaves et al. (2001). Reproduced by permission of Edward Arnold (Publishers) Limited.

The rhythm of the pulse is the pattern in which the beats occur. In a healthy person, the pattern or rhythm is regular because the chambers of the heart are contracting in a coordinated manner, producing a regular pulse beat. In children and young adults the pulse is regular but there is a slight acceleration during inspiration and a slight deceleration during expiration, known as sinus arrhythmia. This is uncommon over the age of 40 years (Houghton and Gray, 2007).

Irregularity of pulse rhythm can be divided into three types: occasional irregularity, regular irregularity and irregular irregularity. An occasional irregularity may be perceived as a missed pulse or 'dropped beat' and is often the result of an occasional ectopic (an extra beat, followed by a compensatory pause). This should be noted, but ectopics are a common finding, and are often of little consequence. A regularly occurring irregularity may be detected as a cyclical event and may be the result of a heart block. Again, this should be reported as it may well compromise the circulation, sometimes with catastrophic effects. An irregularly irregular rhythm is often a result of atrial fibrillation (AF). Although AF is a common irregular cardiac rhythm, the Department of Health (2008b) recognises that it is under diagnosed and under treated, and thus it is important to report AF when noted.

Apical pulse rate measurements (heard through a stethoscope placed over the apex of the patient's heart) are advocated in infants, and should be counted for one minute (Glasper et al., 2007). The apical pulse rate is also incorporated into the assessment of adults who have an irregular heart rate and/or when a measurement of **pulse deficit** (the difference between the apical and peripheral pulse rates) is required.

pulse deficit
the difference between the apical heart rate and the peripheral pulse rate

Blood pressure

Blood pressure is the pressure exerted by the blood on the walls of a blood vessel. Each blood vessel has its own pressure, the pressure in the vessels falling continuously from the aorta to the end of systemic circulation. This pressure gradient or fall needs to exist for blood to flow. During contraction of the ventricles of the heart, blood is ejected into the systemic and pulmonary circulations, causing a distension of the arteries and an increase in arterial pressure. When contraction ends, the arterial walls recoil passively and blood is driven further through the arterial circulation. Arterial pressure therefore rises and falls during the contraction and relaxation of the heart. The maximum pressure is known as the **systolic pressure**, the minimum pressure that occurs during relaxation of the heart being known as the **diastolic pressure**.

A number of factors determine blood pressure, including peripheral resistance, intravascular blood volume, and the **stroke volume**.

systolic pressure
the blood pressure relating to the contraction of the heart

diastolic pressure
the blood pressure relating to the resting phase of the heart

stroke volume
the amount of blood ejected from the ventricle during each heart beat

- Peripheral resistance is the opposition to the blood flow and is determined by:
  - *Blood viscosity ('stickiness'):* the greater the viscosity, the greater the resistance.
  - *Blood vessel length:* the longer the vessel, the greater the resistance.
  - *Blood vessel diameter:* the smaller the tube, the greater the resistance.
  - *Elasticity of the vessels:* the greater the stretch, the less the resistance.
- Reductions in intravascular blood volume can directly and dramatically decrease blood pressure, especially if the blood loss (such as haemorrhage) or fluid loss (as in burns or dehydration) is rapid. In these circumstances, the body attempts to rectify the problem via the sympathetic nervous system. For example, vasoconstriction of the peripheral circulation redirects blood to the major arteries and vital organs such as the brain, heart and kidneys. Treatment for blood volume loss involves the replacement of blood, plasma or fluid at a rate determined to be appropriate to the patient's condition.

- The stroke volume plays an integral part in the cardiac function. Indeed, the cardiac output (ml per minute) is equal to the stroke volume (ml per beat) multiplied by the heart rate (beats per minute).
  Cardiac output = Stroke volume × Heart rate
- Normal cardiac output is approximately 5 litres per minute (Marieb and Hoehn, 2010). The stroke volume is in turn affected by factors such as the venous return to the heart, the resistance against which the heart is pumping, and the contractility of the heart. Thus, patients who develop cardiogenic shock following myocardial infarction have a decreased stroke volume due to the decreased strength of the heart beat, and the blood presure falls.

For a more detailed explanation of the physiology of blood pressure, see Marieb and Hoehn (2010).

A routine component of the cardiovascular assessment is the measurement and recording of blood pressure. The most frequent, non-invasive method of measuring arterial blood pressure employs a sphygmomanometer. The frequency of recording will depend on the patient's condition, the reason for admission and the results of the reading. It is therefore essential that the technique is performed accurately, on the same arm each time, and that the patient is prepared prior to the procedure. Other factors which should be considered when undertaking an accurate blood pressure measurement are detailed in Chart 10.3. The effects of anxiety should also be considered, and ideally patients should be as relaxed as possible prior to a blood pressure recording. However, it is notable that in some groups of patients a phenomena known as 'white coat **hypertension**' or the 'white coat effect' can occur (Williams et al., 2004). In these circumstances, anxiety relating to an anticipated recording results is a stress effect which artificially raises the blood pressure. This effect therefore needs to be considered, and can be overcome via repeated measurements, especially with the use of ambulatory blood pressure monitors in a community setting.

hypertension
high blood pressure

Chart 10.3 Technique for accurately measuring blood pressure

- Use a properly maintained and calibrated device. This may be automated or manual.
- The patient should be comfortably seated; tight clothing around the arm removed; and the arm supported at heart level.
- An appropriately sized cuff should be used.
- If a manual manometer is used, the observer needs to be at eye level with the device, and the cuff deflated slowly. The blood pressure should be read to the nearest 2 mmHg.
- The diastolic value should be measured at the disappearance of sounds (Korotkoff phase V – see Table 10.3).
- On initial assessment, blood pressure should be recorded for both arms, as patients may have differences between arms. On subsequent measurements, the arm with the higher reading should be chosen.
- Document findings.

Source: Williams et al. (2004); Dougherty and Lister (2008).

✹ Activity 10.3

Measure a colleague's resting blood pressure. Ask them to complete 20 sit-ups. Note the blood pressure again. Note the difference and consider the physiological changes that have occurred.

Normal values for blood pressure readings are shown in Table 10.4. A persistently high blood pressure reading is known as hypertension. Williams et al.

Table 10.3 Korotkoff sounds with examples of pressure values

Phase	Sound	mmHg	Pressure
1	Tapping that is sharp and clear	120	Systolic
2	Blowing or swishing	110	
3	Sharp but softer than phase 1	100	
4	Muffled and fading	90	
5	No sound	80	Diastolic

hypotension
low blood pressure

(2004) identify that hypertension exists when the systolic value is greater than 139 mmHg, and/or the diastolic value is greater than 89 mmHg. It is estimated that 40 per cent of adults in England and Wales have hypertension, which is of concern due to the correlation between hypertension and coronary heart disease and stroke (British Hypertension Society/Royal College of Physicians, 2006). A low blood pressure reading is known as **hypotension**, and exists in adults when the systolic blood pressure is lower then 100 mmHg (Marieb and Hoehn, 2010).

Hypotension may result from shock, or may be a normal finding for certain individuals. Elderly patients in particular may be affected by orthostatic hypotension (O'Brien et al., 2003). In this condition the sympathetic nervous system is slow in its response when patients stand from a sitting or lying position, resulting in a syncopal (fainting) episode. If orthostatic hypotension is suspected, postural blood pressure should be undertaken, being performed on the same arm with the patient first lying and then standing. If a difference exists between the two systolic pressures, the patient is said to have a postural fall in blood pressure, which is especially significant if the difference is 20 mmHg or more. Care is necessary when undertaking this procedure, as it may provoke a syncopal episode.

Table 10.4 Average systolic blood pressure values

Age (years)	Systolic pressure (mmHg)
<1	70–90
1–2	80–95
2–5	80–100
5–12	90–110
>12	100–120

Source: Advanced Paediatric Life Support: The Practical Approach. 4th Edition. Advanced Life Support Group (2005). Reproduced with permission.

Peripheral perfusion

oedema
an excessive accumulation of fluid in the tissue spaces

Peripheral perfusion is assessed by considering the colour, texture and temperature of the skin, the presence of peripheral pulses or **oedema** and the capillary refill time.

When assessing the colour of the skin, any pallor and/or cyanosis should be noted. Pallor may indicate shock, haemorrhage or poor perfusion. The conjunctiva of the eyes can also be inspected as a lack of their usual reddish colour indicates anaemia. Cyanosis, which is a bluish tinge to the skin or mucous membranes, can be central or peripheral. Central cyanosis, such as blue lips, is an indicator of poor gaseous exchange, and reflects decreased oxygen levels in the blood (Jarvis, 2003). Peripheral cyanosis is an indicator of decreased blood flow and perfusion, reflecting decreased oxygen delivery to the tissues (Jarvis, 2003). This can be noted in the extremities and the nail beds.

The texture and temperature of the skin will reveal any localised or generalised warmth or coolness and any signs of sweating. A localised heat reaction may occur following a bite or sting, whereas generalised heat may be present with an underlying pyrexia or sepsis. Sweating (diaphoresis) may indicate that the patient is pyrexial; and the skin may become cold and clammy in situations such as circulatory shock and pain, reflecting peripheral vasoconstriction secondary to the action of the sympathetic nervous system (Marieb and Hoehn, 2010).

Palpation of the peripheral pulses (see Figure 10.2), will indicate the presence of arterial blood flow to the extremities and both limbs should always be checked for pulses or blood flow as this may vary considerably from limb to limb. If an area of tissue is not adequately perfused, it becomes ischaemic, the metabolic function of the tissue deteriorates and the damage eventually becomes irreversible (necrosis). Arterial insufficiency may lead to the following signs: ulceration of skin; thickening and slow growth of the nails; and skin which is shiny, scaly and hairless. Oedema and pain may also be present in the limb. Characteristically the patient will awake in pain at night and hang the limb over the edge of the bed to increase the blood supply, thus alleviating the pain. Clinical investigations can include Doppler testing, which utilises non-invasive continuous-wave ultrasound.

A capillary refill test (CRT) can be utilised when assessing the adequacy of tissue perfusion. This can be assessed peripherally by applying firm pressure for five seconds on a fingertip held at heart level (Resuscitation Council (UK), 2006), or centrally by pressing for five seconds on the centre of the sternum (Advanced Life Support Group, 2005). This cutaneous pressure squeezes the blood out of the capillaries, and the length of time taken for the skin to turn pink again indicates the speed of capillary refill. A CRT greater than two seconds may be an indicator of decreased tissue perfusion, but a prolonged CRT may also occur if the patient is cold. This finding should thus be used in conjunction with other clinical signs, and a central CRT is considered to be more reliable than a peripheral CRT when assessing for circulatory shock (Advanced Life Support Group, 2005).

Peripheral oedema may result from changes in osmotic pressure (for example decreased protein levels in the blood, which might occur in liver failure), congestion (for example in congestive heart failure), or if there is poor lymphatic drainage. Oedema is usually gravitational and may be observed in the feet or legs, or even in the genital area or sacral region if it is excessive. Patients may be taking diuretic therapy, so fluid balance and/or daily weights should be accurately ascertained to determine fluid loss.

Pulmonary oedema is characterised by acute breathlessness, often with frothy sputum, and is caused by acute left-sided heart failure. These patients are often seriously ill and are frequently unable to talk, feeling as if they are 'drowning'. Urgent medical assistance is necessary, and the patients will usually be prescribed oxygen and diuretics.

✷ Activity 10.4

Try performing a capillary refill test on yourself and then on a colleague. Read the text to ascertain the normal values.

⬭ Link

Chapter 9 also discusses cyanosis.

⬭ Link

Chapter 8 reviews urinary elimination in more detail.

Frances Riteur is an 80-year-old lady with known congestive heart failure. Her diuretic therapy has been altered, and the practice nurse is monitoring the effects of her new treatment.

What will the nurse be monitoring?

- Frances will probably be weighed weekly. A weight loss of 1 kg per day represents a loss of 1 litre of fluid per day.
- Any reduction in peripheral oedema will be noted.
- Any reduction in breathlessness will be noted.

- Any improvement in exercise tolerance, sleep pattern, and appetite will also be noted as it may indicate a lessening of her cardiac failure.

Fluid balance

A fluid balance record may be requested for patients who have circulatory compromise. An accurate recording of all forms of input and output is essential as it will compare total input and output and show whether these are optimal. Urinary ouput for an adult normally ranges from 1.5 to 2 litres per day (> 0.5 ml/kg per hour), but this depends on normally functioning kidneys, the kidneys receiving an adequate blood supply and a lack of obstruction to urinary flow (Smith, 2000). Problems with any of these three mechanisms can therefore affect urinary output. If, for example, a patient becomes hypovolaemic post surgery, the decreased cardiac output will result in decreased renal perfusion, and hence the urinary output will drop. A reduced urinary output may thus be an early indicator that a patient's condition is deteriorating, and **oliguria** should be reported. Oliguria is said to exist when the urine output is less than 0.5 ml/kg/hour in adults (Smith, 2000), 1 ml/kg/hour in children and 2 ml/kg/hour in infants (Advanced Life Support Group, 2005).

oliguria
inadequate production of urine

Fluid charts can also reveal the effects of diuretic therapy, which is used to improve urinary output. Additionally, patients may be weighed daily or twice weekly as a method of assessing the weight/fluid balance, as 1 kg of weight is equivalent to 1 litre of water.

Total fluid balance figures are often transferred onto a cumulative fluid balance chart, which allows several days or weeks of recording to be easily viewed. Continuous fluid balance over a longer period of time is vital in some groups of patients, for example those with renal failure or cardiac failure.

⚭ Link

Chapter 1 explores pain assessment methods.

Pain

The ability to assess and effectively manage a patient's pain is an essential nursing skill, and this section specifically details the assessment, recording and monitoring of pain arising from circulatory problems. As part of the pain assessment, the nurse should identify the location, severity and description of a patient's pain, and consider whether there are any precipitating or alleviating factors.

An individual may be able to state the location of their pain (for example central chest pain) or point to it, but a site may be difficult to establish in individuals if there is a language barrier, for example young children, and those who do not have English as their first language. Anatomical diagrams and multilanguage tools may be helpful with such patients. Some departments use graphical tools to chart a patient's pain, and these can be referred to again in subsequent reviews and evaluations.

It is important to establish the severity of the pain, and different types of scale exist to assist with this process. In the case of verbal descriptor scales (Chart 10.4), an individual is asked to select a word that describes their pain. These scales are quick and easy to use, but do require an understanding of English or translation to other languages. A second tool is the visual analogue scale (Figure 10.3) which is usually a straight line with either numbers or descriptors along it. These are quick to use, but they require abstract conceptualising by the patient, which may be difficult in young children or those with learning disabilities. The third type of scale is the pain behaviour tool. This relies on the principle that patients who are in pain exhibit certain types of behaviour (Chart 10.5), which can be objectively assessed.

Chart 10.4 Verbal descriptor pain scale

- None
- Slight
- Moderate
- Severe
- Agony

No pain					Moderate pain				Worst pain imaginable	
0	1	2	3	4	5	6	7	8	9	10

Figure 10.3 Visual analogue pain scale

An ideal pain assessment tool should allow for a quick but comprehensive pain assessment, which combines the patient's subjective interpretation of their pain with an objective assessment by the nurse of the effects of this pain on the patient's behaviour. Such a tool should also facilitate the ongoing assessment and evaluation of pain and pain control. Figure 10.4 shows a pain ruler that meets these criteria. The Manchester Triage Group has designed a pain ruler aimed at emergency departments, but with obvious value to other clinical environments (Mackway-Jones et al., 2006). The Manchester tool combines the verbal descriptor, visual analogue and pain behaviour tools, which facilitates both patient and practitioner assessment.

★ Activity 10.5

Identify the pain assessment tools used in your clinical area. Ascertain whether pain scores are linked to an analgesic protocol, for example a pain score of 8 out of 10 equates to the need for opiate analgesia.

Do nurses make their own judgements of what pain clients are experiencing? Do particular clients express more pain than others?

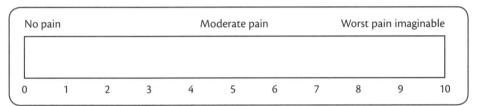

Figure 10.4 A pain ruler

Normal activities		Able to do most activities		Prevents some activities		Stops most activities		No control	
0	1	2	3	4	5	6	7	8	9	10
No pain		Mild pain		Moderate pain		Severe pain		Excruciating pain	

Chart 10.5 Pain behaviour scale

- Verbal response
- Body language
- Facial expression
- Behavioural change
- Conscious level
- Physiological change

It is important to remember that patients frequently understate the amount of pain that they are in. This may be especially true with older clients specifically those who have lived with chronic pain, and have found ways of adapting to and coping with pain. Children may also understate pain, possibly because of fear of the consequences, such as having to go to hospital.

A description of the pain is necessary to clarify and confirm its location and severity, and may also indicate its probable cause. For example, a client who describes leg pain that is cramping and excruciating, being worse on walking, may have intermittent **claudication** secondary to arterial insufficiency. Investigations obviously need to be performed to confirm the initial suspicion, but the description helps the practitioner to prioritise the management of these patients.

Precipitating factors such as exercise, stress, movement, respiration, position, time and duration are helpful in determining the probable cause and possible effects of the pain. Chest pain on respiration, particularly inspiration, may, for example, arise from the pleura or pericardium.

Alleviating factors such as heat, cold, rest, analgesics, position and distraction may again indicate the cause of pain but may also help with pain management strategies. A patient with angina, for example, who complains of chest pain when walking in the cold can be advised to alter her walking habits or try prophylactic vasodilators such as glyceryl trinitrate prior to exercise.

The physiological effects of pain may be minimal, but on occasion marked tachycardia and hypertension might develop in response to the stress effect; while vagal stimulation might result in bradycardia, hypotension and syncope. Chronic pain can certainly curtail a patient's activities or lifestyle, and health education advice may be appropriate. For further information, see Macintyre and Schug (2007) or Park et al. (2000).

Nursing Interventions

Cardiopulmonary resuscitation/defibrillation

Cardiac arrest is a medical emergency which every health professional needs to be prepared for. The most common cause of cardiac arrest is the sudden onset of either **ventricular fibrillation** (VF) or pulseless **ventricular tachycardia** (VT) secondary to coronary heart disease. These **arrhythmias** lead to a sudden cessation of cardiac output, and hence in these instances the chain of survival is necessary to maximise the chances of successful resuscitation (Resuscitation Council (UK), 2006). The four links in the chain are:

1   Early recognition of both the patient at risk of cardiac arrest, as well as of the patient who has arrested. Early call for help, for example summoning help from the ambulance service in the community, and cardiac arrest team in-hospital.
2   Early cardiopulmonary resuscitation (CPR).
3   Early defibrillation if the rhythm is VF or pulseless VT.
4   Post-resuscitation care.

The emphasis is upon early intervention, as time delays will worsen brain hypoxia, as well as lessen the chances of successful defibrillation. Good basic

---

claudication

pain in the lower limbs due to insufficient arterial blood supply

ventricular fibrillation

the ventricular activity of the heart is chaotic, and thus the heart is unable to pump

ventricular tachycardia

the ventricular activity of the heart is fast, which decreases the cardiac output. VT is not always pulseless, but cardiac arrest is more likely when the heart rate is very fast

arrhythmia

a deviation from the normal (sinus) heart rhythm

life support is thus fundamental to ensuring that oxygen continues to circulate to the brain and other vital organs despite the absence of a pulse, thereby helping to slow the speed of patient deterioration while advanced life support techniques are instituted. It is thus imperative that nursing staff ensure that they are equipped with the skills and knowledge to adequately perform good basic life support when necessary.

When VF/pulseless VT are the cause of the cardiac arrest, defibrillation is required to restore a spontaneous circulation. With the advent of both fully automated and shock advisory biphasic difibrillators, it is increasingly common for nursing staff to be responsible for the early provision of shocks, especially in the hospital setting. This reflects that nursing staff are a constant presence on the wards, and are thus in a prime position to act as first responders.

Other cardiac arrest rhythms include **asystole** and **pulseless electrical activity** (PEA). In PEA the cardiac monitor demonstrates electrical activity which is compatible with a cardiac output, and yet there is no mechanical activity to propel blood around the body. There are various causes of PEA (and indeed cardaic arrest in general) including **hypovolaemia**, hypothermia, hypoxia, hypo/hyperkalaemia and other metabolic disorders, tension pneumothroax, cardiac tamponade, toxic/therapeutic disorders and thrombo-embolic and mechanical obstruction (otherwise known as the 4 Hs and 4 Ts; Resuscitation Council (UK), 2006). These non-shockable rhythms are generally less prevalent than the shockable rhythms (VF/pulseless VT), and yet in hospital both asystole and PEA become much more prevalent. This reflects the fact that hospital patients unsurprisingly often have signficant health problems, and hence cardiac arrest may follow a period of gradual clinical deterioration from conditions such as sepsis, haemorrhage or respiratory disease. Cardiac arrests in such sitautions have a worse prognosis than those related to sudden cardiac arrest secondary to VF or pulseless VT, and hence the emphasis is again upon the early recognition and management of the sick and deteriorating patient prior to cardiac arrest (NICE, 2007).

Full guidance pertaining to CPR can be found on the Resusciation Council (UK) website: www.resus.org.uk. These guidelines are frequently revised, and it is therefore necessary that both health-care organisations and employees monitor and implement any changes.

asystole
absence of any electrical activity from the heart

pulseless electrical activity
absence of a cardiac output, and hence a pulse, for a heart rhythm which appears as if it could generate a pulse

hypovolaemia
an abnormally low circulating blood volume

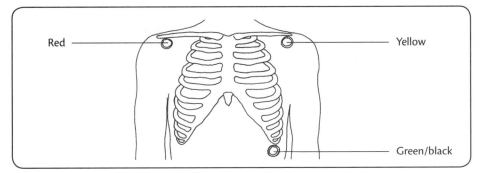

Figure 10.5 ECG chest lead placement

Cardiac monitoring

A cardiac monitor displays a graphical representation of the electrical activity occurring within the heart. It is a useful tool to assess a patient's heart rhythm and also provides information about their condition and progress. Whereas cardiac monitors were once the domain of specialist units, they are now increasingly used in a variety of clinical settings. Chart 10.6 outlines hints on using cardiac monitors.

Chart 10.6 Hints on using a cardiac monitor

- Ensure that the cardiac monitor is situated in a safe and observable position.
- Switch it on at the wall and on the monitor (if appropriate).
- Set the monitor to lead 2 unless told otherwise.
- Attach the electrodes to the client's skin surface as shown in Figure 10.5.
- The electrodes need to be firmly attached to the patient's skin. This may be difficult if the patient is shocked and sweating. If the leads do not adhere, the following may be useful: shave the chest if necessary (in the area where the electrodes need placing); abrade the skin lightly (most electrodes have a rough edge to achieve this); and dry the skin.
- Ensure that the rhythm tracing is visible and observe it regularly.

It is important to always match what is seen on the cardiac monitor to the patient's condition. For example, leads dislodged from a patient may mimic asystole. Likewise, it is also important to note that the cardiac monitor may appear to show a near normal ECG rhythm during PEA cardiac arrests. The guiding principle is to look at the patient first and the monitor second.

sinus rhythm
the normal rhythm of the heart

The normal cardiac rhythm, or **sinus rhythm**, has a characteristic waveform (Figure 10.6), and an understanding of this, in addition to the physiology of

---

Casebox 10.3

Joseph Smith, a 65-year-old gentleman, develops central chest pain while digging in the garden. His wife dials 999, and he is conveyed to the Emergency Department.

What information should the nurse aim to obtain from the handover from the ambulance crew?

- The time of the onset of the pain.
- The location of the pain – is it central, does it radiate into the jaw or into the arms?
- The characteristics of the pain e.g. a verbal description, and pain score.
- Associated features e.g. shortness of breath and nausea.

- Any ambulance treatment en-route e.g. aspirin, oxygen, opiates.

What should the nurse's priorities be when assessing Mr Smith?

- Undertaking an ABCDE assessment (primary survey); summoning assistance; and recording a 12 lead ECG.

The ECG, as well as the history, indicate that Mr Smith is having an ST elevation myocardial infarction.

What are some of the nursing roles in this situation?

- Support and reassurance for the patient, as well as for any family members present.

- Involvement with the administration of any further treatments. The patient may receive thrombolytic drugs to dissolve the thrombus in the coronary artery. Increasingly, however, patients such as these receive primary percutaneous coronary intervention, involving angioplasty and stents (DoH, 2008b). The patient will thus need to be transferred from the Emergency Department to a cardiac catheter lab.

normal cardiac conduction, helps the observer to note any deviations from the normal ECG. What follows is a basic introduction to ECG interpretation; for a more detailed approach, see books such as *Making Sense of the ECG* (Houghton and Gray, 2007).

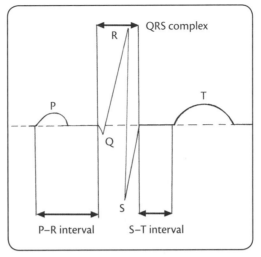

Figure 10.6 Normal ECG waveform

The isoelectric line, or baseline, is seen as a straight line. The first wave of the ECG is the P wave, representing the **depolarisation** of the atrial myocardium. Atrial depolarisation leads to atrial contraction (systole), during which blood is expelled from the atria into the ventricles. The P wave is followed by the QRS complex, which represents ventricular depolarisation. The Q wave is the first downward (or negative) deflection after the P wave, but is not always present in normal conduction. The R wave is the first upward (or positive) deflection after the P wave, and the S wave is the downward deflection that follows an R wave. Following ventricular depolarisation, ventricular systole occurs, resulting in blood being expelled into the systemic and pulmonary circulations. The next deflection on the ECG is the T wave, representing ventricular muscle **repolarisation**, which corresonds with ventricular diastole. It is in this period that the ventricles fill with blood prior to the next systolic contraction. Atrial repolarisation occurs during ventricular depolarisation, but the waveform is masked by the greater electrical activity occurring in the ventricles. A normal or sinus beat therefore has a P wave, a QRS complex, a T wave, and an S–T segment which is on the isoelectric line. Alterations to these waveforms indicate cardiac arrhythmia, disease or damage.

When analysing the ECG rhythm, various pieces of information are required to ascertain whether the rhythm is sinus in origin or whether there is an arrhythmia. What follows is a six-stage process that can be used for the basic analysis of an ECG rhythm:

1   Heart rate.
2   Regularity of heart rhythm.
3   Presence/absence of P waves.
4   P–R interval.
5   QRS complex duration/width.
6   Rhythm interpretation.

Heart rate

The heart rate can be obtained in several ways. The paper speed for most ECG machines is 25mm/second, which gives 5 large squares per second. Thus, if the rhythm is regular, count the number of large squares between two consecutive R waves and divide the number into 300 to determine the heart rate, as there are 300 large squares occurring in one minute. For example, 5 large squares

depolarisation
loss of the polarised state of the plasma membrane, involving a loss or reduction of the negative membrane potential

repolarisation
return to the resting state of the plasma membrane in which the inside of the cell is negative relative to the outside

between two R waves divided into 300 gives a heart rate of 60. However, if the heart rate is irregular, such as with atrial fibrillation, this method is clearly unreliable. In such situations an alternative method is necessary, which involves counting the number of QRS complexes that occur in a six-second period on an ECG strip (that is 30 large squares). The resultant number of QRS complexes is then multiplied by 10, which indicates the number of complexes that occur in a 60-second period.

Regularity

The regularity of the rhythm should be noted. If this is not obvious, it can be ascertained using a ruler or ECG rule, or merely by marking a piece of paper at the top of two complexes and moving it along the rhythm strip to see whether the other complexes fall regularly. Irregular rhythms are unlikely to be sinus in origin except for **sinus arrhythmia**, in which acceleration and deceleration occur with respiration.

sinus arrhythmia
an irregular heart rhythm following the pattern of respiration

P waves

The presence of a P wave should be noted, as it is an essential component of **sinus rhythm**.

P–R interval

The P–R interval is measured from the beginning of the P wave to the beginning of the QRS complex. It can be measured in either time (0.12–0.20 seconds) or squares (3–5 small squares on the ECG paper). For the rhythm to be sinus rhythm, the P–R interval must fall within this duration. If the P–R interval is greater, it may indicate atrio-ventricular heart block.

QRS complex

The QRS duration is measured from the beginning to the end of the QRS complex. Again, it can be measured in time (less than 0.12 seconds) or squares (less than 3 small squares on the ECG paper). Beats that are sinus in origin and are conducted normally through the conduction system will fall within these parameters.

Rhythm interpretation

Having followed the processes outlined above it should be possible to decide whether or not the rhythm is sinus in origin. Further skills are then necessary to determine which other rhythm it might be, but these are beyond the scope of this section.

Anti-embolic precautionary measures

The British Thoracic Society (2003) identify that the classification of venous thromboembolism (VTE) includes both deep vein thrombosis (DVT) and pulmonary embolus (PE). As stated at the beginning of this chapter, PEs are associated with significant morbidity and mortality, and hospital patients are at particular risk. It is for this reason that the prevention of VTE is vitally important.

Anti-embolic stockings, heparin, and foot pumps

Ball and Phillips (2001) identify that thigh-length graduated compression stockings should be used in situations where patients have a risk of developing VTE, such as those patients undergoing major surgery, and those who have poor mobility while in hospital. Meta-analysis has revealed that when these stockings are worn until discharge they significantly reduce both DVT and PE (Ball and Phillips, 2001). Agnelli et al. (1998) also demonstated the value of pharmacological agents such as heparin, and low molecular weight heparins in particular are regularly administered subcutaneously as part of thrombo-prophylaxis. Furthermore, the House of Commons Health Committee (2005) has recommended the use of mechanical foot pumps to improve the circulation for those patients unable to mobilise promptly post surgery, especially if the use of heparin is contraindicated due to the risk of bleeding complications.

Exercises

Passive/active exercises are an important measure to promote venous return and decrease venous stasis in order to prevent a DVT. Preoperative and bed-bound patients can be taught and encouraged to combine deep breathing techniques and active leg exercises to achieve this. Exercises can be performed passively for unconscious or immobile individuals. Further measures to encourage blood flow are regular changes of position, the use of bed cradles to relieve pressure on the limbs and ensuring that the top sheets are not tightly tucked in.

> **✳ Activity 10.6**
>
> Consider clients of any age who are immobile and at risk of developing a venous thromboembolism. What precautionary measures can be adopted to prevent this?

Blood transfusion

A blood transfusion involves the administration of either whole blood or one of its components from one person to another. The types of blood or blood product commonly used are whole blood, concentrated (packed) red cells, platelets, fresh frozen plasma and cryoprecipitate (which contains high levels of factor VIIIc, von Willebrand factor and fibrinogen, all of which are useful when clotting is deranged – McClelland, 2007). In the transfusion process, however, it must be remembered that problems can arise.

Safety precautions prior to transfusion are detailed in the *Handbook of Transfusion Medicine* (McClelland, 2007), which is a national guide issued online by the UK Blood Transfusion and Tissue Transplantation Services (www.transfusionguidelines.org.uk). Blood products should only be removed from controlled temperature storage (CTS) when needed – red cells need to be used within 4 hours of removal from CTS, and cannot be returned to the blood bank stock if they have been out of CTS storage for longer than 30 minutes. Each hospital will have a local procedure for checking blood, but the core requirement is that the trained nurse responsible for the transfusion needs to confirm the patient's name, date of birth and hospital number, the expiry date of the blood, the blood groups of the donor and recipient, and the serial number of the unit of blood. Traditionally two members of staff have been involved in these checks, but some NHS Trusts are now introducing policies placing the responsibility solely upon one trained clinician. A permanent record of the transfusion episode needs to be entered in the clinical notes, including the signed prescription sheet. The unit should also be checked for signs of deterioration or damage. If there is any doubt, the blood should not be given but returned to the laboratory and advice requested. The transfusion should be prepared aseptically, and a specific blood administration set with an integral in-line filter should be used. In addition, some units use additional filters, and local policies must be checked.

Observations during transfusion are an integral and essential part of the patient's care and should commence with a set of baseline observations prior to the commencement of the transfusion (pulse, blood pressure, temperature and respiratory rate). Local policies vary, but McClelland (2007) indicates that a further set of observations should be undertaken 15 minutes after the commencement of the unit; and again once the unit has been transfused. Transfusion reactions can occur very rapidly and are most likely to occur during the initial administration of each unit. The pattern of observations should be repeated for all new units of blood.

Transfusion complications

Circulatory overload occurs from an excessive intravascular volume that usually results in pulmonary oedema. This is most likely to occur in chronically anaemic patients who require the additional oxygen-carrying capacity of red blood cells but not the volume. The problem is prevented by using packed cells and giving diuretics. If circulatory overload occurs, the patient should be seated upright and reassured, the transfusion should be discontinued immediately and medical advice should be sought.

agglutination
the clumping of foreign cells due to an antigen–antibody reaction

Haemolytic mismatch is one of the most serious complications of a blood transfusion, and clinical problems can arise rapidly following as little as a 10–15 ml infusion of incompatible blood. Problems are caused by antigen–antibody reactions, leading to acute intravascular **agglutination** and **haemolysis**. Early symptoms include fever, shivering, tachycardia, wheeze, rash and hypotension. Further complications are chest tightness, loin pain, shock and disseminated intravascular coagulation (DIC). DIC results in inappropriate clumping of platelets in the microcirculation, which results in tissue ischaemia secondary to these thrombi, as well as bleeding due to the over-consumption of coagulation factors (Barkin and Rosen, 2003). The degree of the haemolytic reaction therefore ranges from mild to severe, with shock and death in some instances. The transfusion should be stopped immediately and any remaining blood sent for analysis. Contact medical help immediately, as aggressive treatment may be necessary.

urticarial hives
a skin condition that manifests as red wheals causing intense irritation; it is usually a result of hypersensitivity

Allergic reactions are fairly common, ranging from mild irritation to anaphylactic shock. Symptoms include flushing, **urticarial hives**, wheezing, chest tightness, laryngeal oedema and peri-orbital oedema. Anaphylaxis is potentially fatal and requires urgent treatment. This may include intra-muscular adrenaline, intravenous chlorphenamine (an antihistamine); intravenous hydrocortisone (acting as an anti-inflammatory agent), and nebulised salbutamol (acting as a bronchodilator).

Disease transmission is theoretically possible following transfusion and has occurred in the past, but today all blood in the UK is routinely screened for HIV and hepatitis. It is also extremely rare for blood to be contaminated with other micro-organisms, although Gram-negative bacteria can reproduce at 4°C. Reactions include pyrexia, rigor, chest and abdominal pain and the development of septic shock.

Cold blood can cause hypothermia when given in large quantities, and this can provoke further coagulopathies (disorders of coagulation – Greaves et al., 2001). In most instances active blood warming is not indicated, especially as a temperature greater than 38°C can cause **haemolysis** of red cells (Dougherty and Lister, 2008). However, if large amounts of blood are to be transfused in an emergency then blood should be warmed to 37°C.

haemolysis
the disintegration of red blood cells, causing severe anaemia and possibly jaundice

Intravenous fluid therapy

A patient may receive intravenous fluid therapy if they are unable to maintain their fluid balance orally. Causes include dehydration due to inadequate oral intake, severe vomiting or diarrhoea, sepsis, excess urine output or perspiration, severe burns, surgical procedures and unconsciousness. Intravenous fluid therapy is common in acute hospital settings, but it must be remembered that such therapy needs to be administered by a trained nurse in accordance with local policy; and is an invasive procedure with many potential complications. These include:

- infection
- inflammation
- thrombophlebitis
- extravasation (infiltration of fluid into the surrounding tissues)
- septicaemia
- air or particle embolism
- circulatory overload
- anaphylactic reaction.

The nurse's role is described in Chart 10.7.

Chart 10.7 Hints for intravenous therapy

- Ensure that whoever sites the cannula selects an appropriate position and uses an aseptic procedure.
- When sited, the cannula should be firmly secured.
- The cannula should be regularly inspected (at least twice a day) for signs of infection and inflammation.
- If fluids are being delivered via the cannula, it is essential to ensure that the right fluid is given to the right patient via the right route at the right time at the correct rate (the five Rs).
- Most hospitals operate a policy whereby intravenous fluids need to be checked prior to delivery by two nurses, one of whom is a qualified nurse. To ensure that fluids are delivered at the correct rate, electronic pump devices are frequently used in many clinical settings. If these are not

available, a formula for calculating the number of drips per minute is required. One such formula is described in Chart 10.8.
- The system that is used for delivering the fluid must be inspected for damage and sterility.
- It is essential to ensure that the system is free of air bubbles when primed with fluids and during the process of fluid delivery.
- All contact with the intravenous system should be aseptic to reduce the risk of infection.
- You may also see drugs added to the fluid system. The additives may be prepacked or require adding. In most hospitals, this is a procedure for a trained nurse.

Chart 10.8 Formula for drip rate calculation

$$\frac{(\text{Number of ml} \times \text{drops per ml})}{(\text{Number of hours} \times 60)} = \text{drops/minute}$$

The following example represents a client who is prescribed 1000ml (1 litre) of fluid over 4 hours. The giving set in use delivers 20 drops per ml. The figure 60 is a given constant representing 60 minutes in 1 hour.

Therefore

$$\frac{(1000 \times 20)}{(4 \times 60)} = 83.3 \text{ or } 83 \text{ drops/minute}$$

Note: The giving set package must be carefully inspected for the number of drops per ml as this may vary.

Chapter Summary

An adequate circulation of blood is necessary to ensure homeostasis. Circulatory disease, however, is common. It is thus imperative that nursing staff are able to undertake a circulatory patient assessment, and implement interventions in response to problems found. It is particularly important that nursing staff are able to detect life threatening situations such as cardiac arrest and shock, and are able to summon help and initiate resuscitative measures.

? Test yourself!

1   Name the stages of the nursing process.
1   List five common causes of shock.
2   What are some of the early physical signs of shock?
3   What is the normal range for the adult heart rate?
4   Name three key factors which affect blood pressure.
5   List five physical features which may be noted if a patient suffers from peripheral vascular disease.
6   What is a normal capillary refill time?
7   What is the normal urine output (mls/kg/hr) for infants, children and adults?
8   What are the 8 reversible causes (4 Hs and 4 Ts) considered in cardiac arrest?
9   Describe the types of pain assessment tool available.
10 Describe five complications of a blood transfusion.

References

Advanced Life Support Group (2005) *Advanced Paediatric Life Support: The Practical Approach*, Mackway-Jones, K., Molyneux, E., Phillips, B. and Wieteska, S. 4th edn. Blackwell Publishing, Oxford.

Agnelli, G., Piovella, F. and Buoncristiani, P. (1998) Enoxaparin plus compression stockings compared with compression stockings alone in the prevention of venous thromboembolism after elective neurosurgery. *New England Journal of Medicine* **339**: 80–5.

American College of Surgeons Committee on Trauma (2008) *Advanced Trauma Life Support*, 8th edn. American College of Surgeons, Chicago.

Ball, C.M. and Phillips, R.S. (2001) *Evidence Based on Call: Acute Medicine*. Churchill Livingstone, Edinburgh.

Barkin, R.M. and Rosen, P. (2003) *Emergency Pediatrics*. Mosby, Philadelphia.

British Hypertension Society/Royal College of Physicians (2006) *Hypertension. Management in Adults in Primary Care: Pharmacological Update*. http://www.nice.org.uk/nicemedia/pdf/HypertensionGuide.pdf (accessed 10 May 2009).

British Thoracic Society (2003) British Thoracic Society guidelines for the management of suspected pulmonary embolism. *Thorax*, **58**: 470–84.

Camm, A.J. and Bunce, N.H. (2005) Cardiovascular disease. In Kumar, P. and Clark, M. (ed.) *Clinical Medicine*, 6th edn. Elsevier Saunders, Edinburgh.

DoH (Department of Health) (2007) *The Coronary Heart Disease National Service Framework: Building for the Future – Progress Report for 2007*. The Stationery Office, London.

DoH (Department of Health) (2008a) *Impact Assessment of a National Screening Programme for Abdominal Aortic Aneurysms*. The Stationery Office, London.

DoH (Department of Health) (2008b) *The Coronary Heart Disease National Service Framework: Building on Excellence, Maintaining Progress – Progress Report for 2008*. The Stationery Office, London.

Dougherty, L. and Lister, S. (2008) *The Royal Marsden Hospital Manual of Clinical Nursing Procedures*, 7th edn. Wiley-Blackwell, Chichester.

Glasper, E.A., McEwing, G. and Richardson, J. (2007) *Oxford Handbook of Children's and Young People's Nursing*. Oxford University Press, Oxford.

Goldhaber, S.Z. (1997) Pulmonary embolism. In Braunwald, E. (ed.) *Heart Disease: A Textbook of Cardiovascular Medicine*, 5th edn. W.B. Saunders, Philadelphia.

Greaves, I., Porter, K. and Ryan, J. (2001) *Trauma Care Manual*. Arnold, London.

Houghton, A.R. and Gray, D. (2007) *Making Sense of the ECG: A Hands on Guide*, 3rd edn. Hodder Arnold, London.

House of Commons Health Committee (2005) *The Prevention of Venous Thromboembolism in Hospitalised Patients*. The Stationary Office, London.

Jarvis, C. (2003) *Physical Examination and Health Assessment*, 4th edn. W.B. Saunders, Philadelphia.

Macintyre, P.E. and Schug, S.A. (2007) *Acute Pain Management: A Practical Guide, 3rd edn*. Elsevier Saunders, Edinburgh.

Mackway-Jones, K., Marsden, J. and Windle, J. (2006) *Emergency Triage, 2nd edn*. Blackwell Publishing, London.

Marieb, E.N. and Hoehn, K. (2010) *Human Anatomy and Physiology*, 8th edn. Pearson Education, San Francisco.

McClelland, D.B.L. (2007) *Handbook of Transfusion Medicine*, 4th edn. The Stationery Office, London.

NICE (National Institute for Health and Clinical Excellence) (2006) *Atrial Fibrillation: The Management of Atrial Fibrillation (Clinical Guideline 36)*. NICE, London.

NICE (National Institute for Health and Clinical Excellence) (2007) *Acutely Ill Patients in Hospital: Recognition of and Response to Acute Illness in Adults in Hospital (Clinical Guideline 50)*. NICE, London.

O'Brien, E., Asmar, R., Beilin, L. et al., on behalf of the European Society of Hypertension Working Group on Blood Pressure Monitoring (2003) European Society of Hypertension recommendations for conventional, ambulatory and home blood pressure measurement. *Journal of Hypertension* **21**: 821–48.

Park, G., Fulton, B. and Senthuran, S. (2000) *The Management of Acute Pain*, 2nd edn. Oxford University Press, Oxford.

Resuscitation Council (UK) (2006) *Advanced Life Support*, 5th edn. Resuscitation Council (UK), London.

Smith, G. (2000) *Alert: A Multi Professional Course in Care of the Acutely Ill Patient*. University of Portsmouth, Portsmouth.

Swanton, R.H. (2003) *Cardiology*, 5th edn. Blackwell Science Ltd, Oxford.

Verdecchia, P. (2003) European Society of Hypertension recommendations for conventional, ambulatory and home blood pressure measurement. *Journal of Hypertension* **21**: 821–48.

Williams, B., Poulter, N.R., Brown, M.J., Davis, M., McInnes, G.T., Potter, J.F., Sever, P.S., and Thom, S. (2004) Guidelines for management of hypertension: report of the fourth working party of the British Hypertension Society. *Journal of Human Hypertension*, **18**: 139–85.

Chapter

PAM JACKSON, LYNN TAYLOR AND NADIA CHAMBERS

11 Wound Management

📖 Contents

☑ Learning outcomes

The purpose of this chapter is to explore the prevention of pressure ulcers and the nursing management of wounds. After working through it, you should be able to:

- Define the terms 'chronic and acute wound' and pressure ulcer
- Discuss the use of risk assessment tools in your current area of work
- Identify the different grades of pressure ulcer
- Discuss ways in which pressure ulcers can be prevented
- Outline the stages of the healing process
- Discuss the factors affecting wound healing
- Describe the optimum environment for wound healing
- Outline the elements of wound assessment
- Identify different types of dressing and other wound management strategies and discuss their appropriateness for different wounds and stages of healing.

The chapter contains a number of activities that will help to deepen your understanding of this complex topic. Some of these activities require you to access and read more specialist textbooks in anatomy and physiology or wound management.

What Is a Wound?

The exciting topic of wound healing is continually evolving as research identifies new knowledge. To play a part in prevention of pressure ulcers and wound management it is necessary to understand why pressure ulcers occur, what is meant by the term 'wound' and identify the different types that may be encountered.

Any kind of breach in the integrity of the skin or underlying tissues is commonly described as a wound. Wounds can be classified according to how they are caused, whether they are acute or chronic, how deep they are, the stage of healing, or the method by which they are expected to heal.

The Healing Process

The ability to support the maintenance of tissue viability, prevent pressure ulcers and manage wounds effectively is underpinned by a sound understanding of the structure and function of normal healthy skin and the normal healing process. Normal wound healing is a complex, well-coordinated, multiphase process. The phases of this process are usually described separately to facilitate understanding, but it is important to remember that each phase overlaps with the next, often running concurrently, and each phase may vary in duration or may be reversed or become static in certain circumstances.

The phases of wound healing

Four main phases have been identified and these are discussed in more detail.

Haemostasis or coagulation

Haemostasis involves vasoconstriction leading to the formation of a clot. This is essential to stop bleeding and limit exposure to contaminants. This results in wound contraction, which decreases the surface area of the wound. This process is part of the physiological response to blood **extravasation**. Platelets are activated by exposure to extravascular collagen, releasing growth factors that stimulate tissue regeneration, and then become sticky and aggregate, getting trapped in a fibrin mesh which forms the bulk of the clot (Hunt et al., 2000).

Inflammatory phase

This phase usually occurs over 3–7 days and is initiated by the release of chemical mediators, such as histamine and **prostaglandins** which attract neutrophils, monocytes and fibroblasts to the injured area by a process called **chemotaxis**. These mediators cause blood vessels to become more permeable and to vasodilate, allowing **wound exudate**, containing protein, nutrients and growth factors to leak out of the capillaries and bathe the injured area. This inflammatory response is a normal response to injury and is not to be confused with infection. This phase is delayed in patients who are immunosuppressed or have infected wounds.

The primary functions of this phase are:

extravasation
leakage of fluid from a blood vessel

prostaglandins
hormone-like substances that affect vasomotor and smooth muscle tone, capillary permeability, platelet aggregation, endocrine and exocrine functions and the nervous system

chemotaxis
a signalling process involving movement of cells in response to a chemical stimulus

wound exudate
a translucent, yellow-tinged fluid, rich in proteins and antibodies, produced during the inflammatory phase of the healing process

- *To combat potential infective organisms:* neutrophils are activated in the inflammatory response and clear the site of contaminating organisms by phagocytosis, aided by the macrophages.
- *To cleanse the area of debris:* monocytes enter the area and transform into activated macrophages to clear the debris through phagocytosis. This debris is often seen as creamy yellow **slough**, particularly in chronic wounds.
- *To initiate* **angiogenesis** *and* **collagen synthesis** macrophages stimulate the production of a variety of angiogenic **growth factors and cytokines** such as interleukin. This process initiates the growth of capillary buds (angiogenesis) as well as the regrowth of sympathetic nerve fibres. The process of angiogenesis is stimulated by a hypoxic environment. Fibroblasts, activated by these mediators, migrate to the wound site, initiating the early stages of the proliferative phase.

Proliferative phase

This phase of the wound healing process occurs over a variable time span and is characterised by the formation of **granulation tissue** which has a dense network of capillaries fibroblasts and collagen fibres. The fibroblasts produce an **extracellular matrix**, which is a framework of collagen fibres, elastin and proteoglycans, anchored by fibronectin, that support and sustain the products of angiogenesis. The successful progress of this phase is dependent upon the oxygen and nutrient supply.

The growth of capillary buds forming a network of loops within the wound is crucial to the level of oxygen available during the proliferative phase, as fibroblast activity is sensitive to oxygen supply. These capillary buds give granulation tissue its characteristic knobbly or granular appearance.

Two other major processes occur concurrently within the proliferative phase of wound healing – epithelialisation and contraction. The granulation tissue filling the wound bed is gradually resurfaced by epithelial cells, which migrate in from the wound margins or regenerate as 'islands' from hair follicles or glands. Epithelial cells regenerate and migrate by sliding over one another across the wound surface, and their eventual contact with one another inhibits further migration. This process is facilitated by a moist, warm and oxygenated environment. The process of contraction, initiated during the inflammatory phase, is largely controlled by the activity of myofibroblasts, which develop from fibroblasts and their activity reduces the surface area of the wound. Granulation, contraction and epithelialisation mark the completion of the proliferative phase.

Maturation phase

This final phase in the wound healing process is concerned with the remodelling and strengthening of the collagen fibres within the wound. The collagen produced during earlier stages is relatively soft, type III collagen, which is deposited fairly randomly during granulation, resulting in a low tensile strength (about 25 per cent of normal tissue) in the newly healed wound. During maturation, this is replaced with stronger type I collagen, which is organised through cross-linking

slough
soft dead tissue and bacteria resulting from injury or inflammation

angiogenesis
the production and growth of new blood vessels

collagen synthesis
the production of supportive, protein based, fibrous connective tissue

growth factors and cytokines
small molecular weight proteins that regulate cell proliferation and differentiation

granulation tissue
red, moist, fragile connective tissue that is characteristic of the proliferative phase of the healing process

extracellular matrix
a gel-like matrix produced by fibroblasts, composed of various polysaccharides, collagen fibres and water

of the collagen fibres into bundles lying at right angles to the wound margins. This increases the tensile strength of the wound to about 80 per cent of normal tissue: it will never become as strong as uninjured tissue. This ongoing process, facilitated by the activity of fibroblasts and characterised by a gradual reduction in vascularity of the wound site, shrinkage and paling of the scar tissue, can continue over a number of years.

Table 11.1 Comparison of the acute and chronic wound environment

Acute	Chronic
• Vasodilation with increased capillary permeability	• Defective remodeling of the extra cellular matrix (ECM)
• Increased cellular activity	• Inflammation is prolonged
• Neutrophils and macrophages engulf and destroy bacteria	• Chronic wound fluid biochemically differs from acute wound fluid. It slows or can stop the proliferation of cells and is detrimental to wound healing (Schultz et al., 2003)
• Macrophages stimulate the proliferation of fibroblasts needed for the formation of collagen	
• Matrix Metalloproteinases (MMPs) are released and degrade the damaged extra cellular matrix (ECM)	• There may be hyperproliferation at the wound edges preventing re-epithelialisation
• Growth factors and cytokines regulate the wound environment by stimulating and inhibiting the actions of inflammatory cells	• Growth factor activity is altered. Some fibroblasts become senescent affecting their mitotic activity and ability to promote the production of collagen
• Angiogenic factor stimulates the growth of the new capillary network	• Macromolecules scavenge growth factors and growth factors are inactivated stopping or delaying healing in the wound
• Increased mitotic activity	• The release of Tissue Inhibitor Metalloproteinases (TIMPs) is reduced allowing the number of Matrix Metalloproteinase (MMPs) to increase and cause degradation of the ECM
• Epithelial cells migrate from the wound edges or hair follicles within the wound and reinstate the integrity of the wound	
	• High bacterial content usually of more than one type
	• Wound healing is delayed or static

senescence
the cells have lost the ability to proliferate and become less responsive to growth factors

Acute wounds may have achieved re-epithelialisation in 21 days. The maturation of the wound may continue for up to 1 year or longer. In the case of a chronic wound the process of normal healing has been interrupted. Healing may occur over weeks, months or in some cases years. When managing a chronic wound the practitioner will attempt to reverse the chronic wound status to that of an acute wound. The chronic wound is 'stuck' in the inflammatory or proliferative stage of wound healing and cannot progress to the formation of healthy granulation tissue and epithelialisation. The molecular and cellular environment of the acute and chronic wound are different (see Table 11.1).

The progression of a wound to healing will be affected by the patient's general health. This includes factors such as low oxygen tension, ischaemia, metabolic disease, infection, autoimmune diseases and certain medications (see the section on factors affecting healing).

Surgical wounds and minor traumas are usually acute wounds. These wounds may become chronic if they become infected. Without complications these wounds will heal by primary intention. In the case of a surgical wound the opposing skin edges are brought together and sutured or stapled. There is no open cavity to be filled with granulation tissue. Chronic wounds are open wounds in which healing has been delayed for a significant period of time. These wounds are encouraged to heal from the base of the wound by the production of granulation tissue and epithelialising from the skin edges or hair follicles.

Modes of healing

It is common to refer to the healing process as occurring by one of three modes: primary intention, secondary intention or tertiary intention.

Primary intention

Healing by primary intention occurs in wounds where there is only partial thickness tissue loss and the skin edges can be brought together, usually by sutures, staples or glue, to ensure an absence of dead space in the wound. The four phases of wound healing occur, but there is little granulation tissue produced and minimal wound contraction, epithelial cells migrating along the suture line. Superficial wounds heal by regeneration of tissue similar to the tissue lost/damaged in the injury. Where the wounding results in scar formation the wound will have healed by a process of repair. Remodelling of the collagen fibres in scar tissue takes place, as previously described, and there is usually minimal defect.

Secondary intention

Healing by secondary intention refers to wounds where there has been full thickness tissue loss and the skin edges remain apart. Again, the wound will progress

> **★ Activity 11.1**
>
> What types of wound have you seen in practice?
>
> Using Table 11.2, try to identify the cause and mode of healing of each type.
>
> Discuss with your mentor the differences in management of acute and chronic wounds.

Table 11.2 Examples of wound classification

Description of wound	Cause	Expected mode of healing
Surgical excision	Removal of skin and underlying tissues during surgery	Secondary intention
Surgical incision	Precise cut made during surgery	Primary or delayed primary intention
Burn	Thermal, electrical or chemical	Secondary intention
Laceration (cut), abrasion (graze) puncture (stab wound)	Trauma	Primary intention
Venous ulcer	Pathology (intrinsic), for example chronic venous insufficiency	Secondary intention
Arterial ulcer	Pathology (intrinsic), for example atherosclerosis	Secondary intention
Diabetic ulcer	Pathology (intrinsic), for example diabetes	Secondary intention
Pressure ulcer	Pathology (extrinsic), for example pressure, friction or shear	Secondary intention
Fungating wound	Pathology (intrinsic), for example carcinoma	Neither

through all four phases of healing, but the wound will heal by a process of repair rather than regeneration and it will be necessary for the wound bed to fill with granulation tissue, to become resurfaced with epithelium and to contract before and during scar formation. The new tissue is different from the original tissue and has less tensile strength or elasticity. Pressure ulcers, leg ulcers and burns are all examples of wounds that will heal by secondary intention.

Tertiary intention

Healing by tertiary intention or delayed primary closure is when a wound that may be infected or contaminated is left open to facilitate the drainage of **pus** and the formation of granulation tissue. When the complicating factor has been excluded, the wound can be surgically closed, and healing by primary intention can take place. This needs to be achieved within a short timescale, for instance a week.

A Professional Perspective

Tissue viability, including **pressure ulcer** prevention and wound management are high-profile areas of nursing activity that are important both in terms of patient comfort and care, and the economic strain placed upon service providers (Cullum and Dealey, 1996). All nurses are expected to seek out best evidence and apply it in their everyday practice (DoH, 2000) Evidence-based education and clinical guidelines, such as those developed by NICE (2005), and bench-marking processes such as those outlined in *Essence of Care* (DoH, 2003) are key elements in establishing sound, client-focused, **evidence-based practice**. You may have noticed journal articles and websites concerned with tissue viability and wound management, and you may be familiar with multidisciplinary asso-ciations such as the Wounds UK, the Tissue Viability Society, and the European Pressure Ulcer Advisory Panel(EPUAP). Many NHS Trusts employ clinical nurse specialists or nurse consultants for tissue viability with the distinct remit of developing a strategy for tissue viability which will involve the management and coordination of care, teaching and research in wound management and pressure ulcer prevention. It is, however, important to remember that this area of nursing practice is one that most, if not all, practitioners will encounter, both pre- and post-qualification.

Accountability in wound management

Inherent in the concept of professionalism is the notion of service and with this the 'duty of care' that is entered into during practice, for which the professional practitioner is held accountable (NMC, 2008). Whenever a professional nurse assesses, plans, implements or evaluates a care intervention, a duty of care arises. The nurse can be held to account for the knowledge base upon which such an intervention is founded and must be able to demonstrate practice within the limits of such knowledge (NMC, 2008).

✷ Activity 11.2

Visit the European Pressure Ulcer Advisory Panel website at www.epuap.com to review its contents and identify any additional relevant websites. Download any potentially useful information.

pus
characteristic fluid composed of exudate, dead tissue debris, macrophages and bacteria

tissue viability
the sustained health, growth and repair of body tissues

pressure ulcer
a pressure ulcer is an area of localised damage to the skin and underlying tissue caused by pressure, shear, friction or a combination of all of these (EPUAP, 2009). 'The critical determinants of pressure ulcers are believed to be intensity and duration of applied pressure. Extrinsic and intrinsic factors influence tissue tolerance' (Cullum and Clark, 2006, p. 427)

evidence-based practice
the conscientious, explicit and judicious use of current best evidence in making decisions about the care of individuals (Sackett et al., 1996)

★ Activity 11.3

Find out if any **clinical audits** of pressure ulcers or wound management practice are undertaken in your current placement. What audits are carried out? How frequently are they done? Where are the results recorded and how is action taken?

∞ Link

Chapter 3 explores accountability in more detail.

clinical audit

a process for measuring outcomes of care and levels of performance against explicit criteria, with the aim of improving the quality of care

∞ Link

Chapter 3 also deals with clinical governance.

The duty of care defines the minimum standard of practice that a patient can expect. In professional nursing practice, this is informed by *The Code* (NMC, 2008) as well as national standards such as NICE Guidelines and *Essence of Care,* by professional associations such as the European Wound Management Association (EWMA) and local policies, guidelines, protocols and procedures. If the duty of care is breached, the individual practitioner will be held accountable for the nursing care involved and may be penalised by their professional body (the NMC).

Accountability and responsibility are similar concepts that are often confused. A distinction can be made in that in order to be held accountable for something, you must have authority over it. This means that you must be in the position to make a decision about a particular course of action. If you are not in such a position, it is your responsibility to say so.

Clinical governance is a framework for professional effectiveness and accountability in all aspects of health-care provision which helps all health-care practitioners to continuously improve quality and safeguard standards of care (RCN, 2003; DoH, 2000). We can consider wound management in terms of the clinical governance framework, as illustrated in Table 11.3.

See Activity 11.4 to review how clinical governance impacts on wound management.

Table 11.3 Clinical governance framework

Key elements of the clinical governance framework	Relationship to wound management and pressure ulcer prevention
Evidence-based practice	Ensuring that wound management interventions and pressure ulcer prevention strategies are based on best evidence
Clinical effectiveness	Ensuring that we do the 'right things, for the right people, with the right knowledge and skills and at the right time'. Clinical supervision and reflection on practice are ways in which we can ensure that we learn from our experience in order to provide best practice
Risk management	Ensuring that we assess all possible risks and plan care to minimise these and learn from adverse events to prevent future problems
Monitoring clinical practice	Ensuring that we undertake regular audits of pressure ulcer incidence and prevalence and wound management practice, using published gudelines as benchmarking tools
Continuing professional development	Ensuring that we keep our knowledge and skills up to date with current developments
Professional self-regulation	Ensuring that we are always able to account for our practice and take responsibility for our actions
Dissemination of good practice	Ensuring that we share and learn from examples of good practice with other members of the interprofessional team
Patient involvement	Ensuring that patients and carers are involved in their management
Quality improvement	Ensuring that we act on results of audits to improve practice

Activity 11.4

Problem: The incidence of pressure ulcers has increased in your clinical area.

- Discuss this problem with your mentor
- Find out if an audit has been implemented
- Have these pressure ulcers occurred in your clinical area or have the patients been transferred to your care with the pressure ulcer?
- What are the grades of the pressure ulcers? What is the anatomical location?

- How easy is it to access pressure relieving equipment?
- Do you have up to date knowledge about pressure ulcer care?
- Does the audit identify similarities or areas of practice that require change and improvement?
- Has the audit data been analysed? Discuss with your mentor how improvements could be made to raise the standards of care in the prevention of pressure ulcers

- Feed back the results to your ward manager.

This scenario demonstrates:
- Leadership
- Personal development
- The need for audit and standard setting
- The need to include clinical and organisational risk
- That nursing should be about maintaining and improving the quality of patient care.

Assessing the Risk

A number of wounds, particularly chronic wounds, are associated with underlying pathology: for example, venous ulcers are often caused by chronic venous insufficiency, arterial ulcers by peripheral vascular disease, fungating wounds by carcinoma and pressure ulcers develop due to a number of contributing factors such as direct pressure, shear, friction or excess moisture. Deterioration in the patient's physical condition increases the risk of developing a pressure ulcer. The likelihood of certain wounds developing as a result of underlying pathology can be assessed and there are a number of risk assessment tools available to assist nurses and other health professionals in their clinical judgement. However, the validity of many of the tools is still questionable and they should not be used in isolation. They include pressure ulcer risk assessment tools, such as the Braden Scale (Bergstrom et al., 1987), Waterlow Scale (Waterlow, 2005), and diabetic foot ulcer risk assessment tools (Farndon et al., 2001). See Table 11.4 for examples of risk assessment scales. Once a patient has been identified as vulnerable and at risk of developing a pressure ulcer, preventative measures should be put in place. Bergstrom et al. (1998) state that assessment on admission is not as predictive as subsequent assessments, probably because clinicians acquire additional knowledge of patients with time. It is important to reassess patients' risk at regular intervals.

Activity 11.5

Try to locate the quality standard(s) for the prevention and management of pressure ulcers in your workplace. How many of these assessment criteria are reflected within them? Discuss your findings with your colleagues.

Table 11.4 Examples of pressure risk assessment tools (a) the Waterlow Scale and (b) the Braden Scale

(a)

WATERLOW PRESSURE ULCER PREVENTION/TREATMENT POLICY
RING SCORES IN TABLE, ADD TOTAL. MORE THAN 1 SCORE/CATEGORY CAN BE USED

BUILD/WEIGHT FOR HEIGHT	◆	SKIN TYPE VISUAL RISK AREAS	◆	SEX AGE	◆	MALNUTRITION SCREENING TOOL (MST) (Nutrition Vol.15, No.6 1999 - Australia		
AVERAGE		HEALTHY	0	MALE	1	A - HAS PATIENT LOST WEIGHT RECENTLY	B - WEIGHT LOSS SCORE	
BMI = 20-24.9	0	TISSUE PAPER	1	FEMALE	2	YES - GO TO B	0.5 - 5kg = 1	
ABOVE AVERAGE		DRY	1	14 - 49	1	NO - GO TO C	5 - 10kg = 2	
BMI = 25-29.9	1	OEDEMATOUS	1	50 - 64	2	UNSURE - GO TO C AND	10 - 15kg = 3	
OBESE		CLAMMY, PYREXIA	1	65 - 74	3	SCORE 2	> 15kg = 4	
BMI > 30	2	DISCOLOURED GRADE 1	2	75 - 80	4		unsure = 2	
BELOW AVERAGE		BROKEN/SPOTS		81 +	5	C - PATIENT EATING POORLY	NUTRITION SCORE	
BMI < 20	3	GRADE 2-4	3			OR LACK OF APPETITE	If > 2 refer for nutrition	
BMI=Wt(Kg)/Ht (m)²						'NO' = 0; 'YES' SCORE = 1	assessment / intervention	

CONTINENCE	◆	MOBILITY	◆	SPECIAL RISKS				
COMPLETE/ CATHETERISED	0	FULLY	0	TISSUE MALNUTRITION	◆	NEUROLOGICAL DEFICIT		◆
URINE INCONT.	1	RESTLESS/FIDGETY	1					
FAECAL INCONT.	2	APATHETIC	2	TERMINAL CACHEXIA	8	DIABETES, MS, CVA		4-6
URINARY + FAECAL INCONTINENCE	3	RESTRICTED	3	MULTIPLE ORGAN FAILURE	8	MOTOR/SENSORY		4-6
		BEDBOUND e.g. TRACTION	4	SINGLE ORGAN FAILURE (RESP, RENAL, CARDIAC,)	5	PARAPLEGIA (MAX OF 6)		4-6
SCORE		CHAIRBOUND e.g. WHEELCHAIR	5	PERIPHERAL VASCULAR DISEASE	5	MAJOR SURGERY or TRAUMA		
10+ AT RISK				ANAEMIA (Hb < 8)	2	ORTHOPAEDIC/SPINAL		5
15+ HIGH RISK				SMOKING	1	ON TABLE > 2 HR#		5
20+ VERY HIGH RISK						ON TABLE > 6 HR#		8
				MEDICATION - CYTOTOXICS, LONG TERM/HIGH DOSE STEROIDS, ANTI-INFLAMMATORY MAX OF 4				

© J Waterlow 1985 Revised 2005*
  Obtainable from the Nook, Stoke Road, Henlade TAUNTON TA3 5LX
* The 2005 revision incorporates the research undertaken by Queensland Health.

Scores can be discounted after 48 hours provided patient is recovering normally

www.judy-waterlow.co.uk

REMEMBER TISSUE DAMAGE MAY START PRIOR TO ADMISSION, IN CASUALTY. A SEATED PATIENT IS AT RISK
ASSESSMENT (See Over) IF THE PATIENT FALLS INTO ANY OF THE RISK CATEGORIES, THEN PREVENTATIVE NURSING IS
REQUIRED A COMBINATION OF GOOD NURSING TECHNIQUES AND PREVENTATIVE AIDS WILL BE NECESSARY
ALL ACTIONS MUST BE DOCUMENTED

PREVENTION
PRESSURE
REDUCING AIDS
Special
Mattress/beds: 10+ Overlays or specialist foam mattresses.
15+ Alternating pressure overlays, mattresses and bed systems
20+ Bed systems: Fluidised bead, low air loss and alternating pressure mattresses
Note: Preventative aids cover a wide spectrum of specialist features. Efficacy should be judged, if possible, on the basis of independent evidence.
Cushions: No person should sit in a wheelchair without some form of cushioning. If nothing else is available - use the person's own pillow. (Consider infection risk)
10+ 100mm foam cushion
15+ Specialist Gell and/or foam cushion
20+ Specialised cushion, adjustable to individual person.
Bed clothing: Avoid plastic draw sheets, inco pads and tightly tucked in sheet/sheet covers, especially when using specialist bed and mattress overlay systems
Use duvet - plus vapour permeable membrane.

NURSING CARE
General HAND WASHING, frequent changes of position, lying, sitting. Use of pillows
Pain Appropriate pain control
Nutrition High protein, vitamins and minerals
Patient Handling Correct lifting technique - hoists - monkey poles Transfer devices
Patient Comfort Aids Real Sheepskin - bed cradle
Operating Table
Theatre/A&E Trolley 100mm(4ins) cover plus adequate protection

Skin Care General hygene, NO rubbing, cover with an appropriate dressing

WOUND GUIDELINES
Assessment odour, exudate, measure/photograph position

WOUND CLASSIFICATION - EPUAP
GRADE 1 Discolouration of intact skin not affected by light finger pressure (non-blanching erythema)
This may be difficult to identify in darkly pigmented skin
GRADE 2 Partial thickness skin loss or damage involving epidermis and/or dermis
The pressure ulcer is superficial and presents clinically as an abrasion, blister or shallow crater
GRADE 3 Full thickness skin loss involving damage of subcutaneous tissue but not extending to the underlying fascia
The pressure ulcer presents clinically as a deep crater with or without undermining of adjacent tissue
GRADE 4 Full thickness skin loss with extensive destruction and necrosis extending to underlying tissue.

Dressing Guide Use Local dressings formulary and/or www.worldwidewounds

IF TREATMENT IS REQUIRED, FIRST REMOVE PRESSURE

Source: Waterlow Scale (2005) with permission of Waterlow (www.judy-waterlow.co.uk)

(b)

SENSORY PERCEPTION Ability to respond meaningfully to pressure related discomfort	**1. Completely Limited** Unresponsive (does not moan, flinch, or grasp) to painful stimuli, due to diminished level of consciousness or sedation OR Limited ability to feel pain over most body surfaces	**Very Limited** Responds only to painful stimuli. Cannot communicate discomfort except by moaning or restlessness OR Has a sensory impairment which limits the ability to feel pain or discomfort over half body	**3. Slightly Limited** Responds to verbal commands but cannot always communicate discomfort or need to be turned OR Has some sensory impairment which limits ability to feel pain or discomfort in 1 or 2 extremities	**4. No Impairment** Responds to verbal commands. Has no sensory deficit which would affect ability to feel or voice pain or discomfort
MOISTURE Degree to which skin is exposed to moisture	**1. Completely Moist** Skin is kept moist almost constantly by perspiration, urine etc. Dampness is detected every time the patient is moved or turned	**2. Very Moist** Skin is often, but not always moist. Linen must be changed at least once a shift	**3. Occasionally Moist** Skin is occasionally moist, requiring an extra linen change approximately once a day	**4. Rarely Moist** Skin is usually dry. Linen only requires changing at routine intervals
ACTIVITY Degree of physical activity	**1. Bedfast** Confined to bed	**2. Chairfast** Ability to walk severely limited or non-existent. Cannot bear own weight and/or must be assisted into chair or wheelchair	**3. Walks Occasionally** Walks occasionally during day, but for short distances, with or without assistance. Spends majority of each shift in bed or chair	**4. Walks frequently** Walks outside of room at least twice a day and inside room at least every 2 hours during waking hours
MOBILITY Ability to change and control body position	**1. Completely Immobile** Does not make even slight changes in body or extremity position without assistance	**2. Very Limited** Makes occasional slight changes in body or extremity position but unable to make frequent or significant changes independently	**3. Slightly Limited** Makes frequent though slight changes in body or extremity position independently	**4. No Limitation** Makes major and frequent changes in position without assistance
NUTRITION Usual food intake pattern	**1. Very Poor** Never eats a complete meal. Rarely eats more than a third of any food offered. Eats 2 servings or less of protein (meat or dairy products) every day. Fluids taken poorly. Does not take a liquid dietary supplement OR Is NBM and /or maintained on clear fluids or IVs for 5 days	**2. Probably Inadequate** Rarely eats a complete meal and generally eats only half of any food offered. Protein intake includes only 3 servings of meat or dairy products per day. Occasionally will take a dietary supplement OR Receives less than optimum amount of liquid diet or tube feeding	**3. Adequate** Eats over half of most meals. Eats a total of 4 servings of protein (meat, dairy products) each day. Occasionally will refuse a meal, but will usually take a supplement if offered OR Is on tube feeding or TPN regimen which probably meets most of nutritional needs	**4. Excellent** Eats most of every meal. Never refuses a meal. Usually eats a total of 4 or more servings of meat and dairy products. Occasionally eats between meals. Does not require supplementation.

FRICTION AND SHEAR	1. Problem	2. Potential Problem	3. No Apparent Problem
	Requires moderate to maximum assistance in moving. Complete lifting without sliding against sheets is impossible. Frequently slides down in bed or chair, requiring frequent repositioning with maximum assistance. Spasticity, contractures or agitation leads to almost constant friction	Moves freely or requires minimum assistance. During a move skin probably slides to some extent against sheets, chair restraints or other devices. Maintains relatively good position in chair or bed most of the time but occasionally slides down	Moves in bed and in chair independently and has sufficient muscle strength to lift up completely during move. Maintains good position in bed or chair at all times

Note: The lower the score in Braden the higher the risk.
Source: Braden scale, with permission of Braden and Bergstrom.

☀ Activity 11.6

Find out which pressure ulcer risk assessment tool is in use where you work. What risk factors are included in it? If different compare it to the Waterlow scale and Braden scale illustrated here. Ask your clinical mentor the following:

How are the risk assessment tools used? How often is each assessment carried out? Who carries it out? How are the results documented and acted upon? How is the client involved in this?

Casebox 11.1

Mrs B is 52 years old. She has been admitted to hospital 2 days ago following a stroke. She is 5' 2" and weighs 10 stone (63.5 kg). She is conscious but is struggling to communicate verbally. She has a diminished swallow reflex and a hemiplegia and is constantly sliding down the bed. She needs assistance to reposition in bed. She is incontinent of urine and faeces. Her skin is intact. She suffers from hypertension and takes antihypertensive medication. She takes non-steroidal anti-inflammatory medication to treat her osteoarthritis. Mrs B gave up smoking 2 years ago.

Use the Braden and Waterlow risk assessment tools to assess the risk of Mrs B developing pressure ulcers.

- What level of risk did you find?
- Was there any difference using each scale?
- Reflect on this and discuss with your mentor in practice.

Factors Affecting Wound Healing

Wounds do not heal in isolation, and it is important to consider the whole person by completing a holistic assessment, which should aim to identify any existing or potential problems that will adversely affect wound healing. The numerous factors to be considered during an assessment are illustrated in Figure 11.1 and include local, systemic and contextual factors. Some of the key factors are discussed here. By reviewing each element the nurse will be able to develop an effective wound care strategy.

Nutrition

Good nutrition is essential for wound healing. There is a relationship between protein-energy malnutrition and delayed healing, reduced tensile strength, reduced immune-response to infection and development of pressure ulcers. There is also evidence, in a recent Cochrane review, that nutritional supplements reduce the number of new pressure ulcers (Langer et al., 2003). Proteins are

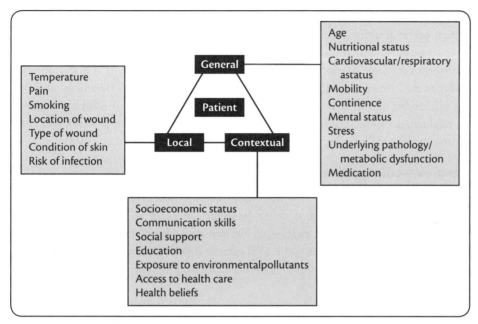

Figure 11.1 Factors affecting wound healing

essential for collagen synthesis, angiogenesis and cell reconstruction (Wells, 1994) and contribute to osmotic equilibrium and the immune response. In malnourished patients, proteins may also be a source of energy. Low blood protein levels (measured in terms of serum albumin) and negative nitrogen balance have been linked to impaired wound healing and increased vulnerability to pressure ulcers (Green et al., 1999).

Lipids, provided from the dietary fat intake, are vital components of cell membranes. Dietary fat is also the largest source of energy required for wound healing, as well as providing a source of fat-soluble vitamins. Essential fatty acids (polyunsaturated fatty acids) are precursors of prostaglandins and hence have a role in the inflammatory process. There is some evidence that **essential fatty acids** improve wound healing (Declair, 1997) and reduce wound infection (Gottschlich et al., 1990).

Carbohydrate, in the form of glucose, is the primary energy substrate required for cellular metabolism. If glucose from carbohydrate is unavailable, amino acids will be oxidised to meet the energy requirements of healing, thus depleting the pool of amino acids available for reconstruction and tissue repair.

Vitamin C is involved in the metabolism of many amino acids and is required for the synthesis of collagen and cross-linking collagen fibres, facilitating the **hydroxylation** of proline and lysine which are essential components of collagen (Lewis and Harding, 1993). Iron (as well as providing the primary component of haemoglobin, which facilitates the transport of oxygen in the bloodstream) is a co-factor in this process. Vitamin C, a strong antioxidant, together with vitamin E, also limit tissue damage by inhibiting potentially harmful **free radicals** from the surfaces of cells and facilitate the movement of white blood cells into

⊗ Link
See Chapter 7 for further information related to nutrition.

essential fatty acids
simple lipids, including the omega-3 and omega-6 fatty acids

hydroxylation
the formation or addition of a hydroxyl (OH) group

free radicals
unstable, highly reactive compounds containing an unpaired electron or proton

wounds and therefore reduce the risk of infection. The B vitamins are involved in enzymatic activity (as co-factors) and are also active in collagen cross-linkage, as is vitamin A, which also influences epithelial growth and acts on lymphocyte proliferation. Zinc is another co-factor in the enzymatic activity associated with collagen and protein synthesis and cell growth. Zinc also has beneficial stabilising effects on membrane structures and formation and has an inhibitory action on bacterial growth. There is some evidence to suggest that, in patients with low serum levels, oral zinc improves healing (Wilkinson and Hawke, 2008).

Cardiovascular and respiratory status

🔗 Link

Chapters 9 and 10 explore issues related to cardiovascular and respiratory status.

Anything that interferes in any way with oxygen delivery will tend to increase susceptibility to infection and delay healing. There is an inverse relationship between infection risk and perfusion (Jensen and Hunt, 1991). Ischaemia and poor blood supply lead to unstable collagen and poor re-epithelialisation as well as tissue necrosis and gangrene. Venous insufficiency can result in venous leg ulcers.

Smoking

Nicotine has a marked negative effect on peripheral blood flow, immune activity, epithelialisation and contraction and carbon monoxide reduces the available oxygen (Siana et al., 1992). This will lead to delayed healing.

Pathophysiology

Poorly controlled diabetes mellitus impairs glucose metabolism, which retards healing and increases the risk of infection, as insulin is essential for fibroblast activity and hyperglycaemia interferes with macrophage activity, collagen synthesis and re-epithelialisation (Barbul and Purtill, 1994). Abnormal leucocytes can affect the immune system – there is a decreased chemotactic and inflammatory response as neutrophils' ability to phagocytose is decreased (Mulder et al., 1998). High blood glucose levels with a low oxygen content is an ideal medium for bacterial growth.

Age

Wound healing complications are more common in the elderly, due to the body's reduced capacity to repair and slower cellular activity. The elderly are also more likely to have an associated pathology or be undernourished.

Pain

🔗 Link

Chapters 10, 12 and 13 also discuss pain.

Pain can have a detrimental effect on recovery and healing. The European Wound Management Association, in a position paper on pain stated that dressing removal, especially if adherent to new tissue, has been identified as the most painful experience associated with a wound (EWMA, 2002). Pain needs to be assessed, in terms of intensity, duration and frequency and the effect it is having on the patient's mental state.

Stress

Stress is implicated in poor healing due to reduced efficiency of the immune response. Carers of relatives with Alzheimer's took significantly longer to heal from a punch biopsy, compared to other carers (Kiecolt-Glaser et al., 1995).

Complications of Wound Healing

There are occasions when the wound healing process is interrupted and healing does not progress as anticipated. Some commonly observed complications in the wound healing process are now discussed.

Infection

Infection can significantly delay healing and increase hospital stay. There are three factors that influence the development of an infection: the number of bacteria, the virulence of the bacteria and the state of the patient's immune system (host resistance). Nearly all wounds are **contaminated** and many are **colonised** but this will not affect the healing process, indeed many chronic wounds can tolerate high levels of bacteria and still heal normally but an overwhelming number of bacteria (10^5 organisms per gram of tissue) will usually result in a clinical **infection**, interfering with the healing process by prolonging the inflammatory phase and depleting resources (Robson, 1997). This is generally characterised by localised cellulitis, spreading erythema as the infection spreads from the wound into the surrounding tissues. Signs of inflammation may also be present (heat, swelling, redness and pain) and an increase in wound exudate (often purulent in nature). In chronic wounds, cellulitis may be absent and other signs, such as a darkening in the appearance of granulation tissue, a change in pain or odour or an increase in wound exudates may be the only indicators. When a chronic wound appears to stop improving and is not healing, it may be because it is **critically colonised.** Some bacteria are more virulent than others, and may lead to infection, even if the number of bacteria is not that high. Biofilms (see Chart 11.1) may be present in the wound. These micro-colonies have a high resistance to antibiotics and antimicrobials. If the patient has a poor immune system due to immune deficiency or compromise, their resistance will be lower and they are more likely to develop an infection.

contamination
all wounds are contaminated as the breach in the skin allows normal skin flora to populate the wound

colonisation
contain multiplying bacteria but there is no systemic host reaction

infection
multiplication of bacteria in tissue with an associated host reaction, e.g. cellulitis, raised white cell count and C-reactive protein

critical colonisation
high levels of bacteria and unresponsive to treatment, although no clinical signs of infection (Schultz et al., 2003)

Chart 11.1 Biofilms

Note: In some wounds it is difficult to treat the infection due to the presence of biofilms

- Biofilms consist of a mixed species of bacteria that are grouped together and form a protective coat around themselves called a glycocalyx. This increases their resistance to antibiotics and antimicrobials. They cannot be seen with the naked eye, but the presence of biofilms may be suspected when there is a slime present in the wound bed or the wound is slow to heal. Some wound product manufacturers now claim that their products will break down and rid the wound of these biofilms.

Dehiscence

'Dehiscence' is the term used to refer to the 'splitting' open of a closed surgical wound. If the collagen fibres that have been laid down are not strong enough to withstand the internal and external tensions applied to the wound, the newly formed layers of the wound will separate. The dehiscence of a wound is often associated with infection and/or the presence of a haematoma or poor nutrition. The dehisced wound is often left to heal by secondary intention. The dehiscence will significantly increase the time to heal and the risk of complications.

Haematoma

Haematoma is the name given to a localised collection of blood and plasma trapped within the skin or an organ, which can become a breeding ground for bacteria and interfere in collagen deposition.

Haemorrhage

Primary haemorrhage (severe blood loss during surgery) and intermediary haemorrhage (severe blood loss immediately following surgery) can affect wound strength by interfering with the function of the fibroblasts. Secondary haemorrhage (blood loss up to 10 days post-operatively) commonly results in haematoma formation and subsequent infection.

Abnormal healing

★ Activity 11.8

Can you think of certain measures that could be taken to prevent any of these complications of healing? Discuss your ideas with your colleagues.

Abnormal healing is characterised by abnormalities in scar tissue formation and includes:

- *Hypertrophic scarring*, common in young patients. A large amount of scar tissue is laid down along the incision line, resulting in a raised, fibrous wound site.
- *Keloid scarring*, more common in patients with heavily pigmented skin. Again, a large amount of scar tissue continues to be laid down, but in this case the scar tissue infiltrates the surrounding skin, resulting in bulbous growths over and around the wound site.
- *Overgranulation* occurs when granulation tissue progresses beyond the normal wound bed (Dunford, 1999). It is often associated with a prolonged inflammatory phase and results in delayed re-epithelialisation.
- *Contractures*: hypercontraction of the wound during the maturation phase can result in excessive shortening of the associated muscle tissue, which, combined with the presence of fibrous scar tissue, inhibits muscular extension.
- *Malignant disease*: because of the intense cellular activity within a wound, there is the potential for chronic wounds to undergo malignant change. Failure to heal over an extended period of time can be associated with such a process. Tumours can also break through the surface of the skin, resulting in a fungating wound.

The Optimum Environment for Healing

Wound bed preparation, through the creation of an optimum environment for wound healing, is essential. Careful planning is required to choose the most appropriate wound care products and to involve the patients wherever possible to increase compliance with treatment. One glance through a hospital formulary, or a look around a modern treatment room will give an indication of the numerous products currently available to facilitate wound management. Such an array can create a certain amount of confusion when deciding which product will be best suited to which wound. In order to avoid this situation, it is important to make a thorough assessment of the patient and their wound (see Casebox 11.1), and plan the best wound care strategy. Basic principles of wound care include cleansing or debridement, management of exudate and moist interactive healing (Schultz et al., 2003). Morgan (2008) described the characteristics of an 'ideal dressing' although few, if any, of the dressings available conform to every criterion. Thus, the optimum environment at the wound–dressing interface will be:

- *Moist:* research conducted over 40 years ago (Winter, 1962) indicated that re-epithelialisation was enhanced when a moist environment was maintained, both within the wound bed and at the wound–dressing interface. This means that the body must be well hydrated and dressings should promote high humidity.
- *Free from excess exudate:* although wound exudate, containing leucocytes, neutrophils, nutrients and growth factors, is essential to moist wound healing, excess wound exudate will interfere with the healing process, contributing to wound bed oedema. It will also leak on to the surrounding skin, resulting in the **maceration** of healthy tissue.
- *Protected from bacterial contamination:* the wound needs to be protected by a physical barrier, to prevent bacteria entering the wound and thought must be given to potential sources of infection, such as hands, and other body fluids. Strike-through of exudate, when wound fluid leaks through the wound dressing, allows the passage of bacteria both into and out of the wound and thus increases the risk both of contamination of the wound and cross-infection.
- *Protected from particulate or toxic contamination:* foreign bodies, such as fibres causing granulomas can act as a focus for bacteria. Again, a physical barrier is required that will not shed fibres into the wound.
- *Thermally insulated:* the length of time a dressing stays on a wound between changes is an important factor. Not only should any dressing used maintain a stable temperature, but also practices such as frequent, unnecessary exposure of the wound, the use of cold cleansing solutions and changes in the ambient temperature must be avoided, as any persistent drop in temperature will lead to vasoconstriction, reduced cellular activity for several hours and shift the **oxygen dissociation curve** to the left, resulting in a decrease in the amount of oxygen delivered to the tissues (Morgan, 2008). Wounds heal more slowly in cold environments: if skin temperature drops from 20 °C to 12 °C, tensile strength reduces by 20 per cent.

maceration
the softening and detexturising of tissues due to prolonged exposure to moistness

oxygen dissociation curve
the plotted curve that demonstrates the release of oxygen from haemoglobin in capillaries into the interstitial fluid in areas of low oxygen tension

- *Well perfused:* gaseous exchange may take place at the wound–dressing interface, but it is more important that there is a good blood supply to ensure that the oxygen and nutrient demands of the wound are met, as well as removing waste products from the wound site.
- *Protected from mechanical trauma:* new epithelial cells and capillary buds are extremely delicate and can be easily damaged during dressing changes (especially if the dressing material adheres to the wound surface or the surface is rubbed during wound cleansing). Studies have shown that these cells can also be damaged by the use of antiseptic solutions, for example hypochlorite (Leaper, 1996). Thus, the environment must be assessed for potential hazards that could cause further trauma.
- *Undisturbed:* frequent dressing changes, however 'wound environmentally friendly' the dressings are, will interfere with the healing process and may be associated with an increase in pain.

As well as promoting the optimum environment for wound healing, the 'ideal dressing' should be cost-effective, perform in such a way as to maximise the achievement of treatment objectives, be acceptable to patients and carers and be readily available in both hospital and community settings.

Different types of dressing vary in terms of their suitability to absorb exudate, aid debridement, facilitate granulation or re-epithelialisation, and reduce infection or odour. Not all dressings of a similar type have the same characteristics and you will need guidance in making the best choice. There are a large number of different dressings available (see Table 11.5) and new ones are constantly being added to the formulary (Morgan, 2008). Many Trusts have developed their own wound formulary or guidelines to help the nurse in her decision-making.

Table 11.5 Generic types of wound dressings

Modern wound dressings	Examples
Foams	Lyofoam® (SSL), Allevyn® (S&N)
Hydrocellular	Allevyn® compression (S&N)
Hydrogels	Purilon Gel® (Coloplast), Intrasite Gel® (S&N), Geliperm®
Semi-permeable films	Opsite® (S&N), Tegaderm® (3M)
Hydrocolloids	Comfeel® (coloplast), Granuflex® (ConvaTec)
Alginates	Sorbsan® (Maersk), Kaltostat® (ConvaTec), Algisite M® (S&N)
Fibre-hydrocolloids	Aquacel® (ConvaTec)
Low-adherent	N.A Ultra® (J&J), Mepitel® (Molnlycke)
Silver dressings	Avance® (SSL), Acticoat® (S&N), Arglaes® (Maersk)

Deciding on the most suitable products for use in wound management is bewildering due to the number of different wound dressings on the market. If your Trust has its own wound formulary you can decide on the most suitable product using this list.

First you must have a rationale for your choice of product.

1   Wound management has to be teamwork. Underlying medical conditions and factors affecting wound healing must be addressed.

2   Identify the tissue in the wound bed. For example, is there any slough or **necrotic** tissue? Is there good granulation tissue?

3   Do you suspect infection? Is there any odour?

4   How much wound exudate is there?

5   What is the condition of the surrounding skin?

necrotic
dead, devitalised tissue

Is the wound painful? Is this continuous or intermittent? Is the pain occurring at the dressing change only? The nurse has to decide on the most beneficial treatment plan.

If the wound is necrotic or sloughy a decision would be made to debride or deslough the wound. (A decision is often made to leave hard black **eschar** intact to use it as nature's own dressing by allowing the underlying tissue to heal naturally). If infection is suspected this tissue must be removed. This is called debridement and may be done by a specialist nurse or surgeon using a scalpel (sharp or conservative sharp debridement). Some dressing products will also promote autolytic debridement. These products aid the body's physiological processes to break down this tissue. At the same time the level of exudate will need to be managed. If the wound is dry the wound will need to be rehydrated. If the wound has a high level of exudate a dressing will be required to manage the level of exudate. The cause of the high exudate should be investigated.

eschar
dead tissue, characterised by its dry, crusty, black appearance, which adheres to the wound bed

If infection is suspected an antimicrobial will be used. If there is damage to the surrounding skin this will need to be protected. If the patient is experiencing pain this will need to be investigated. The patient may require analgesia to be given prior to the dressing change or if the pain is caused by the dressing removal another product could be used. Most practitioners would opt to use none or low adherent dressings.

It is important to listen to what the patient says. Having a wound can be a frightening experience so keep the patient informed of the intended dressing plan and include them in the decision making about their care.

Many wound dressing products are suitable for more than one type of wound (see Table 11.6). The tissue within the wound bed should be identified: is it necrotic, sloughy, granulating, epithelialising? Are there indications that the wound is infected? There may be more than one tissue type in the wound bed.

There are also a growing number of non-dressing alternatives for managing wounds. Larval therapy uses sterile maggots on sloughy, infected or critically colonised wounds to aid debridement. Manuka honey has antibacterial and anti-inflammatory properties and appears to aid healing in a wide range of wounds (Molan, 1999). The use of negative pressure through Topical Negative Pressure stimulates angiogenesis and growth of granulation tissue, controls oedema at the wound bed, reduces infection and other functions and hence reduces healing time (Collier, 1997). There are various systems in use such as vacuum-assisted closure (VAC). These systems are expensive but are widely used as they greatly reduce the time to wound healing. The therapy is often used in the management of large or complex wounds.

✳ **Activity 11.9**

Find a copy of the *Morgan Formulary* (2008) or your Trust's formulary of wound management products. Note that the dressings listed are divided into groups, for example hydrocolloids.

Identify the particular characteristics of as many groups as you can and compare them with the elements described in the text. See if you can identify an example (by trade name) for each group.

Table 11.6 Examples of possible dressing choices and rationale for use

Level of exudate	Tissue type	Action required	Primary dressing	Secondary dressing	Comments
Low	Necrotic	Rehydrate and promote autolytic debridement. Protect from bacterial contamination	Hydrogel	Gauze and film dressing	The secondary dressing should have a high moisture vapour transmission rate (MVTR) to maintain the moisture balance at the wound bed and prevent maceration of the surrounding skin
		Removes medium for bacterial growth and allows assessment of wound depth.	Hydrocolloid	None required	
Moderate to high		Unless infection is suspected eschar is left intact to separate naturally	Alginate or Hydrofibre / Topical Negative Pressure (TNP)	Adhesive foam dressing	
	Sloughy	Manage as for necrotic wounds	As for necrotic wounds / Larval therapy		Slough in the wound may prolong the inflammatory phase of healing
Low	Granulating	To maintain healthy granulation tissue and promote epithelialisation. Maintain the moisture balance at the wound bed	Hydrogel / Low adherent dressing / Hydrocolloid	Gauze and film dressing / None required	New granulation tissue is fragile and may bleed easily.
High		Protect from bacterial contamination	Hydrofibre / Alginate / TNP	Adhesive foam dressings	
Low	Infected or critically colonised wounds	To reduce the number of bacteria in the wound. To promote healing. To protect from further bacterial contamination	Impregnated iodine dressing / Silver antimicrobial dressings / Silver sulphadiazine / Cadexomer iodine / Silver antimicrobial dressings / Honey dressings / TNP with antimicrobial foam / AMD dressings	Gauze and film dressing / Depending on the mode of delivery secondary dressings may not be required / Film	If the wound is clinically infected systemic antibiotics will be required / Check for raised temperature, pulse, white cell count and C-Reactive protein cellulitis, odour, pus, increase in exudate, friable granulation tissue
High				Adhesive foam dressings	
Low	Epithelialising	To protect fragile tissue. Protect from bacterial contamination	Film dressing / Hydrocolloid	Not required	
	Leg wounds		Do not use adhesive dressings on leg ulcers or fragile sensitive skin	If the dressings are being secured with a bandage a secondary dressing will not be required	

Care-planning in Wound Management

An effective method for designing a programme of care interventions is the nursing process. The stages of the nursing process form the framework for a systematic and holistic review of nursing care, based around a problem-solving approach. One of the benefits of adopting a systematic approach such as this is that you will be able to demonstrate clearly through documentation not only the decision-making processes involved in designing care interventions, but also – and most importantly – the effectiveness of those interventions.

A good way of exploring care planning in detail is to use a client profile. The profile described in Casebox 11.2 will form the basis for a detailed analysis of planning care in wound management.

> **⌘ Link**
>
> Chapter 1 explains the nursing process in more detail.

Casebox 11.2

Mr Hartley is a frail, elderly gentleman of 88 years, who is a widower. He has arterial disease and type II diabetes mellitus and has had two toes on his left foot amputated. He now lives in a residential home but maintains regular contact with his family. He recently had a fall resulting in a fracture of his femur. He was admitted to hospital where he developed pneumonia and a Grade 3 pressure ulcer over his sacrum. His condition has improved and he is ready to return to his residential home. We now need to plan his transfer back to his residential home.

Whilst in hospital, he appeared rather agitated at times and complained of pain related to the pressure ulcer over his sacrum but was reluctant to 'make a fuss'. He tired easily and on admission to hospital his clothes appeared loose. He had gained some weight since his admission. His Body Mass Index is now 18.5. He had a history of occasional incontinence prior to admission to hospital. He can stand using a frame but needs some help to walk to the toilet.

Whilst in hospital he has been nursed on a profiling bed with an alternating pressure relieving mattress. The sacral wound has improved. It now measures 3 cm × 4 cm × 1 cm deep. It has a moderate serous exudate requiring dressing changes on alternate days. The wound bed tissue is 100 per cent granulation. The wound is no longer infected. The surrounding skin is healthy and intact.

> **✳ Activity 11.10**
>
> Using the information presented in Casebox 11.2, write an assessment of Mr Hartley and identify any actual or potential problems using the assessment framework in the text. Using Table 11.4 see if you can write a wound management plan for Mr Hartley.

Wound Assessment

Morison (2000) suggests that a holistic assessment should take into account environmental and social factors as well as physical and psychological factors in order to develop a sound wound management strategy. A number of frameworks exist for wound assessment (for example Morison et al., 2004).

You will now need to take into account the factors affecting wound healing described in Figure 11.1 above, to enhance the data you have already gathered.

You will probably have identified many of the problems described below.

General physical condition

Actual problem

Mr Hartley appears tired.

Mental function

Mr Hartley appears rather agitated.

Mobility

Actual problems

Mr Hartley is unable to mobilise independently without help. His mobility is hampered by having two toes missing on his left foot and the presence of a pressure ulcer on his sacrum.

Nutritional status

Actual problems

- Mr Hartley has gained some weight but still has a low BMI.
- Mr Hartley has enhanced energy, protein, vitamin and mineral requirements due to the pressure ulcer.
- Mr Hartley has type II diabetes that is not very well controlled, which increases his risk of infection and impaired wound healing.

Continence

Actual problems

- Mr Hartley may have urinary incontinence.
- Mr Hartley needs help to get to the toilet independently.

Potential problems

- Mr Hartley may suffer skin excoriation from leakage of urine and his wound may be contaminated by leaking urine.
- Mr Hartley may suffer from constipation as a result of immobility.

Cardiovascular status

Actual problems

Arterial disease, which has led to the amputation of two toes on his left leg. Arterial disease implies an impaired blood flow to wound sites and impaired healing.

Pain

Although Mr Hartley has complained of some pain related to his sacral pressure ulcer it might be worse than he is saying.

Actual problems

- Mr Hartley appears to be in pain but may not be voicing the extent of his pain.

- Mr Hartley appears rather agitated and may be frightened, but may be reluctant to cause a fuss. Pain is often associated with stress and anxiety that will delay healing.

Potential problems

Increasing pain may further limit Mr Hartley's mobility.

Skin

Mr Hartley has a pressure ulcer on his sacrum.

You may be surprised at how much information can be gathered from the careful reading of a client profile, but certain areas need clarification so that problems can be better identified.

> **Link**
> Chapter 12 explores mobility issues.

Continence

You will need to establish if Mr Hartley is suffering from urinary incontinence and, if so, how long he has been suffering from it. In order to promote continence and prevent constipation, you will need to establish Mr Hartley's normal bladder and bowel habit.

A continence chart can be used to assess this. The Residential Home and Mr Hartley's District Nurse will need this information.

> **Link**
> Chapter 8 explores issues related to continence.

Nutritional status

It is important to use a nutritional screening tool, such as MUST (Elia, 2003) to identify if Mr Hartley is undernourished or is at risk of protein energy malnutrition. This will include weight, height and calculation of his Body Mass Index, in addition to identifying any recent unintentional weight loss. You should ask Mr Hartley if he can remember what he has eaten and drunk over the past 24 hours and what his favourite foods are and try to establish the reason for his ill-fitting clothes. Talking to the staff at the Residential Home will also be able to help with this information. You will also need to establish how much he understands about diet and diabetes. There are a number of nutritional guidelines for pressure ulcer prevention that you can use to help in your assessment, such as the EPUAP one (Clark et al., 2004).

Concurrent disease

In order to enhance your information relating to Mr Hartley's diabetes, it will be necessary to establish a pattern of blood glucose level over a period of time, starting with a baseline level on admission. You will also need to know whether Mr Hartley is excreting glucose in his urine. How is his diabetes being managed? It is important to share this information with the Residential Home and District Nurse.

> **Link**
> Chapter 10 explores cardiovascular issues.

★ **Activity 11.12**

Using Chart 11.2
and the wound
assessment outlined
in the text, assess the
wound of a patient
with a pressure ulcer.

How easy was it to
assess the grade of
pressure ulcer?

How did you assess
the size of the wound?

How are wound
details documented?

Visit the PUCLAS
(pressure ulcer
classification) site on
the EPUAP website for
detailed assessment
with photographs.

Pain

You will need to establish whether Mr Hartley is experiencing pain and, if so, its nature, intensity, location, duration and precipitating factors (for example movement or wound dressing changes). You will also need to ascertain Mr Hartley's feelings about pain control and prevention.

Look at the wound and surrounding area. What can you see?

Assess the quality of the skin in terms of hydration, elasticity, colour, temperature and integrity. Establish exactly how and where the integrity of the skin has been breached, assessing each wound individually and recording:

- *Wound site:* anatomical location.
- *Wound dimensions:* measure wound surface area by tracing around the edge of the wound or by recording length/width and depth. Digital photography is often used to record wound size.
- *Pressure ulcer grading:* a numerical value relating to their severity (EPUAP, 2009; or Reid and Morison, 1994). See Chart 11.2 for classification of pressure ulcers.
- *Wound bed status:* what percentage of the wound bed is occupied by necrotic tissue (eschar), slough, granulation tissue and epithelial tissue? Try to establish the stage of wound healing and presence of oedema (although this is not always possible).
- *Exudate:* how much exudate is there? How can you quantify the amount? Is the level high, medium or low? Is it increasing or decreasing? What does the exudate look like? Is the exudate purulent or bloodstained?
- *Infection:* are there any signs or symptoms to indicate a wound infection?
- *Odour:* present/absent?

Chart 11.2 Classification of pressure ulcers

- **Grade/Category 1**: Non-blanching erythema of intact skin. Usually over a bony prominence. Discolouration of the skin, warmth, cold, oedema, induration or hardness may also be used as indicators, particularly on individuals with darker skin.
- **Grade/Category 2**: Partial thickness skin loss of dermis. Presents as a shallow open ulcer with a pink wound bed without slough or bruising. May present as an intact or ruptured blister.
- **Grade/Category3**: Full thickness skin loss involving damage to subcutaneous tissue that may extend down to, but not through, underlying fascia. Can be shallow or deep depending on adiposity (fatty tissue). Bone or tendon are not exposed. Slough may be present but does not obscure the wound bed.* Bruising may indicate deep tissue damage.

- **Grade /Category 4**: Full thickness tissue loss with exposed bone, tendon or muscle. Slough or necrosis/eschar may be present. Often includes undermining and tunnelling. (The bridge of the nose, ear and malleolus do not have adipose tissue and these ulcers may be shallow; if bone *is* visible these ulcers would be categorised as grade 4).

Source: EPUAP/NPUAP (2009). Used with permission of the National Pressure Ulcer Advisory Panel (October 2010).

- *Edge of wound*: is it well defined? Is it raised or rolled? Is there any **undermining** of surrounding area indicating that the actual wound size is larger than apparent?
- *Surrounding skin*: is it intact? Well perfused? Macerated? Inflamed? Eczematous? Oedematous?
- *Expected mode of healing*: will this wound heal by primary or secondary intention?

What do you think the primary problems are? Does the wound need to be rehydrated/debrided/protected?

- What wound management strategy do you suggest?
- What is your rationale for choice of product?

Risk assessment

It will be necessary for the District Nurse to repeat a pressure ulcer risk assessment when Mr Hartley returns to the Residential Home. If you are working on a community placement you could do this together. Use a risk assessment tool, such as the Braden scale (Bergstrom et al., 1987) or Waterlow scale (Waterlow, 2005) to provide a framework for professional judgement when assessing Mr Hartley's level of risk of further pressure injury. The initial risk assessment must be completed as soon as possible after admission or transfer so that preventive measures can be taken. Some areas have particular quality standards relating to the prevention and management of pressure injury, and these will often specify the timeframe within which risk assessment should take place, for example, *Essence of Care* benchmarks (DoH, 2003). There are a number of national and international pressure ulcer prevention guidelines now available, such as those developed by NICE (2005) or the European Pressure Ulcer Advisory Panel (EPUAP, 2009).

Assessment in wound management can be summarised thus:

- Assessment is an ongoing process.
- Actual and potential problems are identified to provide the knowledge base for planning care interventions.
- The client is recognised as the primary source of information and secondary sources of information include relatives, carers, friends, other members of the multidisciplinary team, documentation and electronically stored data.
- The primary aim is to assess the client and his or her environment in terms of conduciveness to wound healing and to establish and record wound status, including any factors that may complicate or impair the healing process.
- The second aim is to establish the goal of treatment.

Planning Nursing Care

You will now be ready to enter the planning stage of the nursing process.

It is important to ensure that, whenever possible, you involve the client in agreeing the broad aims, setting objectives and identifying appropriate

undermining
an extension of the wound under the intact skin that cannot be visualised. It is important that this dimension of the wound is identified. This area of the wound needs to heal before the visible wound area or this may result in the formation of an abscess. It may appear that wound healing is slow. This is not the case if the undermining is undergoing healing

interventions. You will now be starting to understand the complexity of nursing care in wound management. The interventions that relate directly to the wound itself form only part of a range of activities that are vital to supporting wound management. Chart 11.3 describes Mr Hartley's wound status on admission to hospital. It is now possible to design a nursing care plan for the management of this wound, based upon your assessment and informed by a sound knowledge base of the principles of wound management. Following the previously outlined stages, the plan of care will develop as follows.

Chart 11.3 Mr Hartley's wound status on admission to hospital

Wound 1

- Cavity wound, located over left ischial tuberosity
- Diameter 6 cm, depth 6 cm
- Grade 3 pressure ulcer
- Wound bed composed of 70 per cent slough, 30 per cent necrotic eschar
- Moderate exudate level
- No signs of clinical infection or odour
- Well-defined edge with undermining for 2 cm to the left of wound

- Surrounding skin excoriated and poorly perfused
- Expected mode of healing – secondary intention
- Primary goals
- Relief of pressure
- debridement of slough and necrotic eschar
- control of exudate
- protection of surrounding skin
- pain management

Identifying the broad aim will be carried out in conjunction with Mr Hartley, asking him what he hopes will be the outcome of his stay in hospital and to what extent he is willing to participate in his care and carefully establishing how realistic these hopes may be. In this case, the broad aim may be identified as:

> To create a local environment that will be conducive to and promote wound healing. The expected outcome is that the necrotic tissue and slough will be removed and there will be formation of granulation tissue.

Specific objectives negotiated with Mr Hartley will include:

- Relieving pressure to prevent further deterioration of pressure ulcer or development of new pressure ulcers.
- Debriding the wound to encourage the **autolysis** of necrotic tissue and slough and its removal from the wound bed.
- Controlling exudate to avoid leakage and maceration of surrounding skin.
- Protecting the surrounding skin to prevent further breakdown.
- Pain management.

autolysis
the natural breakdown of dead, or foreign, organic material by leucocytes and rehydration

Next, *appropriate interventions* should be devised. Having already established that each objective is a statement of intention, or a 'what we want to do', the next step involves identifying nursing interventions, the 'how we are going to do it'. This can be done by reviewing each objective and identifying what action needs to be taken and what resources might be required.

1 *Specific objective*: Relieve pressure to prevent further deterioration of pressure ulcer or development of new pressure ulcers.

Nursing intervention:

- Install an alternating pressure, or constant low-pressure device and chair cushion. (different trusts have different policies about use of support surfaces: check with your mentor).
- Encourage Mr Hartley to move from side to side at regular intervals, to redistribute weight while in bed, and support position with the use of pillows, using the 30 degree tilt (Clark, 1998) if appropriate.
- Limit sitting times.
- Mr Hartley may not be able to get out of bed unaided if an alternating pressure system is used and will need assistance.
- Mr Hartley to agree to participate and use the prescribed equipment.
- Record interventions on a repositioning chart (refer to NICE Guidelines, 2003).

2 *Specific objective*: Protect the surrounding skin to prevent further breakdown.
   Nursing intervention:
   - Wash and dry surrounding skin sparingly, if contaminated, to avoid removing natural skin barriers (Hall, 2007).
   - Avoid friction and shear to skin by use of appropriate manual handling techniques.
   - Choose a skin barrier to protect the skin from further excoriation, which may be caused by proteolytic enzymes in the exudate digesting the corneal layers of the skin. Do not use creams, as this will make it difficult for the dressing to adhere to the surrounding skin. A skin protectant layer such as Cavilon (3M) could be used.

3 *Specific objective*: debride the wound to encourage the autolysis of necrotic tissue and slough and its removal from the wound bed.
   Nursing interventions:
   - Select the appropriate dressing, using the data from your wound assessment and the hospital/local wound formulary, documenting the selection and giving a rationale, for example:
   - Hydrogel selected to instil into wound bed to rehydrate the wound and promote the removal of necrotic tissue by autolytic debridement. Adhesive foam dressing selected to cover the hydrogel in the wound bed, to absorb excess exudate and protect the wound from contamination.

4 *Specific objective*: Control exudate to avoid leakage and maceration of surrounding skin.
   Nursing interventions:
   - Select a dressing that has a high absorptive capacity.
   - Consider applying a skin protectant such as Cavilon to prevent maceration of the surrounding skin.

Implementing Care

⚡ Activity 11.13

Review your assessment for Mr Hartley.

Select one of the actual problems identified and discuss how care may be planned, explaining how each nursing intervention will affect wound healing and identifying which other members of the interprofessional team may be involved.

The implementation stage of any wound management plan is critical in that:

- You ensure that planned care is given.
- You actively involve the client and other members of the interprofessional team.
- You record which elements of the care plan have been carried out, when and by whom.
- You begin to evaluate *as you implement care*, noting the length of time taken to complete an intervention, the ease with which it was undertaken, the degree to which the client was able (or willing) to participate, any associated teaching activities and any changes that occurred while you were implementing care.

Evaluation of Care

By focusing and reflecting on what is happening, both during and after the implementation of a nursing intervention, and then recording your findings, the nursing documentation not only serves as a record of events, but also becomes a dynamic working tool. The description of interactions between client and nurse will provide additional information. This may lead to:

- Further assessment
- Revisions to the care planned.

The key to success in making a care plan a 'working' document is your ability to evaluate the effectiveness of the nursing interventions you have designed. In the management of wounds, you will need to:

- Review the factors affecting wound healing
- Review the wound status
- Evaluate the agreed nursing interventions.

⚡ Activity 11.14

With your clinical mentor, and following the local guidelines for aseptic technique, select a hydrogel and a polyurethane foam dressing from the treatment room of your clinical area or ask the District Nurse how dressings are obtained in the community.

Prepare everything you would need to implement the wound dressing element of Mr Hartley's care plan.

🔗 Link

Chapter 1 identifies ways of evaluating nursing care.

Chapter Summary

The effective nursing management of wounds and the prevention of pressure ulcers is a complex area of activity involving integrated and systematic assessment, the identification of problems, and the planning, implementation and evaluation of nursing interventions. This chapter has given you an overview of the elements underpinning the principles of wound healing and management, highlighting the importance of ongoing, evidence-based education to inform decision-making in practice, the value of reflection as a way of evaluating your experiences, the wide range of tools, frameworks and guidelines available to assist in making a professional judgement and the central role of the nurse in managing care.

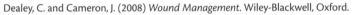
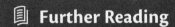

? Test yourself!

1 What are the main causes of pressure ulcers?

2 What preventative measures can be taken to avoid development of pressure ulcers?

3 What are the four main phases of wound healing?

4 The factors affecting wound healing have been described in terms of local, systemic and

contextual. How many of these factors can you list?

5 What are the criteria identified to provide the optimum environment for wound healing?

6 What specific wound characteristics would you include in your assessment of the patient?

Vuolo, J. (2009) *Wound Care Made Incredibly Easy*. Lippincott, Williams & Wilkins, London.

Dealey, C. and Cameron, J. (2008) *Wound Management*. Wiley-Blackwell, Oxford.

📖 **Further Reading**

For live links to useful websites see: www.palgrave.com/nursinghealth/hogston

References

Bale, S. and Jones, V. (2006) *Wound Care Nursing: A Patient Centred Approach*. Elsevier, Philadelphia.

Barbul, A. and Purtill, W. (1994) Nutrition in wound healing. *Clinical Dermatology* **12**: 133–40.

Bergstrom, N., Braden, B., Laguzza, A. and Holman, V. (1987) The Braden Scale for predicting pressure sore risk. *Nursing Research* **36**: 205–10.

Bergstrom, N., Braden, B., Kemp, M., Champagne, M. and Ruby, E (1998) Predicting pressure ulcer risk: A multisite study of the predictive validity of the Braden Scale. *Nursing Research* 47(5): 261–9.

Bethell, E. (2005) Wound care for patients with darkly pigmented skin. *Nursing Standard* **20**(4): 41–9.

Clark, M. (1998) Repositioning to prevent pressure sores-what is the evidence? *Nursing Standard* **13**(3): 58–64.

Clark, M., Schols, J., Benati, G., Jackson, P., Engfer, M., Langer, G., Kerry, B. and Colin, D. (2004) Pressure ulcers and nutrition: a new European guideline. *Journal of Wound Care* 13(7): 267–72.

Collier, M. (1997) Know-how: a guide to vacuum-assisted-closure. *Nursing Times* (suppl. January) **93**(5): 32–3.

Cullum, N. and Clark, M. (2006) Intrinsic factors associated with pressure sores in elderly people. Online *Journal of Advanced Nursing* **17**(4): 427–31.

Cullum, N. and Dealey, C. (1996) Presentation given to the all party group on skin at the House of Commons. *Journal of Tissue Viability* **6**(1): 20–3.

Cullum, N., McInnes, E., Bell-Syer, S. and Legood, R. (2004) Support surfaces for pressure ulcer prevention. *The Cochrane Database of Systematic Reviews Issue* 3.

Declair, V. (1997) The usefulness of topical application of essential fatty acids to prevent pressure ulcers. *Ostomy/Wound Management* **43**(5): 48–54.

DoH (Department of Health) (2000) *The NHS Plan*. The Stationery Office, London.

DoH (Department of Health) (2003) *Essence of Care: Patient-focused Benchmarks for Clinical Governance*. The Stationary Office, London.

Dunford, C. (1999) Hypergranulation tissue. *Journal of Wound Care* **8**(10): 506–7.

Elia, M. (2003) *The MUST Report*. BAPEN, Redditch.

EPUAP (European Pressure Ulcer Advisory Panel) (2009) *Pressure Ulcer Prevention and Treatment Guidelines*. EPUAP, Oxford. www.epuap.org

EPUAP/NPUAP (European Pressure Ulcer Advisory Panel and National Pressure Ulcer Advisory Panel) (2009) *Prevention and Treatment of Pressure Ulcers: Quick Reference Guide*. NPUAP, Washington DC.

EWMA (European Wound Management Association) (2002) *Position Statement on Pain* at *Wound Dressing Changes*. EWMA Medical Education Partnership Ltd, London.

Farndon, L., Henderson, M. and Wright, V. (2001) Conflict to consensus: development of a regional risk assessment tool. *Diabetic Foot* **4**(1): 35–42.

Gottschlich, M., Jenkins, M. and Warden, G. (1990) Differential effects of 3 enteral dietary regimens on selected outcome variables in burn patients. *Journal of Parenteral and Enteral Nutrition* **14**: 225–34.

Green, S., Winterberg, H., Franks, P., Moffatt, C., Eberhardie, C. and McLaren, S. (1999) Dietary intake of adults, with and without pressure sores, receiving community nursing services. *Journal of Wound Care* **8**(7): 325–30.

Hall, S. (2007) A review of the effect of tap water versus normal saline on infection rates in acute traumatic wounds. *Journal of Wound Care* **16**(1): 38–41.

Hunt, T.K., Hopf, H. and Zamirul, H. (2000) Physiology of wound healing. *Advances in Skin and Wound Care* **13** (Suppl. 2): 6–11.

Jensen, J. and Hunt, T.K. (1991) The wound healing curve as a practical teaching device. *Surgery, Gynecology and Obstetrics* **173**(1): 63–4.

Kiecolt-Glaser, J., Marucha, P., Mercado, A., Malarkey, W. and Glaser, R. (1995) Slowing of wound healing by psychological stress. *Lancet* **346**(8984): 1194–6.

Langer, G., Schloemer, G., Knerr, A., Kuss, O. and Behrens, J. (2003) Nutritional interventions for preventing and treating pressure ulcers. *The Cochrane Database of Systematic Reviews*, issue 4.

Leaper, D. (1996) Antiseptics in wound healing. *Nursing Times* **92**(39): 63–8.

Lewis, B.K. and Harding, K.G. (1993) Nutritional intake and wound healing in elderly people. *Journal of Wound Care* **2**(4): 227–9.

Molan, P. (1999) The role of honey in the management of wounds. *Journal of Wound Care* **8**(8): 415–18.

Morgan, D. (2008) *The Formulary of Wound Management Products*. Euromed Communications, Haslemere.

Morison, M. (2000) *The Prevention and Treatment of Pressure Ulcers*. C.V. Mosby, London.

Morison, M., Ovington, L. and Wilkie, K. (2004) *Chronic Wound Care: A Problem-based Learning Approach*. Mosby, Edinburgh.

Mulder, G.D., Brazinsky, B.A., Faria, D., Harding, K.G. and Argren, M.S. (1998) *Factors Influencing Wound Healing.* In Leaper, D.J. and Harding, K.G. (eds) *Wounds Biology and Management*. Oxford University Press, Oxford.

NICE (National Institute for Health and Clinical Excellence) (2005) *Clinical Guideline: Prevention and Treatment of Pressure Ulcers*. September. www.nice.org.uk/cg029quickrefguide

NMC (Nursing and Midwifery Council) (2008) *The Code: Standards of Conduct, Performance and Ethics for Nurses and Midwives*. NMC, London. www.nmc-uk.org

Reid, J. and Morison, M.A. (1994) Towards a consensus: classification of pressure sores. *Journal of Woundcare* **3**(3): 157–60.

Robson, M. (1997) Wound infection. *Surgical Clinics of North America* **77**(3): 637–50.

RCN (Royal College of Nursing) (2003) *Clinical Governance: An RCN Resource Guide*. http://www.rcn.org.uk/__data/assets/ pdf_file/0011/78581/002036.pdf

RCN (Royal College of Nursing) (2005) *The Management of Pressure Ulcers in Primary and Secondary Care: A Clinical Practice Guideline*. http://www.rcn.org.uk/development/practice/ clinicalguidelines/pressure_ulcers

Sackett, D., Rosenburg, W., Muir Gray, J., Haynes, B., Scott Richardson, W. (1996) Evidence-based medicine: What it is and what it isn't. *British Medical Journal* **312**(7023): 71–2.

Schultz, G., Sibbald, G., Falanga, V., Ayello, E., Dowsett, D., Harding, K., Romanelli, M., Stacey, M., Teot, L. and Vanscheidt, W. (2003) Wound bed preparation: a systematic approach to wound management. *Wound Repair and Regeneration* **11**: 1–28.

Siana, J., Frankild, S. and Gottrup, F. (1992) The effect of smoking on tissue function. *Journal of Wound Care* **1**(2): 37–41.

Waterlow, J. (2005) *Pressure Ulcer Prevention Manual*. Waterlow, Taunton.

Wells, L. (1994) At the front line of care. *Professional Nurse* **9**(8): 525–30.

Wilkinson, E.A.J. and Hawke, C. (2008) Oral zinc for arterial and venous leg ulcers. *Cochrane Database of Systematic Reviews*. Issue 4. art.no. CD001273.

Winter, G. (1962) Formation of the scab and the rate of epithelialisation of superficial wounds in the skin of the domestic pig. *Nature* **193**: 293–4.

WAYNE ARNETT AND KEVIN HUMPHRYS

Chapter

Moving and Handling

12

☑ Learning outcomes

At the end of this chapter, you should be able to:

- Describe the basic principles of moving and handling
- Recognise the importance of effective communication when conducting moving and handling assessments and interventions
- Outline the importance of anatomy and physiology in relation to moving and handling
- Familiarise yourself with relevant law, policy and guidelines relating to moving and handling within health and social care settings
- Relate the importance of risk assessment within moving and handling situations
- Describe a range of strategies for the optimum safety of staff and patients/clients when moving and handling.

Introduction

Moving and handling, as defined by the Manual Handling Operations Regulations (MHOR) 1992, means 'any transporting or supporting of a load (including the lifting, putting down, pushing, pulling, carrying or moving thereof) by hand or by bodily force'. Moving and handling is not just something we, as health-care professionals, need to consider when we put on our uniforms, it is something that we do every day in our daily activities and requires assessment, reflection and thought. Although humans are designed to lift objects we need to consider the multifaceted implication of our actions and the actions of others under the heading of moving and handling. Therefore this chapter explores the concepts inherent within moving and handling in the health-care arena and in daily life activities.

Statistics

According to the National Health Service (NHS, 2009) and the Health and Safety Executive (HSE, 2009a), the NHS employs more than 1.5 million people across 400 organisations. This figure rises to 2.6 million when the wider social care sectors are included. Of those, just short of half of staff are clinically qualified, including some 90,000 hospital doctors, 35,000 general practitioners, 400,000 nurses and 16,000 ambulance staff. The NHS in England is far and away the biggest part of the system, catering to a population of 50 million and employing more than 1.3 million people. On average, one million clients every 36 hours, that is 463 per minute and almost 8 per second, use the NHS daily.

The budget for the NHS, when it was launched in 1948, was £437 million (roughly £9 billion at today's value) and in 2007/8 it has risen to more than £90 billion. As with any large organisation sickness absence and injury is inevitable, and it has been estimated that it costs the NHS £1 billion a year. It is also inescapable that these absences, whether preventable or not, have implications on the effective delivery of health and social care services within the wider populous. Within the NHS, moving and handing injuries account for 40 per cent of absence from work through sickness; if we look at this numerically, it is reported that each year there are over 5,000 moving and handling injuries occurring within the NHS, with approximately 2,500 occurring while moving and handling patients (HSE, 2009b).

Although these statistics are extremely worrying they do have the ability to provide a broader picture. But we need to bring this figure down to a more personal and manageable figure; therefore, it has been estimated that one in four nurses have, at some time, taken time off sick as a result of back injury sustained at work (HSE, 2009c).

According to the data obtained from the HSE (2008a), the 2007/8 Labour Force Survey (LFS cited in HSE, 2008b) and the Self-reported Work-related Injuries survey, it has been estimated that the combined number of days lost (full-day equivalent) within the health and social work sector, due to workplace injuries and work-related ill health, was 5.1 million. This results in an estimated average annual loss of 1.9 days per worker. This was significantly higher than the rate for all industries which was 1.2 days per worker.

The most common kinds of reported injuries to workers in all industries occur as a result of moving and handling, or slips and trips. These also represent the most common kinds of reported injury within the health and social work sector as a whole. In 2007/8, moving and handling accounted for 41 per cent of reported injuries to workers, and slips and trips 25 per cent.

The HSE (2008b) continued to estimate that 539,000 people in Great Britain, who had worked in the last year, believed they were suffering from a musculoskeletal disorder (MSD) that was caused or made worse by their current or past work/employment. This equates to 1,800 per 100,000 people (1.8 per cent) who worked in the last 12 months in Great Britain. Of these, about a third, 178,000 people, *first became aware* of their work-related MSD in the previous 12 months. This is estimated to be 590 per 100,000 people (0.59 per cent) with a *new* work-related MSD in 2007/8.

The LFS also stated that MSDs, caused by or made worse by work, resulted in the loss of 8.8 million working days (full-day equivalent). On average, each person suffering from an MSD took an estimated 16.4 days off in that 12-month period, which equates to an annual loss of 0.37 days *per worker*.

MSDs and injuries are often seen by health and social care professionals as an occupational hazard. Current statistics clearly show that we must not just accept these so-called 'consequences of the profession', we must strive to amend the clinical culture that we work within, and our own personal and professional thinking and attitudes towards moving and handling and by these actions influence colleagues and clients alike. We must also strive to promote safe moving and handling practices within daily life activities as we really must begin to reflect upon how many work-related MSDs occur as a result of moving and handling incidents caused by poor moving and handling practices at home which are exacerbated by moving and handling practices within the health-care setting.

If we consider what the main contributory characteristics of work-related MSDs are, we will clearly see that they are not exclusive to the workplace environment (Table 12.1). We must then consider, do we only see the practice of safe moving and handling as a work-based activity, or is it so imbedded within our practice we consider the principles of safe moving and handling within our daily life activities? As you see from the LFS they cite MSDs as either being caused by or made worse by work – so an underlying MSD caused by a daily life activity could be exacerbated by a simple and safe procedure/manoeuvre at work.

Law and Legislation – Employer and Employee

Within the interprofessional arena it is apparent that students and qualified members of staff are totally aware and required to consider, at all times, the relevant policies and procedures that are required for the safe and effective

Table 12.1 The main causes and contributory factors of MSDs

Activity	Workplace	Daily life
Repetitive and heavy lifting	Patient handling and inanimate load handling	Moving/carrying babies/children, shopping, gardening, household chores
Bending and twisting	Patient handling and inanimate load handling	Getting into a car, gardening, moving babies/children, accessing kitchen cupboards, getting shopping from the trolley to the car boot
Repeating an action too frequently	Sitting clients forward, getting clients in/out of a chair/bed/wheelchair	Lifting heavy shopping bags. Moving/carrying babies/children
Uncomfortable working/sitting position	Chair in incorrect position, bed height incorrectly adjusted	Kitchen work surfaces, sink heights, lounge chairs, using laptop in a unsuitable chair/couch
Exerting too much force	Lifting a wheelchair in to the back of a car boot. Pushing heavy equipment from one environment to another	Lifting shopping from trolley to car boot and vice versa. Lifting children who appear too small to be heavy
Working too long without breaks	Working in front of a computer for longer than the recommended time. Not taking breaks due to a busy ward environment	Not taking a break during housework. Not scheduling breaks when looking after children and/or working at home
Exerting a force in a static position for extended periods of time	Photocopying, shredding, medication rounds, wound dressing, observations	Washing up, ironing, baby changing
Adverse working environment (e.g. hot, cold)	Working within the community setting; working behind closed curtains; working environments that lack ventilation and/or poor lighting	Small, cramped living environments. Environments that do not allow for independent movement
Psychosocial factors (e.g. high job demands, time pressures and lack of control)	Unreasonable time scales to complete projects. Insufficient time allocation to conduct patient interventions	Collecting the children from school on time. Taking work home to complete. Demands from friends and family
Not receiving and acting upon reports of symptoms quick enough	Ignoring the symptoms of tiredness, fatigue and stress	Ignoring the symptoms of tiredness, fatigue and stress

Source: Adapted from HSE (2008c).

administration of patient medicines. This consideration is heightened by the knowledge and awareness of the subsequent consequences of drug errors to the patient and the administering nurse(s). However, ask the same question in relationship to moving and handling and a very different level of seriousness is apparent. Many students and qualified staff would not consider the administration of an injection to an unknown client without first following, in its entirety, the stated policy or required procedure; however, ask the same health-care professional to assist in standing a patient using a 'drag lift' (placing forearm under the client's axilla), or using a bed sheet to move a patient, and many would oblige without even considering or reflecting upon the consequences to themselves, the patient, and colleague(s) participating in the manoeuvre. This observation is supported by Cornish and Jones (2010) whose study into the factors that affect compliance with moving and handling, from a student nurses' perspective, that arose while in clinical placement, highlighted eight categories of 'poor practice':

- Use of bed sheets to drag clients up the bed
- Non-completion of risk assessments
- No assessment of clients' abilities
- Lifting/using condemned techniques
- Supporting the patient's weight
- Poor communication
- Poor management of equipment
- Non-completion of equipment safety checks. (Cornish and Jones, 2010)

When asked the most serious complication associated with the participation of 'controversial (unsafe) moving and handling technique', most would state 'back pain', 'musculoskeletal injury', 'fall' and laugh openly when informed that *death* is the worst event that can occur. Many health-care professionals will discuss the most serious physical injury without considering the possibility of psychological trauma associated with their actions on the patient or colleague. Disciplinary proceedings, dismissal, court action and even imprisonment are often never contemplated. With this plethora of information, legislation and policies, why then do these types of controversial practices still continue, and why do students who attend their mandatory moving and handling training comply with known controversial practices?

Cornish and Jones (2010) continue to cite student reasons as the feeling of powerlessness alongside qualified staff, and pressure to use embedded cultural practices such as using sheets to lift clients up the bed, which they know are unsafe. Other students found it difficult to say *no* as they felt it was undermining authority, and actively maintain the illusion that qualified staff know what they are doing and can guide the student, even when teaching and promoting unsafe practice. Students also cited the need to fit into the clinical practice areas and to be accepted by the staff as a reason why they comply with unsafe practice. One student stated that they felt mistreated in a placement when they had tried to challenge poor practice. It seems incomprehensible in the twenty-first century that issues raised by students are still apparent within some clinical areas and individual practices. Some qualified individuals continue to place themselves, their colleagues, the students that are under their care and their clients in danger of serious injury and potential loss of life within moving and handling.

As health-care professionals are bound by law and professional accountability we have to acknowledge that we do not have the option of choice, we have a duty to abide by and comply with the regulatory law that has purposefully been embedded into our culture thus ensuring that safe moving and handling is continuously at the forefront of practice. The regulatory law ensures that individuals who disregard the option of practising safe moving and handling should not only be challenged without fear of reprisal but when necessary appropriate disciplinary and/or legal action is taken against those who continue to promote controversial practice. Many NHS Trusts now support disciplinary action when members of staff continue to practise outdated and controversial techniques that contravene their mandatory training and/or law, legislation, policies, procedures and guidelines. As a qualified nurse you are, in accordance with the NMC Code (2008), personally accountable for the actions and omissions in your practice and must always be able to justify your decisions. The NMC also states that as a qualified nurse you must always act lawfully, whether those laws relate to your professional practice or personal life, and failure to comply with this Code may bring your fitness to practise into question and endanger your registration. Under the NMC's 'Guidance on Professional Conduct for Nursing and Midwifery Students' (2005/2009/2010) it states that you, as a pre-registration student, are not professionally accountable in the way that you will be after you come to register with the NMC. Therefore you cannot be called to account for your actions and omissions by the NMC; it is the registered practitioners with whom you are working who are professionally responsible for the consequences of your actions and omissions. This is why you must always work under direct supervision. This does not mean, however, that you can never be called to account by your university or by the law for the consequences of your actions or omissions as a pre-registration student. With this in mind, student and health-care professionals must be aware of current regulations, governing bodies and associated risk/generic assessment procedures to ensure a safe working environment is maintained and strived for at all times. Therefore, an awareness and compliance of these regulations, legislation, law and so on is compulsory, excuses such as 'moving and handling is always done this way', or 'this manoeuvre/technique is necessary for nursing care' are unacceptable. On occasions staff have been heard to refer to the adage 'I have done moving and handling this way for 20 years and not injured myself' or 'If I do injure myself I will get sick pay and then sue for compensation'. One aspect that is recurrent within the statements above is that health-care professionals have referred to themselves and not the consequences of their actions on clients and colleagues or the accumulative damage that is being done to themselves and others. Unsafe or controversial moving and handling can be so inbred within our culture that the rationale for the use of these controversial techniques cannot be provided when challenged.

According to Dimond (2005) a nurse who has injured their back at work, *may* have a claim against the employer for breach of the duty of care owed to them under common law. Employers may also be in breach of duty if they fail to implement the Manual Handling Regulations 1992, which were introduced in January 1993 as a result of a European Community Directive 90/269/EEC (1990) on the manual handling of loads. The MHOR supplement the general duties of the employers and others by the Health and Safety at Work Act (OPSI, 1974) and the broad requirements of the Management of Health and Safety at Work Regulations 1999 (HSE, 2003). In addition to this, the employer may be vicariously liable for harm caused by another employee, and if injured as a result of defective equipment (for example stand-aid, bed, hoist), the nurse *may* be able to bring a case against the supplier under the Consumer Protection Act 1987. One cannot stress the importance of complying with and understanding the relevant law, legislation, policies, procedures and guidelines that relates to nursing and midwifery and moving and handling. It is not simply a case of do what is done, ask no questions and if I become injured or injure someone else I will sue, there is a great deal that needs consideration, understanding and explanation.

The law, as it relates to moving and handling, is regulated by statute principally in the form of the Health and Safety at Work Act (H&SWA) (OPSI, 1974) and the Manual Handling Operations Regulations 1992, the latter introduced under the provisions of the Health and Safety at Work Act to enable the UK to implement the requirements of European Directives on the manual handling of loads. The H&SWA was, according to Hutter (2001) a radical new approach that enabled health and safety to be seen as the everyday concern of everyone at work by becoming incorporated and deeply embedded into everyday organisational and individual activities. It also emphasised the individual responsibilities and the interdependencies' between groups of workers – so rather than seeing your role in isolation it was seen as an interdisciplinary requirement. The H&SWA also highlighted that regulatory law was attempting to constitute structure, routines and procedures for health and safety to penetrate deep into the organisation and become part of the employers' and employees' organisational life.

These regulations can be divided into two categories that provide a clear indication of what is required from both the *employer* and the *employee* and how they work in unison and not isolation (see Table 12.2). Within these regulations, employers have a general duty 'to ensure, *so far as is reasonably practicable* (SFAIRP) [see Chart 12.1], the health, safety and welfare at work of all employees' (OPSI, 1974) and must avoid the need for hazardous manual handling operations. There may be occasions when this is not reasonably practicable, for these the HSE recommends that employers make a suitable and sufficient assessment and take appropriate steps to reduce the risk of injury to the lowest level reasonably possible.

Table 12.2 Example of the comparison between employer and employee responsibilities under relevant regulations

Employers' responsibilities	Employees' responsibilities
Paragraph 167 of the Manual Handling Operation Regulations 1999, Section 2 of the Health and Safety at Work Act and Regulations 10 and 13 of the Management of Health and Safety at Work Regulations 1999	Paragraph 182 of the Manual Handling Operation Regulations 1999, as well as the Management of Health and Safety at Work Regulations 1999
Require employers to provide their employees with health and safety information and training	Require employees to make use of appropriate equipment provided for them, in accordance with their training and the instructions their employer has given them

Chart 12.1 So far as is reasonably practicable (SFAIRP) or as low as reasonably practicable (ALARP)

According to the HSE (2009) these two terms mean essentially the same thing and at their core is the concept of 'reasonably practicable'; this involves weighing a risk against the trouble, time and money needed to control it. Thus, ALARP describes the level to which we expect to see workplace risks controlled.

The definition set out by the Court of Appeal (in its judgment in *Edwards v. National Coal Board* [1949] 1 All ER 743) is:

'Reasonably practicable' is a narrower term than 'physically possible' … a computation must be made by the owner in which the quantum of risk is placed on one scale and the sacrifice involved in the measures necessary for averting the risk (whether in money, time or trouble) is placed in the other, and that, if it be shown that there is a gross disproportion between them – the risk being insignificant in relation to the sacrifice – the defendants discharge the onus on them.

Example provided by HSE (2009d):

- To spend £1m to prevent five staff suffering bruised knees is obviously grossly disproportionate; but
- To spend £1m to prevent a major explosion capable of killing 150 people is obviously proportionate.

Source: Taken from *ALARP at a Glance* (HSE, 2009d). Reproduced under the Open Government Licence v1.0.

Employees also have a duty under the Act to take reasonable care of their own health and safety and that of other people who may be affected by their actions, and it is essential that all health-care workers adhere to these regulations. As a student nurse, preparing to take on a professional role, faced with moving and handling operations throughout your career, you will need to continue to review any relevant new legislation that is published. All employers are required by law to update their employees on the principles and practice of moving and handling operations.

As the safety of the nurse and patient is paramount, nurse education will include instruction on moving and handling operations, and guidance on local practice and the use of moving and handling equipment. Moving and handling trainers have a responsibility to provide the correct information, as indicated by law, and students contracted within a school/university must, also by law, undergo regular updating. Failure to do so may affect their ability to practise (see Chart 12.2).

When considering the abundance of regulations and guidance from regulatory and governing bodies and how it is so deeply embedded within our work culture, it is surprising and sometimes confusing that injuries, incidence, accidents and near misses occur. It is often due to the noncompliance of individuals who, after attending mandatory training, have made the incorrect personal decision not to follow recommendations for safe moving and handling practices within that clinical area. We also often see strong personalities applying incorrect and controversial personal moving and handling ideals upon other individuals, such as making decisions not to use relevant equipment such as hoists and slide sheets that would make the client's transfer more comfortable, and instead

Chart 12.2 Current law, policy and governing bodies that guide health professionals practice

- Risk assessments – Patient and generic
- Health and Safety at Work Act (OPSI, 1974)
- **The Health and Safety (Miscellaneous Amendments) Regulations (OPSI, 2002)**
- Manual Handling Operations Regulations (OPSI, 1992)
- Human Rights Act (1998) Full force October (OPSI, 2002)
- Mental Capacity Act (OPSI, 2005)
- Disability Discrimination Act (DH, 2005)
- Nursing and Midwifery Council (NMC, 2008): **The Code: Standards of Conduct, Performance and Ethics for Nurses and Midwives**
- NMC (2010). **Guidance on Professional Conduct for Nursing and Midwifery Students**

- Royal College of Nursing (RCN)
- Chartered Society of Physiotherapy (CSP)
- The British Association/College of Occupational Therapists
- The Society of Chiropodists and Podiatrists
- Provision and Use of Work Equipment Regulations 1998 (PUWER) (HSE, 1999)
- Lifting Operations and Lifting Equipment Regulations 1998 (LOLER) (HSE, 2002)
- Reporting of Injuries, Diseases and Dangerous Occurrences Regulations 1995 (RIDDOR) (HSC, 2002)
- Management of Health and Safety at Work Regulations (OPSI, 1999)

advocate the use of physical strength and bed linen, ignoring the updated information that should be clearly and legally recorded within the Individual Client Handling Profile. They are then often surprised when disciplined for carrying out unsafe and controversial techniques, for example the drag lift. One must reflect upon the fact, as seen in Chart 12.1, that for every regulation that applies a duty to an employer there is often a duty that ensures the employee works within the safe systems provided.

It has now been recognised that the implementation of a 'no lifting policy' within an organisation is simply impractical to enforce and monitor, especially when we as human beings are designed to move and lift, but it is the excessive weight, frequency, rotation and so on, that often causes MSDs. The MHOR 1992 set no specific requirements such as weight limits; however, an ergonomic assessment based on a range of relevant factors is used to determine the risk of injury and point the way to remedial action. The Regulations, according to the HSE (2009e), establish the following clear hierarchy of control measures:

1   Avoid hazardous manual handling operations so far as is reasonably practicable (see Chart 12.1 definition), by redesigning the task to avoid moving the load or by automating or mechanising the process.

2   Make a suitable and sufficient assessment of any hazardous manual handling operations that cannot be avoided.

3   Reduce the risk of injury from those operations so far as is reasonably practicable. Where possible, you should provide mechanical assistance, for example a sack trolley or hoist. Where this is not reasonably practicable, look at ways of changing the task, the load and working environment. (HSE, 2009e; MHOR 1992)

The HSE (2006), however, have compiled 'guidelines' of zones that provide weights for lifting and lowering that allow the individual to make a quick and easy assessment. As most injuries occur if handling is done with arms fully

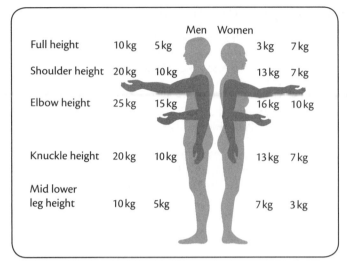

Men Women

Full height	10 kg	5 kg		3 kg	7 kg
Shoulder height	20 kg	10 kg		13 kg	7 kg
Elbow height	25 kg	15 kg		16 kg	10 kg
Knuckle height	20 kg	10 kg		13 kg	7 kg
Mid lower leg height	10 kg	5 kg		7 kg	3 kg

Figure 12.1 Guidelines for lifting and lowering for men and women
Source: Adapted from HSE (2006).

extended or at high or low levels, the guideline weights within these zones have been reduced. The guideline has been designed to allow the individual to assess the task before commencement, to first see which box or boxes the individual hands pass through when moving the load. And secondly you would assess the maximum weight being handled. If it is less than the figure given in Figure 12.1, the operation is within the guidelines. However, if the individuals' hands enter more than one box during the manoeuvre, use the smallest weight, and use an in-between weight if the hands are close to a boundary between boxes. The guideline weights assume that the load is readily grasped with both hands and that the operation takes place in reasonable working conditions, with the individual in a stable, walk-stance body position (see Figure 12.1).

When assessed safe to do so, it may be necessary to assist the patient and/or move an inanimate load; however, it is only acceptable if forces are as low as is reasonably practicable taking into consideration the client's ability to participate, the necessity of the procedure/manoeuvre, alternative methods and equipment required. You must also consider the appropriate plan derived from the appropriate risk assessment. You must also reflect upon what is seen as an emergency. Some may consider an emergency a reason for 'unsafe practices' and 'controversial techniques' to be employed. Any emergency task within the health-care arena should, where possible, have a procedure/policy in place to safeguard all staff and clients which is reflected in the application of a generic risk assessment. This should ensure that appropriate equipment and staffing numbers are available to carry out such manoeuvres in these situations.

Human Rights Act 1998 and the Mental Capacity Act 2005

The Human Rights Act 1998 incorporating the European Convention on Human Rights, came into full force in October 2000 and gives further legal effect in the UK to the fundamental rights and freedoms contained in the European Convention on Human Rights. These rights not only impact matters of life and death, they also affect the rights that individuals have in their everyday life. According to Smith (2005, p. 9) the most relevant aspect of the Human Rights Act 1998 that relate to health and personal injury law are:

- Article 2: Right to life
- Article 3: Prohibition of torture, inhumane or degrading treatment or punishment

- Article 6: Right to a fair trial
- Article 8: Right to respect for private and family life

Before October 2000, individuals, including clients and relatives, who believed that their human rights had been violated had to take their case to the European Court in Strasbourg; however, those rights are now directly enforceable in the UK courts and tribunals. Mandelstam (2002, p. 64) believes that the Human Rights Act will heighten the judicial scrutiny of some health and social-care decision-making, such as whether balanced decisions are being made when, for example, weighing up the needs and wishes of the patient against the local authority's or NHS Trust's limited resources and its concerns about the health and safety of its staff.

The Mental Capacity Act 2005 must also be taken into consideration as the client is an integral part of the individual patient assessment and education process. The client's ability to participate and understand instructions is always fundamental; therefore when assessing a patient for the first time you must ensure that sufficient staffing numbers and equipment are available and that a qualified member of the health-care profession is heading the team. If a client is unable to participate the question 'Why' must be asked; Has the client been fully informed and educated about the task ahead?, Have they given informed consent?, Is the language used confusing and ambiguous?, Do they require communication aids and equipment?, Can the patient do the task unaided and therefore resent your involvement?, Are they frightened?, Are they in pain? and so on. Break the task down into easily explained and demonstrated sequences that simplify the procedure first before you consider the client's overall ability to participate and fully comprehend the forthcoming task.

The purpose of the Mental Capacity Act 2005 is to assume that the client has capacity unless it is established that they lack the necessary capacity. However it is not there to make unfounded judgements about the clients ability to make an informed decision on all aspects of their care. The Act has been written for individual clients who lack the capacity in relation to a given situation at 'one point in time' to which they are unable to make a decision for themselves because of an impairment of, or a disturbance in the permantent or temporary functioning of, the mind or brain.

> **∞ Link**
>
> Chapters 3 and 13 also discuss the Mental Capacity Act.

The client's lack of capacity cannot be established merely by reference to age, appearance or an aspect of their behaviour. An individual client who has the inability to make decisions must be unable to understand the information relevant to the decision about an aspect of care and/or treatment and to retain the relevant information that is pertinent to the objective. Once this information has been provided the client must then be able to use or weigh that information as part of the decision-making process, and then be able to communicate their decision, whether by talking, using sign language or any other means necessary for that client to communicate effectivly and efficiently. However, just because a client is unable to understand an explanation of a task or treatment, given to them in a way that is appropriate to their circumstance and requirements, for example using simple language, visual aids or by any other means, it does

Chart 12.3 Principles of the Mental Capacity Act 2005

The following principles apply for the purposes of this Act.
- A person must be assumed to have capacity unless it is established that he lacks capacity.
- A person is not to be treated as unable to make a decision unless all practicable steps to help him to do so have been taken without success.
- A person is not to be treated as unable to make a decision merely because he makes an unwise decision.
- An act done or decision made, under this Act for or on behalf of a person who lacks capacity must be done, or made, in his best interests.
- Before the act is done, or the decision is made, regard must be had to whether the purpose for which it is needed can be as effectively achieved in a way that is less restrictive of the person's rights and freedom of action.

not mean that they are unable to understand the information relevant to that decision. If the patient can only retain the information relevant to a decision for only a short period of time it does not prevent them from being regarded as able to make the decisions relevant to their care/treatment.

The relevance of the decision-making process must consider the information about the reasonably foreseeable consequences of making a decision which may affect the direction of the chosen pathway of care or indeed the failure to make a decision. It may be necessary, therefore, once the client has been fully assessed in accordance with the Mental Capacity Act 2005, to make a decision in the 'best interests of the client'. When making this decision, however, you must consider whether it is likely that the client will at some time have capacity in relation to the matter in question, and if it appears likely that he or she will, when that is likely to be and at all times, so far as is reasonably practicable, permit and encourage the client to participate in, or to improve his ability to participate, as fully as possible in any act performed for them and any decision affecting them. A decision affecting care/treatment takes into account, if it is practicable and appropriate to consult them, the views of anyone named by the person as someone to be consulted on the matter in question or on matters of that kind, anyone engaged in caring for the person or interested in his or her welfare either family or friend or someone appointed by the court (review Chart 12.3).

Ergonomics

The term 'ergonomics' is derived from the Greek words *ergon*, meaning work and *nomoi*, meaning natural laws. Ergonomics can be defined as the study of the relationship between the working environment and the people within it. It adapts the task to the person – rather than adapting the person to the task; it is important in the prevention of injury resulting from moving and handling activities, ensuring the optimum 'fit' between the people and the work.

Ergonomics puts people first, taking account of their capabilities and limitations, it aims to make sure that the tasks, and equipment, information and the environment suit each worker (HSE, 2007; DoH, 2005).

Ergonomic processes include risk assessment as well as the identification and implementation of measures to reduce the risk. Posture, the types of furnishing used, individual's height, position and manoeuvrability, the tasks undertaken and the environment are all assessed in order to ensure that the job is designed to fit the worker and therefore reduce the incidence of moving and handling injuries.

The HSE booklet, *Understanding Ergonomics at Work* (HSE, 2007) discusses what type of workplace problems ergonomics can solve. By the reduction and elimination of these problems you can begin to reduce MSDs and associated complications that may be attributed to these injuries, such as slips, trips and falls.

Stability – stance, base of support, centre/line of gravity

Stability is a concept that we are all conscisous of and is one that requires very little application. It is a naturally occuring event that humans have mastered to assist mobility, stance and movement. We must, however, within moving and handling, consider the concept more closely, not only for ourselves but also our clients who may need guidance, support and education. We all have a base of support and running through that base of support is the line of gravity (which runs through the centre of gravity). This line of gravity needs to fall within an object's base of support to ensure that the object or person is stable and balanced. Once the line of gravity falls outside the client's or object's base of support, then the object will begin to topple and fall under gravitational forces (Smith, 2005, p. 58).

Stability is one of the key principles of safe moving and handling. One must ensure that you, your client and your colleagues are correctly positioned when carrying out any aspect of safe moving and handling and/or mobility. To maintain a stable base of support you must ensure that while wearing suitable footwear, your feet are shoulder width apart with one foot slightly in front of the other (adjustment of the back foot may automatically occur). This position provides a wide base of support and ensures that you are stable in all directions (see Figure 12.2). If you feel particularly unstable, for example on a moving bus, you will not only widen you stance but to widen your base of support even more you will reach out and hold onto appropriate objects and handles (see Figure 12.3).

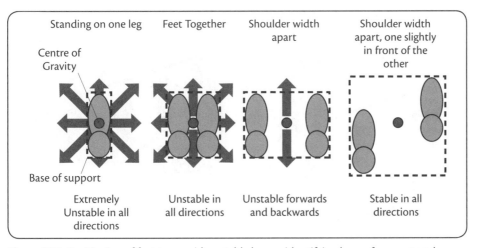

Figure 12.2 Positioning of feet to provide a stable base – identifying base of support and centre of gravity

Consideration and awareness of the importance of base of support and line/ centre of gravity is also necessary when transfering weight from one foot to the other when 'pushing or pulling' in a safe assessed manner, within a manoeuvre. This weight transfer from one foot to the other, allows you to use your body weight to produce movement, rather than the strength in your arms. This again is a process that occurs naturally in daily activities, for example to pull or push open a door we tend to walk up to it, placing one foot in front of the other, with our arms positioned in front and hands ready to make contact with the door. If we are pushing the door open we continue to transfer our weight forward until it is open and if pulling the door open we hold the door handle and transfer our weight backwards (see Figure 12.4).

Leverage – muscles, joints, group actions and lever systems

Muscles, ligaments and tendons have an effect on bones that creates movement. Every skeletal muscle is attached to bone or other connective tissue structures

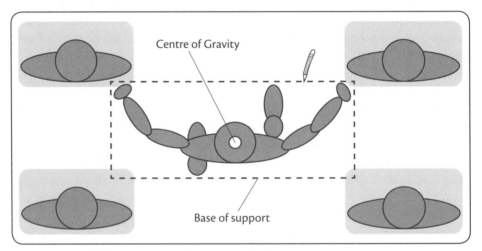

Figure 12.3 Daily life activity – standing on a moving bus

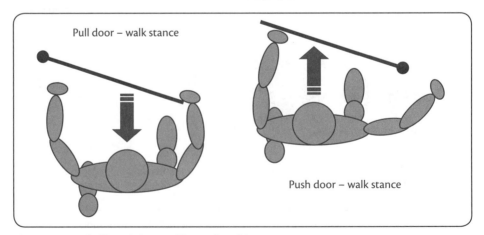

Figure 12.4 Daily life activity – pulling and pushing

at no fewer than two points, these are classified as the origin and insertion. The origin, which is generally proximally located, along with an insertion (generally distally located), are used to create the required action that will produce a range of movement (ROM) that can be created from that joint. The muscle's origin is attached to the immovable or less movable bone, whereas the insertion is attached to the movable bone, and it is this insertion that moves the movable bone to the immovable or less movable bone creating movement. Body movement occurs when muscles contract across joints and their insertion moves towards their origin (Marieb and Hoehn, 2010, p. 253).

Muscles are classified into four functional groups: prime movers, antagonists, synergists and fixators. Joints allow a ROM that is specific for their design, for example the elbow, a hinge joint which allows flexion and extension by the use of muscle group action. Flexion of the elbow is produced by the contraction of the prime mover or agonist, which in this case is the biceps, and relaxation of the antagonist or triceps. Extension is created by the reversal of these forces and roles. No one muscle can function alone, it must be accompanied by another to recreate the initial position of the joint.

In relation to prime movers and antagonists, Marieb and Hoehn (2010, p. 321) state that most movements involve the action of one or more synergists, which help prime movers by adding additional force to the movement and reduces undesirable or unnecessary movement that may occur as the prime mover contracts.

The movement must also be 'fixed' and stabilised to prevent undesirable movement; these muscles are called 'fixators' (Marieb and Hoehn, 2010, p. 321). This working relationship between muscle and bone most often produces actions and movement that involve leverage and lever systems. Tendons anchor the muscle to the connective tissue of the skeletal element (bone or cartilage) or to the fascia of other muscles, whereas ligaments unite bones and prevent excessive or undesirable movement (Marieb and Hoehn, 2010, p. 253).

In your body a 'fulcrum' is produced within the joint, your bones act as levers and muscle contraction provides the effort at the insertion point on the bone. The load is the bone, along with overlying tissue and any other load you are trying to move (Marieb and Hoehn, 2010, p. 323). When carrying a coffee cup this becomes a 'load' along with the bones of the hand, wrist, forearm and surrounding tisue. The elbow joint becomes the 'fulcrum', and the effort is provided by the biceps (see Marieb and Hoehn, 2010, pp. 323–5).

> ✸ **Activity 12.1**
>
> For further reading review the following chapters in Marieb and Hoehn (2010): Chapter 8, Joints (pp. 249–74) Chapter 9, Muscle and Muscle Tissue (pp. 275–319) Chapter 10, The Muscular System (pp. 320–84)

Friction – types and use

Types and use of friction must be considered to aid the effectiveness of normal body movement and the forces produced by muscles. Even the most mundane of tasks, such as getting out of the chair, requires the application of frictional forces to aid normal body movement and assist in the desired outcome.

Frictional forces are present within every daily activity and moving and handling procedure/manoeuvre. We cannot reduce them completely; however, within moving and handling these frictional forces can be equally useful in some situations (for example the frictional coefficient, force of friction between two bodies and the force pressing them together between the soles of shoes and flooring stop a patient slipping when sat on the edge of the bed) and a hindrance in others (for example the frictional coefficient between the client's clothing and the bed sheets prevent a client's independence in moving themselves up in bed).

High frictional surfaces, such as non-slip matting, one-way glide sheets and the rubber soles on shoes/slippers, will be more difficult to move; however, low frictional surfaces, such as slide-sheets, will be easier to move. High and low frictional surfaces are used in normal body movement and may be used in isolation or unison to perform a daily activity or moving and handling procedures/manoeuvres.

To maintain high frictional surfaces, you may place rubber soled slippers/shoes on the client's feet to promote grip and stability, or non-slip matting on a mattress to aid foot purchase when adjusting their position in bed. To encourage a low frictional surface, you may insert a 'slide sheet' under the client to decrease the frictional and shearing forces that will occur when assisting or moving a patient up the bed or when the patient is getting out of bed and their clothing and the bed sheet are causing a high frictional surface. This is also an exemplary example of why bed linin is not used as moving and handling equipment as it increases the frictional surface, reduces movement and increases shearing forces that may result in integumentary damage.

One-way slide sheets will provide both low and high frictional surfaces/forces to aid movement in a chosen direction. Once the desired position is obtained, the material used to provide the low frictional surface (now moving in the opposite direction) produces a high frictional surface. The material used inside the one-way glide is similar to corduroy. If you run your hands across the length of the corduroy strands, they appear smooth and allow your hands to pass over them with ease, but run your hands in the opposite direction and the material's make-up alters and the feel is different. When the material's surfaces are placed together, this alteration in make-up allows the surfaces to run smoothly in one direction and lock in the other.

Communication

An enhanced awareness and understanding of normal body movement and its integration into safe moving and handling will provide you with a sound base to build upon when communicating instructions to your client and/or colleagues. To assess what the client is able to do for themselves, you will be required to 'talk clients through a manoeuvre' using verbalisation and demonstration. But without a holistic awareness and analysis of how you would normally carry out a manoeuvre, safe alternatives and available resources and equipment, nurses often run out of ideas and unsucessfully assist/lift the client into position.

Clear and appropriate communication techniques and terminology are required so as your client understands what the piece of equipment can do to assist. If the client is unclear about what they are required to do and what the equipment does to assist them, ensure that you explain fully and brake down the task into achievable goals. Informed consent must be gained in accordance with the NMC (2005, 2008, 2009, 2010) guidance and Code, ensuring that you have allowed adequate time for questions and answers to be given in full. Praise the client and ensure that they are well and willing to continue at every stage of the procedure therefore ensuring that the client's physical condition has not deteriorated, especially if, for example, this is the first time post-operatively they have mobilised and pain is increasing.

Similar communication should be applied to all colleagues involved in the manoeuvre and opportunities given for alternative techniques/manoeuvres to be discussed. Time should also be allocated to allow adequate clarification of the manoeuvre that is about to be implemented. This open communication should ensure that both the client and the colleagues involved are completely informed of the processes, have had any questioned answered, and discussed procedures/manoeuvres that may not have been considered. Also this open communication should allow an opportunity for anyone who is uncomfortable carrying out the chosen procedure/manoeuvre or who is not trained in this specific procedure/manoeuvre to withdraw from the tasks without judgement or reprisal.

To coordinate the team and the client, who is an integral part of the proceedings and may participate actively, even if it is just being relaxed during the procedure/manoeuvre, the team should use the following instructions: *Ready*; everyone in the team and the patient says... *Yes* (this ensures everyone is paying attention and also provides the opportunity to say No, if something is amiss); *Set*, and *Move* (or *Stand*, or *Turn* or *Sit* etc.). Coordinating terms, such as one, two, three move; ready, steady, move, and two, six turn, are not recommended due to the lack of patient and colleague involvement and the possible confusion of when to action the turn or move.

Humanistic approaches to safe moving and handling

As Davidson and Elliot (2007) point out, nursing is a dynamic and evolving profession, delivered in a wide variety of settings and in a range of models and regulatory frameworks. Furthermore, the authors refer to nursing as being a diverse and multifaceted profession delivered across a range of settings and contexts. Health-care professionals work in many different areas of practice that can include being hospital based or working in clients' homes, or in residential services managed by statutory, voluntary or private organisations. Moving and handling could be practised by health-care professionals under many different circumstances and therefore it has to be considered as an intervention that requires an extensive tool box, enabling them to adapt to any given situation safely and within a legal and ethical framework.

The pressure is certainly on employees to fulfil targets set by government and professional organisations and, therefore, in order to meet these targets, temptation to use moving and handling techniques that can be performed in the shortest possible time may be considered. The danger of this is that practices deemed as 'controversial techniques' and 'high risk for musculoskeletal injury' can be drawn upon. An example of this is the drag lift (placing forearm under the patient's axilla). As Ruszala (2005, p. 276) points out, the danger of using the drag lift is that the person's weight is taken on the relatively narrow and less fleshy areas of the handlers' arms, and may cause pain, soft tissue injury, glenohumeral dislocation and even fracture of the humerus. The sacrum, buttocks and heels can drag on the bed of the chair and contribute to the development of pressure sores [pressure ulcers].

🔗 Link

Chapter 11 explores pressure ulcers in more depth.

Moving and handling interventions must be based on meeting clients' health and social-care needs and of observing their human rights (Richmond, 2005). However, even using evidenced-based interventions they can still be utilised in a very mechanistic manner where the health-care professionals view the client as an 'object to be moved' rather than as a person who has psychological and physical needs. By moving a client in this mechanistic manner negates the client's privacy, dignity and respect and more importantly can violate their right to be treated as an individual. Through a mechanistic approach it is easy for the client and health-care professionals to encounter an injury. It is therefore important that moving and handling is encompassed in a humanistic and person-centred approach which is arguably fundamental to health-care professionals' codes of practice. Kern et al. (2005) identifies humanistic care as being client centred and integrating the psychosocial with biomedical aspects of care. McCormack and McCance (2006) identified four constraints in their framework for person-centred nursing: (1) perquisites, which focus on the attributes of the nurse; (2) the care environment, which focuses on the context in which care is delivered; (3) person-centred processes, which focus on delivering care through a range of activities; and (4) expected outcomes, which are the results of effective person-centred nursing. These constructs could be deemed as being interactive with each other. In every element the client has to take priority and health-care professionals' competence and commitment to the job, the organisational and direct workplace culture are as important as the person-centred processes themselves. It is within the person-centred construct that McCormack and McCance include working with the clients' beliefs and values, engagement, having sympathetic presence, sharing, and decision-making and providing for physical needs.

Central to achieving these would be the utilisation of effective communication skills. The use of such skills is essential to build a therapeutic relationship with the client who is of paramount importance for completing a comprehensive nursing and risk assessment. The nursing assessment should highlight the needs of the client from a holistic perspective and the risk assessment will highlight potential benefits and costs of carrying out an action. These benefits and costs will be for the client, other clients, colleagues and you. In moving and handling, both the nursing and risk assessment will inform the Individual Client Handling profile.

Risk Assessment

Nursing assessments, risk assessment and generic assessments must be completed to comply with current law and legislation as described earlier. Before conducting any assessment, one of the key issues is ensuring that client consent has been obtained. On many occasions the client will be able to give that consent via verbal means, but on some occasions this may not be possible due to levels of consciousness, cognitive ability or mental health needs. In such circumstances the Mental Capacity Act 2005 must be adhered to. It may be that acting in the best interest of the client may suffice, but such decisions must be in accordance with the guidelines outlined within the Act (see Chart 12.3). Ensure decisions, based on best interest, are not taken as 'carte blanche' for any future moving and handling interventions or across to any other intervention for that client. Each time an intervention is required, mental capacity must be reassessed. All these decisions must be documented, and countersigned by a qualified staff member if you are a student.

When conducting a risk assessment it is strongly recommended that you assess and be aware of your own and your client's limitations. It is imperative that relevant supervision and support is sought by you if at any time you are unsure of the situation. Also ensure that you have sufficient staff to assess the client and the situation safely, for example one health-care professional is not enough to assess a client's standing or sitting ability for the first time.

The following five categories are an example of a simple risk assessment and must be remembered and acted upon before actually becoming involved in the facilitation of client or inanimate load moving and handling

E – Environment
L – Load
I – Individual capacity
O – Other factors
T – Task

You should approach the assessment in a non-judgemental fashion, see the client as a person and not by their condition, listen to their story, their preferences and what causes them pain and anxiety. Through our use of moving and handling interventions we want to add positive elements to their story, not negative ones that build on previous pain and anxiety. Avoid coming across as the powerful professional where you could inadvertently make the client feel vulnerable and submissive to the moving and handling process. Part of the nurses' role is to encourage their clients to take an active part in their care.

During the risk assessment think about the way you interact with the client. Try to be reflective on the way that you present yourself. Watch your body language, keep an open posture and use communication appropriate to that client's understanding. Think about cultural, physical and psychological needs. If you feel an interpreter would be appropriate during the assessment then ensure one is present. Recognise that an interpreter is not just available to assist in the translation of the verbal language but also there to assist clients, who use sign language, picture symbols or other forms of communication.

It is important to think about your positioning. The client could be lying in bed or sitting in a chair, therefore when conducting the assessment you need to think about appropriate eye contact. If the client is sitting in a chair and you are in a standing position it could mean that you are peering over the client giving them a feeling of helplessness and lack of involvement in the assessment and care process. Think also about appropriate social distance and the dangers of encroachment into client's personal space. Do not just assume you have permission to touch the client; you need their consent to do this.

Through the assessment consider in more depth:

- Environment: Equipment safety checks. Space constraints within the working area, or the area moving to? Ventilation? Poor lighting? Where the task is to be carried out – indoors or outside? Flooring type and level of surface, Trailing wires, Pets? And so on.
- Load:
  - As an inanimate load: Unwieldy, i.e. size, shape, weight and complexity of the object? Difficult to grasp? Unstable? Sharp, hot, cold? And so on.
  - As a client: Do you actually know the client's weight and when they were last weighed; for example do not take the client's word, actually weigh them when appropriate. Are you aware of weight limitations of equipment and whether in fact the client may well exceed these weight limits and dangers that this presents?
- Individual capacity (the handler and the client): Does it:
  - Require unusual strength? Create a hazard? Require special information, education, training, and demonstrations? Are all the individual members fit and able for the task ahead? And so on.
  - Think about your client, do they have upper and or lower body strength to do the manoeuvre themselves? Check that the client's physical illness is not creating symptoms that can put them at risk if they are moved into a certain position (you would not want to aid a client to stand up if they are feeling dizzy). Does the client understand your communication or do they seem to have difficulty relating to you? How much can the client participate? What are their expectations/wishes? Are they in pain? Are they prone to falls? Have you considered cultural issues? Does their underlying condition prevent or complicate compliance? Are they likely to become agitated and aggressive? And so on.

    Is the client self conscious of their body, are they ashamed to let other people see their body? Do they have low self-concept or low self-esteem and if so how can you reassure them through the moving and handling manoeuvres? Ensure that if the client has any physical disabilities that they are not discriminated against. Ensure that you are familiar with the Disability Discrimination Act 1995.

    Some clients may prefer that only male or female health-care professionals assist them. They may become embarrassed if a health-care professional of the opposite sex is involved in any aspect of their care. Maintain the client's privacy, dignity and respect at all times.

    Given all the options and in accordance with best practice, ask the client how they would prefer to be moved, remember you should be encouraging them to do as much for themselves as possible.

- Other factors and the interaction between these components
  - Resources and equipment. This would include any equipment to be used for the intervention as identified in the risk assessment and in the individual client's handling profile. Remember to check this equipment, ensuring it is in good condition and that where necessary it has been checked by a qualified engineer (Lifting Operations and Lifting Equipment Regulations [LOLER] 1998) and that you have personally checked over the equipment prior to each time you use it (Provision and Use of Work Equipment Regulations [PUWER] 1998 (HSE, 1999).
  - Do you require specialist equipment outside of the equipment available in your area? You may be working, for instance, with a client who is obese and may exceed the weight limit of the equipment available to you. Would you know where and how to get additional equipment if needed?
  - Does clothing of the client impact on the task? Can the privacy and dignity of the client be compromised during the intervention by inappropriate clothing? Can inappropriate clothing affect the moving and handling manoeuvre, for example a theatre gown being held closed by the client, leaving only one hand available to assist the manoeuvre? The wearing of protective clothing such as gloves and aprons which can impede movement.
  - Check to see if the client has a catheter or cannulae in situ, are attached to an intravenous infusion or cardiac monitor etc. These attachments may impede the client's ability to assist in the manoeuvre and in some situations dictate the procedure that can be done – that is, instead of walking while holding a catheter and intravenous stand the use of a wheelchair may be more appropriate.
  - Could a generic assessment save time and still meet the needs? Does the health-care professional undertake regular moving and handling? Do the individual health-care professionals fully understand the task ahead? And so on.
- Task
  - What is the Task – is it clearly defined? What does it involve – twisting, stooping, carrying over distances etc? Does it need to be done – are there alternative measures, does additional time need to be allocated?
  - Explain the procedure to the client and obtain consent. Consider your options if consent cannot be obtained for the client.

ELIOT, being part of a larger risk assessment, must be completed each time a moving and handling intervention is proposed. It does not matter if you have only just left the client, the situation could have changed. During that time the client may have spilt their drink onto the floor, they may have slumped into their chair or down the bed, their condition may be deteriorating and you could now be working with a different health-care professional, with different equipment. Consent issues may also have to be reconsidered as the manoeuvre may have altered and/or been reconsidered.

The 'Risk Assessment or Individual Client Handling Profile' should reflect the client's individual requirements and incorporate the client's ever-changing needs and abilities, that is, can the client participate more after breakfast than before? Does the client require temporary moving and handling equipment following clinical intervention or treatment? For example, while a profiling bed is being delivered, you may decide that to lower the risk, so far as is reasonably practicable, you will use a mattress variator ('V' shape frame that is positioned under the head end of the mattress. The inflation of a cushion opens the frame to bend the mattress to aid sitting) to ensure that the client is able to sit forward in bed with minimal assistance.

Chapter Summary

When assessing the client's ability to assist in any moving and handling manoeuvre, the priority is to encourage and promote independent, normal body movement whenever possible, however insignificant it may first appear. Every time the client is distracted from participating in an independent task, or a task is carried out for them when not necessary the client's rehabilitation may be affected. Without the client actively using muscle groups, joints and so on, they will ultimately weaken and reduce potential mobility and possibly compound underlying conditions, such as diabetes, and affect the delicate balance of the body systems, for example cardiac, respiratory, integumentory, gastrointestinal and so on.

Safe and appropriate moving and handling strategies should be taken into consideration when formulating the individual client's handling profile or risk assessment. These recommended strategies are designed to promote the achievable level of independence and discourage the promotion of dependence.

In essence the assessment should be graduated and build upon acquired knowledge and be conducted in a safe and conducive environment. Whenever possible, education, demonstration and training should take place prior to the manoeuvre; however, this is not always achievable. Ensure that the task in its entirety has been explained to the client and then break it down into achievable goals/task. At safe opportunities throughout the task, and at the end of each stage ensure that the client is well and is not suffering from ill effects of the manoeuvre. Also encourage and praise the client's contribution and obvious effort.

To ensure that this moving and handling task is assessed correctly and graduated a list of moving and handling questions (MHQs; see Chart 12.4) have been designed to:

- Promote safety, for you, your colleagues, your client and relatives
- Promote the application of safe moving and handling techniques
- Demonstrate and apply normal body movement to encourage independence
- Advocate the continual risk assessment of the task
- Prevent controversial techniques occurring
- Guide a logical and sequential process.

> ∞ **Link**
>
> Chapter 9 explores respiratory, Chapter 10 explores cardiac, Chapter 11 explores integumentory and Chapter 8 explores gastrointestinal in more depth.

Chart 12.4 Moving and handling questions (MHQs)

1   What is the normal body movement for the task?
2   Can I teach the client to do this unaided?
   • If yes, then how would this be achieved: verbal/
      non-verbal, demonstration, written?
   • If no, move to Q3.
3   If not completely unaided, is there equipment
      available that would mean the client could do this for
      himself or herself? For example, Jacob's ladder, bed
      lever, bed blocks, slide sheets, profiling bed etc.

   • If yes, then how would this be achieved?
   • If no, then Move to Q4.
4   If unable to perform the task themselves, what is the
      minimum of assistance one and then two health-care
      professionals can give (a) without equipment and (b)
      with equipment?
5   Are there unsafe ways of doing this I must avoid? If so,
      what are they?

Note: It is strongly recommended that you practise these processes under strict supervision until you are deemed safe and/or competent.
Source: Brooks (2008). Reproduced with the permission of the National Back Exchange.

? Test yourself!

1   Identify the key elements of ELIOT.
2   Which part of the legislation identifies the need
      to check moving and handling equipment prior
      to its use?
3   List five contributory factors of musculo-skeletal
      disorders.
4   What is the importance of effective
      communication within moving and handling?

5   What were the key issues that students
      highlighted as being poor practice within clinical
      placements?
6   Why is it important to maintain a good base of
      support while engaging in moving and handling
      interventions?

References

Brooks, A. (2008) *Manual Handling Questions: A Tool for Training, Assessment and Decision Making in Person Handling*. The Column, Severnprint, Gloucestershire.

Consumer Protection Act (1987) *Guide to the Consumer Protection Act 1987: Product Liability and Safety Provisions*. http://www.berr.gov.uk/files/file22866.pdf

Cornish, J. and Jones, A. (2010) Factors affecting compliance with moving and handling policy: Student nurses' views and experiences. *Nurse Education in Practice* **10**(2): 96–100.

Davidson, P. and Elliot, D. (2007) Managing approaches to nursing care delivery. In Chang, E. and Daly, J. (eds) *Transitions in Nursing: Preparing for Professional Practice*. Churchill Livingstone, Australia.

Dimond, B. (2005) *Legal Aspects of Nursing*. 4th edn. Pearson Longman, London.

DoH (Department of Health) (2005) Disability Discrimination Act. HMSO, London.

Health and Safety Commission (2002) *A Guide to the Reporting of Injuries, Diseases and Dangerous Occurrences Regulations 1995*. HSE, Norwich.

HSE (Health and Safety Executive) (1999) *Provision and Use of Work Regulations 1998. Open Learning Guidance*. HSE, Norwich.

HSE (Health and Safety Executive) (2002) *Lifting Operations and Lifting Equipment Regulations 1998: Safe Use of Lifting Equipment. Approved Code of Practice and Guidance*. HSE, Norwich.

HSE (Health and Safety Executive) (2003) *Manual Handling: Manual Handling Operations Regulations 1992. Guidance on Regulations*. HSE, Norwich.

HSE (Health and Safety Executive) (2006) *Getting to Grips with Manual Handling: A Short Guide*. HSE, Norwich. http://www.hse.gov.uk/pubns/indg143.pdf

HSE (Health and Safety Executive) (2007) *Understanding Ergonomics at Work: Reduce Accidents and Ill Health and Increase Productivity by Fitting the Task to the Worker.* HSE, Norwich. http://www.hse.gov.uk/pubns/indg90.pdf

HSE (Health and Safety Executive) (2008a) *Work-related Injuries and Ill Health in Health and Social Work – Days Lost.* http://www.hse.gov.uk/statistics/industry/healthservices/days-lost.htm

HSE (Health and Safety Executive) (2008b) *Labour Force Survey, 2007/8.* http://www.hse.gov.uk/statistics/causdis/musculoskeletal/index.htm

HSE (Health and Safety Executive) (2008c) *What Are the Main Causes of MSDs?* http://www.hse.gov.uk/msd/faq.htm

HSE (Health and Safety Executive) (2009a) *Health and Safety in Social Care Services.* http://www.hse.gov.uk/healthservices/index.htm

HSE (Health and Safety Executive) (2009b) *Musculoskeletal Disorders: Why Tackle Them?* http://www.hse.gov.uk/healthservices/msd/whytackle.htm

HSE (Health and Safety Executive) (2009c) *Musculoskeletal Disorders in Health and Social Care.* http://www.hse.gov.uk/healthservices/msd/index.htm

HSE (Health and Safety Executive) (2009d) *ALARP at a Glance.* http://www.hse.gov.uk/risk/theory/alarpglance.htm

HSE (Health and Safety Executive) (2009e) *Manual Handling Frequently Asked Questions: Is there a maximum weight a person can lift during their work?* http://www.hse.gov.uk/contact/faqs/manualhandling.htm

Hutter, B. (2001) *Regulations and Risk: Occupational Health and Safety on the Railways.* Oxford University Press, Oxford.

Kern, D., Branch, W., Jackson, J., Brady, D., Feldman, M., Levinson, W. and Lipkin, M. (2005) Teaching the Psychosocial aspects of care in the clinical setting: practical recommendations. *Academic Medicine* **80**(1): 8–20.

Mandelstam, M. (2002) *Manual Handling in Health and Social Care: An A–Z of Law and Practice.* Jessica Kingsley, London.

Marieb, E.N. and Hoehn, K. (2010) *Human Anatomy and Physiology.* 8th edn. International edn. Pearson, Benjamin Cummins, London.

McCormack, B. and McCance, T. (2006) Development of a framework for person-centred nursing. *Journal of Advanced Nursing* 56(5): 472–9.

NHS (National Health Service) (2009) *Choices: Your Health, Your Choices.* http://www.nhs.uk/NHSEngland/aboutnhs/Pages/About.aspx

NMC (Nursing and Midwifery Council) (2005) *An NMC Guide for Students of Nursing and Midwifery,* NMC, London.

NMC (Nursing and Midwifery Council) (2008) *The Code: Standards of Conduct, Performance and Ethics for Nurses and Midwives.* http://www.nmc-uk.org/aArticle.aspx?ArticleID=3056

NMC (Nursing and Midwifery Council) (2010) *Guidance on professional conduct for nursing and midwifery students.* http://www.nmc-uk.org/Documents/Guidance/Guidance-on-professional-conduct-for-nursing-and-midwifery-students-September-2010.PDF

OPSI (Office of Public Sector Information) (1974) Health and Safety at Work Act. http://www.opsi.gov.uk/RevisedStatutes/Acts/ukpga/1974/cukpga_19740037_en_1

OPSI (Office of Public Sector Information) (1992) Manual Handling Operations Regulations 1992, No. 2793. http://www.opsi.gov.uk/SI/si1992/Uksi_19922793_en_1.htm

OPSI (Office of Public Sector Information) (1999) Management of Health and Safety at Work Regulations. http://www.opsi.gov.uk/si/si1999/19993242.htm#3

OPSI (Office of Public Sector Information) (2002a) The Health and Safety (Miscellaneous Amendments) Regulations. http://www.opsi.gov.uk/si/si2002/20022174.htm

OPSI (Office of Public Sector Information) (2002b) Human Rights Act 1998, Chapter 42. http://www.opsi.gov.uk/ACTS/acts1998/ukpga_19980042_en_1

OPSI (Office of Public Sector Information) (2005) Mental Capacity Act, Chapter 9. http://www.opsi.gov.uk/acts/acts2005/ukpga_20050009_en_1

Richmond, H. (2005) Legal and professional responsibilities. In Smith, J. (ed.) *The Guide to the Handling of Patients: Introducing a Safer Handling Policy.* 5th edn. NBPA, London.

Ruszala, S. (2005) Controversial techniques. In Smith, J. (ed.) *The Guide to the Handling of Patients: Introducing a Safer Handling Policy.* 5th edn. NBPA, London.

Smith, J. (ed.) (2005) *The Guide to the Handling of Patients: Introducing a Safer Handling Policy.* 5th edn. NBPA, London.

Chapter

Dying, Death and Spirituality

13

📖 Contents

- Awareness of Death
- Health Promotion and Dying
- Choice and Priorities of Care
- The Nurse's Role in End of Life Care
- The Concept of Pain and Symptom Control
- Last Offices
- Ethical Issues in End of Life Care
- Bereavement
- Spirituality
- Chapter Summary
- Test Yourself!
- Further Reading
- References

☑ Learning outcomes

This chapter is concerned with dying, death and loss. It will introduce you to the concept of death and begin to examine some of the principal aspects of palliative care. At the end of the chapter, you should be able to:

- Reflect on the nature of death in today's society
- Discuss the concept of death
- Explore how and when people die
- Identify the key principles of palliative care
- Discuss the principles of pain and symptom control
- Reflect on the nature of communication with patients who are dying and their relatives
- Consider the ethical dilemmas that end of life care can present
- Identify the measures required in caring for a body after death
- Consider your role in bereavement
- Reflect on the spiritual nature of human beings and its importance in health care.

For most of us, death seems a long way off. We hopefully enjoy our lives and are more interested in living life to the full than worrying about dying. It might be argued that we cannot fully appreciate life unless we confront death, and although this may be very true, it might also be argued that with today's healthy lifestyles and an expectation of life until well into our eighties; there is no reason to concern ourselves with death. Whatever the truth of these arguments, you have as a nurse chosen to enter a profession in which you will inevitably be confronted by death. You therefore need to be able to care not only for people who are dying, but also for their relatives through this process and beyond as they are confronted by grief and bereavement. In addition, there is a need to care for yourself and your colleagues. We are after all dealing with one of the most powerful and emotional periods of life – the transition from the living known world to the unknown world of death.

A word of caution here: some of the discussions and exercises in this chapter may be distressing if you have recently been bereaved or have someone close to you who is dying. Feel free to miss out this chapter and revisit it when you feel the time is right for you.

Awareness of Death

The End of Life Care Strategy (DoH, 2008, p. 37) comments:

> There is now much less familiarity with death and dying than in previous centuries. Many people will not have had to deal with a close family member or close friend dying until they are into their mid-life years, and some will not have seen a dead body until this time. Most deaths occur in institutions, for example, hospitals and care homes and are therefore removed from people's direct experience.

Perhaps you have not given death very much thought, or perhaps you have experienced death in your life and it has loomed large in your thoughts. Whichever is true, you are encouraged here to think about how death is viewed by society today.

It is suggested that we live in a death-denying society. In other words, even in the face of the obvious we find it difficult to accept that we will one day die. We rarely discuss the subject and, for many, death takes place hidden away in institutions such as hospitals, hospices and nursing homes. It might be argued that this blind spot occurs partly because very often we have no need to think about death. For most of us, longevity has become the norm and we can be optimistic about achieving our three score years and ten. Modern science and better health care could, it is suggested, leave us with a life span of up 120 years. So if this is the case, why should we concern ourselves with a far-off event? Nevertheless, the knowledge that we will one day die always lurks in the background. Death may face us at any time of life, sometimes suddenly and unexpectedly, sometimes creeping slowly upon us:

> This existence of ours is as transient as autumn clouds.

To watch the birth and death of beings is like looking at the movements of a dance.
A lifetime is like a flash of lightening in the sky,
Rushing by, like a torrent down a steep mountain. (The Buddha, in Sogyal Rimpoche, 1992)

Although most people recognise the inevitability of death, to a large extent it is kept in the shadows. Death rattles away at the edge of our awareness (Yalom, 1980), and in modern Western society we have fewer and fewer reminders that we will one day be faced by the reality of death. The emergence of a life-limiting disease can, however, awaken hidden fears that have lain only in the shadow of our awareness. Society's death-denying approach, in which dying is hidden away in institutions, death is rarely talked about, and funeral rituals and mourning have become minimised, has little power over keeping death at bay (Aries, 1981). As Morgan (1995) comments, 'death refuses to die' – death can strike at any moment and we may be very unprepared for it:

> When you are strong and healthy,
> You never think of sickness coming,
> But it descends with sudden force
> Like a stroke of lightning.
> When involved in worldly things,
> You never think of death's approach;
> Quick it comes like thunder
> Crashing round your head. (Milarepa, in Sogyal Rimpoche, 1992)

Sogyal Rimpoche (1992) suggests that, deep down, we know we cannot avoid facing death forever and that the more we can accept the impermanence of life, the greater freedom we can find in living. It is up to you to decide how far you will explore your own personal living and dying, but you might wish to consider this advice by La Rochefoucauld (in Walter, 1990): 'Death and the sun are not to be looked at steadily', but 'As with the sun, so with death: without staring at it, the wise person lives in its light'. Whatever your personal explorations involve, you have chosen a profession in which you will inevitably be faced with people who are dying and people who are bereaved. Although many people in society never have to face death until middle age or beyond, you will inevitably have to confront it. As Collick (1986) suggests, 'death is a crisis for the dying and for the living for which both are usually wholly unprepared'. A large part of understanding death and dying is achieved by learning through experience rather than being taught, and you might like to start this process by reflecting on some of the losses in your life.

Where and how people die

There is evidence to suggest that most people would prefer to die in their own home (NICE, 2004), although this needs to be carefully interpreted as people's choices change over time and in particular during the course of an illness. It may be more important to meet their aspirations in terms of a good death including:

> ✹ **Activity 13.1**
>
> Think of some of the losses in your life. Don't think just of deaths but of all sorts of loss, such as the loss of security the first time you went to school, or when a brother or sister first left home. What effect did these losses have on you? What did you do to cope?

- Being treated as an individual with dignity and respect;
- Being without pain and other symptoms;
- Being in familiar surroundings;
- Being in the company of close family and/or friends (DoH, 2008).

These aspirations are more difficult to meet in acute settings and yet a significant number of people, whether or not their condition is cancer related, die in NHS hospitals. It is also evident that a considerable number of people with non-cancer-related conditions die in nursing and residential homes. Despite this, many people do spend much of their last year of life in their own home but are admitted when their condition worsens and their families feel that they are no longer able to cope (Barclay, 2001). The patient might feel the need for the security of an acute medical setting or unforeseen emergencies may arise. This clearly has implications for how care is provided and where resources are needed.

It is also useful to reflect on the age at which people die. Mortality tends to be high during the first year of life, decreasing during childhood and then gradually rising with age from 15 years onwards (Victor, 2000). However, unless you are a midwife or a children's nurse, the majority of people you care for will be 65 years or older and dying from a wide range of conditions, of which the cancers comprise just one specific collection of conditions.

When am I dead?

> ✳ **Activity 13.2**
>
> Given most people would like to die in their own homes:
> a) Who should be involved in this decision?
> b) What choice of places of death might be available?
> c) What would your preference be and why?

If nurses are to care for people who are dying in a way that is positive, it is important to recognise that we are alive until we are dead, and that we should have the opportunity, should we choose, to live to our full potential. Life exists on a continuum from conception to death. During this time our health varies and is affected by many factors in our internal body environment and by external influences. Despite efforts to deny death and preserve life, death continues to be the inevitable earthly end and the last stage of life.

This end-point of life that we call being dead is not as easily defined as one imagines. The common understanding of death is the absence of vital signs, that is, a cessation of breathing, a lack of a palpable heart beat and fixed dilated pupils. In most cases of expected death, these remain the usual criteria, but the situation has been complicated by modern technology, which allows people to be kept alive on life-support machines. Establishing the exact moment of death in such circumstances requires different criteria, such as brain death tests, to cope with this technologically supported extension to life (Veatch, 1995). Furthermore, although most Western societies try to make a clear distinction between being alive and being dead, some societies have a much wider differentiation. Some societies consider the person to be alive for a considerable period after most Western cultures would regard them as dead, while other cultures grieve for people as if they were dead in a way that most Western societies would hold to be inappropriate because the person would still be considered to be alive (Rosenblatt, 1997). But have you ever heard anyone in our own society say, 'For me she died a long time ago; now there is just an empty shell'? Perhaps in some circumstances we too have different definitions of death.

Whichever way we look at death, dying has no easily definable point. When does light become dark, and when does day become night? These are arbitrary and manmade divisions. We are all dying until we reach that ill-defined point we call death, or, put in a more positive way, life continues until a decision is made that we have reached that end-point we call death.

When am I dying?

Understanding the point at which someone is defined as dying is itself a grey area. Davis et al. (1996) emphasise that a diagnosis alone is not enough. Someone, whether it is the patient, a carer or the medical staff, needs to reach a position at which they accept the condition as being terminal. Nevertheless, dying and being in a terminal condition is not necessarily the same thing. A prognosis suggesting that there is no obvious curative treatment does not mean that the person does not have much active living to do, and even the terminal phase will differ from person to person. The whole process of dying may take various directions and shapes. Death may be sudden or lingering, expected or unexpected; it may progress slowly and then take a sudden downturn, or the process may move up and down before finally declining to death (Glaser and Strauss, 1968). For some, there may be little opportunity to reflect on the process, but many others have the opportunity for living fully right up until the moment of death. Although dying is a time of crisis, it can also be a time of opportunity for change and positive growth (Yalom, 1980).

The point of this discussion is that if we are to care for people who are dying, we first need to acknowledge that there are many grey areas: just as the person who is dying is facing uncertainty, nurses too sometimes have to face ambiguity and uncertainty. It is important, however, to focus on the fact that people are living until they are dead and that they deserve the highest quality of life that is attainable. One positive way at looking at this is to view care of the dying from a health-promotion perspective.

Health Promotion and Dying

The concepts of health and death rarely fit comfortably together, yet if life exists until death 'health for all' must include all people from birth up to the end of life. The White Paper *Our Healthier Nation* (DoH, 1999) is targeted at helping people to achieve healthier, more fulfilling lives. Although it makes no reference to care of the dying, it might be hoped that some aspects of the White Paper would be interpreted and acted upon within the scope of those who are defined as dying. Good health is described by the White Paper as requiring a confident and positive outlook and being able to cope with the ups and downs of life. Health is not just about how long people live but about quality of life, ensuring

∞ Link

Chapter 18 explores health promotion in more detail.

★ Activity 13.3

Imagine you are asked to look after a 67-year-old woman who is in the terminal stages of an illness. What would be your main concerns over how to care for her?

that they are not robbed of dignity and independence; it is equally important to all people whatever their clinical health status.

Seedhouse (1997) emphasises the importance of allowing people to achieve their maximum potential for health whatever their starting point. This health-promoting perspective thus allows a more positive view of the dying process. It is also a view that gives patients a choice. How they choose to do their dying may be very different from how we might choose to do ours, but their decision should always be respected. This perspective on death and dying fits well with the philosophy of caring for the dying, usually referred to as palliative care.

Definitions of palliative care

'Palliative care' is the term used to refer to the care of patients whose condition is not amenable to curative treatment. Such conditions invariably lead to the person's death, but the length of time involved is extremely variable. NICE (2004) defines palliative care as:

> the active holistic care of patients with advanced, progressive illness. Management of pain and other symptoms and provision of psychological, social and spiritual support is paramount. The goal of palliative care is achievement of the best quality of life for patients and their families. Many aspects of palliative care are also applicable earlier in the course of the illness in conjunction with other treatments.

Palliative care aims to:

- affirm life and regard life as a normal process
- provide relief from pain and other distressing symptoms
- integrate the psychological and spiritual aspects of patient care
- offer a support system to help patients live as actively as possible until death
- offer a support system to help the family cope during the patient's illness and in their own bereavement.

terminal illness

refers to a prognosis suggesting that there is no obvious curative treatment. 'Terminal care' is the term reserved for the care provided to patients in the last days, weeks or sometimes months of their life

The term '**terminal illness**' tends to hold highly negative connotations and can lead to patients receiving appropriate care far too late in their condition, whereas palliative care can and should start at the time of diagnosis, in some cases several years before the person reaches the terminal stages of the illness.

The growth of modern palliative care grew out of the work of Dame Cicely Saunders who opened St Christopher's Hospice in Sydenham in 1967. A former nurse, she moved into the world of medical social work before finally training as a doctor. Through her work, she became very conscious of the poor care and distress of patients who were dying. Her vision was for people to die free of pain and that they should be enabled to live until they died, supported by skilled carers and with their physical, psychological, spiritual and social needs addressed. Dame Cicely Saunders caught the imagination of the country and the world, and by the year 2001 over 93 countries throughout the world had initiated hospice and palliative care interventions (Hospice Information Service, 2001).

Palliative care has now become a speciality in its own right, initially emerging through the work of the **hospice** movement. Specialist palliative care can be provided in a variety of settings, including hospices. These may be independent, voluntary or fall within the NHS. Many hospices also have a day unit providing a range of facilities from symptom control to counselling and complementary therapies.

Palliative care may also be offered in the home, supported by the primary care team, and may involve a Macmillan nurse. Macmillan nurses are invariably clinical nurse specialists funded by the organisation Macmillan Cancer Relief, and although they predominantly work in the community, some may be employed as part of the hospital palliative care team. In addition, Marie Curie nurses offer hands-on care to patients at home, usually spending their whole shift caring for one individual. These nurses are usually part charity and part NHS funded, and range from care assistants who have specialised in this area to highly trained palliative care nurses.

Hospital palliative care teams offer support and symptom control to patients in general hospital wards. This is often where palliative care begins, early intervention usually meaning better managed palliative care.

Whatever the setting palliative care involves a number of specialised professionals including:

- Clinical nurse specialists in palliative care (often Macmillan nurses)
- Consultants in palliative medicine
- Social workers
- Clinical psychologists
- Other supporting professionals, such as physiotherapists, occupational therapists and in some cases complementary therapists.

One of the criticisms of palliative care has been its predominant focus on people with cancer, but although much has been learnt from the experience gained while caring for those with cancer, there is now a desire to make such expertise available in the care of people with other chronic diseases. There is also a considerable need to extend this expertise into other settings including nursing homes, where more and more people will end their lives (Komaromy et al., 2000). The *End of Life Care Strategy* (DoH, 2008) sets out an agenda to meet the needs of people at the end of their life in whatever setting they are in and whatever the condition.

Palliative care should become an integral part of all clinical practice whatever the illness or its stage. So, for example, this would include not only patients with cancer, but also those with dementia, chronic heart disease, stroke and respiratory disorders, meeting the needs of people in nursing homes, hospitals and community.

This approach is very significant to the nurse because it acknowledges the importance of all nurses providing palliative care rather than this just being something left to specialists.

hospice
voluntary or NHS-funded establishments where palliative care is provided. Hospices attempt to provide the best possible quality of life for the final stages of an illness. This includes family support and bereavement services

Choice and Priorities of Care

To meet the needs of patients and families palliative care requires an integrated approach with agreement between different settings, common assessment regimes, treatment and guidelines. This can only be achieved with good communication between professionals and by involving the patient and family.

To help people whose preferred place of care, at the end of their life, is home a framework has been established known as the 'The Gold Standard Framework' (GSF) (Macmillan Cancer Relief, 2005). This was developed by Dr Keri Thomas, adopted by Macmillan Cancer Relief and endorsed by the NHS. The framework was successfully piloted in over 76 GP practices and is now being adopted across the country. It is also being incorporated into care homes and community hospitals. The seven key Gold Standards that underpin the framework are:

1 Communication
2 Coordination
3 Control of symptoms
4 Continuity – out of hours
5 Continued learning
6 Carer support
7 Care in the dying phase

The object is to set up an easy to use and cost-effective system that clearly identifies those in the community with palliative care needs. Where this is done a coordinated multidisciplinary care package can be put in place to care for the patient and the family. In particular this enables the needs of the patient and family to be met out of hours. In the last days of life, when it can be particularly difficult for the family, measures such as the 'The Liverpool Integrated Care Pathway for the Dying Patient' can be initiated (Ellershaw and Wilkinson, 2003). This is discussed in this chapter under the section 'In the last days of life'.

If patients and families are to meet the challenge ahead then it is important to plan for the future and for the care that will be needed. Advance Care Planning (ACP) is an opportunity for patients to consider and discuss a wide range of issues that will help plan for their end-of-life care. This will be an important element in the new *End of Life Care Strategy* (DoH, 2008). The intention is to prepare for end-of-life care in a way that will give health professionals the best opportunity to provide for what the patient wants at a time when they may not be in a position to make those decisions for themselves. An ACP discussion (NHS, 2007) might include:

- the individual's concerns
- their important values or personal goals of care
- their understanding about their illness and prognosis
- their preferences for types of care or treatment that may be beneficial in the future and the availability of these.

Through these discussions, patients' and families have the opportunity to consider where they would want to be cared for at the end of their life, to tell professionals their preferences about how they would like to be cared for, and to make any advance refusal of treatment. They may also choose to discuss funeral plans; wills and other financial matters that can help them put their affairs in order. Consideration needs to be given as to who is the best person to conduct the discussion, and ethnic and cultural differences must be taken into account (Barnes et al., 2007).

It is important to be clear about the difference between a statement of wishes and preferences and an Advance Decision to Refuse Treatment (ADRT). The former helps to inform care-givers of a whole range of possible wishes including treatment and care but also their feelings, values and beliefs. They are not legally binding but must be taken into account when deciding on a person's best interests should they lose capacity to make such decisions for themselves. An ADRT, however, is a legally binding decision made by a person when they have capacity, to refuse a particular treatment such as artificial feeding, the use of antibiotics or artificial ventilation. There are clear guidance and rules to entering into such a decision (see NHS, 2007).

The process of ACP usually takes place in the context of an anticipated deterioration in the individual's condition but clearly the process may start earlier. Small beginnings can be very empowering, giving the patient and family permission to talk about their concerns and wishes and may act as a catalyst for constructive dialogue between the patient and carers as the situation changes. An ACP not only provides valuable information for patient choice, once they have lost capacity, but is very helpful in keeping an open dialogue with the patient and family throughout their care. The discussion should not necessarily be seen as a one-off event but a series of discussions with multidisciplinary team members allowing the patient's wishes to emerge and evolve. All discussions should be documented, communicated to appropriate care professionals and regularly reviewed.

Mental Capacity Act 2005

When making a decision regarding care or the refusal of treatment the person making that decision must have mental capacity to do so. It is the duty of the health-care professional to ensure that the patient is given every opportunity to make decisions for themselves and where they cannot decisions are made in their best interest. The Mental Capacity Act 2005 creates new legislation about the way in which decisions are made on behalf of people aged 16 and over and who lack the capacity to make those decisions for themselves. The Act became law on 1 April 2007.

The five key underlying principles:

1 A presumption of capacity: Every person has a right to make decisions and it must be presumed they have capacity unless it is established otherwise.
2 Individuals should be supported where possible so that they can make their own decisions: Until all efforts have been made to help a person make a decision for themselves they must not be seen as unable to make a decision.
3 People have a right to make decisions whether or not these decisions may seem eccentric or unwise to other people: and they should not be judged merely because their decision appears unwise to others.

4   Best interests: Any decision made on behalf of another individual who lacks capacity must be done in their best interests.

5   A person's rights and freedoms must be restricted as little as possible: Before carrying out any act or decision on behalf of someone who lacks capacity, regard to how that can be achieved in a way that is least restrictive to their rights and freedoms must be considered.

⊗ Link

Chapters 3 and 6 also discusses the Mental Capacity Act.

It is important to bear in mind that capacity can fluctuate over time and depending on the complexity of the decision to be made. Capacity must therefore be decided on a decision-by-decision basis. Guidance on the Act can be found in Chapman (2008).

Meeting the needs of people at the end of their life requires a coordinated and multi-professional approach. For the moment, however, we will reflect on the role of the nurse within this multidisciplinary team.

The Nurse's Role in End of Life Care

The nurse's role in palliative care is about caring for the living, so it is primarily about providing high-quality nursing care. We will focus here on some of the important elements required to provide quality care to people facing death as a result of their illness, but first try to think of the sort of person you would like to care for you or a member of your family; what sort of person would they be, and what sort of skills would you want them to have?

It is always difficult to pin down the specific skills required to be a good nurse, but Saunders (1978) offers some help in this when she talks of 'being with' people when they are suffering. It is as if we walk alongside them offering support as and when it is needed. Saunders identifies the characteristics required for this role:

non-judgemental
accepting the values of others

- Respect the identity and integrity of other human beings
- Be sensitive and **non-judgemental**
- Know when to listen and when to speak
- Have the knowledge and skills to intervene in a way that promotes the best quality of life as perceived by the patient.

⊗ Link

Chapter 4 contains a range of strategies to enable you to develop reflective skills.

The list may appear straightforward, but each item requires considerable skill and expertise. It is perhaps a skill that can be learnt only through experience, coupled with hard work on ourselves, through reflection, and a developing sense of self-awareness.

Davies and O'Berle (1990) also provide a useful framework that encapsulates those elements expressed by Saunders. The dimensions they describe in Figure 13.1 emerged from work interviewing patients and their families, and although the research reflects care delivered by specialist palliative care nurses, these dimensions are relevant to any nurse involved in end of life care.

⊗ Link

Chapter 2 explores therapeutic relationships in more detail.

- *Valuing* – is very much a core element in connecting with another and includes respect and being non-judgmental.

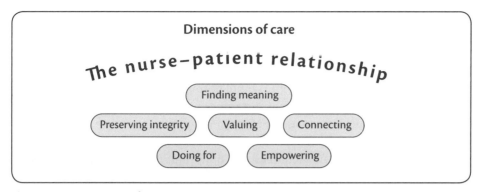

Figure 13.1 Dimensions of care
Source: Adapted from Davies and O'Berle (1990).

- *Connecting* – this relational aspect of caring becomes increasingly important in the care of the dying. It is through this that we connect with patients and their relatives. It is hard to describe what this actually means but it bears similarities to empathy. It is about listening, having a caring attitude that says 'You are important.' It means giving quality time to the person, even if this is only a couple of minutes.

- *Empowering* – one of the great anxieties facing people who are dying is losing control, which easily happens when vulnerable people are faced with powerful professionals and sometimes find themselves in a strange institutional environment. It is therefore important not to disempower people but to allow the person to care for themselves and make decisions for themselves as much as is possible. This can be very difficult, particularly when you are faced with what might appear to you an irrational decision, such as refusing some form of treatment. It is at such times that the need to be non-judgemental, coupled with being supportive, becomes increasingly important.

- *Finding meaning* – facing death may be a daunting prospect and a time when people question why and what life has been about. They seek to sort out their life and the meaning it has for them and for others around them. This is part of the spiritual aspect of our lives and will be dealt with more thoroughly later in the chapter.

- *Doing for* – people who are dying often need a lot of physical care and emotional support; families too may feel inadequate and frightened. At such times, nurses may need to provide much of the care, including pain and symptom control. This may be carried out by an individual nurse but is supported by a team approach. There is an inherent danger here of taking over from the patient and relatives so it is important in '*doing for*' that this is carried out, whenever possible, in negotiation with the person and family to avoid disempowering them.

- *Preserving integrity* – caring for the dying can be a challenging experience and it is important for nurses not to lose sight of their own self, their ability to maintain a positive view of themselves and their capacity to feel valued by themselves and by others. This may mean reflecting on the care given and exploring the meaning of life and death. In maintaining integrity, it is important that the nurse has good support within and outside her professional arena. Becoming emotionally involved with and upset for someone who is dying is not a loss of integrity: it is quite normal sometimes to feel emotional turmoil, just as it is quite normal sometimes not to feel any emotional attachment. Loss of integrity comes about when these emotions incapacitate the nurse and there is a loss of self-esteem and self-worth, perhaps associated with guilt and inadequacy. At such times it is important to seek help and support.

The Concept of Pain and Symptom Control

Pain and symptom control is an important and specialist area when caring for the dying; a detailed and technical discussion will therefore be left to other texts to explore. Nevertheless, it is important to have an introduction to some of the concepts related to pain and pain management and the diversity of potentially unpleasant symptoms that need careful management in those who are dying.

Although not all patients with a life-limiting disease will experience pain, it remains one of the most feared symptoms (Clark, 1993). Pain is not, however, a straightforward sensory experience but an inclusive one that is moderated by emotional, social and spiritual elements as well as physical influences. This is known as the 'concept of total pain'. We can usually tolerate quite intense pain if we know that it will go away and that it is not ultimately associated with our impending death. For individuals with a life-limiting disease, the pain is not only often chronic, but also a constant reminder that it is part of a disease process that will result in their death.

Pain is a highly personal and individual experience and as such requires detailed assessment and management that goes far beyond simply prescribing **analgesics**. As such, good pain management requires a considerable input from the nurse in terms of assessing the non-physical aspects of pain. But the physical aspects are important too. The World Health Organisation (2005) advocates the use of a three-step analgesic ladder (Figure 13.2) when managing pain. This concept is basically simple but is for most patients effective in minimising their pain. It advises that medication should be:

1   Step 1 *By mouth* whenever possible.
2   Step 2 By the clock. In other words the analgesia should be given at regular intervals and not just waiting until the pain is manifest.
3   Step 3 By the ladder.

Non-opioid analgesics for mild pain may include paracetamol; **opioids** for mild-to-moderate pain may include drugs such as dihydrocodeine; and opioids for severe pain may include morphine. You may wish to look these drugs up in your drugs handbook.

This method of pain control has been accepted worldwide as a valuable model. You are not expected to have a full grasp of its prescribing implications

analgesics
pain-relieving drugs – an absence of pain is termed 'analgesia'

non-opioid analgesics
analgesics such as paracetamol and non-steroidal anti-inflammatory drugs, for example aspirin

opioids
drugs such as morphine derived from the opium poppy; these are controlled drugs

but instead to recognise that effective analgesia is available to patients. If the patient is to remain relatively pain-free, pain management should be started early and analgesics given regularly and reviewed regularly. With early intervention, most patients start at step 1, but it is perfectly acceptable to start at step 2. What is essential is to get the patient as pain-free as possible as quickly as possible if that is what the patient wants.

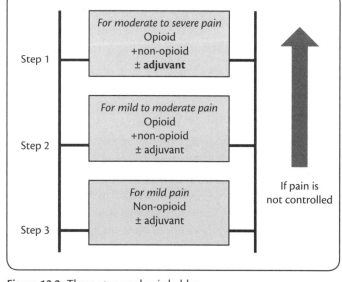

Figure 13.2 Three-step analgesic ladder

Source: Adapted from WHO (2005).

Other symptoms

Other distressing symptoms experienced by the patient are many and varied. Solano et al. (2006) identified 11 common symptoms experienced by people at the end of their life and who were suffering from a variety of conditions including cancer, heart disease, AIDS, respiratory and renal disease. The eleven symptoms identified were:

Chapter 6 reviews administration of medication.

- Pain
- Nausea and vomiting
- Constipation
- Diarrhoea
- Anorexia
- Fatigue
- Breathlessness
- Confusion
- Insomnia
- Anxiety
- Depression.

As with pain, a careful and comprehensive assessment of all symptoms is very important. What might be a minor irritation for a healthy individual can be a huge burden to a person approaching the end of their life, draining their energy, self-esteem and enjoyment of life, and leading to insomnia, fatigue and depression. Each additional symptom adds to the patient's total discomfort, yet with good nursing and medical care many of the symptoms are treatable and/or avoidable. It is thus essential to assess thoroughly and regularly, and never dismiss any symptom of which the patient complains. Although some of the symptoms involved require specialist intervention, many can be managed by good-quality nursing care, including caring therapeutic communication.

Communication

What is special about communication when caring for the dying? Maybe nothing. However, NICE (2004) identifies face-to-face communication as one of the key topic areas and suggests it is fundamental to good quality palliative care, yet is is often reported by patients and carers as being poor. What do you say to someone who is facing death? How do you respond to the relatives and friends? Perhaps part of the difficulty lies in our deep-rooted fears of death, referred to earlier in the chapter. Because these fears lie essentially in our subconscious, we may not even be aware of their existence. There are, however, other more overt fears that may get in the way of open communication. Buckman (1998) identifies the following fears commonly encountered in health-care professionals:

- There is a fear of the pain *we feel* because of patients' and relatives' distress. Sometimes we almost hurt for them.
- We fear being blamed by patients for their condition and ultimate death, as if it were our fault. This blaming does sometimes happen as patients and relatives struggle to understand why nothing can be done to cure them. Nursing and medical staff also struggle with how to manage a condition that is not amenable to treatment.
- We fear not knowing what to say because we have never been taught what to say. Indeed, talking about dying is not like other clinical procedures: although you can have guidelines, there is no script for the right thing to say. But if we always wait for the right thing to say, we may end up with nothing being said, a common scenario. With the right intent and a little courage, we will gain experience and become more confident in effective therapeutic communication.
- In a similar way, our desire always to have the right answer can make it difficult for us to say, 'I don't know.' Yet we may have many unanswered questions, and trying to flannel with patients and relatives will only lead to mistrust. An honest 'I don't know' can lead to a more open communication and a developing trust between the patient and the health professional.
- Talking to patients and relatives can sometimes result in their giving an emotional reaction. This can lead to fears of how to manage this reaction and how to manage other staff members who may feel that you have 'upset' the patient. Nevertheless discussing life and death issues is upsetting, and we need to be prepared for a whole variety of possible reactions and learn how best to manage them.
- Many people have fears about their own death. Some of these lie in the person's awareness and some may be subconsciously held. Health-care professionals are regularly confronted by death, however, it is more difficult for them push such fears aside and out of their thoughts.
- Some nurses wonder how much they should express their feelings and fear that to do so would be unprofessional. Although it is important to remain in control of the situation, it is rare for patients or relatives to see emotion as unprofessional, and indeed a lack of any emotion can be seen as insensitive.
- Finally, there is a fear of the hierarchy. What am I allowed to say? How should I respond when asked questions? Will the hierarchy blame me, especially if they have differing views about talking to patients?

These fears can lead to nurses using blocking or distancing tactics to avoid talking to the patients (Wilkinson and Mueller, 2003). They may avoid the patients altogether, use small talk, give false reassurances, ignore or not pick up on cues, use jargon, deal only with the positive or pass the buck (Jarrett and Maslin-Prothero, 2004). Patients and relatives can be left feeling stranded in an uncertain world; the barriers erected may encourage them to withdraw into themselves and become even more anxious and depressed. In addition, without clear communication patients and families are void of essential information necessary for them to be involved in the decision-making process.

Learning to cope with these fears comes easier to some than others. We all have a unique background that affects how we manage such situations, and it is important that you are gentle with yourself and develop your abilities gradually. Just reading this chapter will certainly not be the answer, and perhaps a good place to start is reflecting on your own thoughts and experiences of death. Some guidelines can, however, help in providing at least a little scaffolding to support you through your learning:

- Listen to patients and their relatives. Don't feel you have to have the answers; just listen and care.
- Remember that not everyone wants to talk about their illness or about dying, so don't force it on people, but do be sure it is not just you that is avoiding the issue.
- Don't deny people their feelings by telling them not to worry or not to be silly. Acknowledge their feelings by saying something like 'It must be worrying' or 'It seems you are very frightened'.
- Offer openings such as 'Is there anything you would like to talk about?'
- Don't distance yourself. Sit with the person and, when appropriate, use touch as a way of connecting with them.
- Be prepared for a variety of emotions, including anger. This is rarely personal but may be an expression of the person's fear, uncertainty and loneliness.
- Don't be offended if they choose someone else to talk to. We can't always be the right person, but this does not mean that you are not a good nurse or not good at communication.

In the last days of life

The final days of a person's life can be difficult for health-care professionals to manage, especially if they do not have specific training in the care of the dying. The 'Liverpool Care Pathway for the Dying Patient' (LCP) is an evidence-based pathway developed in a hospice but able to be adapted and used in the community, acute hospital setting or nursing home. The focus is on providing only the essential care needed to meet the needs of the patient during the last days and hours of their life. This care should be of the highest quality and include caring for the family during this phase of the patient's life and into bereavement. Great emphasis is made of regular assessment of physical, psychological, social and spiritual domains of care (Ellershaw and Wilkinson, 2003). Further information on the LCP can be found at the Marie Curie Palliative Care Institute Liverpool (MCPCIL) website www.mcpcil.org.uk.

Link

Chapter 2 discusses some of the core skills in good communication, including an introduction to breaking significant news. You might wish to review this now in the light of the discussion on communication in death and loss.

Last Offices

'Last offices' is the term used to describe the last elements of care carried out after a person has died. For many nurses, this is their first contact with death, and handled sensitively it can be a positive experience. Much of the procedure is not founded on research, but is based on myth and ritual. Nevertheless, ritual can itself be an important part of caring and should not be dismissed lightly. Much of the laying out of the dead provides an avenue for the nursing staff to offer their last opportunities for care and may for some act as a final closure. Procedures for last offices will vary and also depend on whether the person has died in hospital, at home, in a nursing home or in a hospice. There are, however, some broad, very practical aspects to the procedure, and the following principles outlined by Cooke (2000) need to be followed. Examine your local policy on last offices and reflect on each of these aspects of care:

- Appropriate care should be given to the bereaved relatives. If possible, give them the opportunity to be with the deceased before the body is removed from the ward. Prepare the area by removing as much clutter and as many clinical items as you can. Ensure that there are chairs next to the bed for the relatives to sit on.
- You will need to be guided by local procedures for preparing the body, but in essence individuals can be left in their nightwear; leaving a hand exposed allows the relatives to touch and hold the person. Covering the face with a sheet can make death frightening and unnecessarily mysterious for the relatives. Relatives should not be discouraged from talking to, hugging and kissing the person; this, after all, may be the last time they are close together.
- It is not a necessary routine to wash the patient, but a judgement should be made on whether, for example, a man should be shaved. If nurses choose to wash the patient as a way of saying goodbye, this will often be acceptable as long as it does not infringe any religious or cultural norms for the patient.
- Be careful not to do anything that would have been out of the ordinary for the person when alive, for example, do not put lipstick on a woman who would normally never have worn it.
- Offer to stay with the relatives, but be equally prepared to leave them alone in privacy. Relatives will need to be given advice and help with what to do next. They may wish to talk to the doctor or nurse to ask about the circumstances of the death. It is important for them not to be left with many unanswered questions, and it is helpful for them to have a contact person should questions arise at a later date.
- Ensure that there is appropriate support for the staff. Death will not always be an upsetting experience, which is perfectly acceptable. On some occasions and for some staff, however, it may be an upsetting experience, so be alert to your own feelings and the feelings of the staff around you. Be supportive and if necessary take 'time out' to reflect on what has happened. It is always useful to identify someone in your life whom you can talk to at such a time, even if this is only at the other end of the telephone.

- Provide appropriate support for other patients as they are invariably aware when someone has died. Do not try to hide the facts from them – they have a right to know – particularly in long-stay wards or nursing homes, and they may need an opportunity to talk.
- Provide dignity and privacy for deceased patients, treating them with the respect you would have given when they were alive.
- Protect staff, other patients and relatives from infection and hazards. You should consult local procedures for infection control measures, but essentially those who have died are no more or less infectious then when they were alive. Universal precautions should still, however, be used. Body bags may need to be used for infectious patients.
- Ensure a respect for the religious and cultural beliefs of the patient and family. If possible, find out from the family before the patient dies what specific procedures are required afterwards. Then ensure that these are adhered to.
- Comply with the relevant legal requirements. Always check whether the coroner needs to be informed of the death; if so, drains, catheters, tubes and so on should normally be left in situ.
- Ensure the care and safe custody of patient's property.
- Provide prompt and effective communication with other wards and departments.

Remember that many people are involved – relatives, porters, mortuary staff, doctors, chaplains, infection control nurses and patient administration staff. A procedural approach and rationale can be found in the Royal Marsden NHS Trust Manual of Clinical Nursing Procedures (Dougherty and Lister, 2008).

Ethical Issues in End of Life Care

There are many challenging ethical issues in end of life care. They are difficult for patients, for families, and they are matters that can divide professional staff. It is our responsibility to be open and to listen to everyone concerned. In a good multidisciplinary team most of the concerns can be managed. A few of the ethical issues will be highlighted here and they include stopping treatment, the doctrine of double effect and euthanasia. The latter, of course, remains illegal but that does not mean that the subject is not raised, especially from patients and families.

Withholding and withdrawing treatment

The decision to stop or limit curative medical treatment is not always clear and may present difficulties for the patient family and for health professionals. Frequently patients and families, understandably, cling to hope of cure, remission or just keeping decline at bay. This can be particularly difficult when it is artificial feeding that is withdrawn. However, when medical treatment is no longer serving a purpose and potentially causing more harm, it may need to be withdrawn. This need not equate to withdrawing hope. Making decisions about

✳ Activity 13.4

Ask a children's nurse and a community nurse how they manage last offices. Identify the differences and try to work out a rationale for these.

Look at the Royal Marsden Hospital Manual of Clinical Nursing Procedures (see further reading) for details of last offices and requirements for different faiths.

Look at the Age Concern website (www.ageconcern.org.uk) and search for the information contained in 'What happens when someone dies'.

what is in the patient's best interest requires careful consideration and negotiation. In all cases, supportive treatment and nursing care will still be provided along with the need to help the family reappraise meaning and hope within the current circumstances.

Withholding treatment may also be confused with euthanasia or physician-assisted suicide. It is important that such distinctions are clearly explained to those involved. The former suggests intent to deliberately end the life of a patient whereas the latter is a decision to withhold treatment based on clinical efficacy without intention to end life.

However, the discontinuation of treatment may seem to some as a signal for them to stop living, a turning to the wall as a form of passive suicide. On the other hand, it may be that the physician who is clinging to tenuous hopes of cure or increased life span and may proffer unwise attempts to persuade a family to continue treatment when in reality the patient is ready to relinquish further treatment.

Doctrine of double effect

Sometimes it is necessary to use pain-relieving medication and sedation to ease a patient's suffering. Used in the prescribed manner these therapies rarely end someone's life although they may play a part in hastening the death, for example because the patient may sleep more and therefore take less fluid and food. This principle of double effect is not without its difficulties but if it is used proportionately to the patient's symptoms and where possible is carried out with the full consent of patient, and with consideration for the family then concerns can invariably be allayed.

Euthanasia

✶ Activity 13.5

Further reading on euthanasia can be found at http://www. bbc.co.uk/ethics/ euthanasia/.

The question about euthanasia and assisted dying has had a high profile in recent years, especially with media coverage of people choosing to go to Dignitas (a Swiss assisted suicide group). However, it currently remains illegal in the UK. Nevertheless, patients and families do, from time to time ask health-care professionals to terminate their life and this can be a difficult dilemma for staff to manage. Detailed discussion on euthanasia is beyond the scope of this chapter but some of the definitions and issues are outlined below. Note that the definitions themselves are open to argument.

Euthanasia is the intentional bringing about of a person's death, by killing them (active euthanasia) or letting them die (passive euthanasia) and is done so in the person's best interest. Active euthanasia is brought about by an act, for example administration of a lethal drug. Passive euthanasia is brought about by an omission usually by withholding or withdrawing treatment:

- Withdrawing treatment: such as switching off a ventilator that is sustaining life.
- Withholding treatment: not starting some treatment that might extend a life for a short period of time.

It has been argued that what is commonly referred to as the 'doctrine of double effect' (see above) is euthanasia by the back door. However, the important distinction here is one of intention in that any prescribed medication is aimed at the symptoms and any unwanted side effect (in this case a hastened death) is not intended.

A further important distinction is between voluntary euthanasia where a person requests the termination of their life and non-voluntary euthanasia where the person is not in a position to make such a request, for example an infant, someone who is unconscious, or someone with profound learning disability.

Those who argue in favour of euthanasia suggest that people should not have to endure pain, suffering and loss of dignity, and should if they have capacity be able to act autonomously, deciding for themselves when to end their life. Those who argue against euthanasia may have strong religious reasons for doing. The anti-euthanasia lobby also fear that if it were legalised it would be abused; the slippery slope argument. Others may have no moral objection to euthanasia but find the law inadequate in legislating for such a complex moral scenario.

Unbearable pain is often cited as the main reason for requesting euthanasia but research on patients' and families' concerns at the end of life indicate that it is much broader than physical pain. Physical conditions such as incontinence, paralysis and breathlessness were also cited. Psychological factors including depression, exhaustion, loss of control and dignity, loss of hope and feeling a burden were particularly evident (Hickman et al., 2004; Sullivan et al., 2000).

The current debate in the UK focuses on whether, in some circumstances, a person should be assisted to end their life (**physician assisted suicide, PAS**). In 2005 Lord Joffe attempted to legalise PAS through an Act of Parliament but the Bill was rejected. Such systems exist in Oregon (USA), the Netherlands and Belgium and is decriminalised in Switzerland. In the UK the arguments for and against are well documented by the two main protagonists 'Dignity in Dying' formerly 'The Voluntary Euthanasia Society', who believe in greater patient choice at the end of life and argue that this provides choice and dignity in dying, and 'Care not Killing' who call for the government to reject assisted dying and instead move to better palliative care for all. The arguments put forward by these organisations can be easily accessed via the internet.

The simple answer to a patient who asks for assistance to end their life is to reply that it is illegal, but this minimises the patient's distress. At the very least it is an opportunity to help the patient explore their concerns, to be listened to. In listening to the patient and the family it may be possible to begin to understand the distress they are experiencing and it might be that in asking to die they are looking for a reason to live. Such discussions, however, should not involve advice that might be construed as assisting the patient to end their life; this remains illegal.

Patients and families experience many challenges when faced with the end of their life. At a time when they are feeling stressed it is important not to disenfranchise them but to involve them in the decision-making process. In doing so there is an opportunity to explore different perceptions, and where possible help

physician assisted suicide (PAS) where the physician provides the means (the prescription) but it is the patient who must be the person to administer the medicine that brings their life to an end

✷ Activity **13.6**

Try to be as objective as you can and think of reasons why it would be good to legalise PAS and reasons why it would be detrimental to legalise it.

these to be resolved, or at the very least enable a better understanding for all those concerned. This may be of particular importance where culture, religion and differing value positions are evident.

Bereavement

Death can release a whole variety of emotions. Some people may hardly be affected: perhaps the relationship was not very strong, or the death may have been a relief as it marked the end of suffering. For others, death can be very difficult to come to terms with. C.S. Lewis (1961), tormented by the death of his wife, opens his book with the comment:

> No one ever told me that grief was so like fear. I am not afraid but the sensation is like being afraid. The same fluttering in the stomach, the same restlessness, the same yawning. I kept on swallowing.

What these emotions and feelings relate to and what purpose they serve have been the subject of great debate for many years. Do we have to work through grief in a series of stages, and do we eventually have to let go of the lost person before we can get on with life? The debate remains in a state of flux so only a brief outline of some of the models proposed will be described here.

bereavement
the state of having lost someone significant

grief
a natural human expression and reaction to a loss

Many recent models of **bereavement** stem from the work of Freud and his contemporaries. Freud (1917) saw **grief** as a process to be worked through, something he called 'grief-work'. He hypothesised that, to recover from grief, the person needed to let go of all the energy invested in their loved one before they could invest that energy in another (Freud, 1917). Although most of the bereavement models have since changed and developed, this concept is still central to many of them. One of the models emerging from this tradition is that of Worden (2002), who describes a 'tasks of grief' model in which the bereaved work through a series of tasks. These tasks are:

- To accept the reality of the loss
- To experience the pain of grief
- To adjust to an environment no longer containing the loved one
- To relocate the deceased and memorialise the loved one.

Parkes (1996) describes grief as a psychosocial transition in which the bereaved individual has to readjust to a new world without the deceased person. Every aspect of life becomes changed and they have to adapt to this new and altered world. Parkes also identifies a number of stages involved in the grieving process: shock and alarm; searching; anger and guilt; and finally gaining a new identity. Central to this theory is letting go of the old world and adapting to the new.

A widely published model is that of Kubler-Ross (1969), who also describes a staged model consisting of denial, anger, bargaining and acceptance. Her initial work was in fact based on people who were dying. She talked to many terminally ill patients and observed the way in which they were attempting to adapt to their illness and impending death. The work of Kubler-Ross opened up a whole new way of caring for those who were dying. The stages she observed and described were similar to those which people appeared to pass through when bereaved.

Although the theories described here all add something to the understanding of grief, they are also open to criticism in that people rarely follow such a neat pattern of bereavement and are just as likely to want to maintain a connection with the deceased as to let them go completely (Klass et al., 1996; Walter, 1999). In a study of bereaved parents, Rubin (1993) found that they still maintained a firm attachment to their child up to 13 years after the death, and there is reason to believe that such an attachment may continue for as long as the parent lives.

More recent studies have placed a greater emphasis on people's individual experience of grief, which is in turn considerably influenced by culture and social norms. It is not unusual in our current society for people to expect the bereaved to get over their grief quickly, yet for many it is a long and sometimes painful struggle. So much depends upon the relationship with the deceased, the person's usual coping strategies and the support available. In addition, factors such as the mode of death, for example a prolonged illness, suicide or an accident, can have a profound impact on how the bereaved person manages their grief. The death of a child may be especially difficult to cope with and requires careful and sensitive management.

An alternative approach to the bereavement process has been proposed by Stroebe and Schut (1999). They have suggested a dual-process model in which bereaved people oscillate between working at their grief and expressing their feelings on the one hand, and allowing themselves to deal with everyday tasks and take on new roles on the other (Figure 13.3). This model allows a more individualised approach to bereavement, taking into account gender and to some extent cultural differences. This model acknowledges that people some-times need to be fully immersed in the emotional aspects of their loss, whereas on other occasions they need time to adjust to life without the deceased, manage

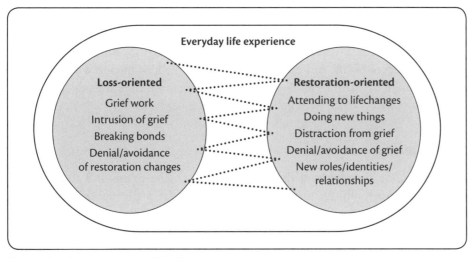

Figure 13.3 Dual-process model of bereavement

✸ Activity 13.7

List the types of loss experienced by someone who has to leave their own home and move into a nursing home. What sorts of positive and negative thoughts and feelings might they experience?

Think of all the types of loss that people might experience through ill-health – psychological, physical and social losses.

day-to-day life and be distracted from their grief. People oscillate between these two, sometimes confronting their grief and at other times avoiding it.

Nurses are for the most part involved with people during the acute stage of grief when someone significant has recently died. However, it is worth remembering that many people, who enter the health-care system, whether in hospital or at home, will have experienced losses during their life. In particular, older people are frequently faced with the death of family and friends, and those who move into nursing home care face many additional losses. Bereavement responses will also be manifest in people who are confronted by a social loss, such as the loss of a job or a relationship, and the associated loss of self-esteem and self-worth. Illness, too, brings with it many losses, including the physical loss of body parts or body function.

Whatever the cause of the loss, it is important to focus on individuals rather than a theoretical perspective. Listen to their story rather than trying to fit them into any model or stage. Accept them and their way of grieving. Helping people through grief and bereavement relies heavily on your ability to communicate effectively through listening, touch, the use of silence and sensitive responding. You might find the 'Ten ways to help the bereaved' (Chart 13.1) a useful starting point for deciding what you can do to help.

Chart 13.1 Ten ways to help the bereaved

• Be there	• Be familiar with your own feelings about loss and grief
• Listen in an accepting and non-judgemental way	• Offer reassurance about the normality of grief
• Show that you are listening and understanding something of what they are going through	• Do not take anger personally
• Encourage them to talk about the deceased	• Recognise that your feelings may reflect how they feel
• Tolerate silence	• Accept that you cannot make them feel better

Source: Adapted from Goodall et al. (1994).

Perhaps you could add to the list 'By recognising the spiritual nature of bereavement' because when someone is bereaved, questions often emerge about the whole nature of life and death. Relatives may need someone who will listen and not judge them but enable them to explore these fundamental questions. The nature of spirituality will be the focus of the next section.

Spirituality

Spirituality is not something that belongs only to the dying and those suffering, but is potentially an aspect of our everyday lives throughout our life. It is, therefore, an important element in all aspects of nursing, and it is discussed here partly out of convenience and partly because it is in times of crisis that many people become more acutely aware of the spiritual nature of life. Sogyal Rimpoche (1992) comments:

Spiritual care is not a luxury for the few; it is *the* essential right of every human being, as essential as political liberty, medical assistance, and equality of opportunity. A real democratic ideal would include knowledgeable spiritual care for everyone as one of its essential truths.

So what is spirituality and spiritual care? It is clearly not easy to define, and the danger of defining it is that in doing so you lose its very essence. Walter (1997) argues that when you begin to examine the various definitions, you are left with the question of how some aspects are any different from 'psychological care', 'social care' and religion. However true this might be, spirituality is perhaps more than the sum of its parts: the diverse elements when enmeshed become something new and very individual. Stoll (1989) captures this sentiment by expressing the relational aspect of spirituality and the religious dimension when she writes:

> Spirituality is my being; my inner person. It is who I am – unique and alive. It is me expressed through my body, my thinking, my feelings, my judgements and my creativity. My spirituality motivates me to choose meaningful relationships and pursuits. Through my spirituality I give and receive love; I respond to and appreciate God, other people, a sunset, a symphony and spring. I am driven forward, sometimes because of pain. Spirituality allows me to reflect on myself. I am a person because of my spirituality – motivated and enabled to value, to worship and to communicate with the holy, the transcendent.

Kellehear (2000) argues that although spirituality is difficult to define, some level of definition is not only possible, but also important. Definitions provide a platform for debate and practice, and are useful providing we recognise they are dynamic and changing, and open to dissent and challenge. It is suggested that human beings seek to understand and transcend suffering, desiring to understand and make sense of their situation; this is no more so than when people are faced with death (Kellehear, 2000). He describes a multidimensional model that incorporates the situational, religious, and moral and biographical aspects of spirituality (Figure 13.4). Although not everyone will access all three areas or all the elements within the areas, they do assume the types of need that co-exist in spirituality. What the areas have in common is that each reflects an attempt at transcendence, in other words an attempt to find meaning from a given life crisis.

I will not attempt to explain all these aspects of spirituality in the model but will try to give a flavour of what Kellehear (2000) is suggesting.

Religious

Religion is for many an important aspect of spiritual life. Through this vehicle many seek to find answers and guidance through prayer, meditation and ritual. It is an almost impossible task to describe the particular practices of the many religions, and even within the same religion people will have different interpretations and depths of devotion. Indeed, there is a danger of trivialising people's

✷ Activity 13.8

Think about the word 'spirituality', making notes about what you feel the term means to you.

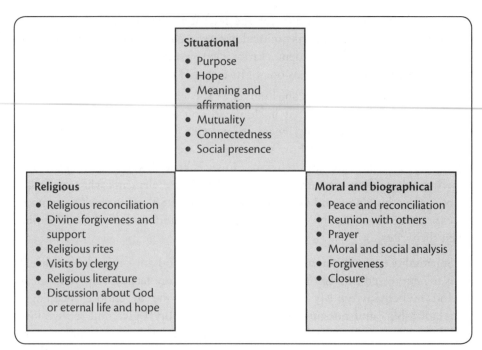

Figure 13.4 Dimensions of spirituality
Source: Adapted from Kellehear (2000).

beliefs if we simply focus on the ritual aspect of their belief system. This makes it even more important to take care in the assessment process.

Rather than simply 'ticking the box', it is important to ask what patients' religion means to them and what they need while they are in our care – do they wish their spiritual leader to visit them, what dietary needs do they have, and so on? If it is not possible to ask the patient, consult the relatives. If the patient is terminally ill, find out what the potential requirements might be in the terminal stages of the illness and after death. Sikhs, for example, may desire to have prayers said to them during the last stages of their life. Muslims may require that only Muslims touch or prepare the body after death.

In summary, be respectful of religious needs, seek advice and guidance early, keep contact numbers for local spiritual leaders and trusted local interpreters, listen to the needs of patients and relatives, and provide support to allow people to practise and meet their religious needs.

Situational

The situational aspect relates closely to trying to understand and make sense of the situations in which people find themselves. It emerges from the immediate situation, with its attendant medical problems, treatment and environment, be this hospital, hospice or their own home. People seek to discover hope and purpose in the place and situation they are in, to seek hope where there sometimes appears to be none. There can be nothing worse than to tell someone that there is nothing more we can do for them. But if we are to 'die living', there is always hope, hope to see a grandchild born, to paint a final picture, to see the sun rise, to be held by those you love, to be angry and express your emotions, to cry and seek solace, to fight and struggle. There is a need for help in this potentially frightening journey and people may seek the closeness, presence and affirmation of others as they seek to find meaning from their situation.

Moral and biographical

This also involves finding meaning in life but more from a biographical perspective – 'What has my life been about?' It is so easy just living life from day to day that we forget to ask more fundamental questions, but people faced with a life crisis frequently reflect on their life and try to make sense of it. It is also a time to seek forgiveness from loved ones, to say the things often left unsaid and to make amends. This may not always be achieved. The nurse can help by using the skills already discussed, giving time, however little, listening, caring, touching, giving a smile, listening to the anger, and providing privacy for visits. For some this may be done through prayer, which may be religious or secular. When faced with death there may be a need to bring about some degree of understanding on the life lived, and if possible sort out and put into perspective their life history.

This section has reflected on the complex nature of spirituality and has suggested that it is concerned with more than religion, being instead something within all of us – even though some may be more aware of this than others. At a time of crisis, however, spirituality may become more central to our thinking. Narayanasamy (2001) suggests that, to develop these skills, nurses need to develop their own self-awareness of spirituality, becoming aware of their own attitudes, values and prejudices and recognising what skills they have and which they are deficient in. Some of the skills needed are listening, trust-building and giving hope, as well as a knowledge of spirituality.

Chapter Summary

Death is the inevitable end to life for all of us. As a nurse, you are in a position to help many people with this transition and to help and care for the bereaved that are left. This chapter is only a brief introduction to this fascinating aspect of nursing; it does not pretend to be comprehensive, and in places you have perhaps been left with more questions than answers. You are encouraged to read widely around the subject and to do so critically, but just as important is your ability to learn from experience through active reflection. You may find it useful to explore a range of sources of information on death and loss, including novels, poetry and the arts; some suggestions are offered in the further reading below.

This chapter has tried to emphasise the individual nature of caring for people who are dying or bereaved. It has not been possible to include every scenario, but whether you are dealing with a dying neonate or a child, an adult or older person, someone with mental health problems or a learning disability, each requires their individual circumstances to be carefully considered.

? Test yourself!

1   List the common cardinal signs of death.

2   What are the dimensions of palliative care described by Davies and O'Berle (1990)?

3   What does the term 'total pain' mean?

4   What does the term 'analgesic ladder' mean?

5   What, according to Solano et al. (2006) are the 11 most common symptoms seen in patients with end stage disease?

6   What does the term 'last offices' mean?

7   What is the principal difference between euthanasia and physician assisted suicide.

8   What are the two elements of the dual process model of bereavement described by Stoebe and Schut (1999)?

9   Identify at least four ways in which you can help bereaved relatives.

10 What are the three elements of spirituality, as defined by Kellehear (2000)?

11 Make notes on your feelings about caring for the dying. What would you like to do to develop your skills and abilities in this area of nursing care?

Further Reading

For live links to useful websites see: www.palgrave.com/nursinghealth/hogston

Buckley, J. (2008) *Palliative Care: An Integrated Approach*. Wiley-Blackwell, Chichester. This text is a valuable resource for any health-care professional involved in end of life care. It is evidence based and takes a holistic and integrated approach to palliative care.

Dougherty, L. and Lister, S. (ed.) (2008) *Royal Marsden Hospital Manual of Clinical Nursing Procedures*, 7th edn. Blackwell, Oxford. A very helpful evidence-based manual on clinical procedures.

Earle, S., Komaromy, C. and Bartholomew, C. (eds) (2009) *Death and Dying: A Reader*. Sage, London. This book provides a wide range of readings of value to anyone exploring death loss and palliative care.

Hill, S. (1977) *In the Springtime of the Year*. Penguin, London. This is a useful novel as it explores how two people experience different reactions to grief, neither fully understanding the other.

Lewis, C.S. (1961) *A Grief Observed*. Faber & Faber, London. The grief journey of the philosopher and writer, well known for his Narnia books. Lewis writes movingly of his feelings following the death of his wife. You might also like to watch the film *Shadowlands*, which is meant to recount the journey experienced by Lewis and his wife as she becomes ill and ultimately dies.

Nyatanga, B. (ed) (2008) *Why Is it so Difficult to Die?* Quay Books, London. A useful and recent book for health-care professionals exploring many aspects of death and loss.

Payne, S., Seymour, J. and Ingleton, C. (eds) (2004). *Palliative Care Nursing: Principles and Evidence for Practice*. Open University Press, Maidenhead. A very comprehensive textbook covering a diverse range of palliative care topics.

References

Aries, P. (1981) *The Hour of Our Death*. Knopf, New York.

Barclay, S. (2001) Palliative care for non-cancer patients: a UK perspective from primary care. In Addington-Hall, J.M. and Higginson, I.J. (eds) *Palliative Care for Non-cancer Patients*. Oxford University Press, Oxford.

Barnes, K., Jones, L., Tookman, A. and King, M. (2007). Acceptability of advance care planning interview schedule: a focus group study. *Palliative Medicine* **21**: 23–8.

Buckman, R. (1998) Communication in palliative care: a practical guide. In Doyle, D., Hanks, G. and Macdonald, N. (eds) *Oxford Textbook of Palliative Medicine*. Oxford University Press, Oxford.

Chapman, S. (2008). *The Mental Capacity Act: Guidance for End of Life Care*. National Council for Palliative Care, London.

Clark, D. (1993) *The Future for Palliative Care: Issues of Policy and Practice*. Open University Press, Buckingham.

Collick, E. (1986) *Through Grief: The Bereavement Journey.* Darton, Longman and Todd, London.

Cooke, H. (2000) *When Someone Dies: A Practical Guide to Holistic Care at the End of Life.* Butterworth-Heinemann, Oxford.

Davies, B. and O'Berle, K. (1990) Dimensions of the supportive role of the nurse in palliative care. *Oncology Nurses Forum* **17**: 87–94.

Davis, B.D., Cowley, S.A. and Ryland, R.K. (1996) The effects of terminal illness on patients and their carers. *Journal of Advanced Nursing* **23**: 512–20.

DoH (Department of Health) (1999). *Our Healthier Nation.* The Stationary Office, London.

DoH (Department of Health) (2008). *The End of Life Care Strategy: Promoting High Quality Care for all Adults at the End of Life.* Department of Health, London.

Dougherty, L. and Lister, S., (2008) *The Royal Marsden NHS Trust Manual of Clinical Nursing Procedures.* 7th edn, Blackwell Science, Oxford.

Ellershaw, J. and Wilkinson, S. (eds). (2003) *Care of the Dying: A Pathway to Excellence.* Oxford University Press, Oxford.

Freud, S. (1917) *Mourning and Melancholia.* Std edn, Vol. XIV, 1957. Hogarth Press, London.

Glaser, B.G. and Strauss, A.L. (1968) *Time for Dying.* Aldine Press, Chicago.

Goodall, A., Darge, T. and Bell, G. (1994) *The Bereavement Training Manual.* Winslow, Bicester.

Hickman, S.E., Tilden, V.P. and Tolle, S.W. (2004) Family perceptions of worry, symptoms and suffering in the dying. *Journal of Palliative Care* **20**(1): 20–7.

Hospice Information Service (2001) *Palliative Care Facts and Figures.* www.hospiceinformation. co.uk (accessed June 2009).

Jarrett, M. and Maslin-Prothero, S. (2004). Communication, the patient and the palliative care team. In Payne, S., Seymour, J. and Ingleton, C. (eds) *Palliative Care Nursing: Principles and Evidence for Practice.* Open University Press, Maidenhead.

Kellehear, A. (2000) Spirituality and palliative care: a model of needs. *Palliative Medicine* **14**: 149–55.

Klass, D., Silverman, P.R. and Nickman, S.L. (1996) *Continuing Bonds: New Understandings of Grief.* Taylor & Francis, London.

Komaromy, C., Siddell, M. and Katz, J. (2000) The quality of terminal care in residential and nursing homes. *International Journal of Palliative Nursing* **6**: 192–200.

Kubler-Ross, E. (1969) *On Death and Dying.* Macmillan, New York.

Lewis, C.S. (1961) *A Grief Observed.* Faber and Faber, London.

Macmillan Cancer Relief (2005) *Gold Standard Framework.* http://www.macmillan.org.uk/ healthprofessionals/disppage.asp?id=2062 (accessed May 2009).

Morgan, J.D. (1995) Living our dying and our grieving: historical and cultural attitudes. In Wass, H. and Neimeyer, R.A. (eds) *Dying: Facing the Facts,* 3rd edn. Taylor & Francis, Washington.

Narayanasamy, A. (2001) *Spiritual Care: A Practical Guide for Nurses and Health Care Practitioners,* 2nd edn. Mark Allen, Dinton Quay, Wilts.

NHS (National Health Service) (2007). *Advance Care Planning: A Guide for Health and Social Care Staff.* http://www.endoflifecare.nhs.uk/ (accessed June 2009).

NICE (National Institute for Health and Clinical Excellence) (2004) *Guidance on Cancer Services: Improving Supportive and Palliative Care for Adults with Cancer.* The Manual. NICE, London.

ONS (Office of National Statistics) (1997) *Mortality Statistics: England & Wales 1996, General.* Stationery Office, London.

Parkes, C.M. (1996) *Bereavement: Studies of Grief in Adult Life.* Routledge, London.

Rosenblatt, P.C. (1997) Grief in small-scale societies. In Parkes, C.M., Laungani, P. and Young, B. (eds) *Death and Bereavement across Cultures.* Routledge, London.

Rubin, S.S. (1993) The death of a child. In Stroebe, M., Stroebe, W. and Hansson R.O. (eds) *Handbook of Bereavement: Theory, Research and Intervention.* Cambridge University Press, Cambridge.

Saunders, C. (1978) *The Management of Terminal Illness.* Arnold, London.

Seedhouse, D. (1997) *Health Promotion: Philosophy, Prejudice and Practice.* John Wiley & Sons, London.

Sogyal Rimpoche (1992) *The Tibetan Book of Living and Dying.* Rider, London.

Solano, J.P. Gomes, B. and Higginson, I.J. (2006). Prevalence of symptoms in advanced disease, based on a systematic review of 64 studies. *Journal of Pain Symptom Management* **31**(1): 58–69.

Stoll, R. (1989) *The essence of spirituality.* In Carson, V. (ed.) *Spiritual Dimensions of Nursing Practice.* W.B. Saunders, Philadelphia.

Stroebe, M. and Schut, H. (1999) The dual process model of coping with bereavement: rationale and description. *Death Studies* 23: 197–224.

Sullivan, A.D., Hedberg, K. and Fleming, D.W. (2000) Legalised physician assisted suicide in Oregon – the second year. *New England Journal of Medicine* **342**, 949–54.

Veatch, R.M. (1995) The definition of death: problems for public policy. In Wass, H. and Neimeyer, R.A. (eds) *Dying: Facing the Facts*, 3rd edn. Taylor & Francis, London.

Victor, C.R. (2000) *Health policy and services for dying people and their carers*. In Dickenson, D., Johnson, M. and Katz, J.S. (eds) *Death, Dying and Bereavement*, 2nd edn. Sage, London.

Walter, T. (1990) *Funerals and How To Improve Them*. Hodder and Stoughton, London.

Walter, T. (1997) The ideology and organisation of spiritual care: three approaches. *Palliative Medicine* **11**: 21–30.

Walter, T. (1999) *On Bereavement: The Culture of Grief*. Open University Press, Buckingham.

WHO (World Health Organisation) (2005) *WHO Pain Ladder*. http://who.int/cancer/palliative/painladder/en/index.html (accessed June 2009).

Wilkinson, S. and Mueller, C. (2003). Communication in care of the dying. In Ellershaw, J. and Wilkinson, S. (eds) *Care of the Dying: A Pathway to Excellence*. Oxford University Press, Oxford.

Worden, W.J. (2002) *Grief Counselling and Grief Therapy*, 3rd edn. Springer, New York.

Yalom, I.D. (1980) *Existential Psychotherapy*. Basic Books, New York.

ANITA GREEN

Chapter

Drug and Alcohol Misuse

14

📖 Contents

☑ Learning outcomes

At the end of this chapter, you should be able to:

- Understand what is meant by the different terms: drug and/or alcohol use, illicit drugs, dependency, harm reduction, motivational interviewing, detoxification and relapse prevention
- Describe the signs and symptoms of the most popular illicit drugs used
- Outline the requirements of a basic drug and alcohol assessment
- Name two pharmacological interventions used for someone who is physiologically dependent on either alcohol or illicit drugs
- Recognise your own feelings and attitudes when caring and treating someone who uses alcohol and/or illicit drugs
- Recognise the significance of your own and other's self-awareness when communicating with someone who is an alcohol and/or illicit drug user.

Introduction

Nurses come into contact with people who use drugs and/or alcohol and therefore play a vital role in the assessment, provision of physical and psychological care, support, guidance and treatment of their presenting health-care needs. The person may be accessing health-care services as a direct consequence of their drug and/or alcohol use, for example, admission to hospital for an alcohol detoxification; they may have a health problem which is indirectly linked to their drug and/or alcohol use, for example a fall at home after drinking alcohol; there may also be the situation where a person is admitted to hospital with a health problem that has no relationship to or is not a consequence of their drug and/or alcohol use. In this situation, the person's drug and/or alcohol use may or may not be immediately apparent to the caring for them. When a person's drug and/or alcohol use is known, nurses involved with their care and treatment have a responsibility to understand drug and alcohol use and recognise the physical, psychological and social needs of the drug and/or alcohol user. The nurse must also acknowledge their own feelings and attitudes when caring and treating someone who uses drugs and/or alcohol in a way that may be perceived as unsafe or harmful to themselves or others. The nurse's understanding of the legalities, national and local policies associated with alcohol and illicit drugs should better inform her practice and decision-making about the appropriate care and treatment required.

Even though nicotine in the form of cigarettes is a drug which when used regularly leads to psychological and physiological dependency, it will not be addressed specifically in this chapter. However, it is acknowledged that as a commonly available legal drug and with the recent changes in law regarding smoking in public places, it has received much attention, and there is not the space in this chapter to address the many health issues associated with smoking nicotine and the implications for nursing practice (please refer to one of the many websites offering information on smoking cessation for example, www.smokefree.nhs.uk).

Definitions of Drug and Alcohol Terms

The terminology used and definitions offered in this chapter have been chosen to reduce language sometimes associated with negative and pre-conceived unhelpful attitudes towards people who use substances. The terms used also attempt to reflect the strong influence of the service user movement present in the statutory and non-statutory services available to those who seek help for drug and alcohol problems. It is also important to avoid the 'overmedicalisation' of someone who uses either or both illicit drugs and alcohol as the person does not necessarily see themselves as 'unwell' or 'ill' and may not have had any previous contact with drug and alcohol services. The terms drug and/or alcohol (or substance) misuse, drug and/or alcohol dependency and substance users will be used and defined for the purposes of this chapter. The term drug or alcohol with be used when referring to specific drug and/or alcohol issues; the term substance misuse will be used to encompass the broad gamut of drugs and substances used which are classed as illicit and included in the Misuse of Drugs Act (1971) and alcohol misuse when it is used in a way that may cause harm to the individual or others. What must also be considered when discussing drug use and misuse is the way prescribed medication is sometimes taken: against the recommendations of the prescription and prescriber; well beyond the guidance and parameters of the *British National Formulary* and when prescription drugs are sold to another person or taken by a person for which the drug was not prescribed. When assessing a person's drug and alcohol use, their use of prescribed medication should always be considered in order to obtain a full pharmacological and psychopharmacological picture, which should also include a person's caffeine use (in the form of coffee, tea, cola and high caffeine soft drinks) and cigarettes. Nurses and other health-care professionals should contact their link pharmacist for advice and guidance on concerns regarding, for example, drug contraindications relating to non-prescribed medication.

Substance Use and Misuse

Drug and alcohol use and misuse can be defined within a socio-political, legal and cultural context. The acceptable use of substances is usually defined by cultures and social norms and can differ from one culture to another. When the use of a substance falls outside a society's norms and culturally defined boundaries which lead to undesirable or harmful consequences for the individual or community it could be regarded as substance misuse (Wilbourn and Prosser, 2003). The term substance misuse will be used in this chapter when the substance being used is classified as an illegal drug (Misuse of Drugs Act 1971) or is causing physical or psychological distress or physical harm which leads to contact with health-care providers and the provision of care and treatment as a direct consequence of the person's substance use.

Addiction is a term used to describe a syndrome characterised by a compulsion to seek out the substance of choice. There is an urge to continue or resume using the substance even after a period of abstinence (which could include pharmacological treatment for physical dependency). When this term is used it is usually associated with the behaviours connected with substance misuse when the substance seeking behaviour has negative consequences and usually serious detrimental effects on the social, psychological and physical well-being of the person (Wilbourn and Prosser, 2003). The terms 'addiction' and 'addict' are inseparable from negative stereotypes and media images and so can be misconstrued. However, some substance users who acknowledge their compulsion to use a substance may call themselves 'alcoholics' or a 'drug addict'. Their use of these terms to describe their substance use or previous substance use may relate to the treatment model or therapeutic approach used as part of their previous experience of treatment and care informed by different theories. The term 'addiction' is sometimes used interchangeably with substance misuse and

✹ Activity 14.1

From your conversations with friends and relatives, what terms or words do they use to describe someone who uses illicit drugs? List the words and consider the reasons for the language used. Are the terms used based on 'slang', stereotypes, images portrayed in the media, personal experience? How have these terms influenced you in your beliefs and attitudes towards someone who uses illicit drugs?

has been defined using different theories and models which include biological, psychological, sociological and behavioural factors. There is also the argument that the interactions between these different factors could determine whether or not a person will develop and continue to use a substance which leads to dependency (Daley and Raskin, 1991). Now try Activity 14.1.

Physiological dependence occurs when a substance is repeatedly taken which has reinforcing properties causing the body to physiologically adapt to the use of the substance (Wilbourn and Prosser, 2003, p. 179). Substances associated with physiological dependence include tobacco (nicotine), alcohol, opiates, benzodiazepines and caffeine. One of the characteristics of physical dependence is the person's need to take the substance to avoid withdrawal symptoms when the substance is not taken. Withdrawal symptoms can differ, ranging from slight discomfort to severe and sometimes life threatening, depending on the drug of dependency, and relates to sympathetic nervous system over activity. For example, alcohol withdrawal can cause symptoms such as seizures. In very severe cases alcohol withdrawal delirium or delirium tremens (DTs) occurs when alcohol withdrawal causes severe symptoms such as confusion, visual hallucinations and delusions. Withdrawal is far more complicated as highlighted by Rassool and Winnington (2006a, p. 29) who state that it is possible to experience withdrawal symptoms without being dependent on a substance and vice versa (Royal College of Psychiatrists, 1987). The use of cannabis would be a good example of this because it is not normally associated with clear physiological dependency symptoms. Other examples of withdrawal symptoms associated with physical dependency include are identified in Charts 14.1 and 14.2.

Psychological dependence could be described as a compulsion or a craving to continue to take a substance for its effects; for example, its hallucinatory or stimulatory properties. The person feels they need the substance to function and feel 'normal'. Even though the person may not experience physiological withdrawal they may experience depression, anxiety, a poor sleep pattern and appetite.

Edwards and Gross (1976) cited in Rassool and Winnington (2006a, p. 29) include the following components when describing the syndrome of dependency:

- Increased tolerance to the substance
- Repeated withdrawal symptoms
- Compulsion to use the substance (craving)
- Salience of substance-seeking behaviour (seen as more important than anything or anyone else)
- Relief of avoidance of withdrawal symptoms
- Narrowing of the repertoire of substance taking (drug use becomes an everyday activity)
- A return to the substance use after a period of abstinence.

The International Classification of Diseases – Classification of Mental and Behavioural Disorders (ICD-10; WHO, 2007; see also the Diagnostic and Statistical Manual of Mental Disorders (DSM-IV-TR)) requires that three or

Chart 14.1 Alcohol withdrawal

- Alcohol withdrawal symptoms usually begin 6–8 hours after the last drink and peak on the second day of abstinence. By the fourth to fifth day some of the symptoms start to subside.
- Early symptoms include: irritability, anxiety, insomnia, tremors, sweating, and mild tachycardia. Rare cases – grand mal seizures or intermittent visual, tactile or auditory hallucinations.
- Alcohol withdrawal delirium (DTs) can occur from day 2 to 3 but can also occur up to two weeks after the last drink.
- Symptoms include: confusion, disorientation, hallucinations, tachycardia, hypertension or hypotension, extreme tremors, agitation, diaphoresis, fever, hyperthermia and cardiac arrest (Fontaine, 2008, p. 433).

Chart 14.2 Opioid withdrawal

- Opioid withdrawal symptoms can occur within a few hours to a few days after the last dose depending on the type of opioid taken. For example if injectable street heroin is taken withdrawal symptoms would occur within a few hours. If a slow release opioid was taken, for example methadone, the withdrawal symptoms would be delayed because of the long half life of the drug. Symptoms can peak in 2–3 days and last up to 2 weeks.
- Symptoms include: muscle aches, backache, severe abdominal cramps, diarrhoea, watery eyes, runny nose, yawning, tremors, feeling cold, sweating and crawling skin sensations (Fontaine, 2008, p. 433).

---

more of the following criteria must be present at any time over a 12-month period in order for drug and/or alcohol dependency to be identified (WHO, 2007, p. 70):

1 Tolerance, as defined by either of the following:
   - A need for markedly increased amounts of the substance to achieve intoxication or desired effect
   - Markedly diminished effect with continued use of the same amount of substance.
2 Withdrawal, as manifested by either of the following:
   - The characteristic withdrawal syndrome for the substance
   - The same (or a closely related) substance is taken to relieve or avoid withdrawal symptoms.
3 The substance is often taken in larger amounts or over a longer period than was intended.
4 There is a persistent desire or sense of compulsion to take the substance or unsuccessful efforts to cut down or control substance use, a great deal of time is spent in activities to obtain the substance, use the substance, or recover from its effects. The person experiences difficulties in controlling substance taking behaviour in terms of the onset, termination or levels of use.
5 Important social, occupational or recreational activities or interests are given up or reduced because of substance use. An increased amount of time is necessary to obtain or take the substance or recover from its effects.

Activity 14.2

What would you define as 'risky' drug/alcohol taking behaviour? Make a list and consider your definition within a social, physical, psychological, economic and political context.

6 The substance use is continued despite knowledge of having a persistent or recurrent physical or psychological problem that is likely to have been caused or exacerbated by the substance (for example, continued drinking despite recognition that an ulcer was made worse by alcohol consumption).

The term tolerance is used when the body physiologically adapts to the repeated presence of the substance being used, usually the substance is being taken regularly and in sufficient quantities for tolerance to develop. Higher doses of the substance are required to reproduce the original desired effects (Rassool and Winnington, 2006a).

The Misuse of Drugs Act 1971

The media and some of the literature on illicit drugs talk in terms of 'soft' and 'hard' drugs. Cocaine, 'crack' cocaine and heroin being classed as 'hard' drugs and cannabis classed as a 'soft' drug. The two terms are used to simplify the level of risk associated with the drug. However, the terms do not consider the complexities associated with the different drugs used and misused and the social, economic, psychological and physical context in which the drug is taken and so the two terms can therefore be misleading. The terms also do not take into account alcohol and nicotine – 'legal' drugs associated with many deaths and prescribed medication which can be misused and lead to accidental or self-induced overdose and in some cases death. A more in-depth discussion can be found at www.drugscope.org.uk.

The Misuse of Drugs Act (MDA) 1971 establishes a legal category of 'controlled drugs' which identifies that if a person is in possession, using, producing or/and supplying a specified drug they are committing an illegal act. The MDA 1971 divides drugs into three classes, A, B and C (see Table 14.1). Each class summarises the penalty for possession of the drug, and dealing and trafficking the drug in the United Kingdom. Drugs under Class A are classified as the most dangerous to a person's health and to society and so carry the highest penalties. Drugs which are categorised under the MDA 1971 are reviewed in light of new research and their categorisation may be changed to reflect the new evidence. Drugs which become popular when previously unknown or there was little evidence of their widespread use and effects can be categorised under the MDA 1971 to reflect new and compelling evidence of increased and more widespread use with recognised physical and/or psychological health risks.

There are a number of prescribed medications that have particular effects which means that they may be misused; for example, they can create physical or psychological dependency. The Misuse of Drugs Regulations 1985 (amended in 2001) subdivides these medications into schedules to reflect the level of potential misuse (Chart 14.3).

Table 14.1 Drug classifications

Class	Drug	Maximum penalties	
		Possession	**Supply**
CLASS A	Cocaine Magic mushrooms (which contain Psilocin) Heroin Morphine Opium Pethidine Dipipanone (Diconal) Codeine prepared for injection Amphetamine prepared for injection Methyl amphetamine (US Methamphetamine) Phencyclidine	7 years prison sentence + fine	Life prison sentence + fine
CLASS B	Codeine Cannabis Amphetamine Barbiturates	5 years prison sentence + fine	14 years prison + fine
CLASS C	Anabolic steroids Dextropropoxyphene (e.g. Distalgesic) Buprenorphine (Temgesic and Subutex) Ketamine Flunitrazepam (Rohypnol) All benzodiazepines Gammahydroxybutyrate (GHB)	2 years prison sentence + fine	14 years prison + fine

Note: The Misuse of Drugs Act is available online at www.drugs.homeoffice.gov.uk
Source: Adapted from the Misuse of Drugs Act 1971.

Chart 14.3 Drug classifications – schedules

- Schedule 1 – contains drugs which are not authorised for medical use and can only be supplied, possessed or administered under a Home Office licence. Examples include drugs in their raw state such as cannabis, coca leaf, ecstasy, LSD, opium and psilocin.
- Schedules 2 and 3 – contain drugs which are used medicinally and are prescribed by a doctor. These drugs only become illegal under the Misuse of Drugs Act 1971 if someone is in possession and the drug has not been prescribed for that person by a doctor. Schedule 2 drugs include, for example: amphetamines, cocaine, dihydrocodeine, heroin and methadone. Schedule 3 drugs include barbiturates, rohypnol and temazepam.
- Schedule 4 – is in two parts to reflect the changes to the law relating to benzodiazepines. Part 1 contains the benzodiazepines (other than rohypnol and temazepam). It is now illegal to be in possession of benzodiazepines without a prescription. Part 2 of the schedule contains anabolic steroids, which can be legally possessed without a prescription but it is illegal to supply.
- Schedule 5 – contains controlled medication that have a lower risk of being misused. The drug comes in a dilute form and taken orally in small doses and sold as over-the-counter medications without a prescription. Included in these schedule 5 preparations are cough medicines and anti-diarrhoea agents.

Source: Adapted from the Misuse of Drugs Act 1971.

Routes of Administration

The different routes for taking illicit substances are as an oral preparation, smoking, sniffing (or snorting), inhaling (or smoking) and injecting (see Table 14.2). Substances can also be taken rectally, though this is a less popular route. Certain substances are associated with a particular route of administration and relates to the experience wanted from the substance and the significance of **titration** for the substance user. Entering the venous system directly by intravenous injecting; via the mucus membranes when 'snorting', or via the lungs when smoking offers a more intense, quicker and more noticeable effect and therefore a more controlled level of titration because of the way the substance enters the body and the blood circulation to directly affect the brain. Substances can also be injected subcutaneously or intramuscularly; the effect is less immediate and the intensity is reduced compared with intravenous injecting. Taking substances orally delays the effect because of the slow absorption via the digestive tract. The process of preparing the substance for use, particularly injecting and smoking, when substance taking paraphernalia is required can become an important 'ritual' and integral to the actual substance taking. For example, 'chasing the dragon' (associated with heroin use), 'rolling a joint' (associated with cannabis) terms inextricably linked with specific substances. For some, the ritual is as difficult to give up as the substance itself. Try Activity 14.3.

What Are the Reasons for People Using Substances?

There may be different reasons for taking a substance the first time. Choosing to continue to take drugs after that first occasion and take amounts at a level that can potentially cause physical and psychological distress or harm which could also lead to dependency may be due to a number of interrelated reasons. Try Activity 14.4.

Young people may choose to use drugs experimentally at a time in adolescence when risky behaviours are more evident and perhaps viewed as a 'rite of passage'; this period of experimentation may be short lived. The adolescent psyche, however, may not consider the added risks of experimenting with substances such as potential overdose, sexually transmitted diseases or other infections contracted, an unplanned pregnancy when intoxicated and may not be aware of ways of minimising the risks. It has been suggested that people who experiment with substances like cannabis may increase their probability of using other more potent substances or increase their usage of their substances of choice so they become a regular or dependent user. The term 'gateway theory' has been used to describe the phenomenon of moving from a 'soft' to a 'hard' substance. However, the use of this term and its meaning has been debated and the general conclusion is that the 'gateway effect' is small and probably not a major factor in the relationship between moving from a substance like cannabis to, for example, heroin. Again, there may be other social, psychological, economic and family circumstances which contribute to a person's shift from one substance to another. See Pudney (2002) for a more in-depth discussion on the 'gateway theory.'

titration
quantity of given substance

☀ Activity 14.3

See the film *Trainspotting* for a vivid, harsh and in the main realistic insight into the life of heroin users who live with drug and alcohol dependency. The film offers a convincing example of withdrawal symptoms using a surreal presentation as the main character, Renton, played by Ewan McGreggor, experiences 'cold turkey' in an attempt to come off heroin in his own way and when 'supervised' by his parents!

☀ Activity 14.4

What reasons can you think of for people using an illicit drug for the first time? What reasons can you think of for people continuing to take drugs when there may be negative implications or consequences? (See Chart for a list of reasons. Rassool and Winnington, 2006a, p 29)

Table 14.2 Usual routes of administration – potential risks and complications

Route of administration	Potential risks	Complications
1. Oral	1a. Non-pharmaceutical preparation (may be contaminated)	1a. Accidental poisoning
	1b. Using a pure formulation of the drug (pharmaceutically prepared)	1b. Accidental overdose
2. Intravenous injection	2a. Contaminated injecting equipment (inc. water, filters, spoons, cooking pots)	2a. Bacterial/viral cross infection from sharing equipment
		2a. Injection using non-sterile equipment (hepatitis, HIV, AIDS, abscesses)
	2b. Poor injecting technique	2b. Trauma to vein, arterial injecting can be fatal, thrombosis, embolism
3. Subcutaneous and intramuscular infecting	3a. Contaminated injecting equipment, poor injecting technique, injecting into breast, penis, neck	3a. Necrotising fasciitis • Embolism • Thrombosis • Nerve damage • Fat necrosis
	3b. Sharing equipment including needles	3b. HIV, Hepatitis, AIDS
4. Inhalation – snorting, sniffing	4a. Volatile substances	4a. Respiratory arrest
	4b. Cocaine	4b. Damage to mucus membrane
5. Smoking	5a. Cannabis burning at a high temperature	5a. Burn damage to lips, mouth and lungs
	5b. Use of plastic bongs or pipes	5b. Toxic fumes inhaled from burning plastic

The term 'binge drinking' has been used recently by the media to describe the high intake of alcohol in one drinking session. The definition of binge drinking is the consumption of more than eight units of alcohol for men and six units of alcohol for women (Drinkaware, 2009). Binge drinking is usually associated with drinking with the intention of getting drunk; drinking to the state of being incapacitated; taking part in drinking competitions, for example drinking as much as possible over a timed period, usually in the form of 'shots'. There have been a number of television programmes offering a vivid picture of the British drinking culture – the cameraperson working alongside a paramedic to capture the 'here and now' drinking habits of the young person out for the evening. There are many physiological risks associated with binge drinking or severe intoxication. Accidents which can include falls and fights, hypothermia, respiratory depression, convulsions and pneumonia and respiratory failure which can occur when someone inhales their own vomit (see the Institute of Alcohol Studies, 2009, for facts sheets). These risks can be further complicated by the use of other substances used in conjunction with alcohol; for example cocaine and benzodiazepines.

Another reason why people may choose to use substances is because they enjoy and gain pleasure from using their substances of choice. It may help them

Chart 14.4 Reasons for continuing to use illicit drugs

The reasons why people take drugs:
- To enjoy the experience
- To achieve the same or a similar experience to alcohol
- To enjoy the short term effects
- To feel confident
- To 'break the rules' – to take part in unlawful activities, go against a culture norm or value
- To be a member of a subculture
- Curiosity
- Accessibility and availability of drug
- Peers' use of drugs
- To lose weight
- To deal with stress
- To avoid unpleasant feelings and thoughts
- To improve work performance
- To improve physique or physical attributes for sporting activities
- Continue using because of attachment to the rituals associated with the drug use
- The drug is an integral part of home or social life
- To relieve boredom
- To reduce or alleviate pain
- To satisfy cravings
- To avoid withdrawal symptoms
- Counteract withdrawal symptoms of other medication (illicit or prescribed) or alcohol
- Counteract side effects of prescribed medication
- A drug taken to enhance the effect of another drug
- Illicit drugs used as an alternative to prescribed medication when a similar drug may not be readily available – for example cannabis use in palliative care.

Source: Adapted from Rassool and Winnington (2006a, p. 29).

relax or give them extra energy required for a particular activity; for example, sports or sex. The substance may be associated with 'weekend' use and separated from 'work' life. There may be no serious adverse side effects; for example drinking alcohol at weekends as part of a social activity. This could change, however, for some individuals if the substance of choice is taken at other times and not associated with recreation. The use of the substance is not 'managed' and the substance user can develop problems associated with the substance use. For example, regularly taking time off work with 'hangovers'; spending more time thinking, seeking out and using their substance of choice. This may lead to a physical and/or psychological dependency when the substance using and activities associated with the substance take priority over daily living routines and move beyond recreational use.

Theoretical Perspectives on Substance Use and Misuse

There are a number of different theories or models provided to help explain why someone continues to use a substance even if it is causing harm to themselves or others, and these may differ from the reasons which contributed to the person's initial use. There does not appear to be a right or wrong theory or model for helping us make sense of substance misuse, but different perspectives informed by our knowledge, understanding and application of biology, psychology and sociology. When a number of different perspectives exist it is important to stay up to date with new research and evidence which can inform treatment and practice. It is also important to understand how the service user perceives and makes sense of their substance use which may be based on, for example, previous experiences of treatment and care, reading literature and research, folklore or family-based anecdotes. It could be deduced that the available evidence suggests a multiplicity of factors that can contribute to and determine why a person develops a substance misuse problem. These factors, underpinned by theories and scientific knowledge, help our understanding of substance misuse and dependency when assessing, treating and caring for someone who has chosen to use substances in a way that goes beyond experimentation and recreational use. These factors include: genetic predisposition; physiological differences such as metabolism, brain chemistry; coping mechanisms; substance availability; the influence of the family, culture and the environment (Daley and Raskin, 1991).

> **∞ Link**
>
> Chapter 16 explores alcohol in relation to genetics.

Alcohol Use

Outside licensed premises drinking alcohol is not illegal for those over the age of 5 years old. Under the age of 5 years old alcohol can only be given under medical supervision (Children and Young Persons Act 1933, Children and Young Persons (Scotland) Act 1937). You can enter a licensed premise from 14 years of age alone as long as you do not consume alcohol. If you are 16 years of age you can consume beer, perry, cider and port in a pub if you are also eating in an area put aside for meals. An adult must purchase the alcohol (Licensing Act 2003). In Scotland no adult needs to be present in order for alcohol to be purchased (Licensing (Scotland) Act 1976). A landlord can, however, decide whether children are allowed anywhere in the licensed premises. In some communities there are by-laws restricting drinking of alcohol on public streets at any age. Police also have the power to confiscate alcohol from those under 18 years of age who drink in public places.

Many of the UK adult population drink alcohol as part of normal recreational activities and associate drinking alcohol with relaxation, socialisation and time off work. Moderate drinking, either at home or in licensed premises fits comfortably with the social norms of society and is not viewed as problematic. The drinking habits of the UK population have changed over the last two to three decades influenced by a multiplicity of factors; for example the increase in disposable income, decrease in alcohol prices, more people drinking in the home, aggressive targeted advertising, the introduction of drinks based on spirits and higher percentage alcohol drinks, changes in drinking rituals which revolve around getting drunk – drinking competitions with 'shots' and 'pre-loading' – drinking to get drunk at home before going out to drink socially. Alcohol is now viewed as a major public health problem affecting people across the age groups (Drinkaware, 2009) and because alcohol is a widely used substance along with nicotine smoking its usage leads to many admissions to hospital.

There appears to be clear evidence that children are drinking at a younger age and drinking to get drunk. Binge drinking is associated with risk taking behaviours including sexual activity which increases the risk of sexually transmitted diseases, for example, chlamydia and gonorrhoea, and unplanned pregnancy.

The Department of Health (2009) has identified what is 'safe drinking' or the safe recommended limits measured in units. The number of units in a drink is related to the concentration of alcohol to the volume of the drink. A unit measurement is the equivalent of 10 mls or 8 grams of alcohol (ethanol). The unit value of a drink can be established using the following calculation:

Strength (ABV) × Volume (mls) ÷ 1000 = Number of units

For example: a pint of strong lager can be approximately 5.2 (ABV) × 568mls (1 pint) ÷ 1000 = 2.95 units (see also Figure 14.1).

The recommended limits of alcohol per week are 14 units (2–3 units daily) for women and 21 units (3–4 units daily) for men. Determining alcohol consumption on a daily basis is more realistic and perhaps reduces the idea that drinking your 'quota' of alcohol in one night is reasonable because it is on the threshold of the Department of Health's recommended limit. The reason for the differences between men and women is because of the way men and women metabolise alcohol in their bodies; even when the woman and man are the same weight and height the woman will usually have a much higher concentration of alcohol in her body.

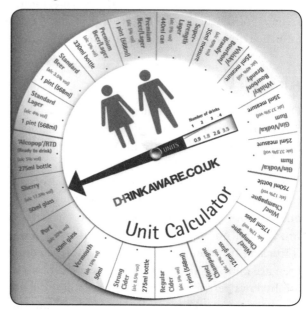

Figure 14.1 Alcohol unit calculator wheel
Source: www.drinkaware.co.uk. Reproduced with kind permission of Drinkaware.

> **✳ Activity 14.5**
>
> If you drink alcohol are you aware of the number of units you drink in a week? Do you drink more alcoholic drinks on certain days of the week? Have you got concerns about the amount of alcohol you drink or has someone suggested that you may be drinking too much? If you have concerns would you consider keeping a drinking diary? Please see www.drinkaware. co.uk for more information on unit measurement.

Alcohol consumed just before bedtime, after an initial stimulating effect, may decrease the time required to fall asleep due to its general sedating properties. Because of alcohol's sedating effect, many people who have difficulty sleeping consume alcohol to promote sleep. However, alcohol consumed within an hour of bedtime appears to disrupt the second half of the sleep period which results in a reduction in overall sleep time The person can feel as though they have not had a 'good night's sleep'. The older person may be at more risk because drinking alcohol prior to going to bed may lead to unsteadiness and if walking is attempted during the night, there is an increased risk of falls and injuries. Try Activity 14.5.

The effects of alcohol on the body

Alcohol is quickly absorbed by the body into the blood system and acts on the central nervous system as a depressant. The symptoms produced by the intake of alcohol depend on the amount drunk, the level of blood alcohol concentration and the interaction with other medication.

There are many physical effects from misusing alcohol. Some are long term and irreversible, others may be temporary and reversible once the person has stopped or reduced their drinking to within the safe recommended limits.

The gastrointestinal tract usually shows the effects of alcohol use (Figure 14.2) early on in the person who is using alcohol well beyond the recommended safe limits in the form of gastritis, oesophageal varices, oesophagitis and gastric ulcers. The person may experience nausea, vomiting, abdominal distention and when internal bleeding has occurred, melaena stools.

Pancreatitis which can be acute or chronic can be caused by long-term alcohol use. The symptoms include severe and constant epigastric pain, abdominal distension, nausea and vomiting. The pain from acute pancreatitis occurs after the first or second day of a heavy drinking episode. Rates of acute pancreatitis have risen significantly over the past 40 years. It is thought that this has been caused by the rise in alcohol misuse, because the excessive consumption of alcohol is a major risk factor for acute pancreatitis, accounting for 36 per cent of all cases (Eby and Brown, 2005).

Alcohol is excreted by the liver and if a person is drinking regularly over the recommended safe limit and/or binge drinking this will increase their chances of developing the first stage of alcoholic liver disease, known as fatty liver. Fatty liver is reversible if drinking is reduced or stopped. Between 20 per cent and

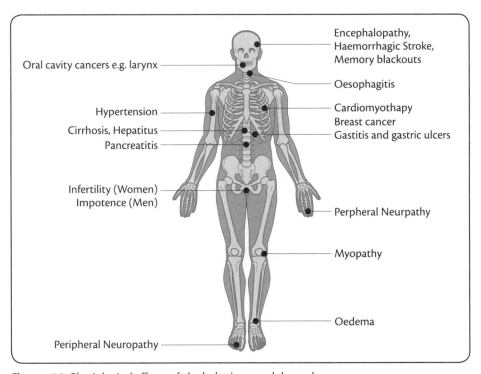

Figure 14.2 Physiological effects of alcohol misuse and dependency

30 per cent of people who are diagnosed with fatty liver and continue to drink excessively will develop alcoholic hepatitis when the liver becomes inflamed and, in its extreme form, is life threatening. The person will experience pain in their right upper quadrant, vomiting, diarrhoea, lethargy, loss of appetite, abdominal pain and may look jaundiced. The abdomen may be distended due to ascites. Around 10 per cent of people with alcoholic hepatitis will develop a permanently scarred and damaged liver called cirrhosis, which causes portal hypertension. The person with alcoholic liver disease may experience very few early symptoms. Not everyone experiences pain because the liver does not contain many nerve endings. Eventually, hepatocellular carcinoma occurs and liver failure when liver damage reaches a more advanced stage. The cardiovascular system is affected; hypertension, tachycardia, oedema, cardiomyopathy and cardiac dysrhythmias (Eby and Brown, 2005). The neurological system can be affected irretrievably if the person continues to drink long term and is either binge drinking or alcohol dependent. Wernicke's and Korsakoff's syndrome usually develop when the person has been misusing or is alcohol dependent for long periods of time. Wernicke's syndrome is a type of encephalopathy associated with vitamin B1 (thiamine) deficiency. The person who drinks heavily will usually present as malnourished with symptoms such as ataxia, nystagmus and confusion. Treated early with parenteral vitamin B1 some of the symptoms may be reversed or reduced. If untreated Wernicke's syndrome can develop into Korsakoff's syndrome caused by a deficiency of B1, B2 (riboflavin) and folic acid (Eby and Brown, 2005, p. 227) and does not generally respond well to parenteral thiamine or vitamin B complex (Wilbourn and Prosser, 2003). The symptoms are: amnesia, peripheral neuropathy – tingling fingers and toes, painful and weak muscles, osteoporosis. The person experiences extreme pain associated with the muscular skeletal system. Drinking alcohol can also affect mental health in other ways and is associated with anxiety, depression, self-harm (NHS Quality Improvement Scotland, 2007), suicide (DoH, 1993) and psychosis (Singleton et al., 2001). Withdrawal symptoms linked to people who drink daily and are dependent, can resemble anxiety, tremors, palpitations and in some cases phobias associated with meeting others, leaving the home and being in crowds.

When assessing someone who uses alcohol and may be dependent or binge, it is important to gather information about other drugs being taken which may

Chart 14.5 Alcohol guidelines for pregnant women

- Pregnant women and women planning a pregnancy should avoid drinking alcohol in the first 3 months of pregnancy because it may be associated with an increased risk of miscarriage.
- If women choose to drink alcohol during pregnancy they should be advised to drink no more than 1 to 2 UK units once or twice a week.
- Although there is uncertainty regarding a safe level of alcohol consumption in pregnancy, at this low level there is no evidence of harm to the unborn baby.
- Women should be informed that getting drunk or binge drinking during pregnancy may be harmful to the unborn baby.

---

also be central nervous system depressants; for example, benzodiazepines, barbiturates, other types of sleeping tablets and opioids. Even if these drugs are taken as prescribed the cumulative effect of alcohol and the medication can lead to respiratory depression and in some cases respiratory arrest. An example of this would be a person who drinks alcohol in the evenings 'medicinally' and has been prescribed night sedation; the additive effect of both drugs even when within normal amounts could lead to respiratory depression.

The National Collaborating Centre for Women's and Children's Health commissioned by the National Institute of Clinical Excellence provided recommendations in 2008 (p. 99) for pregnant women and alcohol use (Chart 14.5).

The Royal College of Midwives responded to NICE and agreed that there was no evidence to suggest that low levels of alcohol are harmful to the baby after the first three months of pregnancy, however, they suggested that women should avoid alcohol while pregnant, and for women to stop drinking alcohol if they want to conceive.

Heavy alcohol intake during pregnancy has been linked to foetal alcohol syndrome, which is characterised by low birth weight, reduced head circumference, congenital and intellectual abnormalities and certain facial features which include: thin upper lip, flattened midface, short **palpebral fissures** and indistinct or **flattened philtrum** (DrugScope, 2005, p. 27).

palpebral fissures
the anatomic name for the eye opening between the upper and lower eyelids

flattened philtrum
the area from below the nose and to the upper lid which is normally grooved

Theories specific to alcohol misuse

The reasons why someone continues to use alcohol when it may be causing physiological, psychological, economic and social harm to themselves and others can be the same as for any drug used. However, there are a number of theories associated with alcohol dependency which need to be considered. The two main risk factors linked with alcohol dependency are genetics and the environment. Those with a family history of alcohol dependency are more likely to become alcohol dependent themselves. Clearly the consumption of alcohol is necessary in order for someone to develop a problem with alcohol which could lead to dependency, therefore the environment does play a part; for example alcohol is readily available to that person and drinking and being drunk is more acceptable within the family and/or community. Evidence suggests that in males and females who are alcohol dependent, 50–60 per cent are genetically determined leaving the remainder due to environmental factors (Dick and Bierut, 2006, p. 151). Genetic predisposition is not necessary to develop alcohol dependency. Similarly, not everyone with a genetic predisposition develops a dependency (Dick and Bierut, 2006). It is an indicator, however, which should be acknowledged when assessing someone with an alcohol problem or is alcohol dependent.

Other Substances Associated with Misuse

There are many substances used and misused which are included in the Misuse of Drugs Act 1971 (see Table 14.3). Further information about the cost of

Table 14.3 Other substances associated with misuse

Drug name	Classification	Street name	Route of administration	Effects	Risks and complications
Benzodiazepines (anxiolitics), diazepam, lorazepam, flunitrazepam, temazepam	Class C POM	Benzos	Oral	Drowsiness, sedation	CNS depression, exacerbated with alcohol, tolerance, dependence, withdrawal can include convulsions
Amphetamine (stimulant)	Class B (Class A if prepared for injection)	Speed, uppers	Oral, IV	Elation, psychomotor agitation, tachycardia	Malnutrition, fatigue, disturbed sleep, anxiety, paranoia
Phencyclidine (PCP)	Class A		Oral, IV, smoked, inhaled	Euphoria, hallucinations vomiting	Violence, hypertension, respiratory depression, convulsions
LSD (lysergic acid diethylamide)	Class A	Acid, dots, tab	Oral	Intensification of perceptions, anxiety, impaired judgement	Unpredictable behaviour, can result in harm to self or others, flashbacks, tolerance
Magic mushrooms (psilocybin, psilocin)	Class A	Shrooms, mushies	Oral (usually prepared – dried, cooked)	Similar to LSD	Similar to LSD – also ingestion of poisonous fungi in error, vomiting, stomach pain
Inhalants, solvents, butane	Not classified under the MDA included in the Intoxicating Substances Supply Act	Glue, lighter fuel	Sniffing, inhaling	Euphoria, light-headedness, excitement	Ventricular fibrillation, decreased cardiac output, brain damage, inhalation of vomit
Alkyl nitrites	Not controlled under the **MDA** or the **Medicines Act**	Liquid gold, amyl, poppers	Liquid which is inhaled	'Rush' sensation, vaso-dilator and muscle relaxant. Associated with enhancing sexual behaviour	Headaches, nausea, tachycardia, dermatitis, excessive use has been associated with methaemoglobinemia
Ketamine	Class C	K, green super K	Smoked, oral, sniffed	Exhilaration, euphoria, out of body experiences, visual distortion, hallucinations when taken in large doses	Taken with alcohol and other depressants – respiratory or cardiac arrest can occur. Anxiety, paranoia, inability to feel pain may lead to the person sustaining an injury without knowing.
GHB – gammahydoxybutrate	Class C	Liquid E, GHB, liquid X	Oral – liquid, powder or capsule	Similar to alcohol – sedation, euphoria, disinhibited	Nausea, disorientation, if taken with alcohol or the depressants – respiratory or cardiac arrest can occur.

substances and the time the substance stays in the body with a more detailed explanation of these substances can be obtained from www.drugscope.org.uk. Cannabis, opiates and cocaine will be discussed in more detail for the following reasons: cannabis is the most popular illicit drug used in the UK and has recently been documented in the media, academic and research papers (see www.drugscope.org.uk for more information) with reference to its reclassification under the Misuse of Drugs Act 1971 and its relationship with mental illness, specifically psychosis, and its use in palliative care. Opiates and opioids, the most popular being heroin, will also be discussed. The National Treatment Agency (NTA, 2009) formulates policy for treatment in England which informs the substance misuse services and the priority of treating and supporting primarily opioid and opiate users. Harm reduction services in the form of needle exchanges were first developed in the late 1980s in response to the rise in blood-borne diseases such as **HIV** and AIDS and **hepatitis** B and C among injecting heroin drug users. Even though the number of heroin users are small in comparison with those who use cannabis the physical problems associated with injectable drug use, particularly heroin are complex and potentially life threatening and require access to harm reduction facilities, which does not necessarily require the person to be part of a treatment programme. Cocaine has, historically been associated with a small percentage of high earners and the 'champagne lifestyle' because it was costly to buy compared with other illicit drugs. More recently cocaine use has increased because its price has fallen and it is now viewed as more accessible to a wider population of drug users. Crack cocaine is a relatively new illicit drug and even though it is related to cocaine pharmacologically it is associated with a different lifestyle and drug taking experience. Recent surveys (UK Focal Point on Drugs, 2008) list cocaine as the second most popular illicit drug next to cannabis (the second most popular illicit drug used to be amphetamine) and for that reason as well as the physical and psychological problems associated with its use among a growing population of users will be discussed under its own heading.

Cannabis

Until recently cannabis was viewed as a 'soft' drug with little consideration given to the psychological and physical implications for its use, particularly when used daily and over long periods of time.

Cannabis is derived from a plant which is now readily cultivated in the UK. Other sources come from Morocco in the form of a resin. One of its psychoactive substances is called tetrahydro-cannabinols (THC) which is concentrated in the flower head with less in the leaves, stems and seeds. Some of the homegrown herbal 'super skunk' varieties give a more intense sometimes hallucinogenic experience (DrugScope, 2009), which may not be the experience required by some, for example those with chronic illness and cancer. Cannabis is usually smoked alone or with tobacco in the form of a 'joint'. The tobacco in a joint helps the cannabis burn more effectively. Cannabis can also be consumed through a bong, eaten as cakes and in stews or drunk as a tea. Cannabis smokers tend to inhale more deeply than a cigarette smoker and hold in the smoke in order to maximise absorption into the lungs. Smoking tends to be preferred because of the rapid absorption after inhalation, which takes effect in minutes; maximum brain concentration is reached within fifteen minutes. The cannabis user is more easily able to regulate the dose and achieve titration through smoking.

Smoking cannabis has stimulant and sedative effects, including increased pulse rate, lowering of blood pressure when standing, bloodshot eyes and increased appetite. Other experiences could also be perceptual alteration, time distortion, short-term memory and poor attention. When taking cannabis a person may be uncoordinated and their short-term memory can also be affected and they may feel less inhibited. Those with a pre-disposition to anxiety, panic attacks and paranoia may find that their symptoms are exacerbated when taking cannabis, particularly, the skunk variety (DrugScope, 2009).

Research and anecdotal evidence has made health-care professionals, service users and their carers more aware of the therapeutic value of cannabis for a number of conditions including asthma, glaucoma, mild to severe pain and muscle spasms, muscular spasticity, multiple sclerosis, motor neurone disease (amyotrophic lateral sclerosis), palliative care and AIDS. Service users, the nursing profession, other health-care professionals and carers need to be aware of the legal, pharmacological, physiological and psychological implications of using cannabis for medicinal purposes and must also be well informed and understand the implications for care and treatment if cannabis is being used medicinally on a regular basis.

Recently cannabis has been related to individuals with mental health issues, particularly those experiencing psychosis. Although the evidence is inconclusive, some research is suggesting that cannabis use can exacerbate or induce an early onset of psychosis in those who may have a predisposition or genetic vulnerability; there is a particular concern for those who start to use cannabis at a young age and links with mental health.

People who use cannabis daily over a long period of time with tobacco expose themselves to illnesses and diseases associated with cigarette smoking including respiratory, heart problems and cancers.

Opioids

Opiates are derived from the opium poppy and include morphine and codeine and come under the broad umbrella term of opioids as a Class A of the MDA 1971. There are also synthetically produced opioids such as methadone, dipipanone (Diconal), temgesic and pethedine. Dilute opioid mixtures can be found in over the counter medicines used for coughs and diarrhoea which are included in the MDA 1971 under Schedule 5. Natural and synthetic opioids are used primarily as analgesics and to aid sleep. Apart from their analgesic effect opioids induce drowsiness, euphoria and sedation. When opioids are injected intravenously or inhaled the level of the drug supplied to the brain is rapid and the user experiences a brief intense sensation sometimes called a 'rush'. This is followed by a period of calmness which lasts longer. Other effects from the drug are: relaxation, sedation, slowed movement, poor attention and memory, euphoria. Opioids are a respiratory depressant and so depress the nervous system including the reflexes which are linked with coughing, respiration and the heart rate and when taken in large doses and alongside other respiratory depressants, for example benzodiazepines and alcohol, have the potential to cause respiratory arrest and coma. Opioids also slow down the gastrointestinal tract. Use of opioids over a long period of time will lead to physiological and psychological dependency. With continued use the body's natural production of endorphins is reduced, which can result in a very low tolerance to pain, and the symptoms of withdrawal (Fontaine, 2008). There are many other complications associated with heroin use, particularly if the user is injecting, as they are more prone to infections, which include hepatitis, HIV and AIDs. Other infections are transmitted via the injection site, which can lead to localised infections, in extreme cases gangrene and blood-borne infections which can lead to septicaemia. Heroin use is also associated with poor nutrition; is some cases malnutrition, general poor physical health, inadequate housing or homelessness. There is also the possibility of overdose which can occur for a number of reasons. For example; changes in the potency of street heroin – there could be an increase in the strength unknown to the heroin user. The heroin user could have had a period of abstinence – for example a prison sentence, have been admitted to hospital or received a medical detoxification. Their tolerance to heroin will therefore be reduced so when they start to take the drug again it is more potent to the body even though the strength may not have changed. If a heroin overdose is suspected, naloxone (Narcan) is given intravenously which is a fast acting narcotic antagonist that reverses respiratory depression.

The main source of street heroin in the UK is from countries of South West Asia, mainly Afghanistan, Iran and Pakistan. 75 per cent of Europe's heroin comes from Afghanistan (DrugScope, 2009). Street heroin is usually an off white or brown powder and 'cut' (contaminated). Generally it is difficult for the heroin user to gauge how much heroin they are taking. Experienced users who have a regular supplier may be able to make a reasonable judgement on the percentage of heroin in a 'bag' (the term for how heroin is supplied). However, there are occasions when a supply of street heroin is contaminated with a harmful additive or may be of a higher strength than usual which can lead to overdose or death. Heroin can be smoked ('chasing the dragon'), snorted or prepared for injection (Shapiro, 2007). Pharmaceutically prepared opioids come in tablet or injectable form (Shapiro, 2007), or as a liquid, for example in the form of methadone which is a thick green liquid and drunk.

Neonatal Abstinence Syndrome (NAS) is a group of symptoms which occur in infants born to mothers dependent on, for example, opioids, benzodiazepines, alcohol and barbiturates. The baby is born with NAS because the drug it was being supplied with in utero is no longer available. NAS symptoms are associated with central nervous system irritability, gastro-intestinal dysfunction and autonomic hyperactivity (DrugScope, 2005, p. 35).

Cocaine and crack cocaine

Cocaine use has received media coverage over the last few years because of its association with a particular life style and the stereotypical personality of someone who is financially well off and famous. However, as the price of cocaine has fallen along with other drug prices, as opposed to other drugs, cocaine use has increased. It is now being used by a wider socioeconomic group.

Cocaine is a powerful stimulant drug still used as a controlled prescribed medication in ear, nose and throat surgery and dentistry for its vasoconstrictor properties which are usually used topically. It is derived from the coca leaf found in Peru and Bolivia. Cocaine can be administered through injection, sniffing or snorting it in powder form which is the most popular route as an illicit drug. By the time it reaches the UK streets it is approximately 20–50 per cent purity after being 'cut' (mixed) with additives such as glucose (Shapiro, 2007). The effect of cocaine taken via the nasal cavity where it is absorbed via the mucus membrane of the nose is usually 2–3 minutes, peaking at 15–20 minutes and lasts for as long as 20–30 minutes. The cocaine user will repeat the dose every 20 minutes to maintain the effect of the drug. Cocaine affects the central nervous system and the short-term effects are similar to adrenalin. There is an increase in the heart and respiratory rate, the appetite is suppressed and pupils dilated. The cocaine user feels they have more energy, confidence, and is euphoric, more alert and excitable. After taking repeated doses of cocaine over a short period of time the person can become agitated, anxious, can experience paranoid feelings and sometime hallucinations. If taken in excessive amounts death can occur through respiratory or heart failure (Rassool and Winnington, 2006b). When someone is using regularly, due to their state of mind and the physiological effects of cocaine, they lose weight and suffer from sleep deprivation. Excessive use can lead to restlessness, hyperactivity and over excitability, talkativeness, anxiety and panic attacks, anger and aggression and in some cases a drug-induced psychosis; the user can experience with this auditory hallucinations. Other physical effects from excessive use include hypertension, nausea, chest pain, confusion and cardiac dysrhythmias (Eby and Brown, 2005). Crack cocaine comes in the form of crystals produced by 'cooking' cocaine in water and soda or ammonia which releases the hydrochloride from the cocaine to form crystals or 'rocks'. Crack is usually smoked in a pipe, glass tube, plastic bottle or in foil or injected (Shapiro, 2007).

When cocaine and other stimulants like amphetamine are taken with other drugs there can be serious consequences. Alcohol taken with cocaine can enhance its effect on the body. The combined effect can cause hypertension. 'Speeding balling' which is when the user injects heroin with cocaine increases the effect of either or both drugs which can lead to an overdose. Cocaine is also contraindicated with other prescribed medications, for example, hypertensive and antidepressant medication. Assessing someone admitted to Accident and Emergency who has used large amounts of cocaine or crack cocaine must include checking for hypertension, tachycardia, cardiac arrhythmias, coronary artery spasm, hyperthermia and seizures which will need to be treated with medication.

Drug and Alcohol Assessment

Assessing someone who is using illicit substances or drinking excessive amounts of alcohol occurs for different reasons. An assessment may take place because the person has become physically or mentally unwell and the deterioration may or may not be directly related to their substance use. It is at this point that knowledge of the signs and symptoms of drug and alcohol use would alert the nurse to any problems which may need to be further assessed and treated (see Chart 14.6). It must be acknowledged that the person may not perceive themselves as having a problem with their substance of choice and for that reason may not be motivated to examine their reasons for using or consider becoming abstinent at the point of assessment. If the person is admitted to hospital suddenly they may feel totally unprepared and could be experiencing anger, humiliation, feeling defensive and/or suspicious. If they do not perceive their substance use as a problem they may be ambivalent about being in hospital and shy away from conversations about their drug use. It is important to establish an accurate picture and understanding of the person's substance use in order to eliminate any medical concerns and to assess the level of risk in relation to their recent substance taking activities so that the most appropriate care and treatment can be offered as soon as possible. Try Activity 14.6.

Chart 14.6 An example of an initial drug and alcohol assessment

---

- An initial assessment of drug and/or alcohol use would include the following:
- A full physiological assessment.
- A detailed history of the person's substance use (including polydrug use and methods of administration).
- An assessment of substance related harm – physical, psychological, legal, financial, social.
- A blood or urine toxicology assessment if appropriate and necessary (for example, if the person is showing signs of overdose or intoxication and is unable to say what drug(s) they have taken.
- An assessment of withdrawal symptoms (to decide if medication is required to reduce the physiological symptoms of withdrawal).
- Is the person being seen by a substance misuse service worker? Are they receiving a prescription from the service or GP?
- Does the person require information? Depending on the circumstances of the person and where the assessment is taking place – for example, the nearest needle exchange service and drop-in counselling services.

A more comprehensive assessment would be completed if the person was accessing mental health services and/or being assessed for a medical/pharmacological detoxification (see Chart 14.7). The information gathered should reflect the substance user's journey of using substances and any relationship between their substance use and any mental health issues. This can be done with the substance user through the use of a parallel time line which maps out the person's earliest memory of drug use and mental health issues up to the time of the assessment. It should include periods or abstinence and treatment. This may be an uncomfortable process for the person and does not have to be perfectly accurate – it is about obtaining the person's own perspective.

✷ Activity 14.6

Think about a practice experience when someone was in hospital with a health problem related to their use of alcohol or illicit drugs. What language or terminology was used by staff during the admission and assessment process? How did this influence your perception of the person and the interactions that took place when you were caring for them?

✷ Activity 14.7

From your practice experiences to date did any of the placements have a resource pack of information about local drug and alcohol services? What are you aware of in your local area? Find out more about local services and put contact details and information about the services together as a resource. This information may be helpful to your future placements that do not have this information readily available.

✳ Activity 14.8

Find specific alcohol assessment tools on websites, for example www.drinkaware.org.uk and www.dualdiagnosis.co.uk. Consider how these could be used in practice to assess someone who is alcohol dependent or using alcohol in a way that may be causing physical health problems.

Chart 14.7 An example of a comprehensive drug and alcohol assessment

A comprehensive drug and alcohol assessment would consist of the following headings:

- Statement of the person's need/problem
- Current drug and alcohol use
- Pattern of drug and alcohol use
- Current use of other substances, including prescribed or over the counter medications
- Level of dependence
- Associated problems – physical, mental health, social (including housing), legal problems, relationship issues (family, partner, friends)
- Level of risk taking behaviour associated with substance use
- Periods of abstinence/relapse – including medical detoxifications
- Sources of help and support
- Personal coping strategies and strengths
- Other professionals/organisations involved
- Previous contact with substance misuse services – for example, details of when this was and name(s) of link health-care workers
- Details of past experiences of treatments – for example, have they previously had detoxifications; rehabilitation, including periods of abstinence.

Source: Adapted from Rassool and Winnington (2006c, p. 181).

It is important that the assessment is carried out in a non-judgemental and empathic way. An understanding of the principles of motivational interviewing can help nurses recognise that individuals who use substances are not always ready to change their behaviour even after experiencing a serious health event leading to admission to hospital. However, they may be receptive to information that will help them reduce the risks involved in their substance misuse. Offering support and guidance which does not necessarily include treatment aimed at abstinence can increase the level of trust, rapport and therapeutic engagement.

Psychological Interventions

Critical to effective care and treatment is the assessment process which should include all the elements indentified in Charts 14.6 and 14.7 and is the time when the therapeutic relationship can be developed to enable the individual to engage with the relevant services which can help to meet their needs. It is important to consider the substance user's concerns and needs which may differ from what the nurse perceives as important.

Motivational interviewing (MI) is a therapeutic approach to working with a person to enable them to feel more empowered and gain insight into their substance use to help develop their motivation to change their behaviour. This method of counselling was developed in the 1980s by Miller (1983) alongside Prochaska and DiClemente's work on 'stages of change' (1983, 1986) (though not necessary in the order presented in the model – Figure 14.3). It is directive in style in order to elicit behaviour change through helping clients to explore and resolve ambivalence. The examination and resolution of ambivalence is the main goal (Rollnick and Miller, 1995). Its circular presentation offers a more

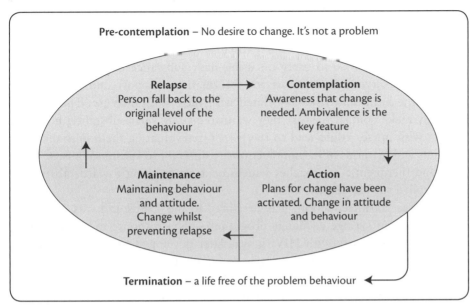

Figure 14.3 The stages of change model

Source: Adapted from Prochaska and DiClemente (1982).

optimistic view to behaviour change, for example, 'relapse' is viewed as part of the cycle of change and can lead to 'contemplation', a state of ambivalence which provides another opportunity for the person to examine their substance use. What makes this model and approach useful to nurses is being able to 'match' the intervention and/or treatment to where the person is on the stages of change model. For example, if the person is pre-contemplative they may not be receptive to offers of treatment and information about working towards abstinence; however, they may accept information about harm reduction strategies. If the person is contemplative they may be receptive to exploring the pros and cons of their drinking/drug taking behaviour.

There are a number of techniques which can be used to build motivation:

- Education about substances and the problems that may be associated with misuse including the effects on mental health
- Presentation of objective assessment data (e.g. liver function test, toxicology reports)
- Balance sheets on which the person lists the pros and cons of continued use/ abstinence
- Exploration of barriers to the attainment of future goals
- Reframe problems or past events emphasising the influence of substance misuse
- Reviewing medication and the use of an optimal medication regime. (DoH, 2002, p. 20).

Harm Reduction

Harm reduction is a strategy and particular stance which accepts that some substance users choose to carry on using their substance of choice and want contact with services and nurses for information, support and guidance on reducing the harm and risks associated with their substance use. They do not primarily make contact because they want to give up their substance; however, contact with nurses could lead to the person re-evaluating their substance use. The aims and methods of harm reduction are different to substance misuse treatment and therapeutic approaches which focus on working towards abstinence or controlled substance use.

The term 'harm reduction' was first used in the 1980s and was associated with needle and syringe exchange programmes as a response to the increasing numbers of drug users with HIV. It was later developed further in the 1990s when outreach workers offered advice to people using ecstasy involved in the dance scene.

Harm reduction covers a number of areas of health care which focuses on reducing risks associated with substance use and there are a number of websites which offer information to support further reading in this area (see further reading section).

Harm reduction interventions:

- Substitute prescribing – methadone, buprenorphine (see Table 14.4)
- Outreach workers
- Needle and syringe exchange services (which may be linked with local pharmacies or substance misuse services in some areas)
- Health-care checks (which may be available through local substance misuse services)
- Harm reduction teams – who offer support and guidance to substance users and health-care professionals working with substance users. This can include advice on safer injecting; teaching cleaning techniques, and encouraging other routes of administration – for example smoking heroin as opposed to injecting it.
- Homeless services
- Sexual health clinics
- Websites which offer advice on safe drinking. For example www. drinkawaretrust.org.uk.

Pharmacological Interventions

There are a number of pharmaceutical interventions available to help someone who wants to withdraw from a substance they are dependent on; this is called detoxification and is used for alcohol, opioids and benzodiazepine dependency. The medications used to help a person detoxify are usually part of a reduction programme, which means that the medication prescribed, for example, methadone or chlordiazepoxide (Librium) are commenced and gradually reduced over a period of time to keep withdrawal symptoms to a minimum. The aim is that the person is drug free after a set time. There are also medications available to help someone once they have abstained from their substance which can help reduce cravings during a period of time when the person is attempting to remain substance free. There is also a maintenance programme approach which is used to help people who need a period of stability on a prescribed medication and not necessarily a total withdrawal from all medication as part of a detoxification process. A methadone maintenance programme would be supervised by a substance misuse service, sometimes including the person's general practitioner and a local community pharmacist. The maintenance programme should provide the street heroin user with enough methadone to avoid withdrawal symptoms and reduce their need to 'use on top' (use street heroin with their prescription). Table 14.4 describes in brief some of the pharmacological interventions used to support someone who is either withdrawing from a substance, is on a maintenance programme or requires help during a period of rehabilitation.

> **⊙ Link**
>
> Chapter 10 discusses hypotension in more depth.

Table 14.4 Pharmacological interventions

Drug	Indications for use	Cautions
Acamprosate	Maintenance of abstinence in alcohol dependence. Treatment commenced as soon as possible after alcohol withdrawal	Side effects are: diarrhoea, nausea, vomiting. Contra-indicated in renal and severe hepatic impairment, pregnancy and breast-feeding
Methadone	An opioid agonist and a substitute for street opioids. It alleviates withdrawal symptoms. Given as a single dose daily. Can be used to help someone withdraw from street heroin or used as part of a maintenance programme	Regular use leads to physiological dependency. It has a street value
Buprenorphine	Partial opioid antagonist. Used in opioid dependency for those who have already reduced their opioid use	The person can experience withdrawal symptoms if on high doses of heroin or methadone and therefore should be reduced before burprenorphine commenced.
Diazepam	Used to assist physical withdrawal from alcohol dependency	Side effects can be drowsiness, lightheadedness. Dependency can develop with regular use. Effects of alcohol are enhanced
Chlordiazepoxide	Used to assist physical withdrawal from alcohol dependency	Same as diazepam
Lofoxidene	Used in opioid dependency to alleviate withdrawal symptoms	Side effects include: dry mouth, hypotension, bradycardia, drowsiness
Naltrexone	Blocks the action of opioids. Used for people who have been opioid dependent as part of a relapse prevention programme	Side effects include: nausea, vomiting, abdominal pain, constipation, diarrhoea, sleep disturbance
Disulfiram	Prescribed for people who have been alcohol dependent.	Extreme reactions when alcohol is taken: headache, palpitations, nausea, vomiting. Must avoid even small amounts of alcohol in mouthwashes, medications etc.

Source: Adapted from the *British National Formulary* (2009).

David is a 47-year-old man who has been admitted to Accident and Emergency after sustaining a head injury from falling over while walking home from his local park. He appears confused and is complaining of difficulty in breathing and has a headache. He does not smell of alcohol, but one of the nurses has reported that there are signs of multiple puncture marks and bruising along both of his arms. Some of the puncture marks are inflamed. When asked, David admitted to using injectable street heroin daily and had injected approximately an hour before being admitted to the Accident and Emergency Department. He states that he has been feeling unwell for a few days.

What would be your immediate concerns regarding David and the way he is presenting?

- David may have a localised infection from one of his injection sites.

- He may have used too much heroin which is affecting his breathing (with the potential of overdosing on heroin).

- He may be suffering from malnutrition, anaemia or a chest infection.

- You would want to rule out other drugs, taken independently of the heroin or used to contaminate the heroin (probably unknown to David).

- Full blood tests to check for infections, anaemia.

What observations and tests would need to be done as part of the assessment?

- Vital signs – hypotension, hypoglycaemia.

- Blood toxicology tests to assess if other drugs have been taken and to assess the level of heroin in his body.

- You would also want to offer harm reduction information to David and find out if he is already in contact with a substance misuse service and if he is receiving any prescribed medication, including medication to help him with his heroin use.

Chapter Summary

People who come into contact with health-care services and have drug and/or alcohol difficulties may have made the contact because they want to stop taking the drug and/or alcohol. They may have found themselves using the service for a number of other reasons which may or may not be related to their substance use. Nurses who care and treat someone with a substance misuse problem must be aware that the person could be feeling distressed, vulnerable, frustrated and even angry depending on their reasons for being in hospital, how they feel about their substance use, and the way health-care professionals communicate with them. Many substance users have a complexity of problems, some of which can be life threatening, therefore the assessment process must be thorough and person-centred. Effective care can only be provided if the person providing the care practises in an antidiscriminatory way (NMC, 2008). The substance user may not be ready to change their substance using behaviour even when they are seriously ill and in receipt of information indicating that their drug taking is very risky and in some cases dangerous. It is important that the health-care professional is able to assess the person's motivation to change their behaviour and to use the most appropriate intervention to 'match' the level of motivation.

Depending on the drug being taken and their level of physical and psycho-logical dependency the person will probably still seek out their drug of choice and continue to want to take it even when they are being cared for in a hospital setting. The health professional must familiarise themselves with the policies and procedures which guide practice in relation to drugs (included under the Misuse of Drugs Act 1971) and alcohol use on hospital premises and be vigilant because visitors (in some cases relatives and carers) may be supplying the person with their drug. There are situations when the police need to be involved because of the challenges faced by nurses and other health-care professionals: when a patient or visitor is intoxicated and aggressive, is openly taking illicit drugs and refuses to cooperate with staff or the visitor is supplying illicit drugs. The team faced with such challenges must work together and adhere to the correct procedures and apply their understanding of drug and alcohol misuse to ensure that the person involved and other patients, visitors and carers are not placed at risk. The nurse should be aware of their own feelings when faced with demanding situations which involve substance misuse and ensure that there is time given in order to reflect on and learn from the situation.

? Test yourself!

1 Using your own words, describe what is meant by the term drug/alcohol dependency.

2 What is meant by the term harm reduction and give three examples of harm reduction strategies.

3 Name two drugs from class A, B and C of the Misuse of Drugs Act 1971.

4 Name six of the physiological effects associated with alcohol misuse and dependency.

Rollnick, S., Mason, P. and Butler, C. (1999) *Health Behavior Change.* Churchill Livingston, Edinburgh.

McWhirter, J. and Mir, H. (eds) (2008) *Guide to Working with Young People about Drugs and Alcohol.* DrugScope, London.

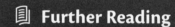

Further Reading

For live links to useful websites see: www.palgrave.com/nursinghealth/hogston

References

British National Formulary (2009) March. http://bnf.org/bnf/extra/current/450035.htm

Children and Young Persons Act 1933 (c.12) http://www.opsi.gov.uk/RevisedStatutes/Acts/ukpga/1933/cukpga_19330012_en_1

Children and Young Persons (Scotland) Act 1937 http://www.opsi.gov.uk/RevisedStatutes/Acts/ukpga/1937/cukpga_19370037_en_1Statutelaw.gov.uk.

Daley, D.C. and Raskin, M.S. (1991) *Treating the Chemically Dependent and their Families.* Sage, London.

Dick, D.M. and Bierut, L.J. (2006) The genetics of alcohol dependency. *Current Psychiatric Reports* **8**(2): 151–7.

DoH (Department of Health) (1993) *Health of the Nation. Key Area Handbook: Mental Health.* HMSO, London.

DoH (Department of Health) (2002) *Mental health Policy Implementation Guide. Dual Diagnosis Good Practice Guide.* DoH, London.

DoH (Department of Health) (2009) http://www.dh.gov.uk/en/public health/healthimprovement/alcoholmisuse/index.htm

Drinkaware (2009) http://www.drinkaware.co.uk/trends/alcohol-in-the-uk

DrugScope (2005) *Substance Misuse in Pregnancy: A Resource Book for Professionals.* DrugScope, London.

DrugScope (2009) http://www.drugscope.org.uk/resources/drugsearch/drugsearch.htm

Eby, L. and Brown, N.C. (2005) *Mental Health Nursing Care*. Pearson, New Jersey.

Edwards, G. and Gross, M. (1976) Alcohol dependence: provisional description of a clinical syndrome. *British Journal of Addiction* **81**: 171–3.

Fontaine, K.L. (2008) *Mental Health Nursing*, 6th edn. Pearson Prentice Hall, New Jersey.

Institute of Alcohol Studies (2009) http://www.ias.org.uk/resources/factsheets/factsheets.html

Licensing (England) Act 2003 http://www.opsi.gov.uk/acts/acts2003/ukpga_20030017_en_1

Licensing (Scotland) Act 2005 http://www.opsi.gov.uk/legislation/scotland/acts2005/asp_20050016_en_1

Miller, W.R (1983) Motivational interviewing with problem drinkers. Behaviour Psychotherapy. 11(2): 147–72.

Misuse of Drugs Act 1971 (including the Drugs Act 2005) http://drugs.homeoffice.gov.uk/drugs-laws/misuse-of-drugs-act/

Misuse of Drugs Regulations (2001) http://www.opsi.gov.uk/si/si2001/20013998.htm

National Collaborating Centre for Women's and Children's Health (2008) *Antenatal care: Routine care for the healthy pregnant woman. Clinical guidelines (commissioned by the National Institute for Health and Clinical Excellence)*, 2nd edn. Royal College of Obstetricians and Gynaecologists, London.

National Treatment Agency (2009) http://www.nta.nhs.uk/default.aspx

NHS Quality Improvement Scotland (2007) *Understanding Alcohol Misuse in Scotland 3: Alcohol and Self-harm.* www.nhshealthquality.org

NMC (Nursing and Midwifery Council) (2008) *The Code: Standards of Conduct, Performance and Ethics for Nurses and Midwives*. NMC, London. www.nmc-uk.org

Prochaska, J.O. and DiClemente, C.C. (1982) Transtheoretical therapy: Toward a more integrative model of change. *Psychotherapy: Theory, Research and Practice* 19(3): 276–88.

Prochaska, J.O. and DiClemente, C.C. (1983) Stages and process of self change of smoking: towards a more integrative model of change. *Journal of Consulting and Clinical Psychology* **51**(3): 390–5.

Prochaska, J.O. and DiClemente, C.C. (1986) Towards a comprehensive model of change. In Miller, W.R. and Heather, N. (eds) *Treating Addictive Behaviours: Processes of Change*. Plenum, New York.

Pudney, S. (2002) *Home Office Research Study 253: The road to Ruin? Sequences of Initiation into Drug Use and Offending by Young People in Britain*. Home Office Research, Development, and Statistics Directorate, London.

Rassool, G.H. and Winnington J. (2006a) Chapter 3. Understanding drug use and misuse. In Rassool, G.H. (ed.) *Dual Diagnosis Nursing*. Blackwell, Oxford.

Rassool, G.H. and Winnington J. (2006b) Chapter 4. Psychoactive substances and their effects. In Rassool, G.H. (ed.) *Dual Diagnosis Nursing*. Blackwell, Oxford.

Rassool, G.H. and Winnington J. (2006c) Chapter 18. Framework for multudimensional assessment. In Rassool, G.H. (ed.) *Dual Diagnosis Nursing*. Blackwell, Oxford

Rollnick S., and Miller, W.R. (1995) What is motivational interviewing? *Behavioural and Cognitive Psychotherapy* **23**: 325–34. http://www.motivationalinterview.org/clinical/whatismi.html

Royal College of Psychiatrists (1987) *Drug Scenes: A Report on Drugs and Drug Dependence*. The Royal College of Psychiatrists. Gaskell, London.

Shapiro, H. (2007) *The Essential Guide to Drugs and Alcohol*. DrugScope, London.

Singleton, N., Bumpstead, R., O'Brien, M., Lee, A. and Meltzer, H. (2001) *Psychiatric Morbidity among Adults Living in Private Households, 2000*. The Stationery Office, London. http://www.statistics.gov.uk/STATBASE/Product.asp?vlnk=8258

UK Focal Point on Drugs (2008) http://www.ukfocalpoint.org.uk/documentbank/UK_FOCAL_POINT_ANNUAL_REPORT_2008_MASTER_DOCUMENT_161208.pdf

WHO (World Health Organisation) (2007) ICD-10 (International Classification of Diseases) 10th Revision. Version for 2007. http://apps.who.int/classifcaitons/apps/icd/icd10online/

Wilbourn, M. and Prosser, S. (2003) *The Pathology and Pharmacology of Mental Illness*. Nelson Thornes, Cheltenham.

Professional
Issues

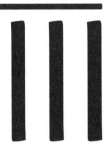

SID CARTER AND ANITA GREEN

15

Body Image and Sexuality

📖 Contents

- Introduction
- What Is Self-image and Normal Body Image?
- What Is Altered Body Image?
- Human Sexuality
- Gender
- Sexual Orientation
- Sexuality and Skilled Care Giving
- Chapter Summary
- Test Yourself!
- Further Reading
- References

☑ Learning outcomes

At the end of this chapter, you should be able:

- Understand the interrelationship between sexuality and body image and your responsibility in understanding these two important aspects of a person
- Recognise the part you play in helping patients and clients when body image and sexuality need to be addressed as an aspect of patient care
- Recognise your own feelings with respect to these areas
- Realise the importance of your own self-awareness when communicating with patients and clients who want support and guidance with their sexuality and altered body image needs
- Understand the importance of interprofessional team working and collaboration when caring for and treating a person with sexuality and altered body image.

Introduction

The expression of sexuality and **body image** appear to be inter-related particularly when associated with physical or mental illness, disease or physical trauma. Sexuality, sexual health and body image when negatively affected can decrease a person's **self-image** and self-esteem. When a person has contact with a health-care setting their illness or disability will probably impact on their sexuality (RCN, 2000) and body image. There can be many adjustments to sexuality and body image, and with these can come changes to self-care (Salter, 1997). It is important that nurses and health-care workers understand the inter-relationship between sexuality and body image and their responsibility in understanding these two important aspects of a person. Nurses and health-care workers need to recognise the part they play in helping patients and clients when body image and sexuality need to be addressed as part of providing care. The nurse and other health-care workers must also recognise their own feelings around these areas and the importance of their own self-awareness when communicating with patients and clients who want support and guidance with their sexuality and altered body image needs. The nurse and health-care workers have a vital role to play here in the physical and psychological care, support and treatment that they offer.

body image
the mental picture we have of our body and feelings towards it

self-image
our own assessment of our social worth

⟳ Link

Chapter 13 briefly discusses spirituality and nursing care.

What Is Self-image and Normal Body Image?

Over the past two or three decades nursing has integrated holistic perspectives and approaches into the care and treatment of patients and clients. We now consider the psychosocial, gender, cultural, spiritual and religious wants and needs of the patient and client when the health-care worker tends to their physical requirements. To perceive the patient and client as a 'whole' and not as a set of components that need separate attention is an important ideal and can help the health-care worker be more receptive to the patient's self-image and self-esteem. According to Price (1990, p. 12) self-image is 'our own assessment of our social worth'. Positive self-image gives us confidence and can increase our self-esteem.

An important element of self-image is body image, the mental picture each person has of his or her body. At birth infants do not have a body image. As babies develop their awareness expands and they begin to explore parts of their body. As they receive sensory stimulation through physical contact with others they become aware of their own separateness (Sundeen et al., 1994, p. 65). Children have a relatively simple view of their own bodies. When children are asked to draw pictures of themselves and the different parts of their bodies, their view of the body and the way it functions will be drawn using elementary shapes to represent organs. Once at school these concepts are developed and become more sophisticated as the child starts to view body image within the context of gender identification (Price, 1998, p. 50). Towards the end of primary education, children's concepts of themselves, their body and its functions are influenced by the attitude of their parental figures through what they say and do and the things that are discussed or not discussed within the family context (Sundeen et al.,

✳ Activity 15.1

Make a list of what you like and dislike about your body. Reflect on what may have influenced your decisions about what you have added to your list.

✳ Activity 15.2

How do you perceive yourself in your later years? List the changes you envisage occurring as you age. Your list could be influenced by how you view your body now and how it functions, your older family members and how they have changed and learned to adapt. Your list could be affected by someone you know who has taken on new challenges as they have aged.

1994, p. 65). Adolescence, a time of rapid physical development can bring with it feelings of awkwardness. Secondary sexual characteristics have to be incorporated into the individual's developing body image. With this go society's expectations of conforming to the social roles of being a man or woman, for example, the different ways we groom and adorn ourselves when in the social arena.

Inevitably, if body image is affected either positively or negatively this will influence the person's self-image. McCrea et al. (1982, p. 226) state that body image as a term, 'Refers to the body as a psychological experience and focuses on the individual's feelings and attitudes towards his own body'. Chilton (1984, p. 158, cited in Salter, 1997, p. 2) demonstrates the links between self-esteem and body image when stating:

> Body image also plays an important part in self-understanding. How a person feels about himself is basically related to how he feels about his body. The body is a most visible and material part of one's self and occupies the central part in a person's perceptions. Body image is the sum of the conscious and unconscious attitudes that the individual has towards his body. Present and past perceptions and feelings about size, function, appearance and potential are included. A person with a high level of self-esteem will tend to have a much clearer understanding of himself.

Added to this complex concept of body image is the element of change. How the individual perceives him or herself can alter depending on external and/or internal influences. These could be psychosocial, cultural, religious or physiological or any combination of these. An example of this is when a woman menstruates. There are hormonal changes occurring in the body associated with the menstrual cycle. These hormonal changes cause physiological changes, for example when the level of progesterone is at its lowest menstruation occurs. This may affect the woman's mood, and also influence how she perceives herself when menstruating. Added to this could be the woman's view of whether or not she wanted to be pregnant and how she associates menstruation with being womanly and feminine. There are cultural differences towards the menstruating woman: historically, the West has used terms like 'the curse' to describe the process of menstruating; this can affect the way women view their menstrual blood and their bodies when menstruating (Kitzinger, 1985, p. 38).

Ageing will also influence body image. As well as physiological changes, which could affect mobility and independent living, society's views on ageing are also an influence on the older person's body image (Price, 1990, p. 31). Changes in body function and appearance are a feature of health as well as illness and can be usefully viewed along an age continuum. To understand how the body is affected by normal physiological change, illness, ageing and hospitalisation and how this influences self-image is important for nurses to understand. Nurses' self-awareness in relation to how they perceive their own bodies and the bodies of others is an important contribution to this process of understanding. Even admission to hospital, before any procedures are commenced, will affect a person's body image and self-image. Removing one's day clothes and getting into bed could bring about feelings of dependency, loss and passivity. Changes to or loss of self-image due to hospitalisation have been well documented and can be linked with the changes or loss of self-identity observed in people who spend more than a few days in hospital (Goffman, 1961; Sanderson, 1985 cited in Savage, 1987). Therefore body image is not a fixed concept, it can change with developmental mile stones and important life experiences (Price, 1990).

Trying to understand an individual's feelings about their body image should also include how they value the different parts of their body. This is very individual. However, the nurse can explore this with the patient when completing the initial assessment. For example, a jockey putting on weight would seriously affect his/her career and an orchestral conductor with a damaged shoulder would be unable to work without suffering pain.

Body reality, body ideal and body presentation

Price (1990, p. 4) defines body image using three fundamental and interrelated concepts: body reality, body ideal and body presentation . This is a helpful starting point for understanding and exploring issues relating to body image.

Body reality

Body reality refers to the body, as it is, an objective representation, for example stating the height of someone, the colour of their hair and the colour of their eyes. Body reality is dynamic; our bodies undergo constant physiological change. Some of these changes we may be more aware of than others; for example, the physiological changes that occur during puberty, such as developing pubic hair, and breasts or facial hair. These will have a dramatic effect on body reality and inevitably affect body image, self-image and self-esteem. From birth to older age there are clear examples of how the body reality changes.

Body ideal

Body ideal represents how we believe our body should look like and perform. Our body ideal is influenced by the beliefs, norms and attitudes that we develop from early childhood as part of primary socialisation. During adolescence the body ideal appears to require constant updating in the light of new trends, with the media offering examples of the most recent 'role models', for example, popular music bands and the accompanying style of dress. The adolescent age group more than any other has to adjust body reality in light of new changes in fashion and social behaviour. Both conventional and non-conventional body piercing and tattooing have increased (Langford, 1996; Larkin, 2004), are attractive to young people and may be considered as permanent body reality change. These body changes may be viewed as a rite of passage and may also have cultural value. There may, however, be implications for the person when body piercing and tattooing are no longer part of their body ideal following changes in fashion or a change of view of these types of body decoration as the person ages.

Body ideal also includes how we think we should smell, age, what we should weigh, and how our body should be proportioned, for example the size of the breasts or penis. Body ideal is also influenced by cultural standards, for example

✹ Activity 15.3

Think about how you present your body to others. Write down what you do, for example through the use of make-up, clothes and hairstyles in order to 'face the world' when you go out to meet others. Does this change depending on who you are meeting, where you are going or what you are doing?

body reality
the body as it actually is in terms of its objective physical characteristics

body ideal
how we believe our body should look and perform, this being influenced by our beliefs and attitudes and by changes in fashion

over the past two decades exercise and fitness leading to a slim, toned body has led to a 'body conscious' society (Sundeen et al., 1994, p. 67). Body ideal may also be influenced by how 'plastic surgery' is portrayed in the media. More information is now available, with 'live' surgery on television and adverts for plastic surgery clinics in magazines which may persuade someone to seek surgical interventions to enhance their bodies. Women approaching the menopause and ageing in a society which appears to value slender, taut skinned youthful looks may choose medical or surgical interventions to temporarily postpone the open and concealed physical changes which are associated with being 'post-menopausal'; conforming to a certain image portrayed by society about how a woman should look. There has also been an increase in the use of tanning beds, particularly among young women who may also be experiencing 'intense personal celebrity worship' (Maltby et al., 2005, p. 17). The formation of para-social relationships (Maltby et al., 2005, p. 17) with media figures where the celebrity is perceived as having a good or healthy body image sometimes associated with having tanned skin could negatively influence the body image of young women (Maltby et al., 2005). Maltby et al. (2001 and 2004) found evidence to suggest that intense-personal celebrity worship could be linked to higher levels of stress, depression and anxiety.

Body presentation

Body presentation is linked with body ideal and represents how we present our body to others in a social context and in intimate situations. Body presentation includes the way we dress, adorn our body, groom, use posture and gesture (Price, 1990, p. 10; 1998, p. 50). Body image can include how we smell. Whether or not we choose to wear deodorant and/or perfumes and if we do the type of perfumes we want others to smell on us can play an important part in how we want to be perceived and the association society places on particular smells and perfumes. We have a level of control over how we present our body to others. We are also influenced by what is expected of us, for example policies regarding the wearing of uniform and how it should be worn, and policies for those who are not required to wear a uniform to work but have guidelines for what is acceptable as 'non-uniform'. We are also aware of the limits and boundaries of how we can present our body to others when, for example when working in the community as a community psychiatric nurse or district nurse.

Being unhappy with our body image affects the way we behave and inevitably affects those around us, even if this unhappiness is temporary. When we feel good about our body image and others notice this and offer positive comments to support us, usually this will positively affect our self-image so that we feel good about ourselves, and it is seen as approval.

What Is Altered Body Image?

Early developments, particularly from childhood to adolescence, pregnancy and ageing are evident through visual physiological changes to body reality and are

---

✴ Activity 15.4

Breast and testicular self-examination should be a routine part of every woman's/man's personal health care. Do you examine yourself? List the reasons why you do/do not regularly practise this self-examination. Ask your close friends the same question. What reasons do they give for regularly self-examining? What reasons are given by those who do not?

---

body presentation

how we present our bodies to others in a social context, including our clothes, make-up and hairstyle perceived as part of normal human functioning. **Altered body image** may not be evident through obvious physiological change to the normal body; however, it may still have a devastating effect on the person even though there may be no external evidence to the observer. Price (1995, p. 2) defines altered body image as:

> A state of personal distress, defined by the patient, which indicates that the body no longer supports self-esteem, and which is dysfunctional to individuals, limiting their social engagement with others. Altered body image exists when coping strategies (individual and social) to deal with changes in body reality, ideal or presentation, are overwhelmed by injury, disease, disability, or social stigma.

This definition appears to recognise the importance of the person in their social and cultural environment and their spiritual and religious awareness and its significance to how they perceive their altered body image.

Loss of Self Model

Blackmore (1989, p. 36) applies Watson's (1980) description of 'loss of self' using the **loss of self model** to explain altered body image: loss of psychological self, loss of socio-cultural self and loss of physical self.

Loss of psychological self is when a person's self-concept and self-esteem is diminished. Loss of socio-cultural self is when a person experiences loss of social identity, social role, family groupings or linkages with cultural background. Loss of physical self refers to the loss of bodily function or functions, a body part or parts or quality of physiological functioning. 'Loss of self' will affect the person in different ways depending on the disease, illness or trauma and the treatment involved, how the person perceives these and their significance to the person's life. An example using this model could be a man who has experienced ostomy surgery. The mutilation and relocation of a body orifice could have a serious effect on body image.

Loss of psychological self

Loss of psychological self would include the patient feeling as though they have returned to an infantile stage of development unable to control their excretory functions. This could affect how the man views his masculinity and his sexuality. He may question his sexual role and functioning. He may ask questions such as 'Do I smell?', 'Am I still attractive?', 'Will my partner still find me attractive?', 'Will people be able to see my ostomy bag?', 'Will I still be able to have sex?' and 'Will my partner still want to have sex with me?' A man involved with sporting activities may question how other men perceive him; is he seen as disabled?

Loss of socio-cultural self

Loss of socio-cultural self arises because society has particular attitudes towards excretion. For adults, urination and defecation usually occur in private and are not usually discussed with others. There is also the stigma attached to having a disease of the bowel. Post-operatively, there may be a degree of unpredictability

altered body image
the state of distress and lowered self-esteem that occurs when coping strategies to deal with changes in body reality, ideal or present are overwhelmed

loss of self model
a model that aims to understand altered body image by considering loss of psychological self, loss of socio-cultural self and loss of physical self

🔗 Link
Chapter 8 explains ostomy surgery.

as the body adjusts to the physiological change and the person adapts to using an appliance. During this time the person may choose to socially isolate himself. Family relationships can also be affected. Apart from the change in role within the partnership or family, to that of patient, which may or may not be temporary, the man has to decide how to include his partner and other family members in the knowledge of his illness and its effects on his day-to-day life. Added to this is any cultural and religious attitude towards excretion. This can be a problem when caring for a stoma site, for example keeping the right hand clean for preparing and eating food (Bell, 1989).

Loss of physical self

Loss of physical self can occur in different ways after surgery. The loss of the normal way of defaecating can be difficult and having to adapt to having a bag on your abdomen can affect how you view your body. Physical changes could include the effects of other treatments after surgery for a stoma formation, such as radiotherapy, which could cause fatigue, sore skin, and nausea and vomiting. Chemotherapy can lead to hair loss, skin discolouration and infertility. Sexual problems and a decreased libido can be suffered by a high percentage of patients (de Marquiegui and Huish, 1999). The general quality of body functioning can be affected (Blackmore, 1989).

Examples of altered body image

There are many different types of altered body image. Some of the examples given in Table 15.1 can be placed in either an **open** or **concealed altered body image** category. A woman who has recently developed anorexia nervosa may not be seen as experiencing anorexia nervosa by others; however, if the illness progresses, and her eating patterns change along with weight loss and other physiological changes associated with anorexia nervosa, then her illness will become 'open' and evident to others.

Along with the idea of altered body image being open or concealed within the categories identified is the consideration of whether or not an injury, illness or disease is permanent or temporary. The person may not know this in the early stages of their condition as a prognosis may not have been given. Once the person is aware of both a diagnosis and prognosis they will have an idea of whether or not there is any permanence. Being given this information will influence how the person adapts and manages any alteration to body image. Another consideration is that those who have sustained extensive or severe disfigurement will not necessarily have more problems and greater psychological distress than people with minor body image changes (Robinson, 1997).

The role of the nurse and other caring professionals

Assessment

It is important to assess how a person perceives their body and how this influences their self-image and self-esteem. Observing the way someone presents, for

---

Activity 15.5

Think of a patient you have cared for who was experiencing altered body image. Write down what you observed and found out about this patient.

'open' altered body image

an alteration in body image that can be clearly seen by others

'concealed' altered body image

an alteration in body image that is hidden from others

Table 15.1 Examples of altered body image

Congenital	Hereditary	Degenerative	Trauma
Open			
Muscular dystrophy	Huntington's chorea	Parkinson's disease	Facial burns
Cleft palate/lip	Retinitis pigmentosa	Multiple sclerosis	Amputation
Spina bifida	Hair loss	Arthritis	
Facial birthmarks	Acne	Ageing	
	Psoriasis, eczema		
Concealed			
Hypospadias	Diabetes mellitus	Conduction deafness	Burns to main body
			Body scarring (abuse) and bruising

Psychological	Surgical	Medical	Miscellaneous
Open			
Anorexia nervosa	Mastectomy	Medication	Tattoos
Schizophrenia	Reconstruction	– Chemotherapy	Body piercing (non-exotic) –
Obsessive disorders	Amputation of limb	– Psychotropic	ears, eyebrows, nose
Alzheimer's and other	Miscarriage	– HRT	Limb prothesis
dementias	Disfigurative surgery, for	Alopecia	Pregnancy
	example for cancer of the	Halitosis	Obesity
	neck	Liposuction	Use of wheelchair
	Breast reduction/	Catheter (short term)	Birthmarks
	enhancement	Lymphoedema	Intravenous infusion
		Naso gastric tube	Body scarring (cultural)
			Facial burns
			Achondrophasia
Concealed			
Nasogastric tube	Circumcision	Sexually transmitted diseases	Crohn's disease
Body dismorphic disorder	Hysterectomy	Medication	Body piercing (exotic) –
Body scarring (cutting)	Orchidectomy	Peri-anal abscess	tongue, nipples, clitoris, penis
Bulimia nervosa	Lumpectomy	Caesarian section	
	Stoma	Impotence	
	Termination	Sterility	
	Male and female	Premature ejaculation	
	genital enhancement –	Catheter (long term)	
	blepharoplasty		

Source: Adapted from Salter (1997) and Price (1990).

example, their posture, hair, dress and make-up, can give important information. Conversations about the patient's cultural background, religion, sexual orientation, age and occupation can further help the nurse make sense of the patient's body image and self-image. The nurse may ask the patient specific questions about their body image and body ideal, for example the importance the patient places on their appearance and physical functioning. The nurse will then start to understand the significance of health and illness for the patient. If a body image change has occurred from being ill or is to occur, for example from surgery, what effect could this have on the patient's body image, self-image and self-esteem in the future? The loss of self model (Watson, 1980) could be used as a framework to assess the significance and context of the altered body image for the patient.

During the assessment process the nurse could have contact with relatives, partners, carers and friends of the patient. Other professionals should also be involved in the assessment process, for example, the GP and counselling services. Assessing the perception and expectations of the patient and carers is important and the nurse needs to be aware of how they are managing the situation. How well informed are they? What strategies are they able to use to manage their own feelings about the patient's altered body image? Are they able to continue supporting the patient? (Price, 1990, p. 75). If the altered body image is permanent, how will this affect the relationship on a psychological, socio-cultural, and physical level? It is important to recognise the needs of the relative/partner/carer/friend and be proactive with the support and information they require. It is also important to be aware of issues of confidentiality for the patient; ideally communication with relatives, partners, carers and friends should only be done with the patient's permission. Some of the areas considered above could be discussed with the patient and relatives, carers, partner and friends together.

Nurses must be aware of, particularly in relation to 'open' or visible disfigurement leading to unfavourable views of the self (Rumsey, 2002; Koo and Young, 2002), negative effects such as lowered self-esteem, depression and anxiety (Kent and Thomson, 2002) and unfavourable reactions from others. Engaging in social activities with those close to the patient is less of a threat than being exposed to those unknown (Rumsey et al., 2004), and encourages the patient to develop strategies in a safer environment to be used when in unfamiliar situations.

Caring skills

Any change in body image, particularly when the change is viewed as negative, requires time for adjustment. For some patients this adjustment may be too difficult to contemplate or totally accept. The patient can feel vulnerable and not in control of their situation. The nurse should be available for the patient to articulate their concerns and fears when the patient feels ready. It may be that the patient is only able to manage hearing small amounts of information about their illness at one time.

As discussed previously, an alteration in body image is a loss and can affect the patient in different ways depending on what the altered body image signifies to the person. The manifestation of this loss is to experience a grief reaction. The patient may experience anger or denial as part of this reaction to their altered body image.

Once the patient has experienced the altered body image there should be a period of rehabilitation. This time could include access to specialist practitioners, for example the stoma care nurse and breast care nurse. This could also include psychologists and physiotherapists. Provision of information about support organisations and self-help groups can also be helpful for the patient and carers. There may also be separate carers' groups available. The adaptation to any change in body image will be influenced by a number of factors including gender, age, altered body image severity, pre- and post-operative preparation,

Link

Chapter 13 provides further information on bereavement.

including patient/client education, beliefs and values, coping mechanisms and sexual functioning. Anyone in a position of caring will be observed by the patient for their reactions and acceptance to the change in body image (Salter, 1997). The qualities and skills of the nurse will help the patient adjust and find their own way of coming to terms with the alteration to their body image. The nurse must not underestimate the challenge this brings to the patient. The nurse must value and respect this process of adjustment. In turn, the nurse has a responsibility to ensure that she or he is able to work with the patient in a meaningful way on both a physical and psychological level. Insight into her or his own emotions about her or his body may help when trying to understand the distress the patient may be experiencing when they have to face a radical alteration to their appearance and body function (Price, 1998). To ensure this, she or he should access regular clinical supervision with someone who is able to help her make sense of the caring relationship she has formed.

> **Link**
>
> Chapter 2 looks at therapeutic communication and working in groups.

Casebox 15.1

Sally is a 24-year-old married mother of two young children, who was admitted to an acute mental health unit for treatment of her depression. She has been resident on the unit for three weeks. She has been treated with anti-depressants and has attended counselling sessions with her care coordinator. Sally is being prepared for discharge home to her supportive family and will receive regular visits from a community psychiatric nurse. Sally has stated to her care coordinator that she is worried about sleeping with her husband in case he wants to be intimate with her. She also stated that she does not feel very attractive and believes that she is 'right off sex'.

What could be the main reasons for Sally feeling this way?

- Any long stay in hospital can influence how someone feels about themselves. Not being able to attend to our 'body presentation' in our normal way could mean that we become dissatisfied with the way we look as the gap between body presentation and body ideal widens.

- The antidepressants that Sally has been prescribed could affect her sexual functioning and libido. She may have become more aware of this as the depressants start to work and she begins to focus her attention on being back at home.

- Sally's body weight and appearance may have changed during the period of time she has felt depressed. This could affect how she perceives and feels about her body.

Casebox 15.2

Janice is a 38-year-old woman who has been living with her partner, Lisa for 11 years. Janice has been diagnosed with Crohn's disease after suffering with chronic diarrhoea, abdominal pain and weight loss for nearly a year and a number of admissions to hospital. She has been taking medication to treat the diarrhoea and analgesics to reduce the pain. Her physician has informed her that she has a partial obstruction of her small bowel. He has referred her to a surgeon who has informed her that surgery may be necessary to remove the obstruction. Janice was also told that she will require a temporary stoma. Janice is devastated and has asked if she can discuss this with Lisa before she agrees to surgery.

List some of the concerns that Janice may have concerning the formation of a stoma.

- How the stoma will look. How it will function. How she will manage the appliance. How it will affect her everyday life. How to broach the subject with Lisa and the effect this will have on their relationship. One of Janice's worries could be whether she may require a permanent stoma in the future. Janice will also be working out how to cope with social situations and any other activities that could involve others becoming aware of her stoma.

Human Sexuality

✵ Activity 15.6

If you had to choose just one sexual behaviour that you would want entirely forbidden, what would it be? Ask a few other people what they would forbid, then ask yourselves, why? What is so bad about these examples of sexual behaviour? The reasons are usually complicated!

Sexuality is an issue that health professionals are often uncomfortable with, although it is part of everyday life. For various reasons, individuals who cope reasonably well with the uncertainties of sexuality in their own lives find this more difficult when in a professional role. In this section we will be looking at why sexuality can create difficulties generally, and can be even more complex in the context of health care. The most common responses to the challenges of understanding human sexuality are either to ignore it and hope it goes away, or to make some hard and fast rules in an attempt to make it easier for everyone. Neither of these approaches has proved to work particularly well in the past, and so we will be advocating a different way. This is to accept the intricacies and paradoxes of human sexuality, try to understand them, and work with them.

Dos and don'ts

✵ Activity 15.7

Think about how important sexuality is to you – your gender, your sexual orientation, fancying people, being fancied, being a parent, dreading being a parent, your body and how it feels, your wardrobe, your haircut ... the list is endless. Now think about services you have participated in, and service users you have worked with. Is any of this richness expressed in what is written or said about them, the buildings the services are provided in, the materials promoting the service? Do the services have specific policies or guidelines to help workers deal with sexuality issues?

Sex and sexuality are fundamental to what humans are, so if nurses ignore this part of people's lives, they are missing a large chunk of the whole person. It is also potentially harmful to the person not to have their sexuality acknowledged. Michel Foucault, a French philosopher, has written extensively about sexuality, and talks about the 'triple edict of taboo, nonexistence and silence' surrounding sexuality (Foucault, 1978, p. 5). What does he mean by this? By using the word 'taboo' he is referring to the largely unwritten rules on sexual behaviour, the beliefs and myths that have developed over time. These appear to be real, but a closer examination reveals that humans have created these systems to guide their behaviour. We will be exploring the derivations of some 'common sense truths' in the history of sexuality section further on in this chapter. Try Activity 15.6.

'Nonexistence' is Foucault's way of expressing one of the ways that sexuality is dealt with, that is, by totally denying its existence, by repressing any mention of sex and sexuality. Many health-care practices appear to be attempting to do this, and it was only relatively recently in Western societies that this approach has reduced. Foucault's mention of silence is linked to the idea of non-existence, but conveys subtle differences. Silence conveys a notion that sex and sexuality exist, but are not to be talked about, just accepted as given, suffered in silence. To get a better idea of these concepts, try Activity 15.7.

The skill of the nurse in dealing with sexuality is to balance the biomedical realities of sexual function, sexual health and the reproductive process with what sexuality means to the individual person. This personal meaning is to do with the sorts of issues we looked at in Activity 15.2. It has to do with the way a person was brought up, current thinking in society in general, their race, culture or religion. The Nursing and Midwifery Council (NMC) makes it plain in the Code (2008), and the competencies required to register as a nurse (NMC, 2004), that nurses must respect each individual's point of view. It is also a requirement that the individual's views be actively included in care planning.

The nurse's role

The ways in which nurses will encounter sexuality could be divided into two. The first is where a patient/client's condition is likely to have a direct and obvious effect on their sexual functioning and sexuality. Examples might be a young woman having a hysterectomy, a man having prostate surgery that may lead to impotence, and a girl with extensive burns to body and face. More positive examples could be orthodontic treatment, cosmetic plastic surgery and IVF. To take this thinking further, spend a little time considering Activity 15.8. (It is interesting to note that many of the examples of health interventions that 'obviously' relate to sexuality are also linked to the person's body image.)

A second way that nurses encounter sexuality is in the sense that everyone has one! Many writers believe that sexuality is a fundamental component of the person, that you are not you without it. Nurses routinely have access to people's most intimate details, but are open to criticism for often ignoring this crucial component of any individual's life. This is an appropriate moment to make it clear that we are not advocating prying unnecessarily into an individual's private life. It is rarely necessary for a nurse to know any details of a patient/client's sexual functioning and relationships. However, we are advocating that nurses should be sensitive to this crucial aspect of their patient/client's lives, and that they should be confident and competent in discussing sexual issues if they arise.

✳ Activity 15.8

Divide a piece of paper into two columns, labelling one column 'Health interventions with a negative impact on sex and sexuality' and the other 'Health interventions with a positive impact on sex and sexuality'. Carrying on from the examples given in the text, write as many examples as you can think of under each heading. Having done this relatively quickly, reconsider the interventions you have chosen. Are they as clearly good or bad as you first thought? For example, IVF is a positive intervention to help couples achieve their need to have children. However, the difficulties that couples having infertility treatment can experience are well known, to the extent that they appear regularly in television documentaries, popular novels and dramas.

Casebox 15.3

Rob is 33 years old and has a learning disability. Until recently he lived in his family home, but chose to move to a housing association flat to live on his own. He visits his local health centre regularly for a minor health problem, and the nurses have got to know him quite well. Rob has started talking to the health centre nurses about how he would like to have a girlfriend, but is starting to feel down because he is still on his own.

Sant Angelo (2000) suggests some likely features of the lives of people with learning difficulties that may well apply to some degree to Rob:

- High incidence of sexually abusive experiences
- Multiple experiences of bereavement and loss
- Difficulties in talking about emotions
- Limited sex education
- Limited expectations and low self-esteem
- A lack of assertiveness about sex and relationships
- A lack of privacy

What simple interventions could be made with Rob to empower him to achieve his desired lifestyle?

- Rob could be encouraged to talk about his feelings. If Rob's needs were simple advice and education, the health centre nurses could perhaps provide this intervention. If Rob's needs went beyond this, he could be offered access to other services, for example, self-help groups run by people with learning disabilities, learning disability community nursing, a range of independent and voluntary services to do with increasing his social network, counselling or other services as appropriate. Most importantly, Rob needs to be listened to with respect and sensitivity, so that he can find the best way to achieve his goals.

Sexuality and self-awareness

✴ Activity 15.9

Consider the following ideas, where do you think they originate from? We are not suggesting that any of them are either right or wrong, but you may find yourself agreeing or disagreeing. Asking yourself 'why?' is working towards self-awareness.
- Gay and lesbian individuals should have freedom of sexual expression.
- Anal sex is unnatural.
- Women are passive receivers of male sexual advances.

Self-awareness is an important attribute for nurses generally, but is perhaps especially so in the case of sexuality, given its possible sensitivity. It is perfectly acceptable for nurses to have strong views on issues to do with sexuality, but potentially harmful to blindly impose them on patients/clients. Being a nurse does not mean having to subscribe to a particular set of beliefs about sex and sexuality. However, it does mean appreciating that there are many viewpoints, yours being simply another version. It is an essential skill to know what your standpoint is, and how that relates to other people. Whatever our views are, they did not come out of nowhere. It can be helpful to our understanding to know where our beliefs originated from, giving us a chance to look at them a bit more closely. Two important issues within sexuality are gender and sexual orientation, which will be explored next. Gender and sexual orientation have both been hugely influenced by ancient cultural, historical, political and religious viewpoints. As a result, views vary widely and can be hotly contested. Before reading the following sections spend some time on Activity 15.9; it should make the material more relevant.

Gender

✴ Activity 15.10

Read round some aspect of the history of sexuality that particularly interests you, using sources such as Nye (1999), Johnson and Ryan (2004), and Stearns (2009).

gender

a social group's interpretation of being a man or a woman. It concerns the status and role of the sexes rather than their physical characteristics

✴ Activity 15.11

Read Chapter 1 in Corrêa et al. (2008) and Chapter 1 in Miers (2000).

Gender is a crucial issue in health care and nursing, going way beyond the physical characteristics of being male or female. The study of gender is the study of how being a man or a woman has an impact on how much money you have, how well educated you are, what diseases you are most likely to have, your life expectancy, your mental health, diet and weight. The literature on gender needs to be studied in its own right (see Activity 15.11, for example) to do it justice. However, nurses can learn from the major finding of the social science of gender. This finding is that gender operates through members of a society learning to make assumptions about the roles and capabilities of the sexes. Most societies are heavily biased to the advantage of men, so the widely held assumptions about women tend to discriminate against them; for example, men are physically and mentally stronger than women, women gossip and men think deep thoughts and so on.

Nurses can contribute towards reducing health inequalities based on gender by challenging the unsupported (and often false) assumptions about the differences between men and women. Study of the historical development of sexuality reveals that women have been regarded as inferior to men since prehistoric times. Records from the ancient civilisations of Egypt, Greece and Rome make it clear that what we now regard as sexism or patriarchy have been considered the norm for many thousands of years (Stearns, 2009). As a result, the principle that men and women are equal is a relatively new one, and still has some way to go before being universally accepted. Nurses can also help by acknowledging that men and women are equal, but often have different attitudes and approaches to health, this acknowledgement being called gender sensitivity (Corrêa et al., 2008).

Casebox 15.4

You are working with a school nurse in a secondary school, and have become involved in the sexual health component of the curriculum. This involves planning and running a series of sessions about sexual behaviour to a group of 12-year-old boys and girls.

- Should boys and girls be taught separately?
- Do boys and girls need to be taught different things?
- Could stereotyped gender differences be avoided?

Sexual Orientation

There is now an enormous amount of material available to explore what is known about sexual orientation, in academic literature, books, films, television, newspapers, magazines and so on. Despite this, gay and lesbian individuals can still experience discrimination in society in general, and health services in particular (Teunis & Herdt, 2007). In recognition of this, the Royal College of Nursing (RCN, 2005) issued a statement guiding nurses in how to combat discriminatory practice, and make positive health contributions to lesbians and gay men. Recent changes in the law have made the legal position of gay and lesbian couples clearer. Couples registering under the Civil Partnership Act 2004 will have a legal status that has parity with married couples, including inheriting property after death. The main difficulties experienced by individuals with alternative sexual lifestyles seem to come from a combination of factors, but you may find it useful to ask yourself these questions:

1   Do I know much about gay, lesbian, transvestite, transsexual, transgender and other lifestyles?
2   Do I really know how I feel about people who have different sexualities to mine?

Your personal answers to these questions really indicate the way to competent and effective nursing practice with people who have alternative sexualities. Make it your business to find out more about the richness and diversity of our sexual lives, and find out if you have some unsupported prejudices that influence your behaviour without you really being aware of it. It is worth noting that attitudes towards homosexual behaviour are very different depending on the culture and the period of history being considered. Ancient Jewish law prohibited sexual contact between men absolutely, whereas ancient Greek civilisations considered love between men as on a higher spiritual plane than heterosexual love (Stearns, 2009). Within the Christian tradition, it was only really in the Middle Ages that the Catholic Church firmly established homosexuality as wrong, while the Eastern Orthodox Churches remained more flexible. The wide range of approaches to being gay or lesbian is further demonstrated by the fact that homosexuality is actually punishable by death in some parts of our world, and yet is totally ignored in others, demonstrating how widely opinion differs. Before getting too complacent, remember that within the last two hundred years, Britain also had the death penalty for homosexuality.

Activity 15.12

Read Chapter 6 of Denman (2004).

This may be starting to feel a bit deep and difficult, so an example of nursing practice told to one of the authors may make the point clearer, see Casebox 15.5.

Casebox 15.5

Dawn has been admitted to a medical ward for some straightforward treatment. Many of the staff were cold and remote towards her because she was a lesbian. Dawn herself did not say much, and was quite bad-tempered in her interactions with all health-care staff. Lucy, one of the nurses noticed this, and found it upsetting, though could not think of a specific intervention that would help. On one occasion, Lucy saw Dawn's partner Julie, walking across the hospital car park. Lucy turned to Dawn, smiled, and said 'Hey, Dawn, that's great, your partner Julie is coming to visit you!' Dawn's demeanour immediately softened, and she started to chat about her and Julie's home life together. From then on, Dawn would talk freely to Lucy, and was more relaxed. The nursing care that Dawn received was more effective, and her treatment was successful.

Why do you think Lucy's simple intervention made such a difference?
Have you had, or heard of, similar experiences?

Desire

Casebox 15.5 demonstrates that being aware of sexuality in your practice does not require superhuman interpersonal skills or encyclopaedic knowledge! It is mainly about listening, observing, and showing some sensitivity to different views. One way of viewing alternative sexualities is to think of all sexuality in terms of desire. Some men like tall women with brown hair who want a family. Some women like men who are reliable and have steady jobs. As far as we know, there are no specific labels for these desires, and the people who practise them are left to do so without interference. However, a man who likes men with brown hair who want a family, and a woman who likes reliable women with steady jobs may well experience interference! We all have preferences in terms of what kind of people and activities arouse us sexually. Use Activity 15.13 to think about your own desires.

It is difficult to avoid the conclusion that society chooses what is acceptable sexual behaviour, but often not clearly, and often based on outdated and unacceptable prejudices. Some of the restrictions are clearly to our benefit, for example laws against rape and sex with children. Others are more difficult to justify outside artificial and misguided belief systems.

✷ Activity 15.13

Describe your ideal partner(s), preferably by writing it down, though imagining will work too.
What do they look like, what are they wearing, what are they interested in, how do they treat you? How would the relationship run: a quick fling, living together, big white wedding, eloping to an exotic destination? Would there be children?

Now think about this ideal scenario you have created. Does it have a specific label that conjures up your desire in complete detail?

Working with vulnerable adults

One area where the sorts of restrictions on sexual behaviour talked about above are justifiable is in the care of vulnerable adults. Just as awareness of the abuse of children grew over a period of time, so it is becoming known that some adults are at greater risk of being abused. This abuse can be sexual, but can take other forms: physical, financial, psychological, neglect, or discriminatory abuse (Penhale and Parker, 2008). Defining who is a vulnerable adult is not precise, but generally a vulnerable adult can be regarded as a person over the age of eighteen who uses community care services, and finds it more difficult than most to protect themselves from harm. This may include some older people, people with learning disabilities, disabled people, and people with mental health problems.

In practice, nurses need to be aware of the potential sexual harm that could befall vulnerable adults. The document *No Secrets* (DoH, 2000) gives guidance on preventing, awareness, and dealing with the abuse of vulnerable adults. Some findings from learning disability research give an idea of the nature of the problem. McCormack et al. (2005) surveyed 15 years of allegations of sexual abuse of people with learning disabilities, finding that just under half were confirmed. Of these, the most common location was the family home, where almost a quarter of the perpetrators of sexual abuse were family members. Most of the abuse was sexual touch, although nearly a third was penetration or attempted penetration. Joyce (2003) conducted a similar survey in a different locality, finding that people with learning disabilities were most at risk from the people they lived with, the people who cared for them, or their family members. Not being taken seriously when reporting sexual abuse was also a feature. To compound the problem, Murphy (2003) found that the sexual knowledge of adults with learning disabilities was significantly lower than non-disabled adolescents, leaving them open to harm through lack of knowledge of acceptable sexual behaviour.

This small selection of the available evidence indicates why nurses have to be vigilant when working with vulnerable adults. Clearly such abuse occurs in a minority of cases, but often enough for nurses to at least be aware of the possibility.

Sexuality and Skilled Care Giving

Even a cursory exploration quickly reveals the complexity, richness and changeability of human sexuality. Further examination demonstrates that if nursing is to take a holistic approach, it can no longer routinely ignore this aspect of human life. But the depth and diversity of human sexuality can make it seem unmanageable at times. A well-known framework that attempts to make sexuality issues more manageable for nurses is the **PLISSIT model** (Fogel and Lauver, 1990). The PLISSIT model categorises a nurse's potential interventions into four levels, each level becoming increasingly intimate and needing more specialist knowledge. The idea behind the model is that all nurses can include sexuality in their practice, but should operate at a level where they feel safe and well informed. The four levels are:

PLISSIT model
a model comprising four levels of nursing intervention to take sexuality and body image into account

- *Permission*: it is suggested that sexual history should be a routine part of assessment. This will raise sexuality as a legitimate concern, and gives patients permission to ask questions about it in their own care. Although this is the most basic level, success is dependent on a non-judgemental accepting approach by nurses.
- *Limited Information*: misconceptions and myths are clarified. Many of the difficulties experienced by people in dealing with their sexuality can be solved quickly, by good quality, evidence-based information. To be told that many people have similar difficulties, and a few simple solutions, can be very liberating, and take very little time. All the nurse needs is a sound (but

not necessarily encyclopaedic) knowledge base, and a straightforward, adult communication style.

- *Specific Suggestions*: can relieve anxiety, promote creativity, and help individuals solve their own problems in partnerships, rather than being the passive receivers of advice.
- *Intensive Therapy*: the person is referred to a specialist sex therapist, who may also be a nurse. It is important if nurses are to make competent interventions that they be clear about the limitations of their knowledge and skill. In some cases, solutions may not be simple, and so expert intervention is needed.

The RCN's (2000) guidance on sexuality promotes the use of the PLISSIT model in nursing practice, and adds further useful advice, such as to ensure privacy and consent to sexual practices. The guidance also encourages nurses to empower patients to develop their sexual identity, and to be careful not to impose their own assumptions on them. Among an extensive collection of useful ideas, the RCN guidance reminds us to respect people's cultural backgrounds, and to be aware that sexuality is still subject to stigma and taboo, as we have discussed earlier in this chapter.

Modernisation of services and sexuality in nursing

The PLISSIT model is a useful tool, and goes a long way to guide nurses to give sexuality much needed importance in nursing practice. The model can potentially relieve anxiety among nurses who are so concerned about not being 'experts' that they ignore sexuality issues altogether. However, it is important to build on the helpful principles established in the PLISSIT model, and take them further by putting them in the context of current and future health care trends.

At the same time, at a national, more structural level, government policy for health-care services is relevant to our discussion. It is clearly the intention that health services in the future will be driven by the people who use them. Lord Darzi's vision for the future National Health Service (NHS) emphasises holistic care, listening to patients, respecting their dignity, and including them in their own health care (Darzi, 2008). Darzi's *High Quality Care for All* report aims to reduce health inequalities, prevent discrimination, help individuals to know more about, and take responsibility for, their own health. All these aims are partly fulfilled by nurses taking account of body image and sexuality, which can have impacts far beyond more obvious biomedical concerns.

As we have seen, sexuality can be about people in different groups having different amounts of power: adults and children, men and women, heterosexual and homosexual. Sometimes these differences in power can lead to abuse, perhaps linked to a powerful person or group not being willing to accept views other than their own. So nurses do need to be sensitive to each individual's notion of body image and sexuality in their face-to-face interactions, as demonstrated in the PLISSIT model, but the broader picture needs to be taken into account, if our care is to be truly holistic.

Chapter Summary

To conclude the chapter, we need to bring body image and sexuality back together again. We examined them separately to make the material easier to absorb, but in our daily lives they are inextricably linked. If we consider our bodies and health, either to celebrate our good fortune, or bemoan an unkind fate, some part of that consideration is to do with sexuality. This could encompass our gender, our sexual orientation, whether we think others will find us attractive, cultural influences, or the physical ways in which we express our sexual selves. This process accelerates considerably when perceptions of our bodies change, as is nearly always the case when we access health services. So, to practise holistic care, nurses need to be aware of body image and sexuality and how they are linked. These links take many forms, but we propose a four-factor analysis that takes account of the complexity of human life, and provides a framework for nurses and other professionals involved in caring.

1   *Intimacy*: nursing can be extraordinarily intimate at times, so to be unaware of the range of potential impacts on a person is unsafe.

2   *Anti-discriminatory practice (ADP)*: without discrimination, body image and sexuality would cease to cause challenges and difficulties in individuals' lives. It is only because humans choose to make judgements about each other, based on particular characteristics, that we might be concerned about how we look, or how we express ourselves sexually. ADP appears regularly in the competencies required for nurses (NMC, 2008), and is an especially important way of working in terms of body image and sexuality. Practising in an anti-discriminatory way means acknowledging the sources of oppression in people's lives, but also actively working towards reducing them (Thompson, 2006). So, you may be accepting of a person who is gay, but you may also have to work to make sure that your colleagues are as accepting as you are.

3   *Empowerment*: this can be an elusive concept (see Thompson, 2007, for a readable overview), but put simply, means focusing your work on enabling the individuals you work with to find their own solutions, and progress independently. Health-care professionals have traditionally had tremendous power over individuals, with a great unwillingness to share it! There is no place for this approach in modern health services; individuals need to regard themselves as having a large say in their own destiny. The issues surrounding body image and sexuality are often related to personal power, so nurses can make a positive contribution by understanding how much power they themselves hold through often being perceived as 'experts'. Patients undoubtedly need us to have expertise, but can do without experts. Also, by practising in an empowering way, nurses can actively demonstrate how power can be shared successfully with patients and include other professionals in providing the best possible care and treatment.

4   *Partnership*: empowerment does not imply that nurses should not actively help individuals. Rather, it means that the care given is within a particular

type of relationship – a partnership. Working in partnership with patients prevents them from relying too much on professionals and services, in other words, from becoming dependent.

This framework applies strongly in nursing practice to do with body image and sexuality. Dealing with these issues may well leave people feeling vulnerable and distressed, for example when facing mastectomy, use of a stoma, disfigurement, and many more. Running the practitioner-patient relationship as a partnership in these high emotion circumstances has several benefits for both parties. Partnership means that a nurse can retain qualities such as warmth and genuineness that are so important, but because they are not 'leading' the process, dependence is avoided. This makes practice safer professionally for nurses, and also for the patient/client, who needs to be able to deal with the world in their own right. You will not always be around, so it is much better for the patient/client to learn to use their existing support networks (family, friends etc.) or be helped to find new ones (specialist support groups, voluntary services and so on).

It would be misleading to suggest that dealing with body image and sexuality issues is always easy. However, a little knowledge and a lot of openness, acceptance and willingness to talk will form a strong foundation for competent practice.

☐ Test yourself!

1   Using your own words describe what is meant by the term 'body image'.

2   What are the three fundamental interrelated concepts used by Price (1990) to define body image?

3   Give five examples of surgical procedures not evident to others (concealed) that could affect body image.

4   Name some factors that may affect the sexual experiences of people with learning disabilities.

5   What does PLISSIT stand for?

6   What are the four principles suggested as a framework for practice in body image and sexuality issues?

Balen, R. and Crawshaw, M. (eds) (2006) *Sexuality and Fertility Issues in Health and Disability: From Adolescence to Adulthood*. Jessica Kingsley, London.

Body Image: An International Journal of Research (first published in 2004).

Bolin, A. and Whelehan, P. (2009) *Human Sexuality: Biological, Psychological and Cultural Understandings*. Routledge, London.

Carlowe, J. (1997) Face values. *Nursing Times* **93**(42): 34–5.

Grogan, S. (2007) *Body Image: Understanding Body Dissatisfaction in Men, Women and Children*, 2nd edn. Routledge, London.

Johansson, T. (2007) *Transformation of Sexuality: Gender and Identity in Contemporary Youth Culture*. Ashgate, Farnham.

Mottier, V. (2008) *Sexuality: A Very Short Introduction*. Oxford University Press, Oxford.

Walker-Hirsch, L. (ed) (2007) *The Facts of Life...and More: Sexuality and Intimacy for People with Intellectual Disability*. Paul H. Brookes, Baltimore.

Further Reading

For live links to useful websites see: www.palgrave.com/nursinghealth/hogston

References

Bell, N. (1989) Sexuality and the ostomist. *Nursing Times* **85**(5): 28–30.

Blackmore, C. (1989) Altered images. *Nursing Times* **85**(12): 36–9.

Chilton, S. (1984) Identity crisis. *Nursing Mirror* **158** (13 June): ii–iii.

Corrêa, S., Petchesky, R. and Parker, R. (2008) *Sexuality, Health and Human Rights*. Routledge, Abingdon.

Darzi, Lord (2008) *High Quality Care for All: NHS Next Stage Review Final Report*. Department of Health, London.

de Marquiegui, A. and Huish, M. (1999) A woman's sexual life after an operation. *British Medical Journal* **318**: 178–81.

Denman, C. (2004) *Sexuality: A Biopsychosocial Approach*. PalgraveMacmillan, Basingstoke.

DoH (Department of Health) (2000) *No Secrets*. Department of Health, London.

Fogel, C. and Lauver, D. (1990) *Sexual Health Promotion*. WB Saunders, Philadelphia.

Foucault, M. (1978) *The History of Sexuality: Volume 1, An Introduction*. Penguin, Harmondsworth.

Goffman, E. (1961) *Asylums: Essays on the Social Situation of Mental Patients and Other Inmates*. Anchor, New York.

Johnson, M. and Ryan, T. (2004) *Sexuality in Greek and Roman Literature and Society: A Sourcebook*. Routledge, London.

Joyce, T.A. (2003) An audit of investigations into allegations of abuse involving adults with intellectual disability. *Journal of Intellectual Disability Research* **47**(8): 606–16.

Kent, G. and Thompson, A. (2002) The development and maintenance of shame in disfigurement: implications for treatment. In Gilbert, P. and Miles, J. (eds) *Body Shame* Brunner-Routledge, Hove.

Kitzinger, S. (1985) *Woman's Experience of Sex*. Penguin Books. London.

Koo, J. and Young, J. (2002) Body image issues in dermatology. In Cash, T.F. and Pruzinsky, T. (eds) *Body Image: A Handbook of Theory, Research and Clinical Practice*. Guildford Press, New York.

Langford, R. (1996) The hole truth. *Nursing Times* **92**(40): 46–7.

Larkin, B.G. (2004) The ins and outs of body piercing. *The Association of Perioperative Registered Nurses* **79**(2): 3330–46. http://gateway.uk.ovid/gw1/ovidweb.cgi (accessed 6 May 2005).

Maltby, J., Houran, J., Ashe, D., and McCutcheon, L.E. (2001). The self-reported psychological well-being of celebrity worshippers. *North American Journal of Psychology* **3**: 441–52.

Maltby, J., Day, L., McCutcheon, L.E., Gillett, R., Houran, J. and Ashe, D. (2004). Celebrity worship using an adaptational-continuum model of personality and coping. *British Journal of Psychology* **95**: 411–28.

Maltby, J., Giles, D., Barber, L. and McCutcheon, L.E. (2005). Intense-personal celebrity worship and body image: Evidence of a link among female adolescents. *British Journal of Health Psychology* **10**: 17–32.

McCormack, B., Kavanagh, D., Caffrey, S. and Power, A. (2005) Investigating sexual abuse: Findings of a 15-year longitudinal study. *Journal of Applied Research in Intellectual Disability* **18**: 217–27.

McCrea, C.W., Summerfield, A.B. and Rosen, B. (1982) Body image: a selective review of existing measurement techniques. *British Journal of Medical Psychology* **55**(3): 225–33.

Miers, M. (2000) *Gender Issues and Nursing Practice*. Macmillan, Basingstoke.

Murphy, G.H. (2003) Capacity to consent to sexual relationships in adults with learning disabilities. *Journal of Family Planning and Reproductive Health Care* **29**(3): 148–9.

NMC (2004) *Standards of Proficiency for Pre-registration Nursing Education*. NMC, London.

NMC (2008) *The Code: Standards of Conduct, Performance and Ethics for Nurses and Midwives*. NMC, London.

Nye, R.A. (ed.) (1999) *Sexuality*. Oxford University Press, Oxford.

Penhale, B. and Parker, J. (2008) *Working with Vulnerable Adults*. Routledge, London.

Price, B. (1990) *Body Image: Nursing Concepts and Care*. Price Hall, London.

Price, B. (1995) Assessing altered body image. *Journal of Psychiatric and Mental Health Nursing* **2**(3): 169–75

Price, B. (1998) Cancer: altered body image. *Nursing Standard* **12**(21): 49–55.

RCN (Royal College of Nursing) (2000) *Sexuality and Sexual Health in Nursing Practice*. RCN, London.

RCN (Royal College of Nursing) (2005) *Not 'Just' a Friend: Best Practice Guidance on Health Care for Lesbian, Gay and Bisexual Service Users and their Families*. www.rn.org.uk/london/downloads/notjustafriend.pdf

Robinson, E. (1997) Psychological research on visible difference disfigurement. In Lansdown, R., Rumsey, N., Bradbury, E., Carr, A. and Partridge, J. (eds) *Visibly Different: Coping with Disfigurement*. Butterworth-Heinemann, London.

Rumsey, N. (2002) Body image and congenital conditions with viable differences. In Cash, T.F. and Pruzinsky, T. (eds) *Body Image: A Handbook of Theory, Research and Clinical Practice*. Guildford Press, New York.

Rumsey, N., Clarke, A., White, P., Wyn-Williams, M. and Garlick, W. (2004) Altered body image: appearance-related concerns of people with visible disfigurement. *Journal of Advanced Nursing* **48**(5): 443–53.

Salter, M. (1997) *Altered Body Image: The Nurse's Role*. Bailliere Tindall, London.

Sanderson, E. (1985) Nursing patience. *Lampada* **4**: 36–7.

Sant Angelo, D. (2000) Learning disability community nursing: Addressing emotional and sexual needs. In Astor, R. and Jeffereys, K. (eds) *Positive Initiatives for People with Learning Difficulties: Promoting Healthy Lifestyles*. Macmillan, Basingstoke.

Savage, J. (1987) *Nurses, Gender and Sexuality*. Heinemann, London.

Stearns, P.N. (2009) *Sexuality in World History*. Routledge, Abingdon.

Sundeen, J., Stuart, G.W., Rankin, E.A.D. and Cohen, S.A. (1994) *Nurse-Client Interaction*. Mosby, St Louis.

Teunis, N. and Herdt, G. (Eds)(2007) *Sexual Inequalities and Social Justice*. University of California Press, London.

Thompson, N. (2006) *Anti Discriminatory Practice*, 4th edn. Palgrave Macmillan, Basingstoke.

Thompson, N. (2007) *Power and Empowerment*. Russell House Publishing, Lyme Regis.

Watson, J. (1980) Altered body image and the self. In Brown, M.S. (ed.) *Nursing and the Concept of Loss*. Wiley, New York.

Chapter

Genetics Knowledge within an Ethical Framework

16

📖 Contents

- Introduction
- An Ethical Framework
- The Human Genome
- Genetic Inheritance
- The Impact of Genotypes in Health Care

- Chapter Summary
- Test Yourself!
- Further Reading
- References

☑ Learning outcomes

The purpose of this chapter is to enhance your understanding of 'genetics' and 'genomics' and to consider the development of genetic knowledge within an ethical framework in relation to the health-care agenda. At the end of this chapter, you should be able to:

- Outline an ethical framework in which to consider the developing genetic knowledge
- Describe some of the issues of the 'human genome' within the health-care system
- Describe the basic structure and function of chromosomes and genes
- Describe the processes of mitosis and meiosis
- Differentiate between genotype and phenotype
- Describe some of the common chromosomal abnormalities
- Utilise a Punnett square to describe patterns of inheritance: dominant, recessive and X-linked.

There are also activities for you to consider and to undertake, and review questions so that you can test yourself.

Introduction

The developments from the human genome project in 2003 have opened up the world of genetics-based health care. It has been recognised by the Department of Health (DoH) that these advances in human genetics will have a profound impact on the health care of present and future generations, not only for people with single-gene conditions such as cystic fibrosis (CF), haemophilia and Huntington's disease, but for common diseases such as heart disease, diabetes, asthma, cancers and mental health conditions (DoH, 2003, p. 5).

To understand the impact on health and ill-health depends upon the knowledge and understanding of some of these genetic developments and this chapter will explore issues such as aspects of inheritance of characteristics and genetic disorders, and the role of genetics and **genomics** in common diseases. Also these genetic developments highlight other ethical issues, such as how genetic information is collected from individuals and then used, and how it is stored so as to preserve the principles of consent and confidentiality.

genomics
this has been described as studying the interaction of all genes with each other and with the environment (National Human Genome Research Institute, 2006).

Developments from the DoH White Paper (2003) have included a competence-based genetics education framework for health-care practitioners. This framework outlines seven competency standard statements for practitioners to achieve at the point of professional registration (Kirk et al., 2003), with each competency standard being underpinned by theoretical and practice indicators. These will enable educational initiatives to consider genetic knowledge (scientific and technical) and the applied human genetics.

From the development of this competence-based genetics education framework (Kirk et al., 2003), further competencies have been developed for all staff (NHS National Genetics Education and Development Centre and Skills for Health, 2007). This competency framework provides a pathway of activities, involving genetics knowledge, skills and attitudes which may be carried out by non-genetics health-care staff. The pathway takes the practitioner through; from identifying clinical practice and individuals where genetics is relevant, to recognising modes of inheritance, to undertaking genetic referrals and to communicating this genetic knowledge to diverse groups, such as other professionals and the general public. This development highlights not only the complexity of roles of all individual practitioners in the present and future genetics era, but the challenges faced by individuals working within an interprofessional context focused upon a constantly developing genetic knowledge base.

The 'standards of competence' set out by the Nursing and Midwifery Council (NMC, 2010) for students to achieve so as to be entered onto the professional register, state

> it requires practitioners to conduct themselves and practise within an ethical framework based fundamentally upon respect for the well-being of patients and clients (NMC, 2010)

These standards of competence must be achieved in the student's field of nursing practice for the part of the nursing register that they are to be entered upon

– adult nursing, mental health nursing, learning disabilities nursing or children's nursing.

A broad concept of 'genetic solidarity and altruism' has been set out (DoH, 2002a), with 'respect for persons' being fundamental within this concept. Four ethical principles underpin this respect for persons: privacy, consent, confidentiality, and non-discrimination (DoH, 2002a). Beauchamp and Childress (2001) advocate that these ethical principles are fundamental to the practitioner-patient relationship. The upholding of these principles pose challenges for practitioners when working with some patient/client groups, such as children and young people, vulnerable adults such as the unconscious person, the person with altered levels of mental capacity, either of a temporary or permanent nature, or the person with a deteriorating condition.

The chapter will explore issues regarding personal genetic information such as consent, confidentiality and protection. The Department of Health has explained this genetic information as

> any information about the genetic make-up of an identifiable person, whether directly from **DNA** (or other biochemical) testing or indirectly from any other source (including the details of a person's family history) (DoH, 2002a, p. 27)

DNA
deoxyribonucleic acid – the double-stranded helix molecule that encodes the genetic information (see Figure 16.3 later in this chapter)

An Ethical Framework

Ethical values or principles influence and guide our thinking, the way we act and as health-care practitioners influence our practice. Four principles have been identified as essential within an ethical framework, when considering health-care practice (Bradley, 2005):

- *Autonomy*: the right of a person to make their own decisions and direct their life
- *Beneficence*: the responsibility of doing good, so providing benefit or beneficial treatment/care to the person
- *Non-maleficence*: the responsibility of avoiding harm to the person
- *Justice*: the responsibility to be equitable and fair in the way we treat others.

Furthermore, the principles of privacy, consent, confidentiality and non-discrimination are intricately bound up with 'respect for persons and their autonomous rights'. A person must be able to fully understand and consider all the issues involved, have adequate information on which to base a decision and must be allowed to do this with no pressure or coercion. If we have respect for persons we must also respect their wishes and the decisions they make about themselves and their health-care choices.

There are challenges when considering autonomy in health-care practice, whereby some situations may restrict the degree of a person's autonomy or their ability to utilise it. Special consideration must be made with vulnerable people such as:

- people with sensory difficulties
- those for whom English is not their first language
- children with developing autonomous ability
- adults with a learning disability or an enduring mental health difficulty
- people with altered levels of ability due to injury or illness.

The issue of 'capacity or incapacity' appears to be the cornerstone of autonomous decision-making. DoH (2002a) highlights that any approach that reflects 'blanket incapacity', whereby a person is deemed to be incapable of any autonomous decision-making, should be rejected and that a preferred approach is to consider each individual decision to be made and then decide whether the person is capable of making that particular decision. It is clearly unacceptable to dismiss a person's decision-making ability without full consideration.

It is clear, therefore, that to uphold these principles, information must be provided to people in a clear, simple and understandable way, and in an objective and unbiased manner, whether written or spoken – provide it in a form that facilitates their understanding (NMC, 2010; Nuffield Council on Bioethics, 2006b). According to the Royal Society (RS), this requirement poses a challenge for health-care practitioners when it is recognised that the basic genetic education of practitioners is trailing behind genetic developments (scientific and technical) (RS, 2005a). It highlights that the role of practitioners, including nurses, will evolve further and this will have implications for basic and applied human genetics education (RS, 2005a).

It is clearly recognised (Kirk et al., 2003; DoH, 2005; RS, 2005a) that health-care practitioners require genetic knowledge so as to understand health and ill-health causation, genetic technologies, and associated management and treatment regimes. The competency-based genetics education framework provides a clear structure in which to set out appropriate knowledge and practice outcomes, so that practitioners can competently practice in whatever field of nursing or health-care setting. An NHS National Genetics Education and Development Centre (NGEDC) has been established by the Department of Health to take a central role in the coordination of educational initiatives, so as to facilitate developments regarding genetics in health-care practice.

Benjamin and Gamet (2005) highlight that not all nurses will require a high level of expertise, but that they will need to have a genetics knowledge base to be able to recognise clients who may benefit from a referral to genetic services. Kirk (2005) suggests that the level of knowledge and understanding required for best practice will partly depend upon the professional role and speciality of the practitioner.

This chapter therefore sets out to provide an overview of genetics so that practitioners can utilise this knowledge within health care when working in varied practice settings.

It is crucial that the utilisation of 'new genetics knowledge' needs to be firmly set within an ethical framework so that fundamental principles are upheld, for the sake of the individual, the practitioner and society (DoH, 2002a). The concept of 'genetic solidarity and altruism' has been proposed by the DoH (2002a), and it is suggested that in all situations of an ethical nature, this concept should be considered.

> The concept of genetic solidarity and altruism has been explained thus:
> we all share the same basic human genome, although there are individual variations which distinguish us from other people. Most of our genetic characteristics will be present in others. This sharing of our genetic constitution not only gives rise to opportunities to help others but it also highlights our common interest in the fruits of medically-based genetic research (DoH, 2002a, p. 38)

However, the DoH (2005) has reported that it does not want to perpetuate a view of **genetic determinism**, for example in the context of an individual's health and behaviour, and highlights that many of the causes of differences are social, economic and environmental factors as well as genetic ones. The risk of becoming more medicalised, due to the possibility of genetic profiling at birth, has been highlighted (DoH, 2005).

Principles for handling personal genetic information in a fair and ethical way are therefore set out by the DoH (2002a) within the concept of genetic solidarity and altruism. The principles of privacy, consent, confidentiality and non-discrimination are embedded within the overarching key concept of respect for persons. The DoH advocates that respect for persons recognises that individuals have the highest moral importance or value, and that this should be regarded as a core principle when considering the ethical use of genetic information.

> Respect for persons:
> affirms the equal value, dignity and moral rights of each individual. Each individual is entitled to lead a life in which genetic characteristics will not be the basis of unjust discrimination or unfair or inhuman treatment. (DoH, 2002a, p. 40)

However, the principle of respect for persons does require that we acknowledge the value and dignity of others and that we respect their autonomy. There have been concerns raised regarding genetic information, for example in the case of carrier status, where the risk of passing this onto children can cause worry and stigmatisation, and uncover risks for relatives that preferred not to know (DoH, 2003; Nuffield Council on Bioethics, 2006b). This type of knowledge can have a positive or negative impact on family dynamics. DoH (2005) highlights that some individuals are pleased to be forewarned about a condition so that they can make choices regarding lifestyle and health care, but also reports that others have expressed concern about knowing a genetic status, especially if there is nothing useful they can do.

It is not yet clear what benefits come from forewarning individuals about conditions such as cancers and heart disease, whether they are likely to change their lifestyle and take preventive measures, or whether they will adopt a fatalistic viewpoint and assume they will develop the condition anyway, regardless of any preventive measures. A key finding from a public dialogue was the view that genetic tests were viewed as 'empowering', particularly if lifestyle changes could

genetic determinism
people's health, behaviour, intelligence and so on are determined chiefly by their genes (DoH, 2005)

> ⊘ Link
>
> Chapters 13 and 15 deal with issues of respect.

be made or if drug treatments were available that would improve the prognosis (RS, 2005b). An important aspect of privacy is protecting individuals from being given information they do not want to know. Insistence on disclosure would disregard their autonomy and their entitlement not to know. This highlights the issue of disclosure or non-disclosure in the interest of the patient; however, it is recognised that situations may arise whereby disclosure of genetic information is in the interest of family members or the public (DoH, 2005; Nuffield Council on Bioethics, 2006b).

When considering an individual and their family's medical history, the consideration of genetic information can impact on family relationships, and may reveal unexpected information regarding parentage, such as with paternity testing (DoH, 2002a). Genetic testing for an individual may also reveal genetic information that has significance for other relatives, and this raises issues of consent from these individuals (RS, 2005b; Nuffield Council on Bioethics, 2006b) and their right to know this genetic information, which may have health and lifestyle implications for them. Within the complexity of this human context, the four ethical principles need to be fully considered:

- *Privacy*: every person is entitled to privacy. In the absence of justification based on overwhelming moral considerations, a person should generally not be obliged to disclose information about his or her genetic characteristics.
- *Consent*: private genetic information about a person should generally not be obtained, held or communicated without that person's free and informed consent.
- *Confidentiality*: private personal genetic information should generally be treated as being of a confidential nature and should not be communicated to others without consent except for the weightiest of reasons.
- *Non-discrimination*: no person shall be unfairly discriminated against on the basis of his or her genetic characteristics (DoH, 2002a, pp. 41–4).

Practitioners in health-care settings face demanding and complex situations where ethical principles may not provide a clear solution. However, they are required to work in such a professional manner that reflects an ethical framework and full consideration of accepted ethical principles, so that when decisions are made and acted upon, they are based upon these ethical principles and demonstrate clear decision-making.

The Human Genome

The concept of the human genome consists of two elements, the nuclear genome and the mitochondrial genome (a circular deoxyribonucleic acid (DNA) molecule inherited from the mother). For the purpose of this chapter, the nuclear genome is being considered. To understand genetic inheritance and disease, we must start by considering the structure and function of the **chromosomes** and genes, and explain the two forms of cell division – mitosis and meiosis.

∞ **Link**

Chapter 3 also discusses confidentiality, privacy and consent.

chromosomes
structures composed of DNA that are located within the nucleus of the cell

Chromosomes

The body has two differing groups of cells – somatic cells and **gametes** (sex cells). These sex cells are spermatozoa in males and oocytes in females. All the other cells of the body are called somatic cells. Chromosomes are structures located within the nucleus of cells, with humans having 23 pairs of chromosomes in the somatic cells, a total of 46, and only 23 chromosomes in the gametes.

Somatic cells are referred to as **diploid** – having pairs of chromosomes – and the gametes as **haploid** – only having one half of the chromosome pair.

Chromosomes are arranged in pairs according to their shape and size, with pairs 1 to 22 being called the **autosomes** and pair 23 called the sex chromosomes. These are described as X and Y chromosomes. A female has two X chromosomes, denoted as XX, and the male has one X and one Y chromosome, denoted as XY. Therefore, in humans the **karyotype** (chromosomal picture) shows a chromosomal count of 46, XX (female) or 46, XY (male) (Figure 16.1).

As the gametes are cells that have unpaired chromosomes, the oocyte will contain an X chromosome, while spermatozoa will contain an X or a Y chromosome. It is because of this that the gender of the offspring is determined by the father, with the inheritance of the X or the Y chromosome being from the father. Fertilisation, the fusion of the gametes, results in a single cell (the **zygote**), with a chromosomal count of 46, XX or 46, XY – the karyotype. Later in this chapter you will plot this process by the use of a Punnett square to demonstrate the inheritance of gender and recessive and dominant traits.

The resultant zygote receives one of each pair of chromosomes from each of the parents, so that when the 23 chromosomes in the mother's oocyte are combined with the 23 chromosomes in the father's spermatozoa, the result is a normal karyotype – with one set of chromosomes and therefore one set of genes from each parent.

gamete
a reproductive/sex cell with a haploid number of chromosomes

diploid
a cell with pairs of chromosomes

haploid
a cell having a single set of unpaired chromosomes

autosomes
chromosome pairs 1 to 22 of the total chromosome complement (karyotype)

karyotype
the chromosome complement of a cell or an individual. It denotes the number, size and shape of the chromosomes

zygote
the fertilised oocyte

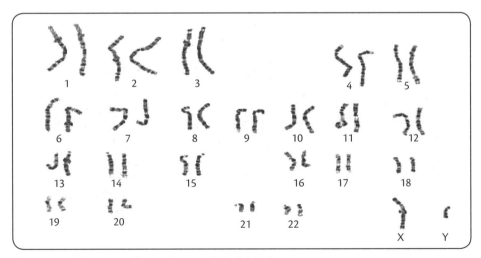

Figure 16.1 A karyotype illustrating a male individual

Chromosomal structure

chromatin

the part of the nucleus that consist of DNA and proteins and forms the chromosomes

interphase

the first stage of the life cycle of the cell during which replication of the chromosomes occurs

mitosis

process of cell division in the somatic cells

meiosis

process of cell division in the gametes

chromatid

the two arms of DNA material that are joined together at the centromere after replication

centromere

point at which the two chromatid arms are held together after replication

The substance called **chromatin** – sometimes referred to as a mass-like substance – is located within the cell structure. It is this chromatin that is seen during the **interphase** or resting stage. Interphase is the first stage of the life cycle of the cell and at this time the cell is undergoing its cellular functions – cell maintenance – by the instructions from its 'housekeeping genes'. During this stage, protein synthesis is also occurring by the processes of transcription and translation, whereby DNA templates are translated from nucleic acid into amino acids for protein production. It is referred to as a 'resting' stage, as it is resting before its cell division stage – **mitosis** or **meiosis**. However, it is important to note that it is during interphase that replication of the DNA structure occurs. This is outlined later in this chapter.

During early cell division (mitosis or meiosis), the chromatin has coiled and forms the structures called chromosomes. At this stage of the cell's life cycle, each chromosome consists of two **chromatids** (arms), joined together by a structure called the **centromere**. These arms are described as short or long, with the short arms being referred to as the p arms and the long arms as the q arms (Figure 16.2). Now do Activity 16.1.

Having done Activity 16.1, you should have noted that the short and long arms of a chromosome are particularly clear with chromosome pairs 4, 5 and 9. The centromere – the location whereby the arms are held together during interphase – can be seen on all the chromosome pairs and is denoted as a white dot.

✳ Activity 16.1

Consider Figure 16.2 of a karyotype and identify examples of the short and long arms of the chromosomes and the centromere.

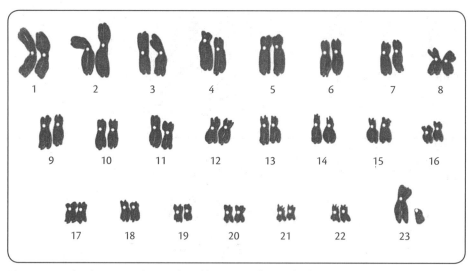

Figure 16.2 The short arms (p arms) and long arms (q arms) of the chromosomes

Deoxyribonucleic acid

DNA has been described as looking like a long spiral staircase – the famous double-stranded helix, first described by Crick and Watson in the 1950s.

Chromosomes are composed of DNA, which is made up of subunits called nucleotides. Each nucleotide in the DNA has three elements: a sugar molecule (deoxyribose), a phosphate molecule, and one of the nitrogen-containing bases – adenine, thymine, cytosine and guanine (Figure 16.3).

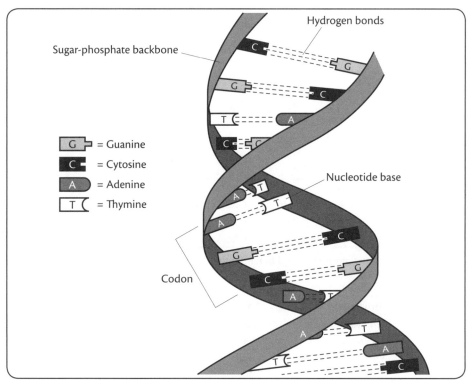

Figure 16.3 DNA molecule demonstrating the backbones and the nitrogen bases (A, T, G and C)

DNA is therefore two long chains or strings of deoxyribose sugar joined with phosphate molecules – producing the uprights of the staircase or ladder – and referred to as the sugar-phosphate backbones. These backbones are connected together – the rungs of the ladder – by the nitrogen-containing bases (nucleotide bases), which are held in place by weak hydrogen bonds. In this DNA structure, these bases demonstrate what is known as the 'pairing rule', with adenine (A) being paired with thymine (T), and cytosine (C) being paired with guanine (G) (a mnemonic for the pairing rule of A-T and G-C is 'All These Genetic Codes').

DNA is described as the genetic code holding all the genetic material for the body and for passing on to the next generation. These processes are undertaken by the action of the genes – segments of the DNA.

Genes

Genes are segments of the DNA that are the inherited genetic code and there are less than 30,000 genes in the human genome. The genetic code is 'read' as three nucleotides at a time, this is referred to as a codon or triplet, with each

Table 16.1 The genetic code: the 'reading' of the bases (A, T, G and C)

First position	Second position				Third position
	T	C	A	G	
T	Phe	Ser	Tyr	Cys	T
	Phe	Ser	Tyr	Cys	C
	Leu	Ser	Stop	Stop	A
	Leu	Ser	Stop	Trp	G
C	Leu	Pro	His	Arg	T
	Leu	Pro	His	Arg	C
	Leu	Pro	Gln	Arg	A
	Leu	Pro	Gln	Arg	G
A	Ile	Thr	Asn	Ser	T
	Ile	Thr	Asn	Ser	C
	Ile	Thr	Lys	Arg	A
	Met	Thr	Lys	Arg	G
G	Val	Ala	Asp	Gly	T
	Val	Ala	Asp	Gly	C
	Val	Ala	Glu	Gly	A
	Val	Ala	Glu	Gly	G

Note: The abbreviations represent the different amino acids, which are given below.

Amino acid abbreviations

Abbreviation	Amino acid	Abbreviation	Amino acid
Phe	Phenylalanine	Leu	Leucine
Ile	Isoleucine	Met	Methionine
Val	Valine	Ser	Serine
Pro	Proline	Thr	Threonine
Ala	Alanine	Tyr	Tyrosine
His	Histidine	Gln	Glutamine
Asn	Asparagine	Lys	Lysine
Asp	Aspartic acid	Glu	Glutamic acid
Cys	Cysteine	Trp	Tryptophan
Arg	Arginine	Gly	Glycine

✹ Activity 16.2

Utilising the genetic code outlined in Table 16.1, identify the codons that code for the amino acids leucine and serine.

codon/triplet acting as a code for a particular amino acid (the building blocks of proteins). The 'reading' of the codon – three nucleotides at a time – is described as reading the first, second and then third position, with each position denoting one of the bases (A, T, G or C). From reading the code, each of the resultant abbreviations, for example Phe (Table 16.1), signifies a particular amino acid. The DNA is arranged in an important pattern and it is this pattern that is the code that carries the protein-building instructions.

You can see from Table 16.1 that some amino acids are coded by more than one codon, such as leucine and arginine. Only a small proportion of an individual's DNA in the chromosomes forms the genes, the remaining is the 'non-coding' or 'junk DNA' and the function of which is not yet understood. Now refer to Activity 16.2.

Having done Activity 16.2, you should have come up with the following answers:

- Leucine is coded by six different codons: TTA, TTG, CTT, CTC, CTA, CTG
- Serine is coded by six different codons: TCT, TCC, TCA, TCG, AGT, AGC.

If the DNA pattern is changed, such as if nucleotides are altered, deleted or inserted, then a different code is read and different amino acids may be produced and a different or altered protein may be produced. These nucleotide mutations or variations can result in genetic mutations such as point mutations, frameshift mutations, and repeat expansion mutations (trinucleotide repeats), which are expanded upon later in this chapter. A point to note is that proteins contribute to various structures within the body or have contributed to the development of structures, such as the colour of the skin, layout of the neurons in the brain, structures such as collagen and keratin, and substances such as hormones, antibodies and enzymes. The effect of mutations or variations can therefore be expressed throughout the body.

The life cycle of the cell

The cell lifespan varies from cell to cell but there are three phases to the life cycle – interphase, cell division (mitosis or meiosis) and **cytokinesis**. For a cell to divide it must replicate the chromosomes so that they are passed onto each of the daughter cells. The first phase of the life cycle is called the interphase or resting stage, where replication of the chromosomes occur. This occurs by the double-stranded helix uncoiling, the hydrogen bonds holding the nucleotide bases together break, and each freed strand then replicates a complementary strand. This structure is held together by the centromere, resulting in double the chromosomal material and hence double the genetic material.

cytokinesis
the division or separation of the cytoplasm of the parent cell following mitosis or meiosis

The second phase is called cell division. In somatic cells (the body cells), this process of cell division is called mitosis and contains four phases: prophase, metaphase, anaphase and telophase. This process involves the centromeres lining up at the centre of the cell, the arms split and are then pulled separately towards the poles (ends) of the cell. This results in half of the chromosome material being placed at each end of the cell.

Cytokinesis, the third phase, commences with a cleavage furrow of the cytoplasm, and continues until the cytoplasm is divided into two separate cells.

Due to the exact replication of the chromosomes in the interphase stage, the process has produced two identical daughter cells – identical chromosomes and hence identical genetic material. The life cycle is a well-regulated process so that the production of new cells is sufficient for body growth and the repair of damaged cells.

The production of gametes is referred to as 'spermatogenesis' and 'oogenesis'. In the development of gametes, the life cycle is made up of the interphase, cell division (meiosis) and cytokinesis. However, it must be noted that the gametes differ from somatic cells, in that somatic cells have 23 pairs of chromosomes and gametes have only 23 chromosomes. This therefore requires a process whereby

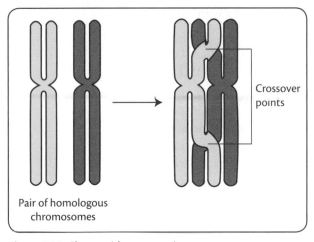

Crossover points

Pair of homologous chromosomes

Figure 16.4 Chromatid arms crossing over

only one from each pair of the chromosomes is distributed to each of the gametes.

Replication of the chromosomes occurs in interphase, as outlined previously. The second phase is the process of cell division (meiosis) involving two nuclear or meiotic divisions. Meiosis I is also called 'reduction division' and meiosis II is also called 'equatorial division', and both divisions have the four phases: prophase, metaphase, anaphase and telophase.

It is during meiosis I that genetic variability occurs so that similarities and differences can be seen within different family members, such as eye colour, personality traits, and genetic diseases. This occurs during reduction division by the crossing (overlaying) of the arms of each pair of chromosomes, these break and rejoin, and hence lead to a mixing of the genes (recombination). This can be seen in Figure 16.4. Therefore the exact DNA sequence varies from person to person, except in identical twins (monozygotic twins).

At the end of meiosis I and cytokinesis, two cells are produced that are different than the parent cell. The second meiotic stage (equatorial division) is undertaken, and along with cytokinesis, results in four cells being produced. Each of these haploid cells has half the chromosome complement, 23, from the parent cell.

Mitosis refers to cell division that is concerned with the development of somatic cells (body cells) as well as with the development of the zygote. At fertilisation, the union of the gametes (sperm and the ovum) produces one cell, called the zygote. This is a cell with a full chromosome compliment that develops by mitosis to become the embryo (first two months) and then the fetus. Processes of 'differentiation and specialisation' occur during embryo/fetal development at recognised times, ensuring that different body cells, tissues and systems are developed for the normal functioning of the human species. Any error occurring while these processes are in action will have consequences for the developing embryo/fetus and these may be evident at birth or in early childhood development.

Chromosomal abnormalities

Four types of mutations or variations can occur during gamete development, zygote development or during an individual's lifetime (body growth and repair), leading to differences in the **phenotype** of the individual. These changes in the DNA sequence, whatever the cause, may have no effect on the function of the gene, may result in an abnormality in the rate of production of a normal protein or may result in the production of an abnormal protein. The resulting phenotype therefore is determined by one of the four following mutations.

phenotype
the characteristics of an individual that are due to both the environment and genetic make-up

Chromosomal numerical

Errors can occur during cell division affecting all or part of a chromosome. Chromosomal numerical errors affect the number of the chromosomes. The most well-known example of a numerical disorder is trisomy 21 (Down's syndrome), where there are three copies of chromosome number 21. This error in cell division is called 'non-disjunction', and is when the chromosomes fail to split at the centromere and separate during the process of cell division, resulting in an extra chromosome (**trisomy**) or in an absence of a chromosome (**monosomy**). A trisomy condition therefore results in extra DNA/genes, and a monosomy condition results in an absence of DNA/genes.

If non-disjunction occurs during mitosis, it can have an impact on body repair and body growth or on the development of the zygote.

If non-disjunction occurs during meiosis, it can have an impact on the production of the gametes, resulting in trisomy or monosomy of the gametes. Hence, if a mutated or faulty gamete is fertilised, it results in a faulty zygote being produced. Other examples of trisomy conditions include trisomy 13 (Patau syndrome), trisomy 18 (Edward syndrome), triple X syndrome, XXY (Klinefelter syndrome in males). An example of a monosomy condition is XO (Turner syndrome in females, denoted as 45, X).

trisomy
having three copies of a particular chromosome

monosomy
having only one copy of a particular chromosome

Chromosomal structural

Chromosomal structural errors are those affecting the structure, and include 'deletion', 'microdeletion' and 'translocation'. A deletion is where there is chromosome breakage and a fragment of the chromosome has been lost. A deletion is indicated by a minus (–) sign on the karyotype, for example 46, XX, 5p- (denotes Cri-du-chat syndrome) or 46, XY, 4p- (denotes Wolf-Hirschhorn syndrome). A microdeletion is a region of chromosome loss that is detected by cytogenetic testing. A translocation is a rearrangement of the chromosome material. This results in part or whole of one chromosome becoming attached to a chromosome from a different pair and so there is no loss or gain of chromosome material; however, these can lead to errors in future generations.

Nucleotide mutations

Nucleotide mutations or variations, affect the nucleotides and are classified at the DNA level – affecting the 4 bases (A, T, G or C). These include 'point mutations' – such as missense and nonsense mutations, 'frameshift mutations' and 'repeat expansion mutations'. A point mutation occurs when a nitrogen base (adenine, thymine, cytosine, guanine) has been substituted for another. The system of reading the codons (triplets) as three at a time is not affected, but in 'missense' the altered codon leads to the coding of a different amino acid than the original – this error is also referred to as a 'spelling error'. In 'nonsense' it creates a premature stop codon and hence leads to a shortened or truncated protein. A frameshift mutation occurs when one or multiple nitrogen bases are inserted or deleted. This mutation affects the reading of the codons (triplets) and hence the sequence of the amino acids is altered and the composition of the final protein is affected.

Repeat expansion mutations (trinucleotide repeats) are where a codon has been repeated over and over many times. An example of this is fragile X syndrome where there is a repeat of the bases CGG (cytosine, guanine, guanine) on the X chromosome at the location of q27.3. Remember that q refers to the long arm of the chromosome and 27.3 refers to the position on the arm. This means that the error has been identified at an exact location (locus). Other examples are Huntington's disease, which is a repeat of the bases CAG (cytosine, adenine, guanine) on chromosome number 4 at the p16.3 location, and myotonic dystrophy, which is a repeat of the bases CTG on chromosome 19.

Mutations of DNA sequence

Cancers can occur due to mutations or variations in DNA sequence (Kirk and Tonkin, 2009). Throughout our lifetime, DNA/genes within the cells of the body are exposed to adverse environmental agents and can suffer mistakes in replication. Most cancers result from these acquired mutations in families of genes called 'oncogenes' and tumour-suppressor genes. These genes are part of the cells' normal machinery for keeping the cell functioning and ensuring effective division (RS, 2005a). When new cells are produced in the body to replace dead or damaged cells, these genes limit the number of new cells to prevent overgrowth of the tissue. These genes therefore have the function of helping to prevent the growth of tumours or cancers. Genetic material is recopied over and over during a person's lifetime with the potential for errors to occur.

Genetic Inheritance

genotype
the genetic composition
of an organism

The **genotype** refers to the genetic make-up of an individual and the phenotype as the expression of this genetic make-up. A change in the sequence of the DNA may affect its function and may have phenotypic consequences.

Regarding the inheritance of traits and disorders, genes that control the same trait and occupy the same locus (position) on the chromosome are referred to as 'alleles'. When alleles code for the same expression of a trait, they are referred to as 'homozygous', and when they code for a different expression of a trait, they are referred to as 'heterozygous'. Table 16.2 uses eye colour as an example.

When one allele masks (suppresses) the one on the other chromosome, it is called the 'dominant' gene, and the one being masked (suppressed) is called the 'recessive' gene. Examples of dominant traits are brown eyes, curly hair and dimples, and recessive traits are blue eyes, straight hair and flat feet. When illustrating recessive and dominant states, then dominant is always indicated by a capital letter and recessive by a lower case one.

Table 16.2 Genotypes expressed as phenotypes, using eye colour as an example

Genotype	Phenotype
BB (homozygous)	Brown eyes
Bb (heterozygous)	Brown eyes
bb (heterozygous)	Blue eyes

The inheritance of single-gene traits and disorders follow simple patterns of Mendel's laws of inheritance, in that they are inherited in a dominant manner, recessive manner or X-linked manner (located on the X chromosome). The **Punnett square** is a method of demonstrating the possible combinations of the genes from the parent (Figure 16.5).

It can be seen from this Punnett square that 50 per cent of children are males and 50 per cent females; however, it needs to be noted that this refers to the genotype of the children – the actual genetic composition. The determination of the male phenotype is determined by genes located on the Y chromosome – the SRY region. All zygotes, male and female, develop identically and then in early embryonic development, the genes in the SRY region activate male development. If this region is absent or mutated, the developing embryo continues to develop as a female, irrespective of having a Y chromosome.

This method of demonstrating the passage of genes from one generation to the next can be used for all inherited traits and conditions. For example, curly (C) hair is dominant and straight (s) hair is recessive. Utilising the Punnett square, it can be seen that two parents with curly (C) hair (phenotype) can have a child with straight (s) hair (phenotype). This is due to the genotype of the parents – the actual genetic make-up (Figure 16.6).

Having done Activity 16.3, you should have the same Punnett square as shown in Figure 16.7. The possible genotype and phenotypes of children are:

- Genotype of Bb: two children with a phenotype of brown eyes (B) and a heterozygous genotype (Bb)
- Genotype of bb: two children with a phenotype of blue eyes (b) and a homozygous recessive genotype (bb)
- Note that a BB genotype would indicate a child with a phenotype of brown eyes (B) and a homozygous dominant genotype (BB).

When an individual is referred to as being of a 'carrier status' for a specific condition, this means that their genotype has one defective recessive gene for the specific condition. However, as it is a recessive gene, it is not expressed in

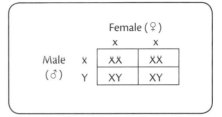

Figure 16.5 Punnett square illustrating the determination of gender

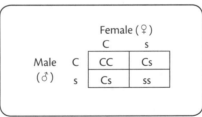

Figure 16.6 Punnett square illustrating the determination of curly and straight hair

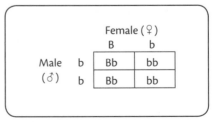

Figure 16.7 Punnett square illustrating the determination of eye colour

Punnett square

consists of a square divided into four, with the possible alleles from the father being placed at the left-hand side of the square and the possible alleles from the mother above it. The possible genotypes of the children are then calculated by combining the alleles in turn

✴ Activity 16.3

Using a Punnett square, plot the eye colour (the phenotype) of possible children from a mother with a Bb heterozygous genotype and a father with a bb homozygous genotype.

the phenotype as it is suppressed by the corresponding gene. Carriers can pass this gene on to the next generation and individuals can be offered carrier testing to determine whether they carry such a gene, for example for CF, phenylketonuria (PKU), sickle-cell anaemia and Tay-Sachs disease. Consent to this type of genetic testing requires consideration of any social and psychological implications for individuals and their relatives and implications for future reproductive decisions. Issues such as prenatal and neonatal screening, diagnostic testing and assisted reproductive technologies are discussed in a report, which may influence reproductive decision-making (DoH, 2006).

The three conditions mentioned in Casebox 16.1 are inherited in different ways and therefore may pose different issues for the family to consider:

- *Cystic fibrosis*: this is inherited in an autosomal recessive manner and therefore has implications due to carrier status of some of the family members. Choices regarding future reproductive choices will need to be considered by other family members and hence ethical consideration will be required when working within an extended family structure.
- *Huntington's disease*: this is inherited in an autosomal dominant manner and is a late-onset disease, in that the symptoms are manifested in later life. As this is inherited in this dominant manner, it will raise issues within the family regarding testing and the purposes of diagnosis. This poses dilemmas for testing in childhood/young adulthood for a late-onset condition.
- *Haemophilia*: this is inherited in an X linked manner, with the gene responsible being located on the X chromosome. This raises gender issues within families, as females have two X chromosomes (karyotype is 46, XX) and may therefore have an unaffected X chromosome as well as an affected one. Males are affected by the condition as they only have one copy of the X chromosome (male karyotype is 46, XY). Choices regarding future reproductive choices will need to be considered by other family members and hence ethical consideration will be required when working within an extended family structure.

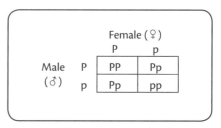

Figure 16.8 Punnett square illustrating the possible phenotypes of children when both parents have a genotype for PKU

The parents of Joseph are informed when he is 12 days old that Joseph, their first child has PKU. They are worried about his health status and that of any future children. They are both from large families and both wish to have a large family in the future.

Using a Punnett square, identify the potential phenotypes of future children using the genotypes of Joseph's parents.

- You could consider how you would inform the parents of this condition, working within an ethical framework upholding ethical principles.

- You could consider the implications of this carrier status in terms of social and psychological impact for family members and in terms of implications for reproductive decisions.

- You might also consider the possible future and implications of gene therapy for conditions such as PKU (12q 24.1) (see Pharmacogenetics later in this chapter).

PKU is an autosomal recessive condition, so is demoted on the Punnett square as lower case p (Figure 16.8).

The possible genotype and phenotypes of children are:

- Genotype of PP: one child with a phenotype of not being affected with PKU and a homozygous genotype (PP).
- Genotype of Pp: two children with a phenotype of carrier status for PKU (p) and a heterozygous recessive genotype (Pp).
- Genotype of pp: one child with a phenotype of being affected with PKU and a homozygous recessive genotype (pp).

The Impact of Genotypes in Health Care

Genetics is clearly recognised in single-gene disorders such as CF, haemophilia and Huntington's disease, but the relevance of the human genome and genomics is being acknowledged in common diseases such as coronary heart disease, diabetes, asthma, cancers, mental health conditions such as schizophrenia and many others (House of Lords Science and Technology Committee, 2009).

The genetics White Paper *Our Inheritance, Our Future: Realising the Potential of Genetics in the NHS* (DoH, 2003) clearly set out the government's strategic vision for genetics and health care. It will have a major impact on how genetic information is fully realised in the health and lifestyle of individuals and in the development of NHS and private health-care systems.

> The secretary of state for health acknowledged that advances in human genetics will have a profound impact on healthcare. Over time we will see new ways of predicting and preventing ill health, more targeted and effective use of existing drugs and the development of new gene-based drugs and therapies that treat illness in novel ways. Above all, genetics holds out the promise of more personalised healthcare with prevention and treatment tailored according to a person's individual genetic profile. *(DoH, 2003, p. 5)*

This governmental position clearly encompasses a number of issues regarding genetics:

- The identification of 'personal genetic information' including genetic disease and predisposition to disease.
- An understanding of how genetics and other factors such as environmental ones interact with each other.
- An understanding of drugs and alternative therapies.
- The development of appropriate educational programmes and initiatives for health-care practitioners.
- The investment and development of appropriate health-care services to meet the needs arising from genetic advances.

Genetics knowledge has the potential to bring extensive benefits for individuals and the genetic advancements will increasingly challenge all practitioners in their daily practice (DoH, 2003, 2008). They will be faced with clinical, ethical, legal and social dilemmas relating to genetics and its impact on the individual. These challenges will not only be faced by all individual practitioners, but need to be brought together through successful team working within an interprofessional context. Developments such as these demonstrate the importance of an interprofessional arena of health and social care.

As part of these developments, an advisory body, the Human Genetics Commission (HGC), was set up in late 1999 so as to 'advise the government on the ethical, legal and social aspects of developments in human genetics as well as their effects on health and healthcare' (DoH, 2006, p. 6). A number of key publications have been published that provide evidence of the debate around these ethical, legal and social influences (DoH, 2000, 2002a, 2004, 2005, 2006; Nuffield Council in Bioethics, 2001, 2002, 2003a, 2003b).

The complexity and challenges faced by practitioners, when considering the upholding of ethical principles, are outlined within reports from the Nuffield Council on Bioethics: *Dementia: Ethical Issues* (2009); *Public Health: Ethical Issues* (2007a); *The Forensic Use of Bioinformation: Ethical Issues* (2007b), and *Critical Care Decisions in Fetal and Neonatal Medicine: Ethical Issues* (2006b). Respecting the individual, family and carers, in terms of their diverse needs, preferences and individuality of those concerned, is paramount in health care.

The *Our Inheritance, Our Future: Realising the Potential of Genetics in the NHS. Progress Review* (DoH, 2008) highlights the development of a number of 'Genetics Knowledge Parks' (GKP) across the country and their influence in the development of policy pertaining to these ethical, social and legal issues arising from genetics.

Genetic profiling

The issue of genetic profiling babies at birth was considered by the Human Genetics Commission and the National Screening Committee (DoH, 2005) so as to consider the potential of all individuals having their own entire genome analysis. This would enable individuals to have personal genetic information that may be important in health care during their lifetime. The government have been provided with an analysis of the 'ethical, social, scientific, economic and practical considerations' of genetically profiling babies at birth (DoH, 2005). They suggested that genetic profiling, along with other health, lifestyle and environmental information, brings the promise of a more accurate assessment of disease status, disease risk and an individual's susceptibility to various environmental exposures (DoH, 2005, p. 10).

This has tremendous implications for an individual's lifestyle and their health-care needs. Individuals may be informed how, based on their genotype, they will interact with factors such as environmental pollutants, foods, and infectious agents (DoH, 2005). Personal choices based on this type of personal genetic and related information are then possible, such as altering one's lifestyle – diet, cessation of smoking, exercise, and the uptake of health and alternative remedies. Health choices are also possible, such as particular drug regimes, targeted to suit the individual's profile.

The Department of Health (DoH, 2005, 2008) acknowledges that many diseases are as a result of the interaction between genetic and environmental factors, with the balance between these two factors varying from disease to disease. But it also highlights that the evidence of the link between most genetic variants and disease is not yet fully clear. This knowledge will progress through research.

However, the Department of Health did reject genetic profiling as a screening tool at this current time, but highlighted that this should not be taken as a rejection of its longer term potential. It suggested that for genetic profiling to be of clinical use, more research must be undertaken about genetic variation and its link with ill-health, and the influence of environmental factors (DoH, 2005). Research is already trying to unravel the complex interactions between nature and nurture that underlie diseases (RS, 2005a). The developing genetic knowledge does facilitate our understanding of how body cells work and how genetic variations and mutations affect normal cell processes and hence disease patterns.

Genetic screening

Genetic screening is offered to members of a defined population who do not necessarily perceive they are at risk of, or are already affected by, a genetic condition or its complications. Genetic screening programmes offer tests to large groups of individuals, by which they may be identified as being at particular risk of a disorder by virtue of their clinical history (or that of relatives), or on a larger scale on the basis of age, gender or ethnic group (Nuffield Council on Bioethics, 2006a). Respect for persons and the associated principles need to be safeguarded when working with individuals involved in genetic screening programmes, as they raise issues such as consent, confidentiality and the counselling needs of the participants.

Genetic testing is used to:

- aid diagnosis where symptoms are already present
- identify whether family members will develop a late-onset disease
- check for carrier status
- in prenatal and neonatal screening programmes.

✵ Activity 16.4

Consider the following implications of genetic profiling babies at birth:

1. The ethical implications and the upholding of ethical principles.

2. The social, economic and practical implications of genetic profiling at birth.

You may wish to consider these from various perspectives, such as families, communities and governmental agencies such as the NHS. (Suggested key publications include DoH, 2000, 2002a, 2002b, 2004, 2005, 2006 and Nuffield Council on Bioethics, 2001, 2002, 2003a, 2003b).

As well as participants in the public dialogue advocating that genetic tests were empowering, the Royal Society identified that even if lifestyle changes were not likely to improve prognosis, around 50 per cent still preferred to have a test, particularly when reproductive decisions were affected (RS, 2005b). However, complex issues arising from genetic testing, particularly relating to family members, was raised by a significant number of the participants (RS, 2005b).

Pharmacogenetics

pharmacogenetics
the study of how people's genetic make-up affects their responses to drugs (RS, 2005a)

The Royal Society has published a comprehensive report into **pharmacogenetics** (personalised medicines), detailing the current position and future possibilities within health-care practice (RS, 2005a).

It is recognised that individuals respond differently to drugs, and that part of this is genetically determined – variations in our genes. Three factors being considered are:

- *Genetic predictor of response* – whether an individual will respond or fail to respond to a drug
- *Adverse drug reactions* – whether an individual will experience any idiosyncratic adverse reactions to a drug
- *Genetic differences in drug metabolism* – whether an individual has a slow or quick metabolic rate for the drug.

This will lead to an individual's genetic difference in drug metabolism and to any adverse drug reactions being considered in the design of their individual treatment regime – 'tailor-made treatments'. Alongside pharmacogenetic testing (the person's genetic make-up), other factors such as gender, age, weight, ethnicity, family history, diet, alcohol consumption and tobacco usage will continue to be considered.

The pharmaceutical industry, in an attempt to take these issues forward through research, is trying to understand the causes of disease and variability of drug responses, drug dosages, why some individuals experience adverse drug reactions, and the fate of drugs within the body – absorption, distribution, metabolism and excretion (ADME) (DoH, 2008). These developments are already evident in cancer care, where an individual's genotype is being utilised prior to the prescribing of targeted drug regimes, for example with the use of Trastuzumab (Herceptin) being developed for some types of breast cancer (RS, 2005a).

However, developments are not restricted to inherited conditions, as many forms of cancer result from changes (mutations or variations) in the genes that occur during our lifetime through errors in cell division (mitosis) in the body's cells (somatic cells) (RS, 2005a). We are dependent upon the process of mitosis during our lifetime, for body growth and repair, and as we continuously encounter adverse environmental agents, these can be detrimental to the process of mitosis and lead to mutations.

Pharmacogenetics is viewed as a promising future in health care; however, it is estimated that it will be more than a decade before their use is widespread

(Nuffield Council on Bioethics, 2006a). The advances in genetics may also lead to further gene-based drugs and gene therapies. In this way, drugs would interact with the individual's genotype, aiming to switch on a helpful gene or to switch off a harmful one. Gene therapy is the introduction of material directly into an individual's cells, and it would aim to replace a defective gene or to alter the activity of gene action (DoH, 2003). The Human Genetics Commission highlights that

> whilst recognising the potential benefits that gene therapy can have, it is only likely to be effective for a few people, and for a very small proportion of the single gene disorders. (DoH, 2006, pp. 80–1)

Many of these therapies are presently being researched, in particular in cancer and coronary heart disease, but promise an evolutionary health-care system based on the human genome.

The ethical debate regarding pharmacogenetics and the principles of consent, privacy and confidentiality, alongside information management, has been outlined by the Nuffield Council on Bioethics (2003a, 2006a).

Chapter Summary

There are a number of issues surrounding genetics that have been considered in this chapter so as to further understand human development, health and disease, mental health and mental disorders, and learning disabilities. This chapter has therefore focused on the structure and function of the chromosomes and genes, the inheritance patterns and the expression of an individual's genotype into phenotype, and the potential impact of mutations upon the developing individual.

The question as to how our genes and other factors, such as social, economic and environmental factors, interact to cause disease or to predispose an individual to disease are highlighted as areas for future research. How our genes can affect our response to drugs has been raised, with developments in pharmacogenetics potentially leading to tailor-made prescribing. Genetic profiling and testing will become a key element of the health-care service, with a more personalised health-care system becoming a reality.

The new genetics knowledge and technology has the potential to bring enormous benefits for patients, such as more personalised prediction of risk, prevention of ill-health, more accurate diagnosis, safer use of drugs and new treatment options. A revolution in health care is possible (DoH, 2003); however, it needs to be underpinned by knowledgeable practitioners and good educational initiatives.

The importance of identifying and resolving any ethical issues such as confidentiality of information, privacy, obtaining valid informed consent, storage and protection of genetic material is fundamental to the developing health agenda.

⸞?⸟ Test yourself!

1   Identify the four secondary principles reflected by the Human Genetics Commission (DoH, 2002a) in the primary principle of 'respect for persons'.

2   Name the four nitrogen-containing bases of the DNA molecule.

3   Describe the pairing rule of the nitrogen-containing bases in the DNA sequence.

4   Name the following conditions: (a) 47, XY+21, (b) 47, XXY, (c) 45, XO, (d) 12q24.1, (e) Xq28.

5   Define the terms: (a) autosomes, (b) trisomy, (c) monosomy, (d) non-disjunction.

6   Calculate the inheritance of a: (a) dominant condition, (b) recessive condition, (c) X-linked condition.

Further Reading

For live links to useful websites see: www.palgrave.com/nursinghealth/hogston

Burke, S., Bennett, C., Bedward, J. and Farndon, P. (2007) *The Experiences and Preferences of People Receiving Genetic Information from Healthcare Professionals,* The NHS National Genetics Education and Development Centre.

Burton, H. (2003) *Addressing Genetics Delivering Health,* Public Health Genetics funded by The Wellcome Trust and the Department of Health. Department of Health, London.

DoH (Department of Health) (2003) *Genes Direct: Ensuring the Effective Oversight of Genetic Tests Supplied Directly to the Public.* Department of Health, London.

DoH (Department of Health) (2003) *Addressing Genetics, Delivering Health.* Department of Health, London.

Gilbert, P. (2001) *Dictionary of Syndromes and Inherited Disorders.* Chapman & Hall, London.

Marteau, T. and Richards, M. (1996) *The Troubled Helix: Social and Psychological Implications of the New Human Genetics.* Cambridge University Press, Cambridge.

NICE (National Institute for Health and Clinical Excellence) (2008) *Antenatal Care: Routine Care for the Healthy Pregnant Woman.* NICE, London.

Royal College of Physicians, Royal College of Pathologists and British Society for Human Genetics (2006) *Consent and Confidentiality in Genetic Practice: Guidance on Genetic Testing and Sharing Genetic Information.* Report of the Joint Committee on Medical Genetics, RCP, RCPath, BSHG, London.

RS (Royal Society) (2003) *Genetics and Health – Visions of the Future.* RS, London.

RS (Royal Society) (2005) *Pharmacogenetics: The Hopes and Realities of Personalised Medicines. A Guide for Health Professionals.* RS, London.

Skirton, H. and Patch, C. (2002) *Genetics for Healthcare Professionals.* BIOS Scientific Publishers, Oxford.

References

Beauchamp, T.L. and Childress, J.F. (2001) *Principles of Biomedical Ethics,* Oxford University Press, Oxford.

Benjamin, C.M. and Gamet, K. (2005) Recognising the limitations of your genetics expertise. *Nursing Standard* **20**(6): 49–54.

Bradley, A.N. (2005) Utility and limitations of genetic testing and information, *Nursing Standard* **20**(5): 52–5.

DoH (Department of Health) (2000) *Whose Hands on Your Genes?* Department of Health, London.

DoH (Department of Health) (2002a) *Inside Information: Balancing Interests in the Use of Personal Genetic Data.* Human Genetics Commission, Department of Health, London.

DoH (Department of Health) (2002b) *Public Attitudes to Human Genetic Information.* DoH, London.

DoH (Department of Health) (2003) *Our Inheritance, Our Future: Realising the Potential of Genetics in the NHS,* Department of Health, London.

DoH (Department of Health) (2004) *Choosing the Future: Genetics and Reproductive Decision-making.* Department of Health, London.

DoH (Department of Health) (2005) *Profiling the Newborn: A Prospective Gene Technology?* Human Genetics Commission, Department of Health, London.

DoH (Department of Health) (2006) *Making Babies: Reproductive Decisions and Genetic Technologies,* Human Genetics Commission, Department of Health, London.

DoH (Department of Health) (2008) *Our Inheritance, Our Future: Realising the Potential of Genetics in the NHS. Progress Review.* Department of Health, London.

House of Lords Science and Technology Committee (2009) *Genomic Medicine. Volume 1: Report.* The Stationery Office, London.

Kirk, M. (2005) The role of genetic factors in maintaining health, *Nursing Standard* **20**(4): 50–4.

Kirk, M., McDonald, K., Anstey, S. and Longley, M. (2003) *Fit for Practice in the Genetics Era: A Competence-based Education Framework for Nurses, Midwives and Health Visitors.* Genomics Policy Unit, University of Glamorgan.

Kirk, M. and Tonkin, E. (2009) Understanding the role of genetics and genomics in health 1: background, *Nursing Times.net,* **105**(45).

National Human Genome Research Institute (2006) *Essential Nursing Competencies and Curricula Guidelines for Genetics and Genomics.* http://research.nhgri.nih.gov

NHS National Genetics Education and Development Centre and Skills for Health (2007) *Enhancing Patient Care by Integrating Genetics in Clinical Practice: UK Workforce Competencies for Genetics in Clinical Practice for Non-Genetics Healthcare Staff.*

NMC (Nursing and Midwifery Council) (2010) *Standards for Pre-registration Nursing Education.* NMC, London.

NMC (Nursing and Midwifery Council) (2008) *The Code: Standards of Conduct, Performance and Ethics for Nurses and Midwives.* NMC, London.

Nuffield Council on Bioethics (2001) *Stem Cell Therapy: Ethical Issues.* Nuffield Council on Bioethics, London.

Nuffield Council on Bioethics (2002) *Genetics and Human Behaviour: The Ethical Context.* Nuffield Council on Bioethics, London.

Nuffield Council on Bioethics (2003a) *Genetics Screening: Ethical Issues.* Nuffield Council on Bioethics, London.

Nuffield Council on Bioethics (2003b) *Pharmacogenetics: Ethical Issues.* Nuffield Council on Bioethics, London.

Nuffield Council on Bioethics (2006a) *Genetic Screening: A Supplement to the 1993 Report by the Nuffield Council on Bioethics,* Nuffield Council on Bioethics, London.

Nuffield Council on Bioethics (2006b) *Critical Care Decisions in Fetal and Neonatal Medicine: Ethical Issues,* Nuffield Council on Bioethics, London.

Nuffield Council on Bioethics (2007a) *Public Health: Ethical Issues.* Nuffield Council on Bioethics. Nuffield Council on Bioethics, London.

Nuffield Council on Bioethics NCB (2007b) *The Forensic Use of Bioinformation: Ethical Issues.* Nuffield Council on Bioethics, London.

Nuffield Council on Bioethics (NCB) (2009) *Dementia: Ethical Issues.* Nuffield Council on Bioethics, London.

RS (Royal Society) (2005a) *Personalised Medicines: Hopes and Realities.* RS, London.

RS (Royal Society) (2005b) *Pharmacogenetics Dialogue.* RS, London.

17 Nursing Practice in an Interprofessional Context

📖 Contents

- What Is Interprofessionalism?
- Moves towards Interprofessional Practice
- Teamwork
- Professional Socialisation
- Good Practice in Teamwork
- Working in Teams
- Moving towards Cooperation
- Responses to Teamworking
- Chapter Summary
- Test Yourself!
- References

☑ Learning outcomes

At the end of this chapter, you will be able to:

- Define the term 'interprofessional practice' and other key elements such as collaboration
- Identify elements of good and bad practice in teamwork settings
- Ensuring the service user is at the centre of teamwork processes and outcomes
- Highlight different professionals' contributions to teamwork
- Describe the role of the primary health-care team as new partnerships are developed
- Discuss the challenges that the changes to primary health-care team present to different professionals
- Plan methods of working in practice that will support effective interprofessional teamwork from a user-centred perspective
- Consider the ethical issues that interprofessional practice may create.

What Is Interprofessionalism?

'**Interprofessional**' is the term most recently used to describe professionals from different disciplines working together. The definition suggests that these professionals are working in collaboration to achieve the same goals for the client, patient or service user. Interprofessional practice can occur in a range of settings, from that of the acute medical ward to community support for older people.

Other terms are also used in place of and in preference to interprofessional: Leathard (2003) notes that, in health care, **multidisciplinary** and interdisciplinary have commonly been used to describe practice. Leathard cites Marshall et al. (1979), who define multidisciplinary practice as the work of a group of individuals with different training backgrounds, for example nursing, medicine, occupational therapy, health visiting and social work, who share common objectives but make a different but complementary contribution. Interdisciplinary has been described by Payne (2000) as work 'where professional groups make adaptations to their role, to take account of and interact with the roles of others'. The term 'multi-agency' is also used to describe the involvement of a range of services and professionals in the delivery of health and social care to an individual. In children's services the term integrated working is used and has been defined as 'everyone supporting children and young people works together effectively to put the child at the centre, meet their needs and improve their lives' (DCFS, 2007, p. 1). The World Health Organisation (WHO, 2010, p. 7) offers a definition of collaborative practice. 'Which happens when multiple health workers from different professional backgrounds work together with patients, families, carers and communities to deliver the highest quality of care. It allows health workers to engage any individual whose skills can help achieve local goals'.

In this chapter, the term 'interprofessional' will be used when describing teamwork that involves working towards the same goal for patients or clients.

Transdisciplinary teamwork (Garner and Orelove, 1994; Batorowicz and Shepherd, 2008) may be a more radical form of practice. It can include working across ordinary professional boundaries to meet the needs of the client or service user. A nurse in the field of learning disability may, for example, give advice on housing or welfare benefits to a young man, although, in day-to-day practice, this would usually be the role of the social worker.

Two key features of interprofessional practice are teamwork and collaboration. Thus, the concept of interprofessional practice may be interpreted in a range of ways, which will be explored in this chapter.

interprofessional
involves a group of different professionals working to achieve mutually agreed goals

multidisciplinary
often used to describe interprofessional teamwork in an academic context

transdisciplinary
working across ordinary professional boundaries to meet the needs of the client, patient or service user

Moves towards Interprofessional Practice

Over the past 30 years, global changes in the delivery of health and social care have placed a different emphasis on the role and work of professionals. Nationally these changes have been created by government policy and concerns about the cost and focus of health and welfare provision. In addition, the developing role of some professional groups and the need to respond in order not to undermine the provision of services has required a new look at practice. Advances in technology that have reduced the time spent in hospital, in addition to the deinstitutionalisation movement, have placed an emphasis on care in the community, along with moves towards personalisation of care and support. This has had an impact on more vocal and questioning consumers and service user groups seeking an understanding of, or participation in, decisions about the treatment and services offered, together with welfare rights. These changes have not occurred in isolation: all can be attributed to one or more of the factors identified. Because this chapter explores interprofessional work, it may be worth reviewing each of these elements separately.

Government policy and the focus of health and welfare provision

Moves to introduce general management structures created by the Griffiths Report (DoH, 1983) refocused the activity and roles of professionals within the NHS, one of the greatest changes being the movement of nurses and clinicians into general management. A second change was the division of the functions of delivering and purchasing care, Owens and Petch (1995) explaining this move as an attempt by the government to control budgets and resources. These changes also occurred in social care and formed part of the NHS and Community Care Act 1990. The separation of the functions of purchasing and providing health and social care was also to influence general practice and the role of the GP. In addition, it offered social workers and nurses new opportunities to support other groups with long-term needs, for example people with learning disability.

The ongoing implementation of the White Paper *The New NHS: Modern, Dependable* (DoH, 1997) and *The NHS Plan* (DoH, 2000a), together with *Primary Care, General Practice and the NHS Plan* (DoH, 2001a), has confirmed the emphasis on primary health care, with the creation of Primary Care Trusts (PCTs). PCTs are responsible for consulting with local communities on healthcare needs as well as commissioning the health care needed from a range of services, for example acute health care. Such changes will continue to affect the way in which professionals work together and will create different partnerships and relationships for practice. In the document *From Vision to Reality* (DoH, 2001b), the government saw PCTs as being pivotal in achieving changes in public health.

In practice, this meant new roles for some professionals. In primary care, for example, practice nurses now take on the responsibility for managing specific elements of chronic disease management, a role traditionally undertaken by the GP. Equally, caring for people who have a terminal illness in their own homes, may now be undertaken by community or district nurses.

Recently there has been an increase in the individualised budget and direct payment funding streams in social care endorsed in *Our Health Our Care Our Say* (DoH, 2006) and in health and social care in *Putting People First* (DoH, 2008a). This emphasis on personalisation where people are active in designing, managing and making choices about their care and support and where it is

∞ Link
See Chapter 18 for more details on public health

delivered is also central to the health-care vision set out in the Darzi Review of the NHS, *High Quality Care for All* (DoH, 2008b).

In other sectors of health care, interprofessional working continues to be an essential part of the NHS's modernisation agenda. New partnerships are emerging with the third sector which includes the voluntary, independent and not for profit groups who provide services (Scragg, 2009). For nurses this can mean working with new groups of staff such as those in Housing Associations and also with personal assistants who are employed by people directly or through an agency to provide individual care.

Role expansion

The Greenhalgh Report (Greenhalgh and Company, 1994) reviewed the role of junior doctors and recommended the reduction of their weekly working hours. One response to this initiative has been that of a broader role for nurses. The document *The Scope of Professional Practice* (UKCC, now NMC, 1992) had already identified several areas in which nurses could take on broader and more autonomous roles, for example nurse prescribing and nurse practitioner roles within community hospitals and nurse-led clinics.

The National Health Service and Community Care Act 1990 also created alterations in the provision of long-term care, which have resulted in a closer working relationship between nurses and social workers. The Medical Practices Committee (2001) notes a need for collaboration across primary care.

Liberating the Talents (DOH, 2002) sets out new ways of working and partnerships in primary care, while the implementation of the new general medical services contract (BMA, 2003) has changed the practice role of GPs and nurses. The National Health Service Knowledge and Skills Framework (DOH, 2004b) brings other priorities including skills in interprofessional collaboration. Clinical commissioning through GP practices mean that more collaborative and integtrated working between acute and primary care will take place especially around long-term care pathways (DoH, 2009a).

Finally, there has been a blurring of the boundaries between health visitors, district nurses and community nurses, although with emphasis on developing specific areas of expertise. All this means a greater emphasis on teamwork and multiprofessional cooperation because clinical work that lay in the domain of the GP or hospital doctor may now be transferred to other professionals. In cardio-pulmonary resuscitation (CPR), a document from the Royal College of Nursing (RCN), the Resuscitation Council (UK) and the British Medical Association (BMA) sets out new guidelines for who can make decisions on resuscitation, which may now be the senior nurse (BMA, Resuscitation Council (UK) RCN, 2007, p. 19 cited in Fisher, 2009).

Changes in service provision

As technology and approaches to treatment have changed, most patients and clients are spending less time in acute hospital settings. Many people are discharged and supported by community or district nurses in their own homes, the majority of care being provided by family members. Running parallel to these developments has been the deinstitutionalisation movement for those who are older or have a learning disability or mental health need.

The transition from institution to community care has seen a shift in the role of professional groups of nurses, occupational therapists, psychologists and speech therapists, which as we have seen has been compounded by an increasing emphasis on voluntary and independent sector provision in the community. The government encourages social entrepreneurship in the provision of health and social care in its commissioning framework for health and well-being (DoH, 2007a).

Work that might once have been undertaken by qualified professionals may now be carried out by support workers or vocationally trained employees. Professional roles have in contrast become more specific because of the different types of support required in community settings.

At the same time, the cost of some roles has been questioned and the need for a professionally qualified individual challenged. Interwoven throughout these changes has been an increased demand for interprofessional collaboration in order to coordinate service delivery in the community.

The rights of service users, clients and patients

The recognition of the changing position of service users with regard to the services offered has gained momentum. An acknowledgement of fragmented services and a need to create a seamless service have built the foundation for change. Responses from service user groups now occur through patients and service user forums called LINks (Local involvement networks). These are underpinned by the Local Government and Public Involvement in Health Act 2007 (DoH, 2007b). Such locally based activity sets the scene for increased partnership between the service user and professional, as well as a greater input into decision-making on the use of resources. Changes in position of the service user or client has meant that the involvement of a large number of professionals in their specific care group is no longer accepted; and greater collaboration within and across professional teams will be needed in order to minimise this and ensure access to the appropriate services.

Why interprofessionalism is important to nurses

For nurses practising in a range of health-care and social-care settings, the need for collaboration to meet service user needs will be a priority, and working together with other professionals and vocational staff will be part of everyday practice. In order to make sense of interprofessional working, and to enhance its success, it is necessary to have a clear picture of how nursing practice in the interprofessional team has evolved over time and what factors have impinged upon its success. A greater understanding of the role of other professional groups may be gained by thinking about interprofessional practice, which may give nurses greater confidence in collaboration.

✷ Activity 17.1

From your recent practice experience, identify all the different professionals you have come into contact with. What is their role and how does it link with yours?

Teamwork

When interprofessional or multidisciplinary work is described, it is usually a function of **teamwork**.

Early writers such as Rubin and Beckhard (1972) and Gilmour et al. (1974) describe it as: 'a team is a group of people who make different contributions towards the achievement of a common goal'. More recently Malin and Morrow (2007, p. 449) describe multidisciplinary teamwork as 'where two or more professionals from different disciplines work together or co-exist alongside each other but separately from each other'.

Others (Cook, 2009, p. 6) would offer a three-strand definition: belonging and being part of something successful and synergy, a common objective or purpose, and being able to achieve more collectively than as individuals outside the teamwork setting.

teamwork
a group of identified professionals working together to achieve a specific outcome or set of outcomes

Collaboration

Collaboration can be defined as being 'A respect for other professionals and service users and their skills and from this starting point, an agreed sharing of authority, responsibility and resources aimed at specific outcomes or actions, and gained through cooperation and consensus' (McCray, 2007, p. 132).

These principles should be clear not just to the individual team members, but also to all those contributing to the team activity. Equally, team members should be working to meet the same goals or objectives for service users, patients or clients.

Effective collaboration requires mutual support and space for disagreement or the exploration of different views to take place. Part of the process of collaboration is deciding when it is needed and when individual team members can make autonomous decisions. In emergency situations, for example, there may be limited time for collaboration, but this does not stop collaboration occurring in emergency or crisis intervention work. Instead, team members may need to develop protocols or guidelines that take into account the decision-making process so that these guidelines can be followed in difficult situations or circumstances.

collaboration
a term to describe working together. The use of the term 'collaboration' often suggests that there may be conflict present and that the work may at times be difficult

Factors affecting teamwork

Although, from the definition, the route to teamwork may seem straightforward, it is in reality a more complicated process. Many factors can influence the ability of a team to practise effective cooperation, all of these occurring in the changing context of health and social-care practice. Important among these factors are financial constraints, team support, endorsement and professional boundaries.

Financial

When budgets and resources are constrained, the issues of cost and who will foot the bill for intervention can create tension within teams. Practitioners at ground level often wish to work collaboratively to solve problems with service users, but the managers who hold the budgets may be constrained and less able to be facilitative, perhaps placing restrictions on the amount of collaboration that takes place.

Team support

A key factor in team development is that of coordination, and resources may once again influence the level of support. Teams need accountable individuals to help the problem-solving process and take practice-focused solutions forward. These individuals may be identified as leaders or coordinators. Those teams lacking leadership or coordination are not as likely to achieve effective outcomes for clients. As a result, the cost in terms of an individual leader's time has to be met. Equally, teams require a physical environment in which to meet, as well as scheduled time to discuss problems, evaluate progress and plan future developments. All these have both obvious and hidden cost implications. Technological changes mean that people may also work in virtual teams with limited face-to-face contact, which can change communication and patterns of interaction. New strategies for leading such teams may be required.

Endorsing teamwork

Team members need to be able to see the benefits of a team-based model of care. When professionals are under pressure to maintain their current workload, finding time for additional means of collaborating and reviewing their current practice may seem yet another, and somewhat onerous, task. However, a review of the outcomes of child protection cases, including Baby Peter (Laming, 2009) show that even more attention to follow up and team collaboration is required by all professionals. The lynchpin of good practice may thus be evaluation as this enables team members to consider the effectiveness of their intervention and whether it has achieved the outcome that was anticipated. Balancing the results of the intervention against the time and cost involved may help team members to decide on the relevance of the team activity they have undertaken. Team members may need to consider the best use of their time together and set priorities, all of which may change following review. As teams work together over a longer period of time, they may be able to make decisions more swiftly, but ongoing evaluation may help them to decide whether such teamwork processes ensure the best outcomes for service users or patients.

Professional boundaries

For teamwork to be centred on clear outcomes for service users, clients and patients, team members need to be clear about the nature of their role within the team and what the boundaries of that role are. In other words, they need to ask what their professional role is, and where it ends and becomes the responsibility of a different professional. Hudson (1999, 2007) notes the significance of professional boundaries and the need for clarity with regard to professional roles and models of care. What practice activity, for example, is defined as core and to be taken on by all members, and what is seen as specific and thus the role of one discipline? Do differing approaches to practice, for example the **medical** versus the **social model** of care, impact on collaboration? Without clarifying the roles, team members may drift towards a common ground, which means that some areas of practice can be neglected.

The changing role of the Registered Nurse for People with Learning Disabilities (RNLD) illustrates this. In practice RNLDs may be the leaders of care when there is physical long-term care to be provided, for a person with learning disabilities. Other professionals, however, working in primary care may not know about the RNLD role or how to access these nurses and may also have statutory responsibility for meeting the needs of this group of people as in the case of social workers. Consequently people with learning disabilities and their families may miss out on a significant resource, and other professionals who could gain from the experience and knowledge of an RNLD might also remain uninformed. McCray's research (2003) has shown that health-care relationships are only one aspect of the role of the RNLDs and collaboration with social workers and social work teams and other professional groups was also important. It is, however, how this collaboration across disciplines takes place that will impact on the final outcomes for people with learning disabilities and their families.

A lack of clarity about the content and nature of other professions' roles can create significant barriers to good practice. These need to be overcome or acknowledged by both those working in teams and those coordinating them. Other elements under the heading of professional socialisation can also inhibit or sustain good working practices.

Professional Socialisation

Individuals' socialisation into and integration within a specific professional group may impact upon their ability to work within an interprofessional team. When a person enters a career pathway with the intention of registering as a professional nurse, for example, a key element of the process is that of **professional socialisation** into the role. This may include guidelines on what clothing to wear in practice, the particular skills and competencies learnt in the common foundation programme and the way in which the client or patient is described, all manifesting themselves in how the learner develops the role or identity of a nurse. Similar processes will occur in all professional groups, a consequence being that when teamwork is practised, such factors may impinge on team integration. Some specific elements of professional socialisation are language, values and professional status.

Interprofessional education

While you may have undergone a significant professional socialisation in your first few weeks in nursing, you may well have also shared formal interprofessional learning about practice in health care with other students in training, for example

medical model
based on a biomedical response to the service user

social model
focusing on the response of wider society to people with disability

★ Activity 17.2

Think again about your recent practice experience. What sort of formal and informal methods of evaluation have you seen? How effective have they been? Consider, for example, reading case notes or care plans, or review meetings within social care agencies.

professional socialisation
the process of taking on a set of values and an identity that are associated with and underpin a particular profession

★ Activity 17.3

Think about your first weeks of nurse education. What activities formed part of the socialisation process? Were you aware of this process at the time?

foundation modules in communication or observed practice of basic support skills. This process enables you to gain insight into how other professionals work and the different and shared challenges they face. The Centre for Advancement of Interprofessional Education (CAIPE) (2007) defines interprofessional education (IPE) as 'occasions where two or more professions learn with and from each other to improve collaboration and quality care'. Studies of IPE undertaken have included attempts to identify the impact of interprofessional education on: preparing for practice, practice outcomes, and how organisations work (Clifton et al., 2006, p. 13). However, these processes are complex to measure and it can be difficult to specify the nature of the effect of an educational experience on patient or service user outcomes. Barr et al. (2005) undertook a systematic review of IPE and found it gave professionals a positive model of interaction, encouraged collaboration and improved patient/ service user care (Howkins, 2008). More evaluation of IPE is being undertaken to attempt to gain further understanding and commonality of good practice in the health-care sector.

Language

A vocabulary of terminology and abbreviations is used continuously within each professional group to communicate information, and the language involved may be unique to that profession. When teamwork is undertaken, the meaning of particular words and expressions will need clarification. If clarity is not sought, assumptions may be made about the meaning of specific language and actions, one result being conflict or conflicting views when language is interpreted in different ways by those who do not belong to that particular professional group.

Personal values

value
something that an individual holds at the centre of his or her being, developed over time and from experience

A **value** is something that individuals hold at the centre of their being. Values are developed over time and from experience, and personal values may reflect an individual's culture, moral stance or lifestyle. Values may be a product of age or historical tradition. Such values may be translated into action through the development of specific views or attitudes, either positive or negative. Values held may suggest that all individuals have the right to the same opportunities, for example that all people with learning disability should be part of ordinary community life. In this case, attitudes, shown in terms of behaviour, could be acting as an independent advocate for an individual when the person needs help with communicating his wishes. In contrast, attitudes may remain observable only in terms of how positively or negatively an individual views a person or situation.

Activity 17.4

What do you think the values of the nurse are? What are these values based on? Do they differ from your own?

Professional values

Link

Chapter 1 discusses care planning.

In addition to personal values, individuals who participate in professional education may also develop a further set of values, and there may be assumptions made within teams about the values of the different professional groups. All are working towards similar goals for the service user, ideally in partnership with that person, but values may in reality be different. Social work may, for example, be concerned with interprofessional practice and achieving outcomes for service users based on a recognition of oppression and inequality in society, and the care plan or care management assessment set in place might reflect this. Equally, physiotherapists may be focused on physiological factors that inhibit good health for service users. In working towards collaborative practice, discussion based on values and what they mean to individual professions may work towards an understanding of professional action. Parton and O'Byrne (2000, p. 5 cited in McCray, 2009), observe 'we cannot assume that our ways of understanding are necessarily the same as others'.

Interprofessional values

Loxley (1997) describes the core values of interprofessional work as trust and sharing. She uses the word **utilitarian**, that is, being or having practical worth, to endorse their validity in teamwork. Essential components of trust and sharing are that they must remain two-way. This means not only relying on people's commitment to the team's purpose or task, but also taking on the team members' belief in themselves as being able to deliver the goods or take on the role, and meeting these expectations. Achieving the ability to trust others and to share practice with them will require confidence and a clear understanding of one's own professional role, which may become more complex when individuals are of a different status.

utilitarian
a solution that aims for the greater good, one which has a practical outcome

Ethics

Interprofessional practice may bring to the fore ethical dilemmas in the practice setting. Cranmer and McCray (2009) for example, describe potential areas of conflict between professions. Medical professionals will have as their highest priority respect for the life of the patient, whereas a social worker's major concern will be the wishes of the clients themselves. This could lead to conflict over issues regarding the clinical treatment of individuals and the giving of information particularly if they are already unwell or have a mental illness or learning disability. Child protection work can also create ethical dilemmas if the needs of the child conflict with those of other family members at home. Nurses too can be involved in a range of complex situations, for example when planning discharge for older people. There may be a difference between the wishes of the older person in question and the family members. The older person may wish to go home, whereas the family may think a nursing home more appropriate. As a nurse, whose wishes do you act upon?

Status

For teams to work effectively, mutual trust and a respect for all members' contributions to the team are required. This trust is achieved partly by having a greater understanding of the key role of other professional groups and acknowledging the differences and similarities in language, values and models of practice used by other professions. The team coordinator or leader should facilitate this process as a model for teamwork is developed.

Nurses have traditionally been seen as semi-autonomous practitioners working to guidelines drawn up by medical staff; doctors have been seen as making autonomous clinical decisions and advising other members of the health care and social-care teams on practice. Speech therapists and physiotherapists, although autonomous practitioners, work largely on an individual basis with clients, advising on very specific areas of intervention. Because of these differences, power and status may become an issue when teamwork is undertaken. Equally, models of service delivery are changing and Baxter and Brumfitt (2008) observe that there is a need for new understandings of professional relationships. Interprofessional stereotypes may still remain, however (Mandy et al., 2004) and doctors, for example, may still be seen as having difficulty taking advice from other health-care professionals, whereas nurses may be viewed as lacking the confidence to advise or provide information related to a specific area of practice. Social workers' views of good practice in mental health services may clash with a more medically orientated response from a consultant psychiatrist. All this can influence the way in which teams function and create future stress for team members.

Good Practice in Teamwork

At this point, nursing practice in an interprofessional context may seem complex and to be avoided at all costs! Nevertheless, having realistic expectations of teamwork may help the nurse to prepare for practice with greater confidence and maintain a focus on what is significant to the outcomes for the client or service user. Some reasons for this are as follows.

Knowledge

Knowledge that identifies some probable causes of friction within the teamwork setting can help to make sense of difficulties and begin to shape the problem-solving process; in other words, to help the practitioner to find a workable solution to the situation. Because of the knowledge held, an acceptance of team members' differences and different contributions to teamwork can lead to a gradual mutual trust. This will in turn contribute towards a working environment in which it is safe to air conflict or state different opinions. A further spin-off will be the prevention of isolation and an increased willingness to share information.

Methods of practice intervention

The responses to a client's or service user's needs may differ across a range of different professionals. A medical model approach may favour giving information and a course of treatment to individuals; this model may be used by doctors. Some nurses may also adopt an information-giving role. Increasingly professionals must respond to a more partnership-based model of practice, seen for example, as Oliver (1996) suggests, where the professional is viewed as a resource to be used by the particular service user. In other words, the client or individual service user will direct the professional's approach, personally requesting specific information, action and responses. This approach is developing within social work and care management-type roles and is explored in the service development part of the Green Paper on social care (DoH, 2005b and in *Our Health Our Care Our Say,* DoH, 2006). It is also central to the Personal Health Budget First Steps Pilots in Primary and Community Care (DoH, 2009a) where people opt to plan their own health care and manage their budget themselves or through a support arrangement. The different models of practice of different professional groups can lead to an inconsistency of information for the service user and cause greater confusion. The teamwork process based on collaboration should, however, provide a framework within which issues such as what information should be given and the level of commitment required by each professional are clearly stated and agreed.

Pritchard (1995) adopts Bruce's (1980) 'teamwork for presentation' matrix to identify stages of team cooperation (Table 17.1). Pritchard's matrix illustrates the steps toward the committed team by describing cooperation in a range of teamwork activities. The main use of this tool has been in the assessment or diagnosis of a team's current position. Here it is used to give an example of what could be achieved within the teamwork setting. Moreover, as Pritchard (1995) notes, there is a need to link teamwork performance to outcomes for service users and, as such, to begin to meet need.

> ✳ **Activity 17.5**
>
> What skills are required to share differing opinions with others? How can these be used?

Table 17.1 Stages of team cooperation

Cooperation in:	'Nominal'	'Convenient'	'Committed'
Team goal-setting	No explicit goals	Follow doctors' goals	Shared explicit goals
Role perceptions	Stereotypes common	Some understanding	Roles clearly understood
Professional status	Wide differences	Differences inhibit co-operation	Differences ignored
Referral of patients	To agency rather than individual professionals	Referral by delegation	Easy two-way referral and open access
Interaction within team	Very little and irregular interaction	Some interaction	Close regular interaction, formal and informal
Mutual trust	Lacking	Guarded	Strong and developing
Communication failure	Often	Sometimes	Exceptional
Confidentiality	A problem	Problems partly solved	Not a problem
Advice to patients	Inconsistent	Poor coordination	Consistent
Preventative care	Not possible	Possible	Optimum conditions

Source: Modified from Bruce (1980).

Meeting need

In a team where conflict is aired, different occupational roles are understood and valued, and individual members feel safe to share differing views, steps can be taken towards clear mutual goals. These can help the teamwork forward, preventing obstruction and confronting difficult issues. This is not easy as services change and may become more complex. Anning et al. (2006) note that the impact of changing practice and team roles can make some team members feel unconfident. Payne (2000) suggests that, as a starting point to meeting need, the team must be able to identify agreed objectives and be able to articulate and resolve differences. Finally, the team must be able to manage interpersonal issues – how the team feel about each other – and make a commitment to teamwork. In learning to manage all of these factors, the needs of service users or clients can remain central to the team's purpose.

Working in Teams

So far this chapter has reviewed some of the factors that can affect teamwork, these being generic in setting and content. In this section, the role of the primary health-care team will be explored to provide a specific example of teamwork and multiprofessional practice.

What is the primary health-care team?

primary health care
the continuing health and social welfare care offered appropriately to individuals in need living in private households

In the foreword to the summary of the White Paper *Primary Care: Delivering the Future* (DOH, 1996), **primary health care** was described as 'the NHS most people see – the NHS of the family doctor and their team, community nurses, therapists as well as pharmacists, dentists and optometrists'. It will also include midwives, district nurses and health visitors. Since the implementation of the White Paper *The New NHS: Modern, Dependable* (DOH, 1997), the role of the primary care team has continued to develop and grow: traditional teams based around health centres may now include counsellors and mental health nurses, and social workers will be involved in areas such as child protection and provision for older people. Plans set in place by the 1996 White Paper expanded the role of the nurse in learning further skills, such as prescribing medication. Equally, the role of the practice nurse has expanded to take on referrals from people who would ordinarily have seen their GP. In addition, the new strategy for people with learning disabilities, *Valuing People* (DoH, 2001c and 2009b), highlights the relationship between the primary health-care team and other services in meeting the ongoing health-care needs of this group of people as one means of preventing social exclusion.

How it has evolved

Jeffereys (1995) wrote that, as a result of the Family Doctors Charter (BMA, 1965) in 1966, arrangements were set in place for positive community-based practice. This charter established a positive role for non-hospital-based medicine, a structure for interprofessional work being instigated. Jeffereys identified the elements of this structure as allowances for GPs who worked together on one site, and promoting the employment of receptionists and practice nurses, by providing reimbursement for their services, and offering interest-free loans for more modern premises. The Health Services and Public Health Act 1968 endorsed a health promotion role for general practice that involved the prevention of ill-health and support for families. Thus, the role of the primary health-care team gradually emerged.

Further changes were to occur in the 1980s as the Conservative government set about cutting the increasing public expenditure. Pietroni (1994) reported that the White Paper *Priorities for Health and Social Services in England* (DHSS, 1976) and the *NHS Management Inquiry* (DoH, 1983) were to culminate in the NHS and Community Care Act 1990 (DoH, 1990). These placed further responsibilities for care within the primary care team, making it the first point of call for all referrals. The introduction of the General Medical Services contract (BMA, 2003) has changed the way in which GPs are funded and their quality and performance measured in relation to specific targets for the nation's health. Services have continued to change as GP practices may now both commission services and deliver them as commissioned through their PCT.

These developments maintain the place of the GP at the centre of decision-making within the primary health-care team although increasingly other professionals, such as practice nurses, might take on the direct assessment and management role of patients with chronic disease such as diabetes. Chart 17.1 highlights the key developments within primary health-care nursing practice.

Chart 17.1 Key developments in primary-care nursing

District nursing

1970s	Introduction of attachment schemes
	District nurses based at GP practices. Established primary health-care teams
1972	Report of the Committee on Nursing made recommendations for formal post-basic education, which became law in 1979
1974	Royal College of General Practitioners published *Nursing in General Practice in the Reorganised NHS* (RCGP, 1974)
1990s	Extended role of the district nurse may include the prescribing of medication, previously the task of the GP
	Review of educational requirements of the role as part of the English National Board specialist pathway curricula
21st Century	As professionals in primary care trusts, guidance in the delivery of the NHS plan (DOH, 2002)

- Further development of prescribing role with potential for selection and training as independent prescribers.
- Support for development of palliative care role as part of *NHS Cancer Plan* (DOH, 2001d)
- *Agenda for Change* and NHS Plan and Knowledge and Skills Framework (NHS KSF) offers transparent criteria for professional role development (DOH, 2004b).

Practice nursing

1970s	Nurses attached to GP practice
1986	Cumberlege Report, *Neighbourhood Nursing: A Focus for Care* (DHSS, 1986)
	Recommended development of the nurse practitioner role – taking on direct referrals to ease the pressure on GPs
1987	Government rejected these plans
1990s	Role of practice nurses under review
1996	White Paper *Primary Care: Delivering the Future* (DoH, 1996) advocates major changes to practice nurse education and role within the primary health-care team

1998   Configuration of primary care groups may mean changes in the practice nurse role

21st century   As primary care trust professionals, opportunity to develop specialist clinical skills in primary care settings (DOH, 2003).

- Change in role and responsibility created by the GMS Contract offers opportunity for further specialism (DOH, 2003)
- Potential outcome of *Agenda for Change* and *NHS Knowledge and Skills Framework* (NHS KSF) (DOH, 2004b) for this group of nurses not yet fully developed although may offer positive development opportunities (McCray, 2005).

Health visiting

1976   Court Report identified the health visitor as a major agent of prevention in family work (Orr, 1975)

1970s and 80s Central Council for the Education and Training of Health Visitors continued to assess the role of the health visitor, especially when the focus on child protection and children at risk increased

1980   Standing conference on health visitor education, A Time to Learn, looked at the changing role of health visiting

1990s   Role still unclear. Purchaser concern with cost of health visitor intervention

1998   Configuration of primary care groups may mean changes in the role of the health visitor

21st century   *Agenda for Change* and NHS Knowledge and Skills Framework offers transparent criteria for professional role development (DOH, 2004a) for professionals in primary care trusts.

- Current green paper on children's services, *Every Child Matters* (DOH, 2005a) may further develop collaborative role. Health visitors could be employed in newly configured children's trusts. Quality services in the community

As part of the NHS modernisation agenda, the primary health-care team (PHCT) is continuing to face the challenge of effective teamwork and the need to develop further professional roles. The government's aim to achieve a seamless service remains, in order that clients and patients are not seen by a vast number of different professionals and to prevent their continual assessment and attendance at different clinics. An emphasis on developing primary health care remains a top priority, based on local needs. One of the key quality functions in primary care will be that of *monitoring service quality* using a range of measures including **clinical audit** outcomes to ensure that effective, high-quality care is offered to a specific local population.

clinical audit
measuring the quality of care and services against agreed standards and making improvements where necessary (see www.hqip.org.uk/our-programmes)

Role of the professional within the primary health-care team

There are still decisions to be made about further extended roles for nurses and how these will contribute to the PHCT. Equally, the need to use resources effectively remains an issue. Also unanswered is why there is still an ongoing need to re-emphasise interprofessional teamwork when PHCTs have been in existence for more than 25 years. Teamwork should be seen as an essential part of working together, yet some gaps still exist. Some broad reasons for the difficulties encountered in teamwork were raised earlier in the chapter. If we look specifically at PHCTs, all the factors identified may inhibit good practice, but it is worth looking at this point at some further constraints on teamwork within PHCTs:

- *Location:* It is probable that the core members of the primary health-care team are situated on one site within a local health centre. Other professionals, such as social workers, who provide an input to the team may, however, be based at different locations. As a consequence, they may miss out on informal contact and lines of communication.
- *Team size*: Within the primary health-care team, a range of individual professionals may be involved in both commissioning and providing services,

and the size and extent of this may impact on team development. Too large a team may prevent clear and focused discussion and inhibit the decision-making process. Examples of this may be seen in the child protection and mental health services.

- *Payment*: Individual professionals working as part of the primary health-care team will be employed on different rates of pay and conditions of service. This could lead to a feeling of resentment among some team members.
- *Resource management*: Within the primary health-care team, responsibility for practice and performance may not be clearly identified. In some teams, GPs may be the decision-makers when bidding for funding for the commissioning of services. In contrast, practice nurses and other nurse practitioners may have limited financial or budgetary control. Although individual practitioners may see themselves as autonomous, issues such as payment performance targets and access to resources, can lead to an inequality of status, and individual contributors to teamwork may as a consequence be seen as being of more or less value.

In the changing climate of primary care, in which GPs have greater financial autonomy, the position of other professionals may be under greater scrutiny, for example when making decisions about the effectiveness of the input of various professionals and, in doing so, questioning roles and performance. Part of this process may lead to a narrowing down of certain roles and a limited input of some professionals to primary health-care teams. Such activities may restrict good teamwork.

Moving towards Cooperation

The position of interprofessional work currently remains uncertain. Pockets of good practice are observable, but mutual cooperation and the desires of service users can be in conflict with government policy, the way in which funding mechanisms operate, and the struggle for power of some professional groups (Figure 17.1).

There are more challenges ahead for professionals who must respond to the needs of the population with Alzheimer's disease as part of the National Dementia strategy (DoH, 2009c). New care pathways will bring together primary care, the third sector and intermediate care services and new partnerships will emerge across all sectors in both the delivery and commissioning of services.

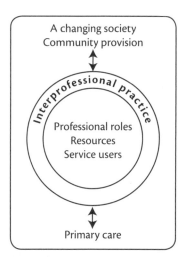

Figure 17.1 Factors affecting interprofessional work

Responses to Teamworking

Research reports and networks

A considerable amount of research and evaluation has been undertaken in the area of teamwork in primary health and social care. In the 1980s many of the findings of studies focusing on primary health-care settings were negative, and the reluctance to collaborate of some specific professional groups, such as doctors, is well documented. More recently, however, the value of interprofessional work has become the focus of research and evaluation. A significant number of international projects and national reports have been published that focus on the value of collaboration, and how to collaborate more effectively. These include:

- *Taking your Partners: Using Opportunities for Interagency Partnership in Mental Health* (Sainsbury Centre for Mental Health, 2000).
- *Towards a Common Cause – A Compact for Care: Inspection of local Authority Social Services and Voluntary Sector Working Relationships* (DoH, 2000b).
- *Securing Better Mental Health for Older Adults* (DoH, 2005c).
- *Creating an Interprofessional Workforce* (CAIPE and DoH, 2006).
- *Walk the Talk* (CAIPE and DoH, 2007). This builds on the 2006 report above. This report examines the culture in which interprofessional work takes place and how to sustain positive practices.
- *The L-Tipp Project* (Lee et al., 2009). This Australian project focused on developing interprofessional capability in the Australian Health and Social Care workforce.

A number of global interprofessional networks exist which focus on all issues related to IPE and notably from a research perspective. These include:

- AIPPEN: Australasian Interprofessional Practice and Education Network
- CAIPE: Centre for Advancement and Improvement of Interprofessional Education (UK)
- EIPEN: European Interprofessional Education Network in Health and Social Care (Europe)
- InterED: The International Association for Interprofessional and Collaborative Practice (International based in Canada)
- RIPEN: Rural Inter-Professional Education Network (Australia)

Educational developments

Education has been one response to the interprofessional agenda. Providers of educational programmes have seen educational activity as a route to a greater understanding of the professional roles of others. Most of the activity that has occurred has been at postregistration or post-qualifying level. Individual professionals have come together to share units of study, an emphasis on problem-solving having been developed during the 1990s. Loxley (1997) reproduces a table from the Centre for the Advancement of Interprofessional Education, Primary and Community Care (1996) that gives a detailed review of the coordinating bodies and their activities.

A number of universities and schools of medicine, social work, pharmacology, nursing and midwifery are also developing units or forums for the development of interprofessional practice initiatives, notably the New Generation project between the universities of Southampton and Portsmouth. A range of online networks are also available, and these are cited at the end of the chapter.

Interprofessionalism as a 'theory' for practice

Many of the elements that form interprofessional practice have been brought together in this chapter. Much of this has centred upon teamwork and collaboration, and a review of roles and professional boundaries. We have seen how the developments in community care have created many of these changes. In reality, interprofessionalism has been seen as a set of skills or competencies rather than a whole new way of informing practice, with a theoretical underpinning. For example, from what knowledge base does interprofessional work come? Loxley (1997) suggests that assumptions are made about what knowledge from a certain discipline might be helpful but that this has not been investigated or studied in a coherent way. It is largely driven by what services need, and because of this, a sound theoretical framework has not yet developed.

A number of academics and practitioners are beginning to study and build a theory for interprofessional practice. As this develops, it is possible that those professionals who have been reluctant to make interprofessional practice a priority may begin to participate. One key area of interest is Activity Theory and its application in multi-agency working. Activity Theory focuses on conflict and how it works in organisations and attempts to explain this within a time of change in services. It is concerned with what happens (processes and communication) in interprofessional practice and how we learn to work together (Hean et al., 2006). Daniels (2005) use Activity Theory to explore the contradictions of interprofessional working. For example, when different professionals may be working towards the same goal, yet be measured on different performance outcomes as part of their performance indicators. They suggest that for interprofessional practice to be effective it may be helpful for professionals to explore together the impact these contradictions might have on their engagement and commitment to interprofessional working.

> ⊂⊃ **Link**
>
> Chapter 4 describes an approach to thinking about reflection in a structured and useful way.

Personal responses

The moves forward outlined above tackle complex issues at a societal service and organisational level. An individual in practice can still, however, begin to create change. For a nurse practising in an interprofessional setting, thinking about individual responses to teamwork and reflecting on their cause or foundation may be helpful. Observing professionals who hold effective team member skills may also provide ideas for the development of personal knowledge and skills.

From this perspective, individual methods of working that can help effective teamwork can be shaped. Part of this exercise should include an active consideration of the changing role of service users in the process. No longer is the service user a passive recipient of care, but will be driving decision making and clinical intervention in order to achieve his or her optimum quality of life.

Chapter Summary

The route to interprofessional practice is a complex one. At times, the agendas of government, service managers, professionals and service users seem to be in conflict, but positive examples can nevertheless be seen in practice. As practitioners, educationalists and service managers design the organisational structures needed to develop further multiprofessional work, professionals can build on their skills in collaboration. The interface of health and social care delivery can then become a positive one.

> ### ? Test yourself!
>
> 1 What does the term 'interprofessional practice' mean?
> 2 Provide examples from your own experience of good and bad teamwork.
> 3 How do different professionals contribute to teamworking?
> 4 What challenges does working in a primary health-care team create for the nurse?
> 5 How will personalisation impact on collaborative practice?

References

Anning, A., Cottrell, D.M., Frost, N., Green, J. and Robinson, M. (2006) *Developing Multi-professional Teamwork for Integrated Children's Services*. Open University Press, Buckingham.

Barr, H., Kopppel, I., Reeves, S., Hammick, M. and Freeth, D. (2005) *Effective Interprofessional Education: Argument, Assumption and Evidence*. CAIPE, Blackwell Publishing, London.

Batorowicz, B. and Shepherd, T.A. (2008) Measuring the quality of transdisciplinary teams. *Journal of Interprofessional Care* **22**(6): 612–20.

Baxter, S. and Brumfitt S (2008). Professional differences in interprofessional work. *Journal of Interprofessional Care* **22**(3): 239–51.

BMA (British Medical Association) (1965) *Family Doctors Charter: A Charter for the Family Doctor Service*. BMA, London.

BMA (British Medical Association) (2003) GP Committee of the BMA and the NHS confederation. *Investing in General Practice: The New General Services Contract*. British Medical Association, National Health Service Confederation, London.

British Medical Association, Resuscitation Council (UK) and Royal College of Nursing (2007) *Decisions Relating to Cardiopulmonary Resuscitation*. A joint statement from the British Medical Association, the Resuscitation Council (UK) and the Royal College of Nursing. BMA, London, October.

Bruce, N. (1980) *Teamwork for Preventative Care*. *Research Studies Press*, John Wiley & Sons, Chichester.

CAIPE (Centre for the Advancement of Interprofessional Education, Primary and Community Care) (1996) *National Coordinating Bodies and their Interests*. CAIPE, London.

CAIPE and DoH (Centre for the Advancement of Interprofessional Education and the Department of Health) (2006) *Creating an Interprofessional Workforce*. CAIPE, London.

CAIPE and DoH (Centre for the Advancement of Interprofessional Education and the Department of Health) (2007) *Walk the Talk: Sustainable Change in Post 2000 Interprofessional Learning and Development*. CAIPE, London.

Clifton, M., Dale, C. and Bradshaw, C. (2006) *The Impact and Effectiveness of Inter-professional Education in Primary Care*. Royal College of Nursing, London.

Cook, S. (2009) *Building A High Performance Team*. IT Governance Publishing, Ely.

Cranmer, T. and McCray, J. (2009) Skills for collaborative working. In Mantell, A. (ed.) *Social Work Skills with Adults*. Learning Matters, Exeter.

Daniels, H. (2005) Introduction. In Daniels, H. (ed.) *An Introduction to Vygotsky*. Routledge. London.

DCFS (Department for Children Schools and Families) (2007) *The Children's Plan*. HMSO, London.

DHSS (Department of Health and Social Security) (1976) *Priorities for Health and Personal Social Services in England*. HMSO, London.

DHSS (Department of Health and Social Security) (1986) *Community Nursing Review. Neighborhood Nursing – A Focus for Care*. Cumberlege Report. HMSO, London.

DoH (Department of Health) (1983) *NHS Management Inquiry* (Griffiths Report). HMSO, London.

DoH (Department of Health) (1990) *Caring for People. Community Care in the Next Decade and Beyond*. HMSO, London.

DoH (Department of Health) (1996) *Primary Care: Delivering the Future*. HMSO, London.

DoH (Department of Health) (1997) *The New NHS: Modern, Dependable*. The Stationery Office, Norwich.

DoH (Department of Health) (2000a) *The NHS Plan*. The Stationery Office, Norwich.

DoH (Department of Health) (2000b) *Towards a Common Cause – A Compact for Care: Inspection of Local Authority Social Services and Voluntary Sector Working Relationships*. The Stationery Office, Norwich.

DoH (Department of Health) (2001a) *Primary Care, General Practice and the NHS Plan*. The Stationery Office, Norwich.

DoH (Department of Health) (2001b) *From Vision to Reality*. The Stationery Office, Norwich.

DoH (Department of Health) (2001c) *Valuing People. A New Strategy for Learning Disability in the 21st Century*. The Stationery Office, Norwich.

DoH (Department of Health) (2001d) *The NHS Cancer Plan: Education and Support for District and Community Nurses in the Principles and Practice of Palliative Care Education Initiatives Funded under the Programme*. The Stationery Office, Norwich.

DoH (Department of Health) (2002) *Liberating the Talents – Helping PCTs and Nurses to Deliver the NHS Plan*. The Stationery Office, Norwich.

DoH (Department of Health) (2003) *Practitioners with a Special Interest in Primary Care: Implementing a Service for Nurses with a Special Interest in the Programme. Liberating the Talents*. The Stationery Office, London.

DoH (Department of Health) (2004a) *Agenda for Change Proposed Agreement: September 2004*. Final Draft. The Stationery Office, London.

DoH (Department of Health) (2004b) The National Health Service, Knowledge and Skills Framework (NHS KSF) and the Development review process. Draft Document. The Stationery Office, London.

DoH (Department of Health) (2005a) *Every Child Matters*. Green Paper. The Stationery Office, London.

DoH (Department of Health) (2005b) *Independence Well Being and Choice: Our Vision for the Future of Social Care in England*. Green Paper. The Stationery Office, London.

DoH (Department of Health) (2005c) *Securing Better Mental Health for Older Adults*. The Stationery Office, London.

DoH (Department of Health) (2006) *Our Health Our Care Our Say*. The Stationery Office, London.

DoH (Department of Health) (2007a) *Commissioning Framework for Health and Wellbeing*. The Stationery Office, London.

DoH (Department of Health) (2007b) *The Local Government and Public Involvement Health Act*. Department of Health, London.

DoH (Department of Health) (2008a) *Putting People First*. Department of Health, London.

DoH (Department of Health) (2008b) *High Quality Care for All*. NHS Next Stage Review Final Report. The Stationery Office, Norwich.

DoH (Department of Health) (2009a) *Personal Health Budgets: First Steps*. The Stationery Office, London.

DoH (Department of Health) (2009b) *Valuing People Now: A New Three Year Strategy for People with Learning Disabilities*. The Stationery Office, Norwich.

DoH (Department of Health) (2009c) *Living Well with Dementia: A National Dementia Strategy*. The Stationery Office, London.

Fisher, R. (2009) Multi-professional practice in primary care nursing. In McCray, J. (ed.) *Nursing and Multi-professional Practice*. Sage, London.

Garner, H.G. and Orelove, F.P. (1994) *Teamwork in Human Services. Models and Application across the Life Span*. Butterworth Heinemann, Boston.

Gilmour, M., Bruce, N. and Hunt, M. (1974) *The Work of the Nursing Team in General Practice*. Council for the Education and Training of Health Visitors, London.

Greenhalgh and Company (1994) *The Interface Between Junior Doctors and Nurses: A Research Study for the Department of Health*. HMSO, London.

Hean, S., Macleod Clark, J., Adams, K. and Humphris, D. (2006) Will opposites attract? Similarities and difference in students perceptions of the stereotype profiles of other health and social care professional groups. *Journal of Interprofessional Care* **20**(2): 162–82.

Howkins, E. and Bray, J. (2008) *Preparing for Interprofessional Teaching: Theory and Practice*. Radcliffe, Oxford.

Hudson, B. (1999) Primary health care and social care: working across professional boundaries. *Managing Community Care* **7**(1): 15–22.

Hudson, B. (2007) The Sedgfield Integrated Team. *Journal of Interprofessional Care* **21**(1).

Jeffereys, M. (1995) Primary health care. In Owens, P., Carrier, C. and Horder, J. (eds) *Interprofessional Issues in Community and Primary Health Care*. Macmillan, Basingstoke.

Laming, The Lord (2009) *The Protection of Children in England: A Progress Report*. The Stationery Office, London.

Leathard, A. (2003) *Interprofessional Collaboration from Policy to Practice in Health and Social Care*. Brunner and Routledge, Hove.

Lee, A., Dunston, R., Nisbet, G., Matthews, L. and Pockett, R. (2009) Interprofessional developments in Australia – L-TIPP (Aus) and the Way Forward. *Journal of Interprofessional Care* **23**(4): 315–17.

Loxley, A. (1997) *Collaboration in Health and Welfare*. Jessica Kingsley, London.

Malin, N. and Morrow, G. (2007) Models of interprofessional working within a Sure Start 'Trailblazer' programme. *Journal of Interprofessional Care* **21**(4): 445–57.

Mandy, A., Milton, C. and Mandy, P. (2004) Professional stereotyping and interprofessional education. *Learning in Health and Social Care* **3**(3): 154–70.

Marshall, M., Preston, M., Scott, E. and Wincott, P. (eds) (1979) *Teamwork for and Against: An Appraisal of Multidisciplinary Practice*. British Association of Social Workers, London.

McCray, J. (2003) *Leading interprofessional practice: a conceptual framework to support practitioners in the field of learning disability. Journal of Nursing Management 11: 387–95.*

McCray, J. (2005) Personal and people development for practice nurses. *BMJ ELearning*.

McCray, J. (2007) Reflective practice for collaborative working. In Scragg, T. and Knott, C. (eds) *Reflective Practice in Social Work*. Learning Matters, Exeter.

McCray, J. (2009) *Nursing and Multiprofessional Practice*. Sage, London.

Oliver, M. (1996) *Social Work: Disabled People and Disabling Environments. Jessica Kingsley, London*.

Orr, J. (1975) Health visiting in the UK. In Hockey, L. (ed.) *Primary Care Nursing*. Churchill Livingstone, London.

Owens, P. and Petch, H. (1995) Professionals and management. In Owens, P., Carrier, J. and Horder, J. (eds) *Interprofessional Issues in Community and Primary Health Care*. Palgrave Macmillan, Basingstoke.

Parton, N. and O'Byrne, P. (2000) *Constructive Social Work: Towards a New Practice*. Palgrave Macmillan, Basingstoke.

Payne, M. (2000) *Teamwork and Multiprofessional Care*. Palgrave Macmillan, Basingstoke.

Pietroni, P. (1994) Interprofessional teamwork. In Leatherhead, A. (ed.) *Going Inter-professional*. Routledge, London.

Pritchard, P. (1995) Learning to work effectively in teams. In Owens, P., Carrier, J. and Horder, J. (eds) *Interprofessional Issues in Community and Primary Health Care*. Palgrave Macmillan, Basingstoke.

RCGP (Royal College of General Practitioners) (1974) *Nursing in General Practice in the Re-organised NHS*. RCGP, London.

Rubin, I.R. and Beckhard, R. (1972) Factors influencing the effectiveness of health teams. *Millbank Memorial Fund Quarterly* **50**(3): 317–37.

Sainsbury Centre for Mental Health (2000) *Taking your partners: using opportunities for interagency partnership in mental health*. Sainsbury Centre for Mental Health, London.

Scragg, T. (2009) Nursing, multi-professional practice and the third sector. In McCray, J. (ed.) *Nursing and Multi-professional Practice*. Sage, London.

UKCC (United Kingdom Central Council for Nursing, Midwifery and Health Visiting) (1992) *The Scope of Professional Practice*. UKCC, now NMC London.

World Health Organisation (2010) *Framework for Action on Interprofessional Education and Collaborative Practice*. WHO, Geneva.

Public Health in Nursing

📖 Contents

☑ Learning outcomes

This chapter will provide a working definition of public health, the underpinning science of epidemiology and health before examining the knowledge and skills increasingly required of the nurse to meet the Health Service agenda of providing a quality health service that aims to prevent ill health and demonstrate that through multi-agency and interprofessional working the public can be supported in leading healthier lives. At the end of this chapter you should be able to:

- Describe the contribution of the nurse to public health activity
- Identify the purpose of a health needs assessment and the contribution of the nurse
- Define policy, evidence-based practice and clinical effectiveness in public health activity
- Have understanding of the skills required to deliver public health activity for health improvement and health protection.

Introduction

The chapter will discuss and analyse the contribution of the nurse to public health within the nine identified areas of public health activity, four core areas and five defined (non-core) areas (Skills for Health and Public Health Resource Unit 2008). These nine areas will be used as a framework for the chapter and related to the public health activities of the nurse. The four core public health areas are those identified as the ones all nurses need and the five defined areas relate to specific contexts within which the nurse may practise (see Table 18.1).

Table 18.1 Core areas of public health activity and defined (non-core) areas

Core areas of public health activity	Defined (non-core areas)
• Surveillance and assessment of the population's health and well-being • Assessing the evidence of effectiveness of health, health care and health-related interventions, programmes and services • Policy and strategy development and implementation • Leadership and collaborative working for health and well-being	• Health improvement • Health protection • Public health intelligence • Academic public health • Health and social care quality

Source: Skills for Health and Public Health Resource Unit (2008). Reproduced under the Open Government Licence v1.0.

Working definition of public health

Wanless (2004, p. 27) defines public health as 'the science and art of preventing disease, prolonging life and promoting health through the organised efforts and informed choices of society, organisations, public and private communities and individuals'. Within this definition public health can be described as the over-arching term for enabling activities that involve interactions around the health of populations, communities, groups of people, families and individuals.

For the nurse this involves all the people they come into contact with during their every day activities. The public health aspect of their role involves the nurse in enabling people to achieve optimum health. This is undertaken through health surveillance, assessment, monitoring, planning, managing and evaluation of the health status. This approach is seen as a fundamental part of good practice with the purpose of improving the health and well-being of the population, preventing disease and minimising its consequences, prolonging valued life and reducing inequalities in health (Skills for Health, 2008).

Working definition – epidemiology

Epidemiology is the science that underpins all public health activity. It is the study of disease in populations rather than individuals (Bailey et al., 2005). It is characterised by the 'study of the distribution and determinants of health, related states or events in specified populations, and the application of this study to control health problems' (Last, 2001, p. 14). An epidemiological approach defines needs in terms of statistics that measure the amount of ill health in the community (**morbidity** and **mortality statistics**).

Working definition – health

The concept of health has been defined in a number of different ways over the last sixty years (World Health Organisation (WHO), 1946; Aggleton, 1991; Ewles and Simnett, 1999; Naidoo and Wills, 2005). The broad concept of health as set out in the WHO constitution in 1946 defines health as 'a state of complete physical, mental and social wellbeing not merely the absence of disease or infirmity'. This identifies the factors that must be considered in assessing health, but it does not identify or acknowledge the levels of health that individuals may experience during their lifespan (Porter and Watkinson, 2007) or explain the criteria for recognising health as a positive human experience.

The socialisation aspects of health cannot be underestimated and typically reflects the wide variations in communities where both young and old live. Each individual has their own idea about health which will be mediated, for example by their own experiences, learnt patterns of behaviour and from key influences on their lives, such as family, school, employment or unemployment. Health is also inextricably linked to the way people live their lives and the opportunities available for choosing health in the communities where they live.

While the WHO definition has been widely criticized as presenting an unobtainable goal it shows the distinction between negative and positive aspects of health: negative in respect of involving the absence of disease or infirmity and positive in respect of entailing the presence of the positive quality of well-being.

Raymond (2005) suggests that definitions of health can be viewed from the following four perspectives:

1   Biomedical – emphasising medical interventions as a way of preventing and treating disease and concerned with an individual's capacity to function.
2   Behavioural – emphasising the individual's responsibility for health influencing behaviour.
3   Social – with a focus on the political and social determinants of health and emphasising social justice.
4   Postmodernist – in which the adequacy of perspectives 1–3 suggests that no one theory can sufficiently explain the health experience.

It is important to remember that health is more than the physical aspects and more than just the absence of disease. It is a multidimensional (holistic) phenomenon, that is, the focus is on the total person and health should be viewed in the context of both internal and external environments. The first challenge for the nurse is in the assessment of the population's health and well-being.

---

morbidity statistics
being number of cases of a specific disease in a specified period of time

mortality statistics
death rate

✦ Activity 18.1

Define what being healthy means for you as:
- A student
- A mother/daughter or a father/son
- A partner/sister/ brother
- Male or female
- A member of the community in which you live.

Surveillance and Assessment of the Population's Health and Well-being: Core Area 1

The surveillance and assessment of the population's health and well-being is a purposeful activity focused on health. It is non-stigmatizing giving the nurse the opportunity to develop insight into people's perception of their health and how they experience it (profiling). There are four main areas of practice where the nurse is involved in profiling the population's health and well-being.

1 Community profiling – an assessment of need within a neighbourhood, district or community hospital.
2 Caseload profiling – an assessment of need within a specific caseload of a nurse (for example long-term conditions, child health promotion, palliative care).
3 A school health profile – a framework to support school-based partnerships (for example drop-in clinics), establish the health profile of the school community.
4 Practice profiling – assessing the need within a general practitioner population.

By developing profiles of the health and well-being of the population the nurse can bring together local information, relevant epidemiological data and needs as expressed by individuals and their local community (see Table 18.2). This approach involves the use of **quantitative** and **qualitative** assessment methods to assess the population's health and well-being and it includes the management, analysis, interpretation and communication of information that relates to the determinants of health and well-being, needs and outcomes. The premise is that this is a purposeful activity focused on the health of the population.

The nurse has contact with different populations while carrying out their work, which provides the opportunity for them to observe and assess the health of people as they experience it (Coles and Porter, 2008). There are a number of populations they could be working with in each of these areas.

The assessment of need

Once the population is identified an assessment of their health and social needs can be carried out. The assessment of need is about finite resources and effective services with a needs assessment being fundamental to planning services for populations, communities, families and individuals.

The assessment of need involves the identification of threats to health and existing health problems, as well as the positive factors that enable people to remain healthy within situations of vulnerability and deprivation. Groups can include some or all of those identified in Activity 18.2. By undertaking a needs assessment, the nurse is able to demonstrate the nature of their difficulties including inappropriate or inadequate services or the lack of awareness of their own health needs. Information gained from this assessment can be used to inform the

---

✸ Activity 18.2

List examples of the populations you could be dealing with? Answer to include:

1. A geographical area (town or an electoral ward, suburb of a city, inner city area, deprived area or housing estate.

2. An institution such as school, nursing home, workplace or prison, a general medical practice or health centre, children in a children's centre, children in a playgroup, adults in a community hospital, people over 85 years of age at a community centre.

3. Social experiences: teenage mothers living in a specific geographical area, homeless families living in bed and breakfast accommodation, travelling families living on allocated caravan sites.

4. Experiences of particular medical conditions: coronary heart disease, strokes, mental illness, cancer.

Table 18.2 Three dimensions of a community

Geographic location	Social construct	Population
Boundaries	Health of the people	Demography
Access to health services	Family structures	Vital statistics
Geographic features	Economic sustainability	Size of population
Climate	Education provision	Density
Ecology	Religions	Composition
Housing	Local government services	Cultural differences
Local Services	Politics	Social class
	Leisure	Occupations
	Communication networks	Mobility

Source: Porter (2005). Reproduced with kind permission of Elsevier.

purchasing and provision of health services for that population, community or individual and to develop an effective programme for a specific target population.

Porter (2005, p. 37) identifies a minimum of three types of information required before the profile is drawn up. These are:

- Information to describe the basic characteristics of the community (for example number of individuals, age, sex)
- Information to describe and monitor the health status of the community
- Information on the determinants of health in the community.

Coles and Porter (2008, p. 3) suggest the assessment of need must also involve 'the identification of threats to health and existing health problems as well as the positive factors that enable individuals, families and groups to remain healthy within situations of deprivation and vulnerability'. This information is collected using a variety of approaches to assessment which will now be outlined. First, a health needs assessment.

Health needs assessment (HNA)

The aim of this approach is to profile health needs of a given population, community, group or family in order to improve their health and reduce inequalities between access to, or availability of, services. It is also about identifying those who need the service most and then designing the service to meet the identified need. A number of tools have been produced, in recent years, to assist the nurse in undertaking a HNA (Hooper and Longworth, 2002; Cavanagh and Chadwick, 2005; NICE, 2005; Haughey, 2008). The process involves collecting data on people and/or services they use so contributing to knowledge of the population's health and well-being. A comprehensive HNA involves an epidemiological (quantitative) and qualitative approach to determine priorities, taking into account the people's perspective, and clinical and cost effectiveness. Black (1994) states that ethical, clinical and economic considerations of need must be factored into this assessment (what should be done, what can be done and what can be afforded). Once information has been gathered nurses can identify any issues arising from the data collection with the Specialist Community Public Health Nurse (SCPHN) or relevant public health practitioner and a plan of

Find a copy of the latest Director of Public Health annual report (Department of Health, Health Authority website, or reference library):

1. Can you identify the incidence of obesity in children of school age within one community?

2. What is the prevalence of obesity among this group?

3. Is there evidence within the report of cost-effective strategies used in reducing the obesity rate in this group?

4. What is the current level of service provision (adequate school nurses, nutrition advice, drop-in centres)?

action can be put in place to address the identified need. In summary, the protection and improvement of the health of populations, communities and individuals (public health) are based on the collection of health and social information and provide the basis for drawing up accurate profiles on the health needs of populations. Table 18.3 adapts and uses the *Principles of Health Visiting* (Cowley and Frost, 2006) to demonstrate the process.

Profiling: An epidemiological approach

The second part of the approach to the assessment of needs is profiling. As with health needs assessment, profiling the population health and social needs enables the nurse to use quantitative and qualitative research methods to collect epidemiological data. Qualitative data can add an important dimension to the nurse's understanding of the complex needs of the population. By analysing existing health data the nurse can predict future health trends which will inform practice. The knowledge gained from the analysis can then facilitate the targeting of health needs using appropriate, available resources.

There are three elements to an epidemiological approach:

- Determining the incidence and/or prevalence of the health problem.
- Identifying the effectiveness (and cost effectiveness) of existing interventions for the issues.
- Identifying the current level of service provision (Haughey, 2008).

Indicators of deprivation are used to identify groups of people who may experience social and economic disadvantage, for example the numbers of those living in poverty or unemployment rates. Measures such as these are used by governments to underpin their health policies (House of Commons Health Committee,

Table 18.3 Health Needs Assessment

Search for health needs: **Getting started**	Scoping: **Identify health priorities (profile)**	Appraisal: **Assess a health priority for action**	The stimulation of an awareness of health needs: **Planning for change**	Influence on policies affecting health: **Developing an action plan**	Facilitation of health enhancing activities: **Moving on and reviewing**
Who is the defined population? Why the assessment? What are the health needs of the given population? How will the HNA happen?	Determine the health needs/ assets of the local population. Identify trends before proposals are put forward for the development and delivery of improved services/ programmes.	Systematically collect, analyse and interpret data in order to create a profile of the local community to provide a local picture of inequalities in describing health needs.	To provide information and implement a programme which enables people to address issues that influence their health. Raise awareness of health needs and facilitate a response if required. Agree who will lead on this.	Findings can be used to inform health equity audits and health impact assessments. A multi-agency team to plan action and interventions and target resources to meet the health need.	Acting as a health agent, mediating between agencies on behalf of individuals, families or community health status. Evaluating the effectiveness of the intervention.

2009) and to enable resources to be targeted to those most in need (DCSF and DoH, 2009b; NICE, 2008). Examples of these can be seen in the development of services for vulnerable children like Sure Start (DEE, 1999), the Family-Nurse Partnership programme (Billingham, 2007), services for those with long-term conditions (DoH, 2005b) and older people (DoH, 2004a, 2005c).

Having knowledge of the links between and relative importance of, social, economic, biological and environmental determinants of health/stressors to health and health needs will help the nurse to identify the need. Figure 18.1 demonstrates health and influences on levels of health (Dahlgren and Whitehead, 2007) and is a helpful reminder of the factors that are important in determining good health. Factors which include health related behaviours, for example obesity, substance misuse, smoking, alcohol and factors from the social environment like employment and education, and factors from the physical environment such as housing conditions, water and sanitation.

For the nurse working in the community they are in a good position to understand the population aspects of health and disease, and participate in helping to prevent the spread of disease. By adopting an epidemiological approach to assessing the health needs of populations they aim to develop knowledge of the causal factors influencing health in order to develop interventions to prevent adverse events before they start (prevent injury or the start of a disease process).

The final and arguably the most important part of the assessment is that resulting from discussion and analysis with individuals on what they perceive their health and social care needs as being.

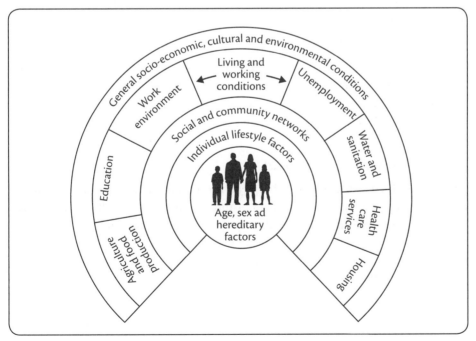

Figure 18.1 Health and influences on levels of health (determinants of health)

Source: Dahlgren and Whitehead (1991). Reproduced with permission of Institute for Futures Studies.

Individual/patient health care needs

Luker and Orr (1992) suggest that a 'health care need' is perceived by an individual when they acknowledge an abnormality which they know should be treated. (A condition that is unrecognised by the individual but is potentially discoverable can be identified through the process of screening.)

Bradshaw (1994) provides a four-point classification of need in his **taxonomy**:

taxomony

laws and principles of classification

1   Normative needs (nurse led)
2   Felt needs (what people really want)
3   Expressed needs (felt needs actioned)
4   Comparative needs (is my need the same as yours?)

Normative needs (nurse led)

Normative needs reflect the judgement of the nurse and these judgements may be different from those of the individual being assessed. Normative needs are defined in accordance with agreed standards and are compared with a standard which already exists. If the individual falls short of the standard then they are identified as being in need.

An example of this is weight and childhood obesity. The evidence is clear that obesity has risen by almost 50 per cent in England since 1979 and the country has the third highest proportion of 13 year olds who are obese, out of 35 developed countries, with children from lower socio-economic groups more likely to be obese (DCSF and DoH, 2007). Even though the risks from obesity are shared with young people, up to 79 per cent of obese young people remain obese into adulthood. The need to address this is evident but the young person does not recognise or chooses not to recognise the need.

Felt needs (what people really want)

The felt needs are identified by the individual and relate to information, services or support which can be translated into service needs. Felt needs alone would provide an incomplete measure of need because it is limited by the perceptions of the individual, but they are useful and necessary as part of a wider assessment strategy.

Expressed needs (felt need actioned)

An expressed need or demand is felt need turned into action. An individual will express a need when they ask for help or information or when they use a service. However it is important to remember that expressed needs should not be taken as an indicator for demand because they exclude needs which are felt but not expressed. As demonstrated by the inverse care law, those members of society who are hard to reach (for example travellers, the homeless, asylum seekers) may not be able to express their needs yet may be the ones who could benefit from the service the most, but are least likely to use it (Tudor Hart, 1971). Reaching out to the most vulnerable people in society and giving them a voice is a key driver in addressing inequalities in health and developing equity in service delivery (House of Commons Health Committee, 2009).

Comparative need (is my need the same as yours?)

This is about the needs of one individual being compared with that of another. For example, if individual A is not receiving a screening service for bowel cancer and individual B is receiving a service then we can say that individual A is in need.

It can also highlight health inequalities. Statistics that measure health inequalities can identify areas where the service needs of individuals are greatest in comparison to others, for example data on socio-economic status and health, including the **decennial** census; government sponsored household surveys, and birth and death records. Most statistics on inequalities are disaggregated by age and gender. National figures on inequalities by disability and ethnicity are not easily available.

In summary, the taxonomy of needs demonstrates the interrelationship between the four definitions of need. The concepts are relative ones and enable individuals to have their say in the allocation and provision of resources and services as part of building a picture of the assessment of their health and well-being.

decennial
happening every ten years

Assessing the Evidence of Effectiveness of Interventions, Programmes and Services to Improve Population Health and Well-being: Core Area 2

The critical assessment of the evidence relating to the effectiveness and cost-effectiveness of health and well-being and related interventions, programmes and services is a central part of the public health role of the nurse. This involves the application of practice through planning, audit and evaluation. Evidence is important to the nurse working in public health because its purpose is to ensure that preventive care, treatment and services are of high quality and improve health outcomes for client groups (Healthworks UK, 2001).

Evidence-based practice is about using the best evidence in making decisions about the patient, based on skills which allow the nurse to find 'and critically appraise, analyse and interpret existing evidence in order to make decisions about best practice for groups of people or populations' (Reading, 2008, p. 170).

Conversely, clinical effectiveness is about providing evidence of what works (DoH, 2000a) and is about doing the right thing in the right way and at the right time for the right patient with the right knowledge and skills (RCN, 1996).

The purpose of measuring effectiveness in the NHS is to ensure treatment, services and public health activity such as preventive care, are of high quality and improve health outcomes for service users (Porter, 2009). Clinical effectiveness links to a political imperative to drive up the quality of the service delivered by the NHS, reduce financial pressures, embrace new technologies and address increasing demands for better services where the emphasis is on improving both the cost-effectiveness and the quality of health services (House of Commons Health Committee, 2009).

⌖ Link

Chapter 3 discusses accountability.

✷ Activity 18.4

Using the framework in Table 18.3, explore the evidence for introducing one of the following:

- Health promoting lifestyle classes to older people (see Kim, 2009)
- Drop-in centre for adults who misuse alcohol (see Harrington-Dobinson and Blows, 2007)
- Cervical cancer prevention by vaccination for 13–17 year olds (see DoH, 2008b)
- The Healthy Start Scheme to all pregnant women (see www.nice.org.uk/PH011)

✷ Activity 18.5

Visit the NHS Library for Health (www.library.nhs.uk) and examine some of the evidence together with examples of good practice and methods of audit and evaluation.

The measurement of effectiveness in the NHS is the business of all nurses and is linked to the political agendas of government. There is a growing concern among nurses and the public about variations in clinical practice and the uptake of research evidence (DoH, 2006c). In addition, financial pressures within the NHS, the development of new health technologies, and increasing demands for more and better services, have led to an emphasis on improving both the cost-effectiveness and the quality of health services (DoH, 2008a). This drive for quality encompasses the twinned concepts of clinical effectiveness and evidence-based practice. These concepts are important for the nurse working in public health as they provide a framework for developing best practice. By adopting them, the nurse is able to make clinical decisions based on and informed by up to date, relevant and robust evidence which can provide professional effectiveness and accountability in all aspects of their public health work (see Chart 18.1). The skills required to accomplish this are those of critical thinking which include searching the literature, critical appraisal, audit and research (Jones-Devitt, 2007).

Chart 18.1 Framework for evidence-based practice to demonstrate clinical effectiveness

1	Identify the practice issue, question current practice and ask what evidence there is to support it
2	Find the evidence through searching the literature, seeking expert opinion and using professional resources and networks
3	Appraise, synthesise and interpret the evidence using critical appraisal skills
4	Put the evidence into practice and implement changes where necessary
5	Monitor and evaluate clinical change, for example through using audit
6	Disseminate and share good practice.

Clinical governance provides the framework through which the nurse and their employers demonstrate accountability for continuously improving the quality of the nursing contribution to public health within the NHS. This is seen as a way to safeguard high standards of care which can be achieved through the creation of an environment in which clinical excellence flourishes (DoH, 2008a).

Governance arrangements bring together all developments relating to clinical effectiveness and quality, with an emphasis on working interprofessionally with practitioners and clinicians from across health and social care, and in partnership with users of the NHS. In order for this to work the nurse must ensure their practice is based on the best available evidence. The National Service Frameworks (NSFs) (DoH, 2002) and the National Institute for Health and Clinical Excellence guidance (NICE, 2008) are integral to a standards-based system and are key in supporting local improvements in service quality. They make this achievable by providing robust evidence and national guidelines upon which practice can be based at a local level.

The framework outlined in Chart 18.1, provides a systematic framework through which the nurse can evaluate their contribution to public health activity. It is an opportunity for them to demonstrate the value of their contribution to the health of the population by revealing the evidence base for practice and clearly identifying health outcomes. Problems are sometimes witnessed with this approach when applying it to practice. In some areas there is robust research evidence to support specific interventions and guidelines for practice are clear (see Barnes et al., 2007). However, sometimes the evidence to support practice is not available or is insufficient (see Feder et al., 2009).

Evaluation of public health activity has to aim at improving health gains. Such a focus provides opportunity for nurses working in public health to demonstrate quality and effectiveness, through the development and use of outcome measures based on broad, holistic models of health and health care. Such measures relate, for example, to improving access to services, or to how they are delivered, and could be illustrated by the inclusion of subjective accounts of clients' experiences.

'The Essence of Care Patient Focused Benchmarks for Clinical Governance' (DoH, 2003, 2006b, 2007) provides support to service improvement by offering patient-focused benchmarks for clinical governance and providing application guidance to practitioners. The benchmarks aim to enable the nurse to work with service users to identify best practice and to develop action plans to improve care. They adopt a qualitative approach, where patients, carers and the health professional work together to agree and describe good quality care and best practice. This can be seen in areas of care relevant to all health and social care settings.

> ⁕ **Activity 18.6**
>
> Seek out a selection of published examples of evaluation of practice which reveal the application of a variety of qualitative and quantitative methods to measure a broad range of health gains and outcomes in public health.

New processes and intermediate health outcome indicators are being developed all the time to measure the effectiveness of interventions by the nurse with service users (see Northrop et al., 2008; Gildea et al., 2009; Hogg and Worth, 2009; McInnes et al., 2000).

In all cases, it is important that the information collected is accurate and comparable.

Public health activities are often long term and health gains may not be visible for many years. The social and environmental setting in the community is very complex, with numerous social, psychological and economic influences on health, and various different health and social care workers involved. The complexity of interventions creates problems with measuring outcomes. The nurse often addresses multiple health and social care needs at an individual, family and community level, and practice is often client led and unpredictable.

These problems have been widely documented within Specialist Community Public Health Nursing (SCPHN) where health visitors and school nurses adopt a broad concept of health, which aims to maintain and improve health in the general population. Such an approach means that changes in health status are more difficult to detect than, for example, health improvements for patients in a community hospital. This is compounded when tests are not available to measure all the varied dimensions of health, and quantitative research methods may not be appropriate. Baseline measurements of health status are also difficult, as outcome measures do not always recognise the wide range of public health nursing skills which may be needed to achieve a particular change in health status. Pressure to concentrate on simple, easily measurable outcomes, could result in the nurse focusing on one aspect of health, such as improving immunisation status, at the expense of trying to improve the overall health of their clients.

Methods of monitoring and evaluating public health nursing performance therefore tend to concentrate on easily measurable outcomes and quantitative statistics such as activity numbers (number and 'type' of clients contacted). The data produced from this can be meaningless and fail to describe the quality or effectiveness of the interventions. Using inappropriate statistics to monitor performance of public health activity may be influencing and changing practice, as activities become restricted to areas which can easily be measured.

It could be argued that a tension therefore exists between the public health activity of the nurse and the dominant approach to, and methods of measuring effectiveness in health care. The scientific method, which emphasises the objective analysis of predictable phenomena, is not always able to capture the complexity of practice. While it emphasises quantitative outcomes it appears to devalue qualitative information which captures the 'processes' of care and consumer perspectives. While the nurse is still required to collect information on biomedical health outcomes and these are evaluated using quantitative statistics, only part of their role and perceived effectiveness is actually measured and recorded. However, policy developments and developments in research and practice reveal opportunities, ideas and strategies that can be adopted and applied more appropriately to measure the effectiveness of public health activity undertaken by the nurse.

Policy and Strategy Development and Implementation for Population Health and Well-being: Core Area 3

This is about supporting policies aimed at improving or protecting the population's health and well-being and participating in strategies designed to implement the policies and assessing the impact of these on the health of the population. The nurse therefore needs to understand what policy is, how it is made and how it is likely to develop so they can appreciate the changes in their working environment as well as changes in the service user perception of their situation.

Toward (2008, p. 124) suggests a number of possible definitions of the term policy and advises the most familiar one is 'policy as government decisions, actions and activities'. She goes on to explain that the areas traditionally included in the definition of social policy encompass policy decisions and actions influencing welfare or intended to combat social problems in society (Toward, 2008). Social policy is about how much welfare the state should provide, how it should be paid for, who should get it and how. It is closely related to economic policy and often constrained by it, for example when the government economic strategy involves reduced public expenditure. Rapid inflation and high unemployment cause hardship and stress to many families and a worldwide recession leads to cutbacks in the financing of public services. And unemployment can lead to increased repossession of homes, due to default on mortgage payment, which in turn puts pressure on social housing and the benefits system.

The nurse has a role to play in influencing the development of policies designed to improve health and well-being and working with others to implement strategies to put the policies into effect. They also have a part to play in assessing the impact of policies on health and well-being.

Policies relating to public health and to services for communities, families and individuals demonstrate a public health approach, which considers public health as 'the science and art of preventing disease, prolonging life and promoting health through the organised efforts of society and informed choices of society, organisations, public and private communities and individuals' (Wanless, 2004, p. 3).

In England over the last fifteen years the development of public health is witnessed in policies, starting with *The New NHS Modern and Dependable* (DoH, 1997), which put public health at the heart of health authorities. Led by a Director of Public Health and Primary Care, public health policies played a leading role in the development of health improvement strategies and strategies developed to reduce inequalities. Where possible Primary Care Trusts work alongside local authorities and their governing boards are made up of different professionals and lay people. *Saving Lives: Our Healthier Nation* (DoH, 1999) identified new, population health responsibilities to improve the health of all and address health inequality in the local community. *The NHS Plan* (DoH, 2000a) aims to improve health and health care for communities. *Shifting the Balance of Power* (DoH, 2001a) installs public health as 'a corporate function' and in *Securing Good Health for the Whole Population* (Wanless, 2004) sees public health identified as requiring a strong leadership and organisation in public health delivery and a national strategy to develop the public health workforce.

Alongside this, the need for new nursing roles in public health are emphasised with the government suggesting that in order to take forward its policies nursing and health visiting has to modernise its role to encompass working across traditional boundaries with voluntary workers and other professionals (DoH, 2006a, 2006b). Policy also outlines new ways of public health working for the health visitor (DoH, 2007) and sets out a vision for Primary and Community Care under four broad themes: people shaping services, promoting healthy lives, continuously improving quality and leading local change (DoH, 2008c).

These and other major policy documents identify the UK Government's commitment to a strong and effective public health workforce with the emphasis on public health practice. This poses challenges to current ways of working for the nurse and in particular, working across traditional boundaries, networking and developing services in conjunction with service users and other professional and voluntary workers. In England policies are increasingly being developed in consultation between government departments and the organisations concerned with their work.

Alongside the policies influencing the development of public health practitioners, the delivery of public health activity in the first decade of the 21st century has become more client and team focused. In the main the drivers for this were identified through the modernisation agenda which put the user of health and social care services at the heart of the reforms (DoH, 2000a). People who use health and social care services have a contribution to make to service provision particularly in identifying their needs (see earlier in the chapter). This core public health value identified by the World Health Organisation (WHO, 1978) and reinforced in 1995 (WHO, 1997), puts community at the centre of the health-care system, defining need, setting priorities and planning and evaluating services, embracing notions of health promotion through community empowerment, participation and self-determination.

By putting the community at the centre of the health-care system we are acknowledging the importance of those social aspects of health problems which are caused by lifestyles and identified within and by the community. *Choosing Health* (DoH, 2004a) and *Healthy Lives, Brighter Futures* (DCSF and DoH, 2009b) recognise the influence of social and economic issues on health and propose to improve the health of the population and reduce inequalities through promoting partnerships between government, local agencies, communities and individuals. This partnership theme is still threaded through government policies designed to support families (NICE, 2006; DoH, 2008d; DCSF and DoH, 2009a). Many of the initiatives build on programmes within which the nurse is regularly engaged. For example, *Choosing Health: Making Healthier Choices Easier* (DoH, 2004a) includes explicit recognition of the preventative work of the specialist community public health nurse (health visitor) 'with communities and families' (p. 48) in particular with reference to children's health, and other health improvement services. *Health Inequalities: Third Report of Session 2008–2009* (House of Commons Health Committee 2009, p. 87) recognises the value of programmes of screening and developmental checks offered by health visitors and their team of nurses over the first year of life, as well as health promotion, parenting support services and immunisations. How policies are acted on will be discussed in the next section.

Leadership and Collaborative Working for Health and Well-being: Core Area 4

This is about turning policies into action through using leadership and collaborative working skills to improve health and well-being by undertaking specific public health activities and tasks. An example of this is seen in the creation and capitalisation of opportunities to involve families in the Early Support project (Heywood, 2009). Funded to promote the implementation of *Together from the Start* (DoH and DfES, 2003), this is an England-wide government programme to achieve child-centred and family-focused services for children aged 0–3 years with a disability or complex need and their families. It is being used in local authorities, hospitals and community-based health services. Families are expected to play a strategic role in the development and monitoring of policy and practice and the service is expected to be proactive in seeking their views. Such an approach requires a strategy whose purpose is to ensure that available resources are used to best advantage to meet the changing needs of the population (Cox and Rawlinson, 2008). Department of Health (2008) provides some tips for success in community involvement (see Chart 18.2).

Chart 18.2 Tips for success in community involvement

- Be clear when you need to involve users of services
- Involve people at the very start of a process
- Be clear with people about what can and cannot be influenced
- Be open, frank and transparent
- Be prepared to listen to what your community tells you.

Source: Department of Health (2008f). Reproduced under the Open Government Licence v1.0.

Formulating a strategy with service users enables the nurse to match the public health activity to the environment in which it is to operate taking into account the broader government strategies (DoH and DfES, 2003; DCSF and DoH, 2009b) and the social indicators of health identified from the profile of the community and health need assessment. As stated earlier in the chapter the nurse is in a perfect position to implement strategies to improve the health and well-being of the community. Once they have profiled the needs of the community and identified high risk individuals they have the skills to target interventions, manage the situation and evaluate the progress of the intervention.

Leadership is about producing change and transformation. The first stage is to review existing public health activity and a SWOT (strengths, weaknesses, opportunities and threats) analysis is useful here. This can be used with the service users as a framework to evaluate current public health activity (Dancar, 2006). Strengths will be those aspects of public health that are delivered well, weaknesses will be those aspects that are not achieving targets or making a difference to the population health and well-being. Strengths and weaknesses tend to be from within the organisation (for example, nursing team). Opportunities and threats relate to those aspects in the external environment (for example, community, school). Once the SWOT analysis is completed opportunities and threats can then be evaluated against the strengths and weaknesses. This is just one of several well-known strategies that can be used as part of collaborative working. Leadership skills are used throughout collaborative working, building relationships within and with communities and organisations and working collaboratively in a multidisciplinary or multi-agency team to improve or protect health and well-being. The skills required to work this way are complex and require both knowledge of how to work collaboratively and the ability to develop and maintain communication with people about difficult matters and or difficult situations (see Chart 18.2). It requires effective communication, orally, visually, written and electronically. The nurse also needs to know how to identify and influence other people and agencies to improve and protect health and well-being and contribute effectively to change within their own sphere of work. Elsey (2008) reminds us that working collaboratively is very challenging and problems of access, resource issues and the culture of health- and social-care organisations can all impact on the level of participation. If fragmentation of health care is to

> ✳ Activity **18.7**
>
> Make a list of the skills you think would help you target interventions, manage the situation and evaluate the progress of the intervention. Compare your list with those skills identified in Table 18.6 at the end of the chapter.

be avoided then all health-care professionals, including nurses, need to embrace creative ways of working (Healthcare Commission, 2008; DoH, 2008a).

In summary, the nurse is required to have knowledge and skills in each of the four core areas. These include the skills of surveillance and assessment of health need and assessment of the evidence to support the effectiveness of their interventions, together with understanding policy strategy and how to use leadership skills in collaborative working with the multi-agency team. With all of these skills in place the nurse is in a good position to participate in improving population health and well-being.

Health Improvement: Non-Core Area 5 (Defined Areas)

Health improvement is about how the nurse identifies and takes advantage of opportunities to improve health and reduce inequalities with people they come into contact with. They use health promotion, prevention and community development approaches to influence the lifestyle and socio-economic, physical and cultural environment of individuals, communities and populations. The importance of health improvement is emphasised in the publication of national standards and guidelines (NICE, 2008; DoH, 2001a) and the nurse's contribution to improving the outcome of health promotion programmes recognised (Netmums, 2008). Health promotion is an important element in current health service provision and aims to enable people to take control over and improve their health (DoH, 2004a, 2006c). Having knowledge of the links between and relative importance of, social, economic, biological and environmental determinants of health/stressors to health and health needs will aid this.

Wigley and Wilson (2009) suggest that effective health promotion requires a multi-pronged approach to improving the health of an identified population where the nurse aims to empower individuals through increasing their knowledge on why and how they should adopt a healthier lifestyle. Whitehead (2001) asserts that to be able to actively promote health, there needs to be a recognition and understanding of health-related behaviour (Whitehead, 2001). Knowledge of the models and principles of health promotion and their application and knowledge of models and approaches to behaviour change help provide frameworks for developing health promoting activity. Theories from health promotion can be used within nursing to provide a structural theoretical framework where concepts can be applied and evaluated. Coupled with an understanding of basic principles of primary, secondary and tertiary prevention (Naidoo and Wills, 2005; Jones and Sidell, 2002), the nurse can be equipped to participate in health promoting programmes to improve health. Table 18.4 gives an example of how a framework for developing health promoting activity can be used to improve quality of life.

Health improvement is not simply something that involves the nurse in doing an activity with the patient, such as in changing a dressing, giving drugs to prevent auditory hallucinations or taking a blood pressure, but instead informs and pervades all aspects of nursing care in enhancing health through:

✹ Activity 18.8

Revisit Figure 18.1 to look at the health and influences on levels of health (Dahlgren and Whitehead, 2007) and this is a helpful reminder of the factors that are important in determining good health. Factors include health-related behaviours (for example substance misuse, smoking) and factors from the social environment (for example employment, education) and physical environment (for example housing conditions, water and sanitation).

- Assessment of health need (see Core Area 1)
- Planning health gain (see Core Area 4)
- Evaluating interventions and strategies for effectiveness and efficiency (see Core Area 2).

Understanding the individual's status in terms of health, beliefs, values and attitudes, along with the structural determinants of health and outside influences, will form a starting point for an assessment of health needs.

In planning health gain, the power that nursing possesses is often very subtle. For health to be improved the nurse must adopt an **egalitarian** relationship that promotes patient input and **autonomy** (Whitehead, 2000). Care must be offered in such a way that it engages people in their own care and encourages and supports them as they commit to fostering their own health gains (Caelli et al., 2003). It is, or should be, the nature of nursing care that empowers the patient. The notion of health gain lies at the centre of health improvement as a core value.

> **∞ Link**
>
> Chapter 3 discusses accountability.

egalitarian
belief that all people are equal and deserve equal rights and opportunities

autonomy
functioning independently

Table 18.4 A framework example for developing health promoting activity

Subject knowledge: Coronary heart disease (CHD)	Subject knowledge: How to reduce incidence of CHD	Models of health promotion	Application of model	Approaches to behaviour change
CHD is a major cause of morbidity and mortality (Stewart and Blue, 2004) Reducing the incidence and prevalence of CHD is a UK priority (DoH, 2000a) Quality of life is poor with congestive heart failure (English and Mastream, 1995) Contributing lifestyle factors to CHD (smoking, alcohol intake, lack of exercise, diet low in fruit and vegetables) (DoH, 2000a). Contributing medical factors to CHD (diabetes, hypertension, abdominal obesity, lipid levels) Yusuf et al., 2004)	Assess the risk of CHD in men and women aged 45–64 in identified at risk populations (e.g. socially deprived areas). Putting prevention first (DoH, 2006a) National, fiscal and legislative changes (smoking ban in public places). Reduce access to alcohol sales (Scottish Government, 2008) Promote voluntary salt reduction targets (Food Standard Agency, 2007). Food labelling Lifestyle changes (British Heart Foundation, www.bcs.com) Don't smoke, eat a balanced diet, exercise	Medical model (risk assessment and disease reduced through treatment) (Naidoo and Wills, 2005) Holistic model (view patient as a whole) (Ewles and Simnett, 1v999) Social model of health (health influenced by determinants: See Dahlgren and Whitehead model, Figure 18.1) Salutogenic model (Antonovsky, 1996) what keeps people healthy	Screening for vascular disease in healthy adults (DoH, 2008e). Statins prescribed for those identified at risk of CHD or stroke Health promotion activity applied to person, their situation and not CHD alone. Empowerment, partnership, involvement (see collaborative working) Activities that strengthen the individual capacity to cope: Advice on lifestyle, money, raising self-esteem	Establish a relationship Negotiate an agenda and assess the importance and confidence in making a change Explore importance and build self-esteem/ confidence Negotiate an action plan, discuss review dates, exchange information, sustain change over a period of time.

Prochaska and DiClemente (1984)

Working in partnership with the service user enables potential to be fulfilled (Tee, 2008). Wigley and Wilson (2009) suggest the main tasks for the nurse are to increase people's knowledge about how and why they should select a healthier route and give them the skills to undertake this.

It is important that the nurse is realistic in terms of what they can achieve within their professional role. Professional dialogue in terms of a discussion with qualified staff and peers often helps to clarify issues before they become problematic.

Reviewing practice is something that all nurses need to do (see Table 18.5). It is particularly valuable for students of nursing as it links very closely with the identification of their learning needs.

Within a supervised capacity, the student nurse should develop ways and means of involving patients and service users in strategies to make health gains. These strategies may be individualised (designed specifically for the person) and form part of their overall care package. Planning for health through raising awareness in an enabling way is crucial.

There should be no place for 'victim-blaming', in which often rushed and ill-informed judgements are made based on stereotypical and partial information. Health improvement strategies will need to be assessed for effectiveness and evaluated in terms of how well they meet the needs of patients/service users and the normative needs of the health professionals involved.

In summary, the nurse develops information and resources to support health improvement and the reduction of inequalities for a number of audiences (for example children, young people, adults with long-term conditions, vulnerable groups, older people). Contact with these groups puts them in a position to provide information and advice on specific measures and approaches to health improvement.

Table 18.5 What to include in a reflection on a health improvement activity

• Introduction	• Reason for selection of the health promotion intervention
• About the health promotion intervention	• Describe the intervention • The relationship between the intervention and yourself as either the participant or observer • The theories that support the concepts you have identified from the intervention (referenced to recent literature) • Relate the concepts and theories back to the intervention and show how these might enhance or alter the intervention • How the intervention relates to the wider organisation, that is, the ward, patient's home, community or society at large • Any ethical or legal implications that can be drawn from the incident
• Analysis of the reflective process	• Did I present the intervention clearly? • Was my reflection on practice supported with evidence from the literature? • Did I offer evidence in support of the incident? • Did I identify issues in the analysis of the situation? • Did I structure my conclusion/summary?

Health Protection: Non-Core Area 6 (Defined Area)

Health protection seeks to protect the public from, or limit exposure to, hazards that may be harmful to health. McCulloch and Prieto (2008) suggest that this field of public health is concerned with the prevention, investigation and control of infectious diseases and environmental hazards. This includes the transmission of communicable diseases and outbreaks and incidents that threaten public health as well as food, water, air and environmental quality and safety. A recent example of this type includes the influenza A H1N1 (swine flu) outbreak across the world where 94,512 cases and 429 deaths worldwide were identified (WHO update, 2009).

By understanding the links between, and the relative importance of, social, economic, biological and environmental determinants of health and stressors to health and health needs the nurse can implement interventions to protect health, while also taking into account inequalities (see Figure 18.1).

For example, knowing that methicillin-resistant staphylococcus aureus (MRSA) can be reduced by effective hand hygiene (Chief Medical Officer, 2006) means that steps can be taken to reduce the incidence of this hospital acquired infection. The introduction of alcohol-based handrub in UK hospitals in the late 1990s has provided a revolution in hand hygiene practice. The 'Clean your hands' campaign initiated by the National Patient Safety Agency in the UK has seen all hospitals in England making alcohol-based handrub available at the point of care (Chief Medical Officer, 2006).

Communicating risks of health and safety and well-being and providing advice on how to prevent, ameliorate or control the risks are all part of the role of the nurse in protecting health.

> **⊂⊃ Link**
>
> Chapter 5 discusses hand hygiene.

Challenges to health may occur in a crude cyclical fashion, whereby diseases pose no real threat until safeguards are removed or 'fail-safe' conditions are disrupted, often through complacency or neglect. This may be true for tuberculosis (TB). TB increased in the UK by 27 per cent between 1994 and 2004 with 13 cases for every 100,000 people in the UK (Chief Medical Officer, 2004). TB has re-emerged in the United Kingdom primarily due to immigration, poverty, loss of public health controls, diagnostic and clinical skills, drug resistance and HIV infection, even though it was never completely eradicated. An opportunistic infection, TB seems to be almost **endemic** where the most vulnerable are at risk because of poor or inadequate housing and diet or substance misuse or as a result of migration from areas of the world where TB is already endemic. These socially excluded groups consist of the disempowered, the frail, the young, the elderly, the single parents with no real chance of escaping poverty and the long-term unemployed.

endemic

a disease that occurs particularly in a specific population, has a low mortality – for example measles

Health, life expectancy, and social circumstances are inextricably linked, TB kills, albeit slowly. Yet if you have a healthy immune system and are adequately nourished and housed, your body will rebuff these disease-causing **pathogens**.

The vicious cycle of ill-health, unemployment and poverty is self-reinforcing and must be tackled. Agreeing standards, using surveillance data and engaging the wider NHS in the management of health protection issues are all techniques that are used in protecting the health and well-being of the population.

Public Health Intelligence: Non-Core Area 7 (Defined Area)

This is about the systems in place and the capacity to deliver intelligence for surveillance, early warning functions, risk to populations, measurement of health and well-being and outcomes. Within the UK, Primary Care/hospital trusts, Strategic Health Authorities feed into the Department of Health in the relevant country (England, Scotland, Northern Ireland or Wales).

The regional Public Health Observatory draws together information from different sources to improve health and well-being. The contribution of the nurse to public health intelligence is in the providing of data on health issues which can be fed into the system as part of developing an overall picture of the problem. For example, the number of people admitted to hospital with swine flu or the mortality rate from a measles outbreak in a local school. The nurse should have an awareness of the qualitative methodologies used in health intelligence and their contribution to the understanding of health and well-being and they also understand the Data Protection Act (1998) and the implications of data disclosure (NMC, 2008).

Academic Public Health: Non-Core Area 8 (Defined Area)

🔗 Link

Chapter 4 discusses reflection in depth.

This is about the teaching of and research into population health and well-being. The nurse develops teaching material, uses mentoring techniques and teaches reflectively in groups and individually. They critique research and use practice to contribute to research. Critical feedback is given through the use of reflective sessions (professional conversations) and learning disseminated with other nurse students within higher education.

Health and Social Care Quality: Non-Core Area 9 (Defined Area)

The nurse acts as a signpost in directing the patient and service user to quality services, on the basis of accessing and analysing relevant information and evidence. They participate in the audit of practice using a variety of audit procedures, including information from patients and service users. They develop an understanding of how health and social care services are commissioned and the principles and processes related to different forms of governance and the systems that support these (DoH, 2009).

Table 18.6 Examples of public health activity for the nurse and some of the required skills for the four core areas and five defined (non-core) areas

	Examples of public health activity for the nurse	Skills required of the nurse
Core areas of public health activity		
Surveillance and assessment of the population's health and well-being.	1. Profiling the community – neighbourhood, school community, community nurse caseload. 2. Health needs assessment – describing the state of health of local people, identify major risks, identify actions needed to address the risks. 3. Population screening – coronary heart disease, stroke, diabetes. Targets individuals for screening or monitoring. 4. Assessment of health needs – common assessment framework (CAF) for children, single assessment process (SAP) with older people.	Collection of data, structure and reading of data, interpretation and analysis, communication and dissemination of findings, report writing on health and well-being (health plans). Screening, monitoring development through health, documenting evidence.
Assessing the evidence of effectiveness of health, health care and health-related programmes and services.	Providing evidence-based practice in public health activity. For example, asthma management, immunisation of children, nutrition advice to young people, lifestyle advice to older person. Collect and collate evidence from different sources, assess and validate evidence. Synthesise and interpret evidence from different sources. Communicate evidence to others and apply evidence to public health activity.	Finding evidence, selecting appropriate evidence, reading evidence, critiquing evidence, validating evidence, consolidating findings, incorporating evidence into practice, evaluating practice.
Policy and strategy development and implementation.	Working with inter-professional and multi-agency team to provide services to different client/patients in a variety of contexts (home, clinic, school, nursing home, community hospital, district hospital. Contribute to and support colleagues in the implementation of policies and strategies within practice arena (for example child health programme, screening for CHD, breast awareness). Provide information on how policies and strategies have affected the population's health and well-being (evaluate success of interventions and modify accordingly). To meet recommendations of practice-based commissioning (for example working in developing services, a minor injuries clinic, drop-in clinic for young people, Chlamydia screening service)	Skills in appraisal, audit, analysis, reviewing, examining, promoting awareness of social responsibility, change management, evaluation and review, monitoring trends, presenting information and arguments to others on how policies affect health and well-being.
Leadership and collaborative working for health	Working collaboratively in a multidisciplinary or multi-agency team to improve and protect health and well-being. Lead and organise others in undertaking specific activities and tasks (health-care assistants, nursery nurses, health trainers). Contribute to change in nursing (modernising working practices), promote the value of health and well-being and the reduction of inequalities in different teams/agencies (Working within the NMC Code (2008), protocols, policies and procedures). Teamwork/partnership approaches with health and social care professionals, voluntary sector within the local community. For example in safeguarding children using the common assessment framework (CAF)	Organisation, management, strategic thinking and action. Effective skills in leadership, communication (oral and written), collaborating with others, consciousness raising, motivation, working with others, skills of analysis, interpretation and use of information, methods of self-appraisal and evaluation. Recognition of caring as a moral imperative. Taking responsibility for self and actions.
Non-core defined areas of public health activity		

	Examples of public health activity for the nurse	Skills required of the nurse
Health improvement	Identify and take advantage of opportunities to promote health and reduce inequalities (for example development of a diabetes awareness event to improve diabetes care for the Asian practice population). Plan, implement and review specific aspects of health promoting and prevention projects (for example developing, managing, evaluating protocols for child health clinics or smoking cessation group. Provide information and advice on specific measures to promote health (for example immunisation, behaviour change). Promoting health: well women and men clinics, school health, addressing sexual health, contraception, menopause, osteoporosis, lifestyle factors such as diet, alcohol use, physical activity, smoking.	Project planning, development, implementation, management and evaluation. Developing, managing, implementing, evaluating health promotion activity. Teaching, advising, facilitating, educating on health issues.
Health protection	Implement interventions to protect health, taking into account health inequalities. Well person checks. Assessment of older people, dietary advice and monitoring, supporting patients with chronic disease Protecting health: immunisation for children, travellers, and elderly.	History taking and physical assessment, identification and management of common medical conditions. Infection control and interpreting codes of practice, giving immunisations and vaccinations,
Public health intelligence	Ensuring data collected is complete before feeding into the system (for example uptake of immunisations by children, young people in schools or flu vaccines in elderly population).	Communicating with people about difficult matters or in difficult situations. Information gathering and analysis and report writing.
Academic public health	Developing teaching materials (for example Powerpoint presentation, posters, handouts), using mentoring techniques (for example supervision of learners), teaching groups (for example relationships to school children), using feedback for critical reflection (for example learning sets with colleagues, groups).	
Health and social care quality	Signpost patients and service users to quality services (for example services in local hospital), Audit services and practices (for example patient survey on value of health improvement programmes). Implement policies, guidelines, protocols and procedures to deliver quality services (for example patient group directives for the administration of vaccines or drugs without prescription. Identify, assess and communicate risks to service quality (for example equipment in need of repair/replacement). Communicate and disseminate information on good practice (for example targets for obesity met).	Medicines management: how to use patient group directives, prescribing for children, adults, older people. Working with risk management systems and evaluation strategies. Maintaining patient safety, dealing with patient feedback, complaints and clinical governance.

Source: Adapted from Skills for Health (2008).

The nurse implements policies, guidelines, protocols and procedures to deliver quality services. They gain feedback from patients and service users using appropriate methods and use it to improve services.

The nurse identifies, assesses and communicates risks to service quality and having knowledge and understanding of the allocation of services, cultural differences between organisations and knowledge of how the quality of services is evaluated enables them to communicate and disseminate information that improves practices and services.

Chapter Summary

This chapter has used the four core areas and five defined (non-core areas) of public health activity to demonstrate the contribution of the nurse to public health activity. It has demonstrated that by working across different care settings in the community (children's centres, nursing homes, rest homes, home visiting services, health centres, general practice and other settings), the nurse is provided with opportunities to come into contact with the well population and to work with people who may never access acute medical services provided by a hospital. This is alongside working with people who are sick and require access to acute services or maintenance of long-term conditions in their homes.

The community setting provides the nurse with the opportunity to work in an interprofessional and multi-agency team and to explore and apply essential public health knowledge and skills. A public health approach enables the nurse to question the perceived relationship between health, health care and disease, all of which have changed over time and is evident in current calls for the NHS to become a 'health' not a 'sickness' service, to provide better prevention services with earlier intervention and do more to tackle inequalities and improve access to services (DoH, 2006b). Finally a public health approach provides the nurse with the opportunity to participate in a range of public health activities (see Table 18.6) carried out by different teams of nurses as part of targeting risk in the population and tackling inequalities in health and improving health in priority areas identified in National Service Frameworks (NSFs) (Porter, 2005).

? Test yourself!

1   Identify the four core areas of public health activity and the five defined (non-core) areas.

2   Revisit the definition of public health (Wanless, 2004) and identify the contribution of the nurse to public health activity.

3   How do government policies influence the development of public health activity for you?

4   What factors must the nurse consider when participating in a health needs assessment?

5   Consider the qualities necessary in the nurse for working with service users in identifying their health needs.

6   What is the role of the nurse in health protection and why is this so important?

Earle, S. (2007) *Promoting Public Health: Explaining the Issues,* In Earle, S., Lloyd, C., Sidell, M. and Spurr, S. (eds) *Theory and Research in Promoting Public Health,* Sage and Open University Press, London.
Ewles, L. and Simnett, J. (2003) *Promoting Health: A Practical Guide,* Bailliere Tindall, Edinburgh.

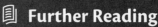 **Further Reading**

For live links to useful websites see: www.palgrave.com/nursinghealth/hogston

References

Aggelton, P. (1991) *Health*. Routledge, London.

Antonovsky, A. (1996) The salutogenic model as a theory to guide health promotion. *Health Promotion International* **11**(1): 11–18.

Bailey, L., Vardulaki, K., Langham, J. and Chandramohan, D. (2005) *Introduction to Epidemiology*. Open University Press, Maidenhead.

Barnes, J., Ball, M., Meadows, P. and Belsky, J. (2007) *Nurse-Family Partnership Implementation Evaluation*. Institute for the Study of Children, Family and Social Issues, Birkbeck College, London.

Billingham, K. (2007) The family nurse partnership programme. http://www.cabinetoffice.gov.uk/upload/assets/www.cabinetoffice.gov.uk/strategy/family_nurse.pdf

Black, D. (1994) A doctor looks at health economics. Office of Health Economics Annual Lecture. Office of Health Economics, London.

Bradshaw, J. (1994) The conceptualisation and measurement of need. In Popay, J. and Williams, G. (eds) *Researching the People's Health*. Routledge, London.

British Heart Foundation (2009) *Lifestyle Changes*. British Cardiovascular Society, Risk factors for coronary heart disease. www.bcs.com

Caelli, K., Downie, J. and Caelli, P. (2003) Towards a decision support system for health promotion in nursing. *Journal of Advanced Nursing* **43**(2): 170–80.

Cavanagh, S. and Chadwick, K. (2005) *Health Needs Assessment: A Practical Guide*. Health Development Agency, London.

Chief Medical Officer (2004) Stopping tuberculosis in England. An action plan for the Chief Medical Officer. DoH, London.

Chief Medical Officer (2006) *On the State of Public Health. Dirty Hands...the Human Cost*. DoH, London.

Coles, L. and Porter, E. (2008) *Public Health Skills: A Practical Guide for Nurses and Public Health Practitioners*. Blackwell Wiley, Oxford.

Cowley, S. (2002) *Public Health in Policy and Practice*. Bailliere Tindall, London.

Cowley, S. and Frost, M. (2006) *The Principles of Health Visiting: Opening the Door to Public Health Practice in the 21st Century*. UKSC, Amicus, CPHVA, London.

Cox, Y. and Rawlinson, M. (2008) Strategic leadership for health and wellbeing. In Coles, L. and Porter, E. (eds) *Public Health Skills: A Practical Guide for Nurses and Public Health Practitioners*. Blackwell Wiley, Oxford.

Dahlgren, G. and Whitehead, M. (2007) *Policies and Strategies to Promote Social Equity in Health*, Background document to WHO, Strategy Paper for Europe. Stockholm Institute for Future Studies, Arbetsrapport/Institutet för Framtidsstudier; 2007:14. http://www.framtidsstudier.se/filebank/files/20080109$110739$fil$mZ8UVQv2wQFShMRF6cuT.pdf

Dancar, A.C. (2006) SWOT analysis. University of St Francis, IL. www.stfrancis.edu/ba/ghkickul/stuwebs/btopics/works/swot.htm

Data Protection Act (1998) www.ico.gov.uk/what_we_cover/data_protection.aspx

DCSF and DoH (Department for Children, Schools and Families and Department of Health) (2009a) *Securing Better Health for Children and Young People through World Class Commissioning*. DoH, London.

DCSF and DoH (Department for Children, Schools and Families and Department of Health) (2009b) *Healthy Lives, Brighter Futures: The Strategy for Children and Young People's Health*. DoH, London.

DCSF and DoH (Department for Children, Schools and Families and Department of Health) (2007) *Children's Plan: Building Brighter Futures*. DCEF, London.

DEE (Department for Education and Employment) (1999) *Sure Start: Making a Difference for Children and Families*. DEE Publications, Sudbury.

DoH (Department of Health) (1997) *The New NHS Modern and Dependable*. HMSO, London.

DoH (Department of Health) (1999) *Saving Lives: Our Healthier Nation*. HMSO, London.

DoH (Department of Health) (2000a) *The NHS Plan*. HMSO, London.

DoH (Department of Health) (2000b) *National Service Framework for Coronary Heart Disease*. HMSO, London.

DoH (Department of Health) (2001a) *Shifting the Balance of Power within the NHS: Securing Delivery*. HMSO, London.

DoH (Department of Health) (2001b) *Modern Standards and Service Models: National Service Framework for Older People*. DoH, London.

DoH (Department of Health) (2002) *National Service Frameworks: A Practical Aid to Implementation in Primary Care*. HMSO, London.

DoH (Department of Health) (2003) *Essence of Care: Patient Focused Benchmarks for Clinical Governance*. DoH, London.

DoH (Department of Health) (2004a) *Choosing Health: Making Healthier Choices Easier*. HMSO, London.

DoH (Department of Health) (2004b) Better Health in Old Age: Report from Professor Ian Philip. HMSO, London.

DoH (Department of Health) (2005a) *Supporting People with Longterm Conditions: Liberating the Talents of Nurses Who Care for People with Longterm Conditions*. HMSO, London.

DoH (Department of Health) (2005b) *Securing Better Mental Health for Older Adults*. HMSO, London.

DoH (Department of Health) (2005c) *Shaping the Future of Public Health: Promoting Health in the NHS*. www.dh.gov.uk

DoH (Department of Health) (2006a) *Modernising Nursing Careers: Setting the Direction*. DoH, London.

DoH (Department of Health) (2006b) *Our Health, Our Care, Our Say: A New Direction for Community Services*. HMSO, London.

DoH (Department of Health) (2006c) *Putting Patients First: Vascular Checks and Risk Management*, DoH, London.

DoH (Department of Health) (2007) *The Government Response to Facing the Future: A Review of the Role of Health Visitors*. DoH, London.

DoH (Department of Health) (2008a) *A High Quality Workforce*. NHS Next Stage Review. DoH, London.

DoH (Department of Health) (2008b) *Arms against Cervical Cancer Immunisation Information*. DoH, London.

DoH (Department of Health) (2008c) *NHS Next Stage Review: Our Vision for Primary and Community Care*. DoH, London.

DoH (Department of Health) (2008d) *The Child Health Promotion Programme*. DoH, London.

DoH (Department of Health) (2008e) *The Coronary Heart Disease National Service Framework: Building for the Future*. Progress report for 2007, DOH, London.

DoH (2008f) *Involving People and Communities: A Brief Guide to NHS Duties to Involve and Report on Consultation*, DoH, London.

DoH (Department of Health) (2009) *Transforming Community Services and World Class Commissioning: Resource Pack for Commissioners and Community Services*. DoH, London.

DoH and DfES (Department of Health and Department for Education and Skills) (2003) *Together from the Start: Practical Guidance for Professionals Working with Disabled Children (Birth – Third Birthday) and their Families*. DoH, London.

Elsey, H. (2008) Collaborative working: organisational development for community participation. In Coles, L. and Porter, E. (2008) *Public Health Skills: A Practical Guide for Nurses and Public Health Practitioners*. Blackwell Wiley, Oxford.

English, M. and Mastream, M. (1995) Congestive heart failure: public and private burden. *Critical Care Nurse* **18**(1): 1–6.

Ewles, L. and Simnett, J. (1999) *Promoting Health: A Practical Guide*, 4th edn. Bailliere Tindall, Edinburgh.

Feder, G., Ramsay, J., Dunne, D., Rose, M., Arsene, C., Norman, R., Kuntze, S., Spencer, A., Bacchus, L., Hague, G., Warburton, A. and Taket, A. (2009). How far does screening women for domestic (partner) violence in different health-care settings meet criteria for a screening programme? Systematic review of nine UK National Screening committee criteria. *Health Technology Assessment* 13(16).

Food Standard Agency (2007) Promote voluntary salt reduction targets. http://www.food.gov.uk/healthiereating/salt/salttimeline.

Gildea, A., Sloan, S. and Stewart, M. (2009) Sources of feeding advice in the first year of life: who do parents value? *Community Practitioner* **82**(3): 27–31.

Harrington-Dobinson, A. and Blows, W. (2007) Part 2: nurses guide to the impact of alcohol on health and wellbeing. *British Journal of Nursing* **16**(1): 47–51.

Haughey, F. (2008) Assessing and identifying health needs. In Coles, L. and Porter, E. (eds) *Public Health Skills: A Practical Guide for Nurses and Public Health Practitioners*. Blackwell Wiley, Oxford.

Healthcare Commission (2008) *Towards Better Births: A Review of Maternity Services in England*. HMSO, London.

Healthworks UK (2001) *National Standards for Specialist Practice in Public Health*. Public Health Register, London.

Heywood, J. (2009) Nothing about Us Without Us: Involving Families in Early Support. *Community Practitioner* **82**(6): 26–9.

Hogg, R. and Worth, A. (2009) What support do parents of young children need? A user focused study. *Community Practitioner* 82(1): 31–4.

Hooper, J. and Longworth, P. (2002) *Health Needs Assessment Workbook*. Health Development Agency, London.

House of Commons Health Committee (2009) *Health Inequalities. Third Report of Session 2008-2009*. HMSO, London.

Jones, L. and Sidell, M. (2002) *The Challenge of Promoting Health: Exploration and Action*. Macmillan, Open University Press, Basingstoke.

Jones-Devitt, S. (2007) *Critical Thinking in Health and Social Care*. Sage, Oxford.

Kim, S.H. (2009) Older people's expectations regarding ageing, health-promoting behaviour and health status. *Journal of Advanced Nursing* 65(1): 84–91.

Last, J.M. (2001) *A Dictionary of Epidemiology*. 4th edn. Oxford University Press, Oxford.

Long, T. (2008) A community health needs evaluation: Improving uptake of services at a children's centre in a deprived and geographically isolated town. *Journal of Children's and Young People's Nursing* 2(3): 108–14.

Luker, K. and Orr, J. (1992) *Health Visiting: Towards Community Nursing*. Blackwell, Oxford.

Macleod-Clark, J. and Maben, J. (1999) Health promotion in primary health care nursing: The development of quality indicators. *Health Education Journal* 58: 99–119.

McCulloch, J. and Prieto, J. (2008) Health protection and the role of the public health nurse. In Coles, L. and Porter, E. (2008) *Public Health Skills: A Practical Guide for Nurses and Public Health Practitioners*. Blackwell Wiley, Oxford.

McInnes, R., Love, G. and Stone, D. (2000) Evaluation of a community-based intervention to increase breastfeeding prevalence. *Journal of Public Health Medicine* 22(2): 138–45.

Naidoo, J. and Wills, J. (2005) *Public Health and Health Promotion: Developing Practice*. Bailliere Tindall, London.

NICE (National Institute for Health and Clinical Excellence) (2005) *Health Needs Assessment: A Practical Guide*. NICE, London.

NICE (National Institute for Health and Clinical Excellence) (2006) *Routine Postnatal Care of Women and their Babies*. NICE Clinical guideline 37, London.

NICE (National Institute for Health and Clinical Excellence) (2008) Improving the nutrition of pregnant and breast feeding mothers and children in low income households. NICE, London. www.nice.org.uk/PH011

Netmums (2008) *Left Fending for Ourselves: A Report on the Health Visiting Service as Experienced by Mums*. www.Netmums.com

Noel, J.S., Parker, S.P. and Charles, K. (1994) Impact of rotavirus in the East end of London. *Journal of Clinical Psychology* 47: 67–70

Northrop, M., Pittam, G. and Caan, W. (2008) The expectations of families and patterns of participation in a trailblazer Sure Start. *Community Practitioner* 81(2): 24–8.

NMC (Nursing and Midwifery Council) (2008) *The Code: Standards of Conduct, Performance and Ethics for Nurses and Midwives*. NMC, London.

Porter, E. and Watkinson, G. (2007) Promoting health. In Hogston, R. and Marjoram, B. (eds) *Foundations of Nursing Practice: Leading the Way*, 3rd edn. Palgrave Macmillan, Basingstoke.

Porter, E. (2009) Measuring effectiveness in community health care nursing and specialist community public health nursing. In Sines, D. (2009) *Community Health Care Nursing*, 4th edn. Wiley, Oxford,

Prochaska, J. and DiClemente, C. (1984) *The Transtheoretical Approach: Crossing Traditional Foundations of Change*. Dow Jones-Irwin, Homewood, IL.

Raymond, B. (2005) Health needs assessment. In Sines, D., Appleby, F. and Frost, M. (eds) *Community Health Care Nursing*. Blackwell, Oxford.

Reading, S. (2008) Research and development: analysis and interpretation of evidence. In Coles, L. and Porter, E. (eds) *Public Health Skills: A Practical Guide for Nurses and Public Health Practitioners*. Blackwell Wiley, Oxford.

RCN (Royal College of Nursing) (1996) *National Health Manifesto*. RCN, London.

Scottish Government (2008) *Reduce Access to Alcohol Sales*. http://www.Scotland.gov.uk/news/realeases/2008/06/17093834.

Skills for Health and Public Health Resource Unit (2008) *Multidisciplinary/multi-agency/multi-Professional Public Health Skills and Career Framework*. Public Health Resource Unit, Oxford.

Stewart, S. and Blue, L. (2004) *Improving Outcomes in Chronic Heart Failure*, 2nd edn. BMJ Publishing Group, London.

Tee, S. (2008) Partnerships for public health; User involvement to improve health and wellbeing. In Coles, L. and Porter, E. (eds) *Public Health Skills: A Practical Guide for Nurses and Public Health Practitioners*. Blackwell Wiley, Oxford.

Toward, S. (2008) Appraising and influencing health policy and strategy. In Coles, L. and Porter, E. (eds) *Public Health Skills: A Practical Guide for Nurses and Public Health Practitioners*. Blackwell Wiley, Oxford.

Tudor Hart, J. (1971) The inverse care law. *Lancet*, 27 February: 1—12.

Wanless, D. (2004) *Securing Good Health for the Whole Population*. HMSO, London.

Whitehead, D. (2000) What is the role of health promotion in nursing? *Professional Nurse* **15**: 257–9.

Whitehead, D. (2001) Health education, behaviour change and social psychology: Nursing's contribution to health promotion. *Journal of Advanced Nursing* **34**(6): 822–32.

WHO (World Health Organisation) (1946) *Constitution*. WHO, Geneva.

WHO (World Health Organisation) (1978) *Alma-Ata Declaration, Primary Health Care*. WHO, Geneva.

WHO (World Health Organisation) (1997) *European Healthcare Reform: Analysis of Current Strategies*. WHO, Copenhagen.

WHO (World Health Organisation) (2009) Update. http://www.direct.gov.uk/en/swineflu/DG_177831 accessed on 16/07/09 at 1315.

Wigley, W. and Wilson, L. (2009) Promoting health and wellbeing. In Childs, L., Coles, L. and Marjoram, B. (2009) *Essential Skills Clusters for Nurses*. Wiley, Oxford.

Yusuf, S., Hawken, S. and Ounpui, S. (2004) Effect of potentially modifiable risk factors associated with myocardial infarction in 53 countries (interheart) case control study. *Lancet* **364** (9438): 937–52. In Kennedy, S. (2008) Assessing cardiovascular risk in the individual. *British Journal of Cardiac Nursing* **3**(8): 358–62.

19

Health Informatics

📖 Contents

☑ Learning outcomes

At the end of this chapter you should be able to:

- Define the term health informatics

- Identify the difference between data, information and knowledge

- Outline how knowledge of issues related to health informatics impacts on patients, care provision, the organisation of care management and the public

- Describe the basic principles of common legislation related to the privacy and use of information

- Identify current health-care policy related to health informatics.

Introduction: What Is Health Care Informatics?

The last 50 years has seen a series of cultural changes that are remarkable in terms of their scale of influence and speed of implementation. Similar periods of change have been noted throughout history and are often connected with technological innovation. These historical periods are commonly dubbed 'ages' or 'revolutions', for example, the 'Bronze Age' or the 'Industrial Revolution'. The latest period of cultural change (which is still ongoing) is associated with the technological development of computing, and is fuelled by a far less tangible commodity – information. The consequences of the information age are easily observed and are taken for granted as change rapidly extends throughout our society. But how do we as a profession define information? And based on this definition, what relevance does information have to health-care provision, the patient's journey through health care, and why should all nurses have some understanding of **informatics**? This chapter hopes to provide some answers to these questions in a way that is easy to read and understand.

informatics
another term for information science, which is the science of the collection, evaluation, organisation and dissemination of information, often employing computers

Broadly speaking informatics relates to the study and processing of information. Health informatics is therefore the study and processing of information related to health care. Protti (1982, cited in Abott et al., 2004, p. 9) defines health informatics as:

> The study of the nature and principles of information and its applications within all aspects of health care delivery and promotion.

Hence, health informatics is a general term with relevance to all the speciality areas of health care and to each branch of nursing. Other definitions such as that offered by Hebda et al. (2005, p. 9) associate health informatics with information and communications technology in the form of computers, and the information systems they help to deliver.

> The application of computer and information science in all basic and applied biomedical sciences to facilitate the acquisition, processing, interpretation, optimal use, and communication of health related data. The focus is the patient and the process of care, and the goal is to enhance the quality and efficiency of care provided.

It is important to acknowledge that computer technology is not always directly involved in the management and processing of health-related information; nor is technology a prerequisite for quality and efficient care delivery. The scale of the modern health service is, however, so great that the development and use of technologically driven systems is required to ensure equity in service provision and efficiency savings on a national level. The result is the Connecting for Health programme in England, Informing Healthcare in Wales and similar programmes in Northern Ireland and Scotland.

Here we will consider why health informatics is, and should be, a rapidly growing concern to all health-care staff. The basic concepts related to informatics will be considered, including what is meant by the terms data, information and knowledge. Systems related to health informatics will be introduced from the perspective of the patient and the patient journey, the health professional, the organisation and the wider public. The role of the internet will be considered within contemporary health care. Consideration to the patient's right to privacy and confidentiality will be briefly explored. Finally, current governmental strategy will be introduced with an explanation of how this strategy has implications for health professionals – whatever their level of expertise.

It is perhaps also important to stress what this chapter does not cover. All too frequently narratives relating to health informatics concern themselves with a focus on computer technology, for example detailing how to search the internet for information. Although computers are essential to health informatics, and therefore such narratives are useful, it is crucial to remember that a computer is nothing more than a tool. No matter how important the tool may be, it is the role of the tool that is of primary importance. This chapter is therefore less concerned with the specifics of how to use computers, and more with the underlying principles of how information is central to care delivery.

Who needs information on health?

Information is central to health-care provision. As an example we will look at a woman with learning disabilities being admitted to a clinic for a pre-arranged investigation. We can see that varying types of information are needed at different levels.

The patient and the patient's family

The patient and/or their primary carer need to have information regarding the admission prior to the event. This might include the appointment details such as the date and time of the admission and any specific details related to the investigation itself. For example, does the patient need to do anything specific prior to the admission, such as avoid certain foods?

The health-care provider

The provider of care requires a variety of information, but not just facts related to the patient's personal details and relevant past medical history. Information and knowledge regarding the best way to care for the patient during their stay is essential if the care to be provided is of the best quality. For example, what evidence exists for the treatments to be used, what local and national guidelines are in place and how are they applicable? Methods are also required for recording and acting on new information gained from the investigation once it is carried out. The provider also needs to supply information on the care it delivers to its purchasers, mainly primary care trusts (PCTs) so that the care and procedures carried out can be paid for. Information will also be made available to other health- and social-care professionals involved in the care and treatment of the patient to ensure continuity of care and to inform decisions on future treatment and interventions by, for example, the GP, community nurse or social care. The organisation also needs to use the information it collects to monitor targets and outcomes as well as plan for the future and compare its performance against other similar organisations.

The Strategic Health Authority (SHA)

The health authority needs information regarding the patient's admission to enable informed decisions relating to the management of resources and health-care strategy at a regional level. This information may involve detailed statistics to be used for the allocation of resources locally, such as staff and materials, and be used nationally by the Department of Health. Equally, the health authority needs information in regard to how care was delivered. In this way, the health authority can monitor the efficiency of care delivery and ensure local and national standards are adhered to. For example, the monitoring of specific staff training and development helps to facilitate the management of risk.

The general public

It may be surprising to learn that the general public also need information regarding the patient's admission. Here the information is much less detailed with no specifics as to patient identity being provided. Examples of this type of information include the waiting times for hospital admission, lengths of stay, mortality and infection rates. This can be used to make judgements on the efficiency of the health authority and wider governmental policy.

Health Informatics and Foundations of Nursing Practice

We are now beginning to gain an impression of the importance of health informatics, but it may still be unclear as to the relevance of informatics to clinical nurses, let alone nursing students. Why does this strange sounding topic represent a foundation of nursing practice? This is a reasonable question to ask, especially as much of this book focuses on the more traditional caring skills. When we consider the scale of modern health care, the reason begins to become apparent.

The National Health Service (NHS) operates on an enormous scale with over 1.6 million patients contacting the NHS per day (Crisp, 2004). The scale of this operation, when combined with modern advances in medical and communications technology, generates a massive quantity and variety of factual data, which must be processed into information before it can become useful. This process requires careful coordination if valuable data is not to become lost or unexpectedly changed (known as data corruption). The need for quality information management within health care has never been higher, and this requires the direct input of nurses at all levels.

All health professionals, no matter what grade, play a crucial role in the management of information and knowledge within any care setting (Hebda et al., 2005). Nurses, representing nearly one-third of the workforce within the NHS, have a potentially massive role in the management of information within the organisation. Nurses are frequently required to act as the hub of patient care – which involves the coordination of patient services including the input of the multidisciplinary team, and the management of a large quantity of information. In this sense, the role of the nurse is complex and nursing knowledge becomes

> **Link**
>
> Chapter 1 has more details on the nursing process.

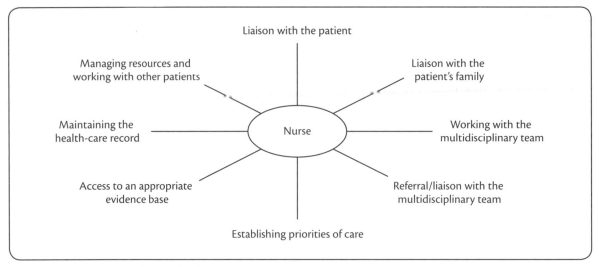

Figure 19.1 The health professional as information manager

central to patient care. Subsequently, it can be argued, one of a nurse's many roles is to act as an information manager for the patients within their direct care.

Consider the information handled by a 'typical' nurse through the application of the nursing process. Bear in mind that this process is not linear, but continuous and multi-faceted. An initial assessment may provide an abundance of data relating to the patient's condition. Indeed the health professional needs to select which assessment to apply in any given context; this may include the use of evidence-based assessment tools such as pain scoring tools. This data must be interpreted, documented and communicated in order to form a diagnosis. The planning of care may involve referral to other members of the health-care team, for example, doctors, specialist nurses, physiotherapists and occupational therapists. Further, the care planned must represent the best possible practice and, wherever possible, relate to an evidence base. Health-care professionals are required to have knowledge of the relevant evidence base in order to ensure they provide the best care possible. Any care provided will need to be considered in the context of the wider caring environment; for example, the priorities of care within a group of patients. This has implications for the management of risk and resources in order to ensure patient safety and promote health. The evaluation of care may also generate new data in need of interpretation and documentation. This may include evaluation of care from others within the multidisciplinary team. The nurse as information manager is illustrated in Figure 19.1.

Data, Information and Knowledge

data
a single item or fact, without any sense of context, for example a number

It is important to consider the central concepts of **data**, information and knowledge in order to gain a fuller appreciation of the role of informatics within health care. This should not be limited to the individual definitions associated to each term, but more importantly on how the terms are connected and interrelated.

Patient assessment

Sarah is 19 months old and has recently been admitted to the children's ward with a suspected infection. Mandy, a student nurse is asked to measure Sarah's body temperature as part of her admission to the ward.

What information does a clinician handle when asked to measure a child's body temperature?

- Perhaps the most obvious information that is handled by the student in this scenario is that relating to the child's temperature, although it should be acknowledged that a great deal of additional assessment information may be gained from such a patient encounter. A single measurement of body temperature when treated in isolation is of little value; however, when compared to known normal values the measurement can help to provide an indication of the patient's general condition. Let us imagine that in this case the temperature measurement is high, indicating that Sarah is **pyrexial**. Mandy now has several items of important information; Sarah's temperature measurement,

the fact that Sarah is pyrexial and the degree of severity of this pyrexia. The knowledge required for Mandy to recognise Sarah's pyrexia is important as this facilitates the extension of knowledge in relation to Sarah's condition.

- Mandy now has a responsibility to ensure that this information is managed properly in order to ensure the correct treatment is provided; but what should Mandy do with the information she now has? It is essential that the information relating to Sarah's temperature be communicated to those who need to know. This requires Mandy to have knowledge of who to contact and how to manage this contact. For example, should Mandy tell the parents, her mentor, the doctor, other patients or everyone? Her choices at this point are central to the patient's care and to that of the family. Mandy should of course document the finding; this may aid both the communication of the result to others and the establishment of a base line from which future temperature measurements can be compared. Now she must

decide where the result should be documented and how. The observation chart is a logical start, but the result should also be documented along with any action taken within the patient's medical record.

- This brief scenario shows how nurses use knowledge to use data and low-level information to help generate newer information at a higher level. In addition, the scenario illustrates how nurses have a responsibility to manage information appropriately. Should Mandy choose not to act on her findings, then the risk of Sarah's condition deteriorating will increase. This is a crucial point: nurses of any level have a central role to play in the management of clinical information. If information is not handled appropriately then the risk of harm increases.

Data is the word used to describe an item of fact without any explanation of how it might relate to other things, in essence, a symbol. If data is inaccurate, lost or unexpectedly changed then the data can be described as 'corrupted'. This represents a significant risk when applying any type of information system, paper or electronic. One accepted method of promoting accuracy is by ensuring the data is recorded at source, for example by the patient's bedside (Abbott et al., 2004).

Essentially, information is the understanding of some kind of relationship between data and the real world. To fully appreciate the dynamic nature of information it is important to understand that the meaning applied to data is dependent on any one individual's interpretation. What represents information

pyrexia
experiencing a raised body temperature or fever

to one person may still represent data to another. Therefore information only exists when an understanding of contextual meaning can be applied to any given data. This understanding of context and meaning can facilitate interpretation of the facts presented. In this sense, information is dynamic – it changes depending on the level of understanding applied. What is information on one level may be just data on another level, depending on the specific context applied and whether that context has any significant meaning to the user. Information therefore is portrayed as an abstract concept; that is, information only exists when the context applied has significant meaning to the individual or system making the interpretation. Information can therefore also be presented as data plus interpretation. Now try Activity 19.1.

Knowledge is the level of understanding required in order to use information constructively and purposefully in the real world. It can be split into three broad classes, procedural, declarative and acquaintanceship. In reality these classifications are largely academic and a degree of overlap is possible. For example, knowing that a sleeve left on the arm will interfere with hearing the Korotkoff sounds when measuring a client's blood pressure (an example of declarative knowledge) may be combined with knowing the correct technical sequence to guide action (procedural knowledge). Within the rest of this chapter knowledge is used as a blanket term to describe any one of the three classifications.

Knowledge is a complex concept (Hebda et al., 2005), yet what links the concept of data, information, knowledge and even the concept of wisdom together is the degree of contextual understanding applied. This is illustrated in Figure 19.2 as a hierarchy in the form of a pyramid.

In Figure 19.2 the bottom level of the hierarchy is represented by data and relates to no understanding of contextual meaning. As understanding and context are increased from a low level to a higher-level, movement through the hierarchy occurs; initially from data to information, then to knowledge and

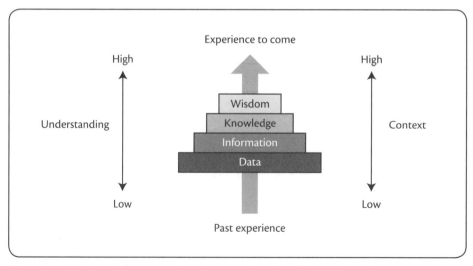

Figure 19.2 The data, information, knowledge and wisdom (DIKW) hierarchy

finally to wisdom. Progression from one level to the next assumes that there is an increased appreciation of context through the synthesis of experience leading to a greater level of understanding. Put simply, the better the understanding of a subject, the more experience can be placed in context to develop new knowledge. As the production of knowledge involves the perception of experience in context, and any given experience may be perceived in a number of different ways, it is possible to see why information may be passed on relatively easily but knowledge needs to be learned by the individual.

Implications for Nursing

The distinctions of data, information, knowledge and wisdom are largely theoretical, and in reality, the boundaries of each category overlap and merge. To a degree this has been illustrated through the description of information – depending on your individual perspective, information may still be perceived as data. Some of you may have experienced this phenomenon as you attempted Activity 19.1 (above). This exercise required consideration of the knowledge required to interpret data into information – a process that is often taken for granted – after all, it is normal behaviour to attempt to make sense of our environment. As we gain new experiences we undergo a process of learning, assimilating data into information and knowledge that then influences the way we interact with our surroundings.

Managing and providing care requires the synthesis of massive amounts of data into information. Knowledge is then required to provide a sense of order to the information, and inform decisions regarding how we go about responding to the infinite variety of experiences that may possibly arise. To help in this process we rely on the use of a variety of information systems. Computer systems are particularly well suited to managing large amounts of data and can be programmed with knowledge-based rules that can trigger an alert or action. For example, drug interactions and doses and normal value ranges for investigations can all be programmed into a computer system to flag a warning should certain conditions be met; such as, the prescription of a dangerous combination of drugs or too high/low a dose, or an abnormal blood result.

Consider the example of an admission form. Regardless of whether the form is paper based or electronic, it is designed to ensure that data is classified into data types, for example name, address, next of kin, doctor/consultant and diagnosis. The form is presented in a structured format and this helps to provide some clue as to the data required. In essence the form is also a knowledge system; the health-care professional can if they so wish, utilise the layout of the form to guide data collection, helping to ensure the assessment is thorough and avoids accidental omissions or errors. There are additional advantages if the form is computer based. It can be programmed with the knowledge needed to identify unusual or incorrect combinations of data, for example, a user may be alerted to the fact they have entered a date for the last menstrual period for a male patient.

A knowledge base can be difficult to define. It is constructed by the assimilation of information and experience and it is used to guide action. Consider as an example nursing; in the past nursing has used tradition, trial and error, personal experience and role modelling to acquire a knowledge base (Hebda et al., 2005). However, more recently there has been an increased pressure for nursing to develop a knowledge base using a foundation of objective research data synthesised into evidence of best practice. National Service Frameworks (NSFs) help illustrate the importance of this knowledge base at a national level.

Nursing knowledge is only one component of a larger knowledge base used to inform patient care. It is therefore essential that this knowledge be underpinned by sound information. This information may relate directly to the individual patient or more generally to guidelines for practice, while further information can be shown to be challenging the very methods in which care is accessed and quality care provided (see Casebox 19.2).

Casebox 19.2

It is 9 pm and Michelle, a new mother, is becoming worried about her son Jack. Jack is 11 weeks old and seems irritable, he is not interested in feeding, feels hot, and Michelle has noticed that his nappies have not been as wet as normal. She decides to check online for information and goes to the self-help section of the NHS Direct website (www.nhsdirect.nhs.uk). There she finds a link on how to recognise the signs of illness in a baby and she notices that several of Jacks symptoms are listed. Growing more concerned she decides to call the NHS Direct helpline.

On contacting the helpline Michelle is asked several questions about the nature of her call by a health adviser before being transferred to a qualified nurse. The nurse asks a further series of questions in relation to Jack and enters Michelle's responses into a computer-based information system. From the responses to these questions the nurse advises Michelle to remove any excess clothing from Jack and to take Jack to see the out-of-hours general practitioner (GP) at her local hospital. The nurse reassures Michelle that this is just a precaution to ensure Jack is not becoming dehydrated. She also informs Michelle that she will contact the out-of-hour's GP service and tell them to expect Michelle with baby Jack.

Casebox 19.2 illustrates how technological development has facilitated new methods to access health-related information. This can be shown to have influenced the perception of health-care provision by both patients and staff alike, and improved the quality of the service provided. The advent of NHS Direct (and the regional variants NHS Direct Wales and NHS 24) has brought immediacy to a patient's ability to access health care. As such, patients benefit from gaining rapid and appropriate advice, while local services benefit from a reduction in unnecessary attendance. The development of new hi-tech health-care systems has in turn challenged the role of the nurse. Casebox 19.2 shows how the nurse uses a form of telephone triage to form an assessment of the patient, and to give appropriate guidance.

In the next section of this chapter we will begin to consider the use of information systems within health care, and how these systems may impact on the patient, the health professional, the health authority and the wider public.

A Systems-based Approach to Health Care

A system can be described as a set of elements that work together to form a whole with an implied or explicit objective (Introna, 1997). For example, this book employs a system to assist you in your learning. It is organised into chapters with a similar structure and feel; it employs uniform conventions within the text to provide information in an ordered way, for example reader activities. The book also has an explicit objective – to support your learning in relation to the fundamentals of nursing.

Large amounts of information are managed through the application of information systems. Information systems are predominantly concerned with an analysis of purpose, design, use and effects of information within organisations (Fitzgerald, 2002, as cited in Paul, 2002). According to the *Dictionary of Computing* (OUP, 1996), information systems represent a multidisciplinary study; the main disciplines involved being those of organisational business and management studies and computer science. Health informatics represents a specialised subset of information systems. Here, the common organisational purpose is connected to health-care provision, and consequently the systems developed relate ultimately to the provision of patient care. This can be argued to be true even if the systems employed are primarily related to management.

Health informatics may involve systems that at first seem far removed from the provision of patient care. However, it is important to remember that each and every system used within the health-care sector can ultimately affect patients or their families. When considering the use of health-care information systems, it is vital to fully consider the impact these systems have on patients and their care.

Casebox 19.3 shows how an information system, primarily related to finance, has the potential to impact on patient care. The use of a financial information system has provided managers with the necessary information to implement change and minimise the threat of overspend. By adding controls to the use of external agency nursing staff, the Trust hopes to cut costs. However, this places ward managers in a challenging position; how do they find appropriately skilled cover if they cannot freely book external agency staff with specialised skills? Additionally, it could be argued that the knowledge of difficulties in finding suitable cover may discourage staff from taking sick leave when it is really needed. The result could potentially impact on the quality of patient care and staff well-being.

Casebox 19.3

From a recent audit using the finance information system it has become apparent that 'Fictional Mental Health Trust' is heading for overspend. Information from the audit indicates that the overspend results from a high sickness rate among nursing staff and the reliance on external agency staff to cover shifts. Fictional Mental Health Trust is consequently suspending the use of all non-essential agency staff in an attempt to limit costs.

Health Informatics: Putting the Patient First

The notion of a patient's journey through the health-care system is central to any consideration of health informatics as this provides an ability to visualise the various information needs that exist. This journey begins with the patient's first contact with the health service and completes at the point of discharge. Casebox 19.4 illustrates a brief example of a patient's journey along with some of the information needs of the patient; however, any one patient's journey may vary from another in a multitude of ways. Figure 19.3 illustrates the journey detailed in Casebox 19.4 by plotting key points on a time line.

Link

Chapter 8 explores urinalysis in greater depth.

Casebox 19.4

Donna suspects that she may be pregnant and arranges for an appointment with her general practitioner (GP). At the surgery, a pregnancy test confirms the pregnancy. The GP explains Donna's immediate options and asks Donna to arrange an appointment to see the local midwife. A referral is sent from the GP to the local general hospital.

When Donna sees the midwife an estimated due date is calculated. One week later Donna receives an appointment through the post for an ultra-sound scan. Three weeks later the scan is performed and this confirms the midwife's initial estimate of dates. Donna is given a picture of her developing baby.

Donna sees her local midwife again two weeks after the scan and a detailed medical history is taken. Four weeks later Donna sees the midwife again and a variety of blood samples are obtained,

these are sent to the laboratory at the local hospital for analysis. Meanwhile an appointment for a 20-week ultra-sound scan is sent through the post. The scan goes well and Donna is given the results from her blood tests. Donna is asked to arrange an appointment with her local midwife in five weeks' time (25 weeks pregnant).

When she sees the midwife she is asked to arrange further appointments every two or three weeks. It is explained to Donna that these appointments are intended to monitor the course of her pregnancy. Measurements of **fetal heart rate**, maternal blood pressure and **urinalysis** are to be recorded in Donna's care record. At 32 weeks of pregnancy Donna and her partner start to attend parentcraft sessions at the local hospital.

At 39 weeks pregnant Donna starts to feel labour pains and decides to contact the

labour ward. The phone call is documented by the labour ward, but at this stage Donna is advised to stay at home. A few hours later Donna's waters break and she contacts the labour ward again. This time she is advised to come into hospital and within several hours Donna has delivered normally a healthy baby boy. Donna is now transferred to the postnatal ward with her son.

Donna remains in hospital for two days and receives daily checks by the midwife. The local midwife visits Donna at home the day after her discharge. Two days later the midwife returns and performs a blood spot screening test from her son's heel. Four days later Donna receives an initial visit from the local health visitor. A week later the midwife make a final visit and Donna is formally discharged from her obstetric care.

fetal heart rate
the measurement of heart rate of the unborn child (fetus)

urinalysis
an analysis of the chemical make-up of urine often used as a method of health screening

Activity 19.2 asks you to map a patient's journey through the health-care system and identify their individual need for information at the various stages. The provision of this information is dependent on numerous elements working together, in other words it is dependent on systems. Consider some of the systems involved in the care of Donna from Casebox 19.4: referral systems, case note systems, antenatal care systems, parent-craft, birth plans, triage systems, admission and discharge systems, postnatal care systems, hospital transport systems, postal systems, hospital support systems. The list could go on and on, but each system has one common connection – it ultimately impacts in some way on patient care. Until quite recently this crucial point was often missed and health-care staff too often perceived themselves as the primary user of health-related systems (Abbott et al., 2004). Remember: any system used in health care is always connected to the patient. Let us now consider one such system in greater depth – the patient care record system.

In the past patient care records have been based on paper documents; however, electronic systems, with their potential for allowing data sharing, are rapidly becoming the norm. Either can be described as being episode-oriented (Hebda et al., 2005). Essentially this means that the record is added to every time the patient undergoes an episode of care; for example, an appointment with the GP. Often, even with computer records, the record of care is normally local to the point of care; hence GPs, hospitals and other associated health-care providers may all retain separate patient records.

Consider the types of data that may be included in a typical patient record (Table 19.1). We can see that the record can be broadly classified into demographics and patient history. The patient history can be said to be episodic, but also longitudinal in that each new episode of care adds to a developing history of past patient contacts. Together, these combine to form a historical continuum of patient contact for the care setting possessing the record.

Paper-based systems have numerous drawbacks. The paper record is a physical resource that can only be in one place at one time. To overcome this problem there is a tendency to use multiple records resulting in the fragmentation and duplication of information. For example, the separation of the primary care record from the secondary care (hospital) record results in the fragmentation of documented care. Often a search is needed to locate a specific care record, and at times these records will be unavailable. Key information relevant to the patient's condition may be buried deep with the paper record and searching through the file can be both difficult and time consuming. **Data integrity** is often compromised through the misfiling of entries and the use of poor handwriting.

✸ Activity 19.2

Within your current practice area, document the progress of a patient from admission to discharge along a timeline as shown in Figure 19.3. What are the information needs of the patient at the various stages?

data integrity
the extent to which stored data is complete and accurate

Table 19.1 Types of information stored in the patient record

Demographic data	Patient history
Name	Family history
Address	Past episodes of care
Telephone	• Previous/current assessment details
Religion	• Past/current diagnosis
Next of kin	• Past/current care plans
	• Evidence of care implementation
	• Evidence of care evaluation G Referrals
	• Results from diagnostic tests
	Discharge/follow-up
	• Discharge letters
	• Referral replies
	• Patient correspondence
	• Other notices, for example legal correspondence

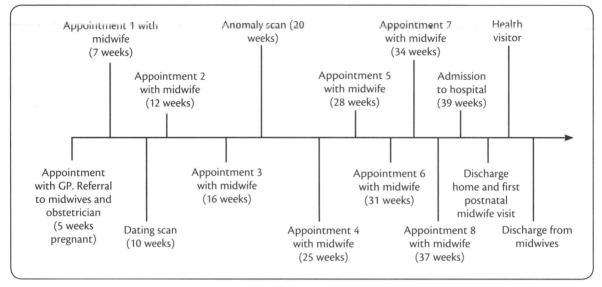

Figure 19.3 A patient's journey

Opposing these limitations are the benefits of an electronic patient record (EPR). These are well documented (DoH, 1998; Abbott et al., 2004; Hebda et al., 2005):

- An electronic record is effectively a virtual record; this means that instead of storing the specifics of any one patient in a paper file, the information is stored in an electronic file located within a central computer system.
- Lack of physical form means that the record's presentation can be changed depending on the needs of each user, thus helping to protect the patient's confidentiality and making the search for relevant information easier.
- Data entry can be subjected to tests for accuracy, even though the integrity of the data entered would still be subject to the individual entering the correct data.
- Information can be presented in a clear and legible format, helping to minimise the risks associated with handwritten texts.
- Searching an individual patient record, or even searching across any number of patient records becomes significantly easier.

These later benefits are dependent on the use of data in a consistent and known format and this has led to the development of clinical coding schemas.

Perhaps one of the greatest potential benefits of an EPR for a patient is the ability to integrate all the disparate health records into one single patient record. This represents a fundamental shift in the concept of patient information, as access to the record is being increasingly granted to the patient. The logic of this is difficult to dispute – the information held in any record does after all 'belong' to the patient and not to the document in which it is detailed. Such integration could be argued to improve patient care through the sharing of relevant information. Abbott et al. (2004) cites the example of an accident and emergency department gaining potential benefit from being able to access GP patient records for relevant drug history. A second benefit is to the individual organisations concerned, as the need for repetitious data collection would be removed and access to information for audit purposes would be increased.

Indeed the benefits of a single integrated electronic patient care record are so substantial that the national NHS strategy for information in health (National Programme for Information Technology in the NHS (NPfIT), 2005) includes the development of just such a health record. This has led to the development and installation of various technological infrastructures from which integrated records can eventually be based. Yet, this type of development is not without its potential problems. For example, integrated care records are dependent on the use of communications technologies to transport information from one system to another. This represents a significant risk to patient confidentiality, integrity of the data and its availability where and when it is needed. Any integrated records system must show that these risks can be safely managed before they are implemented.

The development of an integrated EPR perhaps represents the most important shift in the documentation of patient care since the first medical records were created. Although focus has largely been placed on the like-for-like replacement of paper records with electronic records, the process of integrating these systems is slowly progressing. Certainly the trend for moving to electronic records is set and is likely to continue.

Health Informatics: At the Point of Care

Although the patient remains central in the provision of all health informatics systems it must be acknowledged that care providers can also receive benefit from their use. For example, the patient as the owner of the care record should have direct access to the information within it, but it is the health-care provider who is most likely to use the information as part of care provision. It is therefore the health-care professional who is most likely to access the care record. Yet how does the health professional know what data and information to enter into the care record? What informs their searching of the record or even the questions they ask patients? How do practitioners decide on the care to provide? The answer of course is based on their knowledge.

Data does not generate itself, nor does the resultant information self-generate. Knowledge is required in order to collect data and as such, nurses must be able to access resources to support their individual learning and develop their practice. As emphasis is given within health care to the concepts of 'best practice' and 'evidence based practice' there is a corresponding need to develop knowledge management initiatives to capture, retain, reuse and impart the necessary tools to facilitate understanding in others. To better illustrate how such tools can inform nursing practice let us consider two examples: the National Institute for Health and Clinical Excellence, and the **internet**.

internet
a worldwide network of computers with the capacity to communicate with one another using set protocols

National Institute for Health and Clinical Excellence

Officially launched on 1 April 2005 the National Institute for Health and Clinical Excellence (NICE) is an independent agency providing national guidance on the promotion of health, and the prevention and treatment of ill-health (NICE, 2005). This relatively new organisation has a remit for the provision of guidance in three distinct sub-domains:

- Centre for Public Health Excellence: developing guidance on the promotion of good health and the prevention of ill-health. Guidance will be in the form of recommended interventions (types of activity), for example how specific lifestyle changes can result in a reduced risk of illness.
- Centre for Health Technology Evaluation: developing guidance on the use of new and existing medicines, treatments and procedures within the NHS. Evaluations consider both clinical and economic evidence and recognise that treatment may be both expensive and value for money. In addition this branch of NICE provides guidance on the clinical use of interventional procedures and decision support systems (computer software intended to help health professionals make a diagnosis or treatment decisions).
- Centre for Clinical Practice: intended for the formation of specific clinical guidelines. Guidelines are intended to help clinical staff provide treatment to patients with specific diseases and conditions in order to improve the chances of patients becoming well (NICE, 2005).

Although an independent organisation, NICE is still part of the NHS and consequently any recommendations published have significant impact. According to NICE (2005, p. 9):

> Once NICE publishes clinical guidance, health professionals and the organisations that employ them are expected to take it fully into account when deciding what treatments to give people. However, NICE guidance does not replace the knowledge and skills of individual health professionals who treat patients; it is still up to them to make decisions about a particular patient in consultation with the patient and/or their guardian or carer when appropriate.

From this it is possible to identify two major implications of knowledge management within the NHS. First, the responsibility for being aware of the guidance available is shared by the individual practitioner and the employing organisation. Here the organisation may be expected to ensure that national guidance is incorporated into local policy and that individual employees can gain access to the information provided. The individual practitioner must keep

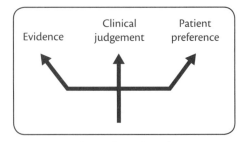

Figure 19.4 The evidence-based practice trident

Source: Adapted from Sackett et al. (1996).

abreast of the guidance published and any potential implications to their practice. Second, that published guidance does not equal rules for practice. The guidance is intended to support practice through the provision of evidence, but this evidence must be considered carefully in relation to the specific circumstances of each individual patient before it is used. Equally, patient preference is seen as an essential factor in decisions relating to treatment. The published guidance of NICE provides support for one prong of the evidence-based practice trident (see Figure 19.4).

The internet

The internets, and especially the World Wide **Web**, have become integral to Western society. The internet is a phenomenon that can be argued to have relevance to health at the organisational level, to individual practitioners, and to patients and their carers alike. At the organisational level NHS Trusts have become truly dependent on the internet, many of their operational mechanisms having been designed around, and having become reliant upon, the use of internet connections. For example; the Web is used for the ordering of stock within a clinical area; email is used for inter- and intra-departmental communications. With the development of integrated health-care records this dependence is only likely to deepen and indeed the list of dependencies offered here could be expanded exponentially. One key aspect of the way the Web is used by health-care organisations is the facilitation of interaction between users and the information presented. Consider the example of a patient wanting to book an appointment with a practice nurse at his local surgery. Most areas within the UK now offer the facility for the patient to book an appointment online. While on one level this service is very welcome, its introduction is not without repercussions. Organisations must consider the equality of the services they offer and a reliance on the use of internet-based appointment services alone is likely to isolate large sections of the society they serve.

Practitioners also benefit from the use of the internet; indeed in the author's opinion, the ability to use the internet has become a core skill of nurses. Of the many possible uses the internet has for individual practitioners the role of information retrieval is perhaps one of the most important. The advantages of having access to quality information are self-evident (see Activity 19.3), yet the access provided by the internet is not without problems. The World Wide Web offers access to a wealth of credible (and not so credible) resources for the practitioner. Practitioners need to be able to search and navigate through a maze of possible sources, evaluate the credibility of any particular source, and critically judge its value to their practice. Indeed, the scale of access that is now available is so vast that the problem of information overload becomes a real possibility. Recognised access points to quality assured content, commonly referred to as portals, can help direct practitioners. The NHS Evidence Health Information Resources (formerly the National Library for Health: http://www.library.nhs.uk/default.aspx) is an example of one such portal. However, any practitioner hoping to find

Web
known formally as the World Wide Web; relates to a network of linked documents (often called pages) stored on computers (called servers) connected to the internet. These documents can be accessed by other computers via the internet.

specific information to support their practice, even from the starting point of a portal, will require a determined attitude, and a core set of dependable search skills (see the Intute website for a range of excellent free tutorials on internet searching: http://www.vts.intute.ac.uk/).

Patients and their carers also use the internet in a variety of ways connected to their health. Searching the internet for health-related information is not uncommon, and while many sources of information are credible, mis-information is not unusual. However, the internet offers the potential to impact on health in more diverse ways. For example, if one accepts that any individual's health has a connection to their social network (Smith and Christakis, 2008), the facilities the internet offers in terms of social networking take on a new context. Social networking sites such as Facebook can be used to form self-help groups which may function through an official organisation, or function unofficially, grown as consequence of 'word of mouth'. Regardless, social networking sites offer a potential means of exposure to a diverse range of social experiences which may influence behaviour. Such influence may be at the detriment to health, as well as to its promotion.

The Management and Organisation of Care

The developments of the NICE and the use of the internet as an information resource represent two examples of how health professionals can seek to develop their knowledge. However, as the limitations highlighted by the RCN survey (Bertulis, 2005) have indicated, the development of resources to support clinicians must be underpinned by appropriate management strategies if patients are ultimately to benefit. This finding supports that of the Wanless Report (2002), an evidence-based assessment of the long-term resource needs within the NHS, that major advances in the effective use of information and communication technologies are required if the NHS is to deliver efficient high-quality services in the future.

The government has published numerous key strategy documents intended to provide a common vision to local authorities on the development of health services and the management of information in England (DoH, 1998, 2000, 2002a). The most recent of these are plotted on a timeline shown in Figure 19.5. Also recognised is the need for increased investment in relation to IT. This is evidenced by a £6 billion investment made to date, and a further £2.3 billion investment set aside for the next three years (NPfIT, 2005). Key to the success of such investment is an understanding of the difference between effectiveness and efficiency (see Casebox 19.4).

Chart 19.1 summarises the key objectives of the current information strategy for England – the National Programme for Information Technology in the NHS (NPfIT, 2005). However, it is possible to identify several central themes from the various strategy documents including:

- Placing the patient at the centre of care and ensuring that the design of care services is not biased towards the needs of the institution providing care.

★ Activity 19.3

Reflect on the way that you prepared for your last nursing assignment. What sources of information did you use? How did you identify these sources? What skills did you require?

∞ Link

Chapter 18 contains more details on the Wanless Report (2002).

Chart 19.1 The National Programme for Information Technology in the NHS (NPfIT) – key objectives

- *New National Network (N3):* to provide a suitable technological infrastruc- ture on which future services can be run
- *A Secure National Email Directory Service:* the development of a centrally managed national email and directory service for the NHS
- 14039_87807_19_cha18 14/9/06 10:02 Page 549
- *NHS Care Records Service:* to develop integrated electronic health records
- *Electronic Booking Service:* for the arrangement of appointments and the management of referrals
- *Electronic Transmission of Prescriptions:* to reduce the risk of prescription errors and make easier the process for issuing and collecting medicines
- *Picture Archiving and Communications Systems (PACS):* to capture, store, distribute and display digital images such as electronic X-rays or scans

- *Secondary Uses Services (SUS):* for the collection and use of anonymous patient-based data for uses other than clinical care (for example incident reporting)
- *National Library for Health:* the development of a library and information resource for all NHS staff
- *Quality Management and Analysis System (QMAS):* national IT system for the provision of objective evidence to GP practices and PCTs for the quality of care delivered to patients
- *GP to GP Service:* the development of a service to electronically transfer the electronic component of a GP care record to a new practice when a patient registers with a new practice.

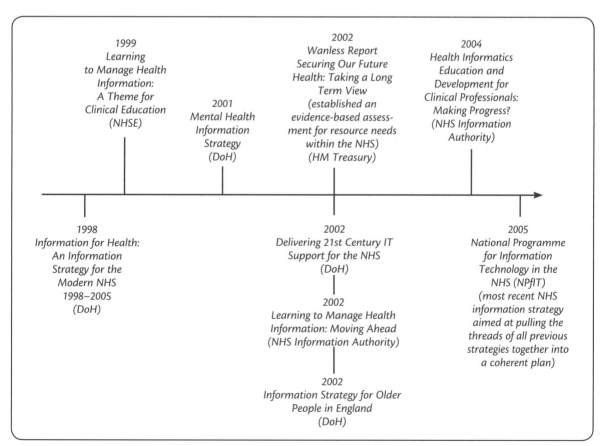

Figure 19.5 A timeline illustrating the publication of health strategies and other related documents to health informatics

Processes that are effective can be defined as those for which a set purpose is achieved whereas processes that are efficient relate to those that limit unnecessary effort and expense. Consider the cases of three identical patients admitted to separate hospital Trusts after suffering a myocardial infarction (MI):

Patient 1: Mr Smith is provided with immediate specialist cardiology care on admission. He remains an inpatient for 12 days and receives excellent treatment including **angioplasty**. On discharge he visits a cardiac rehabilitation clinic three times a week and benefits from the use of a purpose-built gymnasium and hydrotherapy pool, plus expert help in making changes to his lifestyle. He even manages to stop smoking. Within three months he resumes his full-time job. Total cost of NHS resources for three months = £80,000.

Patient 2: Mr Jones is also provided with immediate cardiology care, but in this case it is led by a consultant in general medicine. Angioplasty is unavailable due to budgetary constraints and Mr Jones is discharged home to the care of his GP after five days inpatient treatment. Mr Jones does not make any lifestyle changes and continues to smoke 20 cigarettes a day. He develops angina on exertion and fails his medical to resume work. Total cost of NHS resources for three months = £10,000.

Patient 3: Mr Clarke is provided with the same standard of specialist cardiology care that Mr Smith received. However, Mr Clarke is discharged home to the care of his GP after five days. He attends cardiac rehabilitation classes on a weekly basis and is supported to make changes to his lifestyle by visiting the practice nurse at the GP surgery. He is successful in stopping smoking. After three months Mr Clarke returns to his full-time job. Total cost of NHS resources for 3 months = £40,000.

Which patient received the most effective, efficient care?

- Mr Smith (patient 1) exemplifies effective health care. Specifically, he has made a full recovery and returned to work. However, the cost of £80,000 could be argued to be too high and therefore inefficient. In simple terms Mr Smith's case shows how health care can be effective but also inefficient.

- Mr Jones (patient 2) shows the opposite; in this case the treatment is very cheap, but ineffective – Mr Jones fails to make a full recovery. Here effectiveness has been sacrificed for short-term efficiency gains – indeed the chronic dependency of Mr Jones is likely to become very expensive over the long term.

- Mr Clarke (patient 3) illustrates how care can be both effective and efficient; here Mr Clarke has made a full recovery within the same time period as Mr Smith, but the cost of treatment has been halved by removing wasted effort and expense.

angioplasty
a surgical procedure usually used to unblock a narrowed or occluded artery

- A reduction of inequality in health-care provision (for example equal access to specialist medical services).
- The development of quality through the continued development of national standards and the continued support of NHS employees.

Several of these themes have already been briefly explored throughout this chapter and are confirmed in the recent review by Lord Darzi (2008) – NHS Next Stage Review. Alternative examples can be accessed from the case studies provided by the National Programme for IT in NHS (NPfIT) website. However, in order to provide a more detailed outline of how health informatics is central to the organisation and management of care delivery at both a local and national level, let us now consider the example of National Service Frameworks.

National Service Frameworks

National Service Frameworks (NSFs) are examples of long-term national strategies related to specific areas of health care; they set specific goals and are defined within set time frames. Chart 19.2 details the nine areas of health care currently targeted by NSFs. Primary objectives related to the development of NSFs include: a focus on health promotion and disease prevention, and the reduction of inequality in relation to health-care provision by the development of agreed national standards.

⊘ Link

Chapter 18 further discusses NSFs.

In setting national goals and targets, NSFs become the templates for the development of local strategy and policy, influencing the development of protocols for the care of patients, and becoming a source of evidence on which practitioners rationalise their care. Yet, each of the NSFs published to date also recognises the importance of information management in the implementation of change (Abbott et al., 2004). For example, the NSF on Mental Health was followed by a dedicated strategy for information management (DoH, 2001), as was the NSF for Older People (DoH, 2002b). Therefore, NSFs can be said to emphasise the importance of managing information. For example, at a local level, without the management of information how would any one department, or Trust, assess their performance against the targets set?

Chart 19.2 National Service Frameworks

• Mental Health – launched 1999	• Older People's Services – launched 2001
• Diabetes – launched 1999	
• Paediatric Intensive Care – launched 1999	• Children, Young People and Maternity Services – launched 2004
• Cancer Care – launched 2000	• Renal Care – launched 2004
• Coronary Heart Disease – launched 2000	• Long Term Conditions – launched 2005

Note: All NSFs are available online at http://www.dh.gov.uk.

The Wider Public

So far this chapter has explored the relevance of health informatics, and considered its impact on nursing from the perspective of the patient or carer, the health professional, and the organisation managing the care. Yet the responsibility borne by the health service as a consequence of managing public data has so far received little attention. Issues relating to how data is collected, recorded, used, shared and secured are of key interest to the wider public. Health-related data is sensitive in nature and generic in that some type of health record is kept on each member of the population. Consideration must be given to how information is governed within health care and the development of fair, legal and ethically acceptable methods of managing data. The umbrella term used to describe this process is 'information governance'.

Information governance

Information governance considers how health-related data is: Held, Obtained, Recorded, Used and Shared (HORUS). Specifically it considers:

- The Data Protection Act (1998)
- The Freedom of Information Act (2000)
- Computer Misuse Act (1990)
- The NHS Confidentiality Code of Practice (DoH, 2003b)
- Information security management
- Records management.

A thorough understanding of the various components of information governance is not essential for all clinical staff and is therefore beyond the scope of this chapter. However, having some knowledge of the basic principles involved and how these can impact on professional practice is essential if nurses are to practise in a manner which safeguards the data entrusted to them and protects the confidentiality of the patients within their care.

It is important to note that the Data Protection Act (1998), Freedom of Information Act (2000) and Computer Misuse Act (1990) are legislative Acts. Simply put, this means that they represent the law of the land and are not just applicable to the NHS. A brief description of these key areas of legislation is provided in Charts 19.3, 19.4 and 19.5. Other elements of information governance are broader in their scope than the legislation connected to them. For example, consideration of information security and management should consider, but not be limited by, the scope of the Privacy and Electronic Communications Regulations 2003 – relating to the security of electronic communications – and the Computer Misuse Act 1990, which relates to unauthorised access to computer material.

The five elements of HORUS represent the basis for the principles of information governance. Consideration is now given to each of these areas in turn.

Holding data

A primary concern of the storage of health-related data is the maintenance of confidentiality. Confidentiality has been defined as a duty that arises as one person discloses information to another (DoH, 2003b). It is a requirement of established codes of professional conduct, for example the Nursing and Midwifery Council Code (2008), and it is a legal right for the patient regardless of their competence to extend their trust, for example, to unconscious patients or those detained under the Mental Health Act.

The NHS Confidentiality Code of Practice (DoH, 2003b) examined the nature of confidentiality and put forward a confidentiality model. This model is based on four interconnected principles:

1 Protect – look after the patient's information
2 Inform – ensure that patients are aware of how their information is used
3 Provide choice– allow patients to decide whether their information can be disclosed or used in particular ways
4 Improve – always look for better ways to protect, inform, and provide choice.

⌘ Link

Chapter 3 also discusses the Data Protection Act and Freedom of Information Act.

✳ Activity 19.4

Simple precautions can be used to help promote patient confidentiality. Within your practice environment try to identify how confidentiality could be safeguarded.

For example:
- Avoid careless talk
- Always log off the computer
- Turn the computer screen away from the view of onlookers.

Chart 19.3 The Data Protection Act 1998

The Data Protection Act (DPA) 1998 provides individuals with seven statutory rights in regard to information held about them by a third party. The rights of the individual, known as the data subject, are combined with statutory obligations placed on those who process information, known as data controllers. These obligations are summarised as eight principles of good practice.

The DPA also distinguishes between 'personal data' and 'sensitive data'. Personal data is described as any information about a living individual that can be identified or be derived from the storage or merging of data held by the data controller. Sensitive data is subject to more stringent controls and is directly relevant to health care, in that it is defined as any data that relate to an individual's:

- Racial or ethnic origin
- Political belief
- Religious or spiritual belief
- Trade union affiliation
- Physical or mental health
- Sexual life
- Alleged or actual criminal activity or sentencing

The rights provided to individuals by the Data Protection Act are as follows:

1 The right to subject access: this allows people to find out what information is held about them on computer and within some manual records.
2 The right to prevent processing: anyone can ask a data controller not to process information relating to him or her that causes substantial unwarranted damage or distress to them or anyone else.
3 The right to prevent processing for direct marketing: anyone can ask a data controller not to process information relating to him or her for direct marketing purposes.
4 Rights in relation to automated decision-taking: individuals have a right to object to decisions made only by automatic means, for example when there is no human involvement.
5 The right to compensation: an individual can claim compensation from a data controller for damage and distress caused by any breach of the Act. Compensation for distress alone can only be claimed in limited circumstances.
6 The right to rectification, blocking, erasure and destruction: individuals can apply to the court to order a data controller to rectify, block or destroy personal details if they are inaccurate or contain expressions of opinion based on inaccurate information.
7 The right to ask the commissioner to assess whether the Act has been contravened: if someone believes their personal information has not been processed in accordance with the DPA, they can ask the commissioner to make an assessment. If the Act is found to have been breached and the matter cannot be settled informally, then an enforcement notice may be served on the data controller in question.

The DPA eight principles of good practice are that data must be:

1 Fairly and lawfully processed.
2 Processed for limited purposes.
3 Adequate, relevant and not excessive.
4 Accurate and up to date.
5 Not kept longer than necessary.
6 Processed in accordance with the individual's rights.
7 Secure.
8 Not transferred to countries outside the European economic area unless the country has adequate protection for the individual.

Reproduced with permission from Information Commissioners Office, Data Protection Act Fact Sheet (n.d.).

Chart 19.4 The Freedom of Information Act 2000

The Freedom of Information Act allows individuals to access information held by public authorities in order to develop a culture of openness and accountability within the public sector. The development of such a culture is hoped to increase general understanding about the operation of public sector bodies, how they spend public money and make their decisions. Each public authority must publish an information scheme as a guide to how information can be accessed. Equally, individuals have a general right to access information held by public authorities, subject to certain exemptions. These exemptions are either absolute or qualified. Where the exemption is absolute, the right to know is completely denied, for example requests for personal data. Where the exemption is qualified, the public authority must consider if the release of the information is in the greater public interest

Chart 19.5 The Computer Misuse Act 1990

The Computer Misuse Act of 1990 is a law in the UK that makes illegal certain activities, such as hacking into systems, misusing systems or helping a person to gain access to files on someone else's computer. The Computer Misuse Act is split into three sections and makes the following acts illegal:

- Unauthorised access to computer material
- Unauthorised access to computer systems with intent to commit another offence
- Unauthorised modification of computer material.

The first section in the Computer Misuse Act forbids a person to use someone else's identification to access a computer, run a program or obtain any data, even if no personal gain is involved in such access. You also cannot change, copy, delete or move a program. The Computer Misuse Act also makes illegal any attempt to obtain someone else's password.

The second provision in the Computer Misuse Act is gaining access to a computer system in order to commit or facilitate a crime. You cannot use someone else's system to send material that might be offensive or to send viruses or malicious software. You also cannot give someone your identification so they can use your system for this purpose as this means that you would be facilitating someone else's intent or crime.

Thirdly, unauthorised Modification in the Computer Misuse Act means you cannot delete, change or corrupt data. Access with intent, and unauthorised modification are considered to be very serious and may be punished by heavy fines and/or prison.

Obtaining data

The process of obtaining health-related data should be transparent. This means that the patient should know, wherever possible, what data is being collected, for what reason the data is required, how the data will be used, how long the data will be required for, and how they may be able to access it. It is worth remembering that the information stored within a health-care record is the property of the patient. Under the Data Protection Act 1998 the patient maintains the right to access their own health record. A good example of this transparency in action can be found when contacting the helpline NHS Direct. The automated greeting provided by this service offers to patients an opportunity to find out how their information will be stored and used, and this is further supported by information on the NHS Direct website (www.nhsdirect.nhs.uk).

Recording data

Central to the concept of data-recording is the concept of data integrity. Hebda et al. (2005, p. 65) describe data integrity as a process to 'collect, store and retrieve correct, complete and current data'. Data integrity is essential within health care at all levels of data processing. For example, if any clinical data was inaccurate, out of date or incomplete, it is likely that treatment based on that data would be incorrect. Equally, management or financial decisions based on inaccurate data could be disastrous. Data validity is a key concept to data integrity and is considered briefly below.

Data validity refers to the degree to which data accurately represents what it was originally obtained for. Data validation is therefore a method of ensuring data accuracy and completeness. It is best performed at the time that data is entered and therefore data validation should be a primary concern for all clinical staff. Methods for data validation are commonly applied to computer-based record systems, but data validation procedures should not be limited by the technology used. Validation checks could be as simple as a student asking their mentor if a recorded value is accurate and complete. Timing is essential and data validation should take place at the time data is recorded; realising a previously recorded data value was inaccurate even hours after it was recorded can have potentially lethal implications.

Data use

The main purpose for the collection of patient data may at first appear quite obvious; patients entrust health professionals with information to better inform the care they receive. However, this point of view provides only a narrow perspective and it is important to realise that patient data may be used far more widely. A common method of considering the uses of data is by the classification of primary and secondary use.

Primary use relates to the use of data for the main purpose for which it was originally collected from the individual patient (House of Lords Select Committee on Science and Technology, 2001). Primary use may therefore include those uses of data that relate directly to patient care. However, these may still be fairly broad ranging and can include the use of individual patient data for clinical audit or clinical governance initiatives (DoH, 2003b), for example, adverse incident and near-miss reporting. The primary use of data may require that data is shared with other care agencies within and outside the NHS and it is important that patients are aware of when disclosure of information will be necessary.

Secondary use of data relates to uses of existing data that are not connected to the primary purpose of data collection (House of Lords Select Committee on Science and Technology, 2001). Secondary uses include data used within clinical research, financial auditing, health service initiative reporting, and the formation of diagnosis and treatment trends. In some secondary data processes it may be unlikely that patient confidentiality will be breached. It is therefore uncertain as to whether the patient needs to consent to this use of data.

Sharing data

The concept of data-sharing is closely tied to that of confidentiality. Data should only be shared when absolutely necessary as sharing increases the risk of security breaches and data corruption. Any form of data-sharing must also be lawful. Of particular relevance are the Data Protection Act 1998 and the Privacy and Electronic Communications Regulations 2003 which apply controls on how data may be shared.

The Caldecott Report (1997) represented a milestone in relation to the security of patient-based information within the NHS. In particular it considered the methods of transferring patient-related data between NHS bodies and non-NHS organisations. In the main the committee found that data-sharing was performed legitimately and diversely. In some instances it was found that more patient data was shared than was absolutely necessary. Key recommendations from the report included the need to reinforce confidentiality issues among staff, and the establishment of local accountability for the safeguarding of confidential information through the nomination of Caldecott guardians. The establishment of local accountability was intended to ensure that all methods for data-sharing, including those existing and those yet to be developed, are tested against principles of good practice (Caldecott Report, 1997).

Chapter Summary

This chapter has covered some of the key elements of health informatics theory including the nature of data, information and knowledge. Consideration has been given as to why health informatics should be considered a foundation of nursing practice and how informatics relates to all who are connected with health care. Specifically the impact of health informatics systems has been considered from the perspective of the patient, the practitioner, the health-care organisation and the wider public. Relevant legislation and current national policy has been briefly considered.

? Test yourself!

1 What is the difference between data, information and knowledge?

2 During a day in your placement setting consider all information you come across. Plot the flow of this information: how did it come to you, what happened to it next?

3 Describe a patient journey.

4 What are the differences between an electronic care record and an integrated health record?

5 Compile a list of resources you have found useful in informing your practice.

6 Describe the three basic components of evidence-based practice.

7 What are the main differences between efficiency and effectiveness?

8 What does the acronym HORUS stand for?

9 Can a patient see their own health-care record?

10 What factors should be considered before divulging any patient-related information?

References

Abbott, W., Blankley, N., Bryant, J. and Bullas, S. (2004) *Current Perspectives: Information in Healthcare*. British Computer Society Health Informatics Committee, Swindon.

Bertulis, R. (2005) *Report of Key Findings of RCN's Survey of the Information Needs of Nurses, Health Care Assistants, Midwives and Health Visitors*. Royal College of Nursing. http://www.rcn.org.uk/downloads/news/INA%20report%20external.doc (accessed 11 July 2005).

Caldecott, F. (1997) *Report on the Review of Patient-identifiable Information*. Department of Health, London.

Computer Misuse Act (1990) *Chapter 18*, Crown Copyright. http://www.opsi.gov.uk/acts/acts1990/Ukpga_19900018_en_1.htm

Crisp, N. (2004) *Chief Executive's Report to the NHS*. Department of Health, London.

Darzi (2008) *High Quality Care for All: NHS Next Stage Review Final Report*. http://www.dh.gov.uk/en/Publicationsandstatistics/Publications/PublicationsPolicyAndGuidance/DH_085825

Data Protection Act (1998) *Chapter 29*. Crown Copyright. http://www.opsi.gov.uk/acts/acts1998/19980029.htm

DoH (Department of Health) (1998) *Information Executive: Information for Health: An Information Strategy for the Modern NHS 1998–2005*. http://www.nhsia.nhs.uk/def/pages/info4health/contents.asp

DoH (Department of Health) (2000) *The NHS Plan A Plan for Investment A Plan for Reform*. Cm 4818-I, Accessed online (16/7/05): http://www.dh.gov.uk/assetRoot/04/05/57/83/04055783.pdf

DoH (Department of Health) (2001) *Mental Health Information Strategy*. Department of Health.

DoH (Department of Health) (2002a) *Delivering 21st Century IT Support for the NHS National Strategic Programme*. http://www.dh.gov.uk/assetRoot/04/06/71/12/04067112.pdf

DoH (Department of Health) (2002b) *Information Strategy for Older People in England*. Department of Health. http://www.dh.gov.uk/assetRoot/04/01/98/66/04019866.pdf

DoH (Department of Health) (2003a) *Staff in the NHS 2003*. Governmental Statistics Service. http://www.publications.DH.gov.uk/public/nhsstaff2003.pdf

DoH (Department of Health) (2003b) *Confidentiality NHS Code of Practice*. Department of Health. http://www.dh.gov.uk/assetRoot/04/06/92/54/04069254.pdf

Freedom of Information Act (2000) *Chapter 36*, Crown Copyright. http://www.opsi.gov.uk/acts/acts2000/20000036.htm

Hebda,T., Czar, P. and Mascara, C. (2005) *Handbook of Informatics for Nurses and Health Care Professionals*. Pearson/Prentice Hall, Englewood Cliffs, NJ.

House of Lords Select Committee on Science and Technology (2001) *Science and Technology 4th Report*. House of Lords. http://www.parliament.the-stationery-office.co.uk/pa/ld200001/ldselect/ldsctech/57/5701.htm

Introna, L.D. (1997) *Management, Information and Power*. Macmillan – now Palgrave Macmillan, London.

NICE (National Institute for Health and Clinical Excellence) (2005) *A Guide to NICE*. NICE, London.

NHS Information Centre for Health and Social Care (2007) *NHS Staff 1996–2006 Overview*. http://www.ic.nhs.uk/statistics-and-data-collections/workforce/nhs-staff-numbers/nhs-staff-1996--2006-overview.

NPfIT (National Programme For Information Technology in the NHS) (2005) NHS Connecting for Health. http://www.connectingforhealth.nhs.uk/introduction/ataglance

Nursing and Midwifery Council (2008) *The Code: Standards of Conduct, Performance and Ethics for Nurses and Midwives*. NMC, London. www.nmc-uk.org

OUP (1996) *Dictionary of Computing. Oxford Reference Online*. Oxford University Press, Oxford.

Paul, R.J. (2002) Is information systems an intellectual subject? *European Journal of Information Systems* **11**, 174–7.

Privacy and Electronic Communications Regulations (2003) European Community Directive. http://www.informationcommissioner.gov.uk/eventual.aspx?id=35

Sackett, D.L., Rosenberg, W.M.C., Gray, M.J.A., Haynes, R.B. and Richardson, W.S. (1996) Evidence based medicine: what it is and what it isn't. *British Medical Journal* **312**: 71–2.

Smith, K.P. and Christakis, N.A. (2008) Social networks and health. *Annual Review of Sociology* **34**, 405–29.

Wanless, D. (2002) *Securing our Future Health: Taking a Long Term View*. HM Treasury. http://www.hm-treasury.gov.uk/Consultations_and_Legislation/wanless/

20

Developing Effective Leadership and Management Skills

📖 Contents

☑ Learning outcomes

The purpose of this chapter is to help you to develop your understanding of leadership and management and the skills required to function within these roles. It is not uncommon for nurses to feel that leadership and management is something done by others higher up in the organisation, but many management activities and decisions are undertaken by staff who are not in a management role (Carter, 2009). Indeed good patient care is dependent on a nurse's ability to safely lead and manage delivery of that care (Carter, 2009; NMC, 2008a), and first-year student nurses are involved in the delivery of care to patients, so this chapter is as relevant to them as it is to the registered nurse. At the end of the chapter, you should be able to:

- Define 'leadership' and 'management' and differentiate between the two roles
- Develop a plan for making a change in practice, taking into consideration how a transformational leader would lead change
- Demonstrate ability to plan and organise the work of the team for a shift and delegate activities to members of staff
- Identify sources of power, and reflect on your own sources of power in directing the work of others in the team
- Describe the different leadership styles and

- appreciate the factors which influence the most appropriate leadership style to adopt in order to suit the staff, situation and yourself
- Discuss how knowledge of the expectancy model of motivation and transactional leadership may help you when you are directing the work of the team
- Outline the factors to consider when giving constructive feedback aimed at improving the quality of an individual's performance.

Introduction

This chapter will explore relevant theories in order to shed light on what leaders and managers do, and the skills which are necessary to enable them to achieve the role successfully. The Nursing and Midwifery Council (NMC, 2008a) have outlined the essential skills clusters which every student is expected to attain by the completion of their training, and leadership and management are included within these skills clusters, so this chapter is relevant to students at all stages within their training as well as to registered nurses. For instance: the NMC state that the public can trust a newly registered nurse to 'Provide care based on the highest standards, knowledge and competence' (NMC, 2008a, Essential skills standard 1); this includes working within the limitations of the role and recognising their own level of competency. Thus student nurses right from the start of their training must have an understanding of the concepts of responsibility and accountability when accepting tasks which are delegated to them and the qualified nurse must recognise the knowledge and skills of the team they lead in order to delegate appropriately (NMC, 2008a, Essential skills standard 15). In addition the student nurse needs to observe and develop their own leadership and management skills in preparation for when they become registered nurses and hold responsibility for leading and managing others. Finally, an understanding of the subject of leadership and management will help students to understand what managers are doing and why their role is important.

Fayol (1949) described the role of a manager as someone who plans, organises, directs and controls the work of others. This classical view of management gives a good insight into what it is that managers do. These four aspects of the role of the manager will be explored within this chapter and the leadership and management skills required to achieve each aspect of the managerial role will be investigated.

Leading and Managing in Health and Social Care

The role of the qualified nurse incorporates leadership and management of staff, material resources and services within an increasingly challenging environment. Some of the challenges currently facing nurses include: rising expectations of patients; budget constraints; advances in treatments and information technology; changes in the nature of disease and the way in which services are delivered; and changing expectations of staff working within health care settings (DoH, 2006; DoH, 2008).

The Department of Health (DoH, 2008) has created a vision for the future of the National Health Service (NHS) as a place in which patients and the public are provided with information and choice, and where quality is at the heart of the service provided. To achieve this vision nurses need to focus on the needs of the patient and develop skills in leading and managing care within the rapidly changing arena (Sullivan and Decker, 2005; DoH, 2009).

The role of the leader and manager is extensive and includes developing both qualified and non-qualified staff and ensuring compliance with professional, regulatory and governmental standards of care. In addition they are responsible for facilitating collaborative working between disciplines and departments. Sullivan and Decker (2005) state that the role of the nurse manager is to plan and deliver high quality clinical care by making the best use of human and material resources. In the present arena of health care, the challenge is also to deliver high quality services within tight financial constraints. All of these aspects require good leadership and management skills.

Leadership and Management Defined

Before we begin to examine the roles of leaders and managers we need to define leadership and management; however, leadership and management are difficult to define. The reason for this may be because it is hard to separate the concept of leadership or management from the jobs that they do and the ways in which they do them. The two roles are intertwined and many elements overlap.

Most definitions of leadership originate from researcher's observations of how leaders behave and how people react to these behaviours. Northouse (2004, p. 3) defines leadership as 'a process whereby an individual influences a group of individuals to achieve a common goal'.

On the other hand, a manager is described as someone who gets things done with the assistance of other people (Stewart, 1967). The two descriptions are remarkably similar and the roles of leaders and managers do overlap but there is a fundamental difference between the two roles.

Managers are employed by the organisation and are responsible and accountable for achieving the goals of the organisation. Managers can use their authority (as bestowed by their position in the organisation) to get others to undertake the work which needs to be done. The manager's role is to plan the work which needs to be done and to coordinate resources in delivery of the service (Sullivan and Decker, 2005). In order to achieve this, the manager has to plan, organise, supervise, negotiate and ensure adequate and suitable staffing.

Leaders, on the other hand, may be formal or informal. Formal leaders are those that use the authority bestowed upon them by their position within the organisational hierarchy (Sullivan and Decker, 2009). Informal leaders may emerge at any level within the hierarchy and use their interpersonal skills to influence others to work towards a specific goal. Leaders are skilled at creating a vision that others want to work towards. They empower others by developing their knowledge; communicating and helping them to problem solve (Antrobus and Kitson, 1999).

Finkelman (2006, p. 17) states that 'Leadership and management are not the same...the goal is really to have managers who are also leaders.' Table 20.1 identifies some differences between leadership and management.

Table 20.1 Differentiation of leadership and management

Managers	Leaders
Plan the work to be done in order to achieve goals/objectives and control the budget.	Establish the long-term direction that the service should be heading in and create a compelling vision that staff want to achieve.
Organise the work to be undertaken by ensuring adequate staffing levels and delegating activities. The manager's focus is mainly on *efficiency*.	Align the skills of staff with the work to be done. The leader's focus is mainly on *effectiveness*.
Control the work by checking that activities are going according to plan and problem solving to overcome issues encountered.	Motivate and inspire the staff so they engage with the work to be done.
Ensure that there is a measure of predictability and order in the work undertaken, for example by developing protocols and procedures for staff to follow.	Seek to improve and enhance services and make changes to the way services are delivered.

Source: Adapted from Northouse (2004).

Leadership and management are equally important. A good leader uses their interpersonal skills to clarify what the team needs to work towards and influences others to achieve the task. A good manager plans the work to be undertaken, and ensures the policies and procedures are developed and members of staff are trained so that the team know what is expected of them and have the skills to deliver the service.

In order to be an effective nurse manager some understanding of the role played by leaders and managers is essential. Seminal work undertaken by Fayol (1949) identified four roles of a manager – planning, organising, directing and controlling; each of these will be explored in more depth.

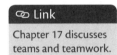

Link

Chapter 17 discusses teams and teamwork.

The Role of the Leader and Manager in Relation to Planning

Planning is described by Sullivan and Decker (2005, p. 56) as a 'four staged process which includes decision making and problem solving in order to achieve specific goals'.

Boddy (2005, p. 169) depicts the four stages of planning as 'the task of setting objectives, specifying how to achieve them, implementing the plan and evaluating the results'.

Planning is an important aspect of managing, whether it be planning the care of an individual patient, or the day-to-day activities in a department, or planning the implementation of a change. Plans help the team to know what needs to be done, by whom and within what timescale. Without plans the work may become chaotic and things could be forgotten. Managers also need to be skilled at contingency planning in order to respond proactively or reactively to problems which arise in the course of the working day such as sudden deterioration of a patient, staff sickness, or an outbreak of infection.

Planning is essential to make the best use of resources, for instance an operating theatre is an expensive resource both in terms of staff and equipment, so it is important that there is a minimal delay between patients within the operating theatre suite. Members of theatre staff plan the order in which operations will be undertaken, and convey this information to the wards so that the patients are prepared for theatre in a timely manner. Without the plan no-one would know what was happening or when, and hence delays would occur resulting in a waste of resources.

Fayol (1949) identified the following four planning stages:

- Establishing goals or direction
- Evaluating the present situation
- Formulating a plan or a means to achieve the goal
- Converting the plan into actions to be undertaken.

Each of these planning stages will be explored in more depth.

Establishing objectives or goals

When planning any activity or change it is important to identify what exactly is to be achieved. This seems obvious, but if the purpose of the activity is not clear then it becomes difficult to plan the details of how to get to the objective. Boddy (2005) recommends that goals or objectives should be Specific, Measurable, Attainable, Realistic and Tangible (SMART) because then progress towards the goals can be reviewed (see 'management control').

Nurses are familiar with planning the care of the patient and the need to set targets or goals to work towards. If targets or goals are not set, then how do we know when we have achieved what we set out to do? An often overlooked aspect of target setting is the impact it can have on motivating an individual or team when they are able to celebrate achievement of the goal.

Evaluating the present situation

This is an important step in the planning process; it is essential to understand the present situation in order to plan what needs to be done next. Nurses review the current condition of each patient on a regular basis in order to ensure that the plans for their care are appropriate to meet their current needs.

When working with a team in delivery of care the nurse should review the skills of the staff and identify any training needs as well as plans for how to address these. This information can be used later in the planning stage when they need to identify who has the skills to undertake certain aspects of the work, and thus will underpin the decision of who to delegate aspects of work to.

When managing a change evaluation of the present situation is important so that the manager recognises what is currently being done well and ensures that they plan the change to incorporate and build upon these strengths.

Formulating a plan or a means to achieve the goal

Good plans are essential because they are a means of communicating what needs to be done in order to achieve the goals/objectives. The nursing process provides staff with a clear plan of what needs to be done for each patient; without these plans the patient's progress towards recovery may be delayed, tests may not be undertaken when they should be and valuable resources may be wasted due to unnecessary delays.

When in charge of a shift the nurse also needs to identify who is responsible for achieving each activity and then should monitor their progress towards the goal, taking corrective action if things are not going according to plan (see 'The managers role in relation to controlling').

Plans are also essential in relation to managing a change. The plan should specify what needs to be done, by whom and within what time scale. This enables everyone involved to know what their responsibilities are; it also makes it possible for progress towards implementing the change to be reviewed.

Converting the plan into actions to be undertaken

Having identified what needs to be done, the manager then needs to allocate work to staff with the skills to carry it out. Those responsible for each task need to be clear about what needs to be done; who else is involved; the resources available to assist them with the activity and the date by which it should be completed.

Planning and change management

The nurse manager is responsible for planning changes and improvements to the service. These plans may be in response to policies and targets set by the government, or in order to improve the quality of service provided. Kotter and Cohen (2002) suggest that when introducing a change the manager needs to first of all develop a sense of urgency for the need to change. This involves making people feel uncomfortable or dissatisfied with the present situation by highlighting where practice is falling short of the desired standard, so that they develop a desire to change.

Kotter (1995) also advocates that the leader of a change needs to develop a compelling vision of the desired future state. To do this the leader needs to demonstrate how the proposed change will bring about improvements in practice. The leadership model which is closely aligned with change management is that of transformational leadership.

Transformational leadership (Burns, 1978 and Bass, 1985)

A transformational leader is seen as someone who questions the status quo and, rather than criticising current practice, they challenge others to think differently by presenting new ideas (Gill, 2006). Transformational leaders are seen as those who motivate staff to do more than they thought they could do, and they do this by gaining the trust, respect and loyalty of the staff (Gill, 2006). The transformational leader uses one or more of the following to achieve performance beyond expectations.

Intellectual stimulation

The leader increases awareness of problems and inspires others to examine difficulties from a different angle (Bass, 1985). This is an important aspect of managing a change because change is often introduced in order to resolve a problem, and as Einstein (1875–1955) once said 'We cannot solve a problem with the same thinking that created it' (Harris, 1995).

Inspirational motivation

The transformational leader creates a compelling vision of the future and in so doing inspires staff to want to work towards making the vision a reality (Yukl, 2006). In addition the transformational leader motivates staff by ensuring that they can achieve their personal goals while working towards the goals of the organisation (Gill, 2006). A third important aspect of inspirational motivation is that the leader models the appropriate behaviour expected from staff (Yukl, 2006). Each of these aspects is important when introducing a change. If members of staff are enthused by the proposed change, they are more likely to get involved with the change process. A leader can help staff to achieve a sense of satisfaction or develop their skills by delegating aspects of the change for them to lead. Finally, staff will watch the leader closely, and if their behaviour indicates they are fully supportive of the change then staff members are more likely to accept the implementation of the change.

Idealised influence

The transformational leader's behaviour is such that they are seen as charismatic and inspire others to follow them (Yukl, 2006; Gill, 2006). The leader gains the respect and trust of others by demonstrating their confidence in the vision and taking responsibility for their actions (Gill, 2006). They exhibit determination and persistence in pursuing the goal and in doing so the transformational leader encourages others to continue working towards the change, even when the going gets tough.

Individualised consideration

The transformational leader gets to know the staff on their team and understands their personal aspirations and their abilities. When introducing a change the transformational leader would try to match individual abilities with the work to be done, so that staff can gain a sense of achievement for their part in bringing in the change.

From the description of the transformational leader above it can be seen that the four 'I's of transformational leadership are applicable to *all* aspects of leading and managing, and can have a positive effect on the team.

Having planned what needs to be done, the nurse manager is then responsible for organising the team in the delivery of the planned care (or change).

The Role of the Leader and Manager in Relation to Organising

Sullivan and Decker (2005) describe organising as the process by which the nurse manager coordinates the work to be done. There are four parts to the process of organising:

1   Identifying what has to be done.
2   Dividing the work up between members of the team.
3   Assigning authority for the work (delegating) and ensuring the team know who to report to regarding the work they are undertaking.
4   Reviewing the use of human and material resources in achieving the work.

Delegation is an important aspect of organising the work. A leader or manager can delegate specific tasks, a range of tasks, projects, roles (such as link roles) or even leadership of the team (Finkelman, 2006).

Delegation

Delegation is defined by Boddy (2005) as giving someone the authority to undertake specific activities. The person delegating the activity remains accountable for the work and so must be certain that they have delegated appropriately. The person undertaking the task is accountable to the delegator for the responsibilities they have taken on (Carter, 2009).

For example a nurse may delegate the task of assisting a patient to wash, dress and move from bed to a chair to a health-care assistant (HCA). When moving the patient from bed to chair, the HCA may not have undertaken a full risk assessment, resulting in them failing to identify that the patient was not well that day and as a result was not able to transfer with the assistance of one person, and the patient falls. The HCA is *responsible* for failing to act appropriately, but the nurse is *accountable* for the decision to delegate that task to them, and for not checking that they knew how to undertake a risk assessment prior to moving the patient. Rather than apportioning blame, the reasons for the accident should be explored and the HCA supported in developing skills in undertaking risk assessments for the future (see 'risk management'). It can be seen from this example that delegation is not just a matter of giving a job to someone else to do, and careful consideration is necessary when delegating to others.

Guidelines for effective delegation

Decide what to delegate

Yukl (2006) suggests that the manager should consider delegating tasks that:

• Can be done better by someone who has more expertise.
• Develop the skills of the person undertaking them.

The task should be challenging, but not so difficult that it puts the person off from trying in the first place. Great care is needed in order to ensure the

---

✷ Activity 20.2

Organising the team to deliver patient care

The next time you are at work consider the following:

• **What** needs to be done
• **When** does it need to be done by
• **Who** is the best person to do it
• **Where** must the work take place
• **Why** does it need to be done?

Plan what and how you will delegate activities to the team.

individual is successful in undertaking the task, as failure could undermine their confidence or ruin their reputation.

Choose who to delegate to

The NMC Code (2008b) highlights the importance of ensuring that the person the nurse delegates to is able to carry out their instructions. The delegator is responsible for selecting the best person to undertake the task (Finkelman, 2006). When considering who may be the best person for the task factors such as their level of knowledge and experience should be taken into consideration. That does not mean that tasks can only be delegated to those with the knowledge and skills to do them, but the manner in which the task is delegated will need to differ accordingly.

How to delegate

The process of delegation is important to ensure ultimate success. Yukl (2006) identifies four steps to the process:

1 *Clarify responsibility.* This involves agreeing what is to be done and to what standard. The individual needs to know of any priorities, and the timescale within which they have to complete the task.
2 *Delegate authority and clarify limits of their discretion.* Boddy (2005) explains that authority is the right that a person has to make decisions about the work they are doing. Authority may include decisions about resources that can be used and decisions which can be made without prior approval. It is the responsibility of the delegator to clarify the amount of discretion the person taking responsibility has for the assignment.
3 *Specify reporting requirements.* When delegating a task to a member of their team the manager's role is to clarify when they want the person to refer to them for advice. For instance, if a nurse manager were to delegate a wound dressing to a third-year student nurse, they could ask the student to inform them if the wound is red, or if there is a discharge from the wound. The manager would then be able to review the wound and advise upon an appropriate wound dressing.
4 *Ensure acceptance of responsibilities.* Within the health-care arena it is important that the person delegating a task feels confident that the person taking responsibility is committed to carrying out the task that has been delegated. The member of staff may be reluctant to admit doubts or concerns about undertaking the task, and in order to provide a supportive environment Yukl (2006) suggests involving them in deciding how much authority they will have and at what point they will refer back to the manager for assistance.

Managing delegation

In addition to deciding what to delegate and how to delegate Yukl (2006) suggests that the manager also needs to:

1 *Inform others that need to know.* Those whose cooperation is essential in order for the task to be undertaken successfully need to be informed who is now responsible for the task. Failure to do this may result in others questioning the authority of the individual and ignoring their requests or directions.

2 *Monitor progress.* In health and social care this aspect is extremely important, the manager needs to be assured that the task is being undertaken safely and to the standard required (NMC, 2008b). When delegating to an inexperienced member of the team who is undertaking the task for the first time close supervision will be necessary, so that the individual is supported and immediate feedback can be given, thus preventing mistakes (NMC, 2008b). Constructive feedback should be provided to the individual, so that they know what they did well, and also how to improve the next time (see 'providing constructive feedback').

    On the other hand more experienced team members who know how to undertake the task may be left to get on with it, but should always report back to the manager so that they know the task has been completed and are aware of any issues encountered while undertaking the task. It is often difficult to strike a balance when monitoring the performance of staff, so the individual does not feel they are constantly being watched, and in order to overcome this agreement can be reached with the individual on how their performance will be assessed.

3 *Ensure all necessary information is passed on.* It stands to reason that if a task is being delegated then the person responsible for carrying out the task should be in possession of all the necessary information. In order to achieve this, the manager should ensure that all those involved pass information directly to the individual, as opposed to them receiving an abridged, second hand version.

4 *Avoid reverse delegation.* When an individual asks for help with the task which they have been delegated the manager needs to avoid taking over, and should elicit the individual's ideas about how to deal with the situation.

5 *Help the individual to learn from mistakes.* Mistakes should be seen by both parties as an opportunity to learn from the situation and avoid similar mistakes in the future. The manager should identify and provide further training or instruction in order to help the individual to develop their skills and ensure success in the future.

The Role of the Leader and Manager in Relation to Directing

Directing is described by Sullivan and Decker (2009, p. 56) as 'the process of getting the organisation's work done'.

A manager's ability to direct activities is dependent on their use of power, authority and leadership style.

Power can be defined as the capacity of an individual to exert their will over others (Buchanan and Badham, 1999) or 'the ability to get others to do what you want them to do' (Clawson, 2009, p. 219).

Authority is defined as 'the right that a person in a specified role has to make decisions, allocate resources or give instructions' (Boddy, 2005, p. 310).

Leadership style is the manner in which the leader behaves towards others.

Power and authority

It is important for an individual leader and manager to recognise their own power and authority and to utilise them appropriately when directing the work of others. French and Raven (1959) classified five sources of power:

1. *Legitimate power* comes from the position an individual holds within the hierarchy of the organisation (also known as *position power*). Their position within the hierarchy gives them authority over those members of staff who are lower down in the hierarchy.

2. *Referent power* (also known as charismatic or personal power), is when the leader or manager is liked by others who want to associate with the leader and support them.

3. *Expertise power* is when members of staff recognise that an individual has specialist knowledge and are therefore willing to follow their suggestions. The specialist knowledge may be about how the organisation operates (knowledge of policies and procedures) or how to perform a task, for example the duty rota or setting up specialist equipment.

4. *Reward power* (also known as *resource power*) can be used at all levels within the hierarchy by praising people for their efforts and celebrating when the team have successes such as bringing in a change in practice. Some levels within the hierarchy are also able to bestow rewards such as enabling someone to move through the Agenda for Change gateway to the next level.

5. *Coercive power* is the ability to get others to do something because they fear reprisal if they do not do it.

A leader has to learn to use their power appropriately in order to achieve the desired outcomes. Table 20.2 outlines some of the pros and cons of the sources of power.

Your answer to Activity 20.3 could discuss how every member of qualified staff has legitimate power and resource power because of their position within the hierarchy, and the ability to give praise to others. The sources of power which can be developed are personal (referent) power and expertise power. To develop personal power the leader needs to be self-aware of the impact of their style and personality on others and to work at building good relationships with their team. Expert power requires dedication and effort to constantly develop knowledge and understanding of the role and the evidence underpinning practice.

✹ Activity 20.3

Recognising personal power: Consider which of the above sources of power you have within your current role. How might you increase the power that you have to influence others with whom you work?

Table 20.2 Pros and cons of sources of power

Source of power	Pros	Cons
Legitimate (position) power	Gives the person the right to direct the work of others	Position in the hierarchy does not equate to respect from staff
Referent (personal) power	Easy to influence others because they like and respect the individual	The holder of this power needs to pay attention to ethical considerations as this power base could be misused to support their own ends.
Expertise power	Enables the holder to improve practice by sharing their knowledge and expertise	It is important to keep updating knowledge or there is a danger of their expertise being out of date.
Reward power	It makes the recipient feel good when they are rewarded for their efforts	Praise needs to be specific if it is to be effective
Coercive power	Effective when someone is not performing at the required level	Has a long-term consequence in terms of how staff members feel about being subjected to coercion.

In order for an individual to use their power to influence others they need to be acknowledged and respected by those whom they are trying to influence (Boddy and Paton, 1998). If the team do not acknowledge and respect the leader they may comply in order to avoid sanctions, but grudging compliance does not necessarily result in satisfactory performance (Cox and LeMay, 2007). In addition to understanding power it is also important to consider the style used by the leader. Leadership style refers to the manner in which a leader relates to others.

Leadership style

The NMC (2008a) essential skills cluster emphasises the need for the registered nurse to demonstrate respect for others and to work in partnership, both of which are important for good working relationships. In addition the manner in which a leader relates to others has a major bearing on how the leader is perceived by others and whether they are respected, and so will ultimately affect the success or failure of the manager in directing activities. Lewin and Lippit (1938) and Lewin et al. (1939) identified three leadership styles: autocratic, democratic and laissez-faire.

Autocratic (or authoritarian) leader

All of the power rests with the authoritarian leader whose primary focus is on getting the work done to a high standard. This leader takes responsibility for planning the work to be undertaken each day. They also make decisions and expect others to follow directions given. In addition the autocratic leader expects staff to feed back on progress of work and to refer/check decisions with the leader.

Democratic leader

Power is shared by members of the team because the democratic leader focuses on developing the team. The democratic leader shares their leadership functions among the team in order to help them develop their skills. They also seek the opinions of staff in the decision-making process and interact with all members of the group. The democratic leader expects staff to take on responsibilities and develop skills.

Laissez-faire

There is a conscious decision to pass power to group members because the leader's primary focus is on enabling others to manage and control their own work. They do this by allowing others to work autonomously and only assisting individuals when required.

It must be noted that this description of the laissez-faire leader contrasts with the view that is often held regarding laissez-faire managers as those who do not care, who leave others to face problems or difficulties and do not get involved (Northouse, 2004).

Having done Activity 20.4 you should have considered how in the authoritarian style, junior members of staff often feel secure with this style of leadership because they are being directed and know that they can turn to someone who will make decisions and guide them. However, if the leader is absent some work may not be undertaken because members of staff are not used to organising their own work and may be unsure about the decisions to be made. As staff develop their knowledge and skills and become more experienced they may find this style increasingly frustrating as they are not learning how to plan and direct work activities and make decisions themselves. The lack of emphasis on developing staff within the team may also result in the team not working well together – especially when the leader is not present to direct activities. With the democratic style, members of staff working with the democratic leader develop skills in decision-making and in leading the team. The emphasis on team working means that the camaraderie develops and the team can function in the absence of the leader. Junior members of the team may require more direction initially. Some members of the team, however, may prefer the leader to make decisions and may feel uncomfortable with this approach, perhaps preferring a more autocratic approach. The laissez-faire style is better suited to working with followers who are experienced and capable of taking on responsibility rather than those who are more junior and still require direction and support.

Most managers have a natural tendency towards one of the leadership styles described, and their style is dependent on their assumptions about their team and their own personality. However, one style of leadership is not appropriate to every circumstance and leaders need to be able to alter their leadership style to suite the circumstances they are faced with and this became known as contingency theory.

Contingency theory

The contingency theory suggests that a leader's effectiveness depends upon their ability to match their leadership style to appropriate situations (Northouse, 2004).

✴ Activity 20.4

Impact of leadership style on the team: Consider the impact that the three different styles of leaders might have on the staff working with them. Draw examples from your own practice to help you.

McGregor (1960), Fielder (1967), Stodgill (1974), House and Mitchell (1974) and House (1996) identified a number of variables which influence the leadership style in any given situation. These variables can be viewed from three perspectives (see Figure 20.1):

1   Subordinates perspective
2   The leader' perspective
3   Variables associated with the organisation and task being undertaken.

In order to achieve a favourable outcome the leader needs to assess each of the variables and identify the most appropriate style which suits the needs of the staff involved and the task being undertaken. In doing so, they also need to take into account their natural style of leading and their power.

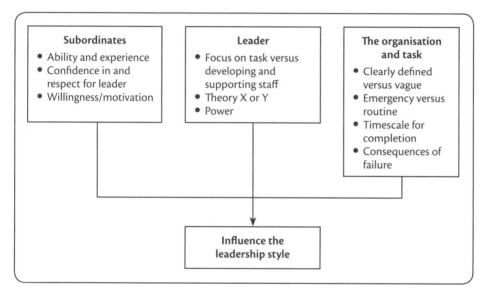

Figure 20.1 Factors influencing the style of leadership

Subordinate variables influencing leadership style

Ability and experience of staff

A team is comprised of individuals who are at varying stages of their career and have different levels of experience. The leader's role is to get the best out of each person (and the team as a whole), and in order to do so the leader needs to take into account the ability of staff members when considering the most appropriate leadership style to use.

Having done Activity 20.5, you should have considered how a first-year student on their first placement will not know what is required of them; they are likely to feel nervous and will need direction. The authoritarian style is therefore most appropriate for them, as the leader will tell them what needs to be done, and show them how to do it. As the responsibility for decision making rests with the leader there is less likelihood of the first-year student making a mistake, and they should feel more secure as they know they have someone to turn to for

✹ Activity 20.5

Choosing an appropriate leadership style to suit the needs of the staff being led: from the descriptions of the autocratic, democratic and laissez-faire leadership styles, consider which leadership style would be most appropriate for the following staff:

- A first-year student on their first placement
- A qualified member of staff who has been working in the department for a year
- An experienced member of staff who has worked in the department for 5 years.

help. The leader's style needs to change as staff members become more experienced in order to help them to develop their own decision making skills, so the democratic style becomes more appropriate for the qualified member of staff who has worked in the department for a year. Experienced members of staff know what work needs to be done, and have developed skills in decision making and organising their own workloads and so the laissez-faire leader's style is appropriate for these staff.

Confidence and respect in the leader

Yukl (2006, p. 216) describes this as 'The extent to which subordinates are loyal and relationships with subordinates are friendly and cooperative'. Members of staff are more likely to comply with requests and direction from the leader when relationships are good between the leader and the team. The team may ignore or undermine the leader if relationships are not good.

House and Mitchell (1974) identified four leadership behaviours which impact on how members of staff feel about the leader and their work:

1 *Supportive leadership:* Creating a friendly work environment in which the needs of team members are taken into consideration.
2 *Directive leadership:* Providing information on what needs to be done and how to do it and ensuring the team follow procedures.
3 *Participative leadership:* Taking the opinions and suggestions of staff into account.
4 *Achievement-orientated leadership:* Setting performance targets and goals which challenge staff to achieve excellence.

A good leader would display each of the above behaviours, and in doing so will engender the support and respect of their team.

Willingness/motivation of staff

If members of staff are willing and feel they have the necessary skills to undertake a task they will respond positively to the leader and allow them to direct their work. The willingness and motivation of staff is closely linked to the degree of confidence and respect individuals have in their leader.

There are numerous theories of motivation – for example Maslow's (1970 [1943]) hierarchy of needs, Herzberg's (1987) two factor theory of motivation – however, there is no one theory that fully explains what motivates an individual. It is clear that motivation is individual (what motivates one person may not motivate another) and that individuals have a choice about whether to act or not. Vroom's (1964) expectancy theory of motivation attempts to explain aspects which influence whether staff will put effort their work.

Expectancy theory of motivation (Vroom, 1964)

The premise of this theory is that people make decisions about how much effort they will put into a job based on their perception of how likely it is that they will succeed in the task. In return they expect to achieve a desirable outcome for doing the job, or avoid undesirable outcomes.

An individual is unlikely to put in the effort required if they are not sure what the job entails, if they feel that they do not have the ability to do the task, or if they do not have the materials they need to do the job well (see Figure 20.2). The leader's role in motivating an individual is to:

- Ensure they know what they have to do
- Develop their knowledge and skills
- Provide the necessary tools, equipment, information and other resources required to do the job
- Alter the individual's perception of the likelihood of success.

A theory of leadership which correlates with the expectancy theory of motivation is that of transactional leadership.

Transactional leadership

With this leadership approach an exchange takes place between the leader and the individual worker where they reach agreement on a reward for undertaking specific duties, for example an individual may agree to work overtime if they are paid extra for doing so.

Gill (2006) describes two elements of transactional leadership:

1 Management by exception which may be passive or active (Bass, 1990). The leader sets work and performance objectives but then may wait for problems to arise and react to mistakes (passive management by exception). Alternatively they monitor progress looking for deviation from procedures and processes, or errors and correcting them (active management by exception).
2 Contingent reward is the provision of rewards (praise, recognition, promotion, financial incentives) for performance which meets expectation.

In order for transactional leadership to work the task needs to be clearly defined and the member of staff has to want the reward being offered or they will not put effort in to their performance.

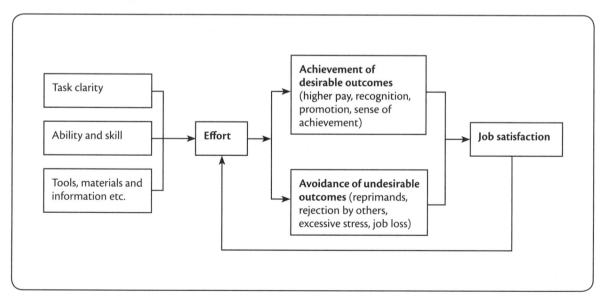

Figure 20.2 Expectancy theory of motivation
Source: Adapted from Vroom (1964).

Leadership variables influencing leadership style

The leaders focus on the task versus developing and supporting people

Stodgill (1974) found that a leader's behaviour depended on whether the leader focused on either organising work, defining roles and responsibilities, scheduling work activities (this was called: initiating structure), or on building camaraderie, respect, trust and liking between the leader and followers (Stodgill called this consideration). Leaders who focus on initiating structure tended to err towards the authoritarian style of leadership, whereas those whose focus was developing the staff and the team tended to be more democratic in their leadership style.

Theory X or Y

McGregor (1960) said that the way in which a manager acts is based upon their assumptions and generalisations. He proposed two sets of assumptions underlying management practice: Theory X and Theory Y.

Theory X was based on the following assumptions:

- People dislike work and will do anything possible to avoid it.
- The average person has little ambition, wants to avoid responsibility and prefers to be directed, they are motivated by security.
- In order to get the work done staff must be coerced, controlled and directed, or threatened with punishment.

Theory Y had contrasting assumptions:

- People apply physical and mental effort in a work situation in the same way as they do when they rest or play.
- Rewarding staff for their achievements generates commitment to the objectives.
- People can exercise self direction and control if they are committed to the objective, so coercion and control are not the only ways in which success may be achieved.

Managers holding the Theory X view of staff are more likely to use an authoritarian style of leadership, whereas, those holding the Theory Y perspective would err towards a democratic style of leadership.

The leader's power

This is described by Yukl (2006, p. 216) as 'The extent to which the leader has authority to evaluate subordinate performance and administer rewards and punishments'. In health and social care environments the leader of a shift is frequently the same grade as the members of staff on shift with them. Hence they do not have the same degree of authority over the staff on the shift as someone who is in a higher grade. However, professional members of staff working in this environment are accountable to their professional body and are responsible for maintaining a safe environment for both patients and staff. In this capacity every qualified member of staff has a responsibility to evaluate and correct the performance of others.

Organisation and task variables influencing leadership style

Clearly defined versus vague task structure

This aspect refers to the extent to which the requirements of the job are spelt out, for example if a procedure exists for a particular task then the leader has more control over the task because they can delegate the activity in the knowledge that staff know how to complete it (or can access the procedure to find out how to do it) and the leader can then monitor adherence to the procedure.

Activities which are vague and unclear reduce a leader's control and influence because there are no set rules to follow and there may be alternative ways to do the job. The leader may not know how to achieve the task and so will need to enlist the help of others within the team. In this circumstance the democratic style would enable the leader to gain input from other members of the team. In addition this style can be used to delegate sections of the work to team members with the appropriate skills to lead on those aspects.

Emergency versus routine work

Emergency situations such as a cardiac arrest require someone to take control and give directions; there is no time for discussion, and decisions need to be made quickly. Therefore the most appropriate style to adopt is the authoritarian leadership style. Routine work, on the other hand, can be delegated to members of the team to complete and in doing so the leader is sharing their responsibility and authority with others within the team.

The time scale in which to complete the task

Often leaders in health and social care are given short timescales within which to make changes. In these situations there is little time for the leader to involve others in decision making and planning the task, hence the style used tends to be authoritarian.

The pace and pressure of work within health and social care environments can also have an impact upon the style of leadership used. Managers often feel under pressure to achieve everything that needs to be done during the shift, and so adopt an authoritarian style as this may be seen as the quickest and easiest option to ensure the work is done. The negative impact of this is that time is not set aside to train and develop staff.

The consequences of not being successful

It is natural for a leader to want to retain control and be prescriptive in circumstances when there is a risk to patients if the task is not carried out successfully. This, however, assumes that the leader has all the knowledge and skills required to direct this situation which may not be the case. In order to minimise the risks involved the leader may need to adopt the democratic style in order to elicit opinions and assistance from others within the team.

The contingency theory highlights that it is not appropriate to use one style of leadership all of the time and that leaders need to be able to adopt the most appropriate style to suit the situation and individual staff members that they are leading.

It can be seen from the above discussion that there are many factors which influence the manner in which a leader and manager directs the activities undertaken by a team.

Throughout this chapter we have examined the role of the manager in relation to planning, organising and directing the work of the team. During the examination of the skills required to function effectively within these management roles the issue of monitoring and evaluating performance has been touched upon, and this relates to the final management role we will be exploring: controlling.

The Role of the Leader and Manager in Relation to Controlling

The idea of controlling may appear outdated and some may feel it is unnecessary or overbearing. Control is often interpreted as someone commanding others by giving orders (Mullins, 2005); however, in management terms, 'control' means to compare performance or results with what was expected (Sullivan and Decker, 2009). The purpose of controlling is to ensure that the work which was planned has been carried out to the standard required. This section will examine three important aspects of control within the health-care environment:

1   Providing constructive feedback in order to improve individual performance
2   Maintaining the quality of services
3   Risk management

Management control

Boddy (2005) outlines the three steps in the control process as:

1   Observing to see what is/has happened
2   Comparing what has happened to what was planned
3   Deciding what actions need to be taken in view of the results and making longer-term plans to overcome problems which have arisen.

Controlling is an essential aspect of the nurse manager's role because the emphasis is on ensuring practice does not fall below the standard required. In order to effectively control the work being undertaken the manager needs to first establish the standards of performance, decide how to measure performance, evaluate the performance and then provide feedback (see Figure 20.3).

When a member of staff is not performing at the level expected then it becomes necessary to give

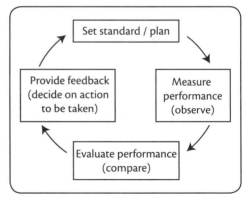

Figure 20.3 Control cycle

constructive feedback to them so that their standard of work (or behaviour) improves.

Providing constructive feedback

Providing constructive feedback is never an easy task for a manager, but it is an essential element of control, so that the member of staff knows what they did well and what aspects of the work need to be improved upon. Yoder Wise (1995) and Finkelman (2006) advocate giving feedback on performance as soon after the event as possible for maximum effect; however, the manager also needs to take time to consider *how* to provide the feedback in a positive way in order to help the individual learn from the situation (Nursing Times.net 2007).

Positive feedback is important because it acts as reinforcement and increases the likelihood of the individual repeating the behaviour/performance again in the future (Nursing Times.net 2007). Positive feedback enables members of staff to know when they are doing the job well and gives the receiver a sense of achievement, which in turn can increase job satisfaction and motivation (Goode and Blegen, 1993).

When giving constructive feedback Finkelman (2006) suggests the following:

1   *Focus on the performance, and not the performer*, remaining objective in this way makes the feedback less threatening to the individual.
2   *Explain the effects of their behaviour.* The reasons why their behaviour needs to change should be made clear.
3   *Specific feedback should be given on what went well with the job they were doing, and what did not go so well.* The feedback should focus on the behaviour that needs to change and include a balance of positive as well as critical comments. To be effective the manager needs to give guidance to help the receiver know what exactly they need to do in order to improve their performance the next time.
4   *Stay calm.* Feedback given in a positive non-threatening manner is easier to accept, and has a higher likelihood of being acted upon.

In addition to controlling the standard of performance of individual staff members, the nurse manager has a responsibility for controlling the quality of the services provided.

The manager's role in maintaining quality

The NMC Code (2008b) requires nurses to provide a high standard of care and practice at all times; control is an important aspect of this, indeed the enquiry into events at the Bristol Royal Infirmary (Kennedy, 2001, p. 352) stated that 'The absence of systems for monitoring the safety of clinical care at national or local level put the care of patients at risk'.

Clinical Governance supports nurses in improving practice and the patient's experience of care (Currie et al., 2003), and one element within clinical governance requires nurses to audit practice in order to ensure the standard of performance is acceptable. In order to audit practice the steps within the control cycle outlined in Figure 20.3 are followed.

While quality management is aimed towards preventing problems from occurring, risk management focuses on reducing the negative impact of problems which have already occurred (Yoder Wise, 1995).

The Manager's Role in Risk Management

The NMC Code (NMC, 2008b) requires the qualified nurse to manage risk and deal with problems. Yoder Wise (1995) asserts that every nurse is a risk manager. Risks within health care fall into five main categories (Sullivan and Decker, 2009, p. 84):

- Medication errors
- Complications from diagnostic or treatment procedures
- Falls
- Patient or family dissatisfaction with care
- Refusal of treatment or refusal to sign consent for treatment.

The nurse manager's role in managing risk is to analyse the situation in order to identify the issues which contributed to the risk occurring. The aim is to prevent similar incidences occurring in the future and reduce the possibility of loss to the organisation through law suits (Pike et al., 2002).

There are four important factors in successful risk management (Sullivan and Decker, 2009):

1 Recognition
2 Action
3 Communication and where possible
4 Immediate restitution.

These four steps correlate closely to the steps within the control cycle (outlined in Figure 20.3). Early *recognition* of a problem is essential in order to ensure that corrective *action* is taken to prevent the situation from becoming any worse. The nurse manager decides what action needs to be taken to correct any issues and *communicates* with staff, providing them with constructive feedback. The nurse manager would also communicate with the client and/or relatives to find out what they want in terms of *restitution*. When handling sensitive situations, such as this, it is important to listen carefully to their responses in order to take appropriate action and prevent a bad situation from escalating to a complaint.

If a medication error, for example, has occurred the nurse managers would initially ensure the patient is observed for any adverse effects and inform the medical staff so that they can administer corrective treatment (if required). The factors which gave rise to the medication error would be need to be explored, and Yoder Wise (1995) suggests the question 'why' should be asked at least five times when trying to ascertain what led up to the problem occurring. For example:

Q: Why was the wrong drug given?

A: I did not check the patient's identity when I gave them their medication.

Q: Why did you not check the patient's identity?

A: I was rushing to finish the drug round.

Q: Why were you rushing to finish the drug round?

A: Because I was late starting the drug round.

Q: Why were you late starting the drug round?

A: The doctor couldn't find the results of a test they had ordered, and asked me to help find them because they were urgent.

Q: Why were they having difficulty finding the results?

A: Because they had not been filed and had got mixed up with another patient's notes.

Q: Why were the results not filed immediately on receipt?

A: The ward clerk is part time and most of the results arrive in the afternoon or evening after she has gone home.

As you can see from the above example there were a number of factors which led up to the incident occurring, and by continually asking 'why?' the nurse manager is able to consider measures which can be put in place to prevent a similar error occurring again. In this example the nurse's failure to check the patient's identity would have to be addressed. In addition the factors contributing to test results going astray would also need attention in order to prevent another incident from occurring. So from this example the interrelationship between risk management and quality management is evident.

Chapter Summary

This chapter has examined the role of the manager in relation to planning, organising, directing and controlling. Each of these functions interrelates with the others, and each is equally as important as the other: *Planning* is essential so that priorities are identified; jobs allocated; and the work progresses in an orderly fashion. *Organising* involves delegating the work to staff and *directing* is about the way in which the leader interacts with, and motivates staff. *Controlling* is essential in order to ensure that the plans have been achieved to the standard required, and corrective action is taken if this is not the case. How these interlink is demonstrated in Figure 20.4.

The focus of the chapter has been on increasing your understanding of leadership and management, which are seen to be equally important. Leaders are seen to be striving to improve services and set the direction, while managers have responsibility for planning and organising how to get there. Many of the theories of leadership examine the way in which leaders relate to others, as well as motivating them. The factors influencing leadership style are explored, by carefully considering these factors a leader can identify the most appropriate style to suite the staff, situation and themselves.

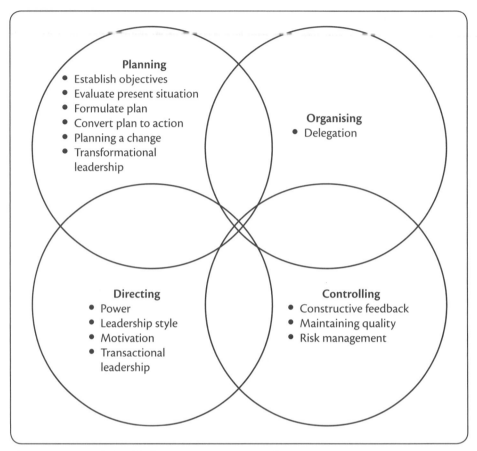

Figure 20.4 Interrelationship between management roles

☐ Test yourself!

1   What are the four roles of a manager as described by Fayol (1949)?

2   Transformational leadership is often associated with change situations but the four 'I's of transformational leadership are key elements in leading and managing a team. What are the four 'I's of transformational leadership?

3   Organising is seen as an important aspect of managing the care of patients, what are the four key elements of organising the work to be done?

4   Outline three aspects which can help a leader to motivate others (Vroom, 1964).

5   What are the three steps in the control process (Boddy, 2005)?

Visit the website http://www.businessballs.com/leadership-management.htm
Boddy, D. (2008) *Management: An introduction.* 4th Edition. FT Prentice Hall, Harlow.
Northouse, P.G. (2010) *Leadership: Theory and Practice.* 5th Edition. London, Sage.

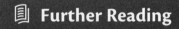 **Further Reading**

For live links to useful websites see: www.palgrave.com/nursinghealth/hogston

References

Antrobus, S. and Kitson, A. (1999) Nursing leadership: influencing and shaping health policy and nursing practice. *Journal of Advanced Nursing* **29**(3): 746–53.

Bass, B.M. (1985) *Leadership and Performance beyond Expectations*. Free Press, New York.

Bass, B.M. (1990) *Bass and Stogdill's Handbook of Leadership: Theory, Research and Managerial Applications*, 3rd edn. Free Press, New York.

Boddy, D. (2005) *Management: An Introduction*, 3rd edn. Prentice Hall, Harlow.

Boddy, D. and Paton, R. (1998) *Management: An Introduction*. Prentice Hall, Harlow.

Buchanan, D. and Badham, R. (1999) *Power, Politics and Organizational Change: Winning the Turf Game*. Sage, London.

Burns, J.M. (1978) *Leadership*. Harper & Row, New York.

Carter, R.H. (2009) Management of care and self. In Childs, L.L., Coles, L. and Marjoram, B. (eds) *Essential Skills Clusters for Nurses: Theory for Practice*. Wiley-Blackwell, Oxford.

Clawson, J.G. (2009) *Level Three Leadership*, 4th edn. Pearson Prentice Hall, Upper Saddle River, NJ.

Cox, Y. and LeMay, A. (2007) Leadership for practice. In Brown, J. and Libberton, P. (eds) *Principles of Professional Studies in Nursing*. Palgrave Macmillan, Basingstoke.

Currie, L., Morrell, C. and Scrivener, R. (2003) *Clinical Governance: An RCN Resource Guide*. RCN, London.

DoH (Department of Health) (2006) *Modernising Nursing Careers: Setting the Direction*. DoH, Belfast.

DoH (Department of Health) (2008) *High Quality Care for All: NHS Next Stage Review*, Final Report. DoH, London.

DoH (Department of Health) (2009) *Inspiring Leaders: Leadership for Quality*. DoH, London.

Fayol, H. (1949). *General and Industrial Management*. Pitman, London.

Fielder, F.E. (1967). *A Theory of Leadership Effectiveness*. McGraw Hill, New York.

Finkelman, A.W. (2006) *Leadership and Management in Nursing*. Pearson Prentice Hall. Upper Saddle River, NJ.

French, J. and Raven, B. (1959) The bases of social power. In Cartwright, D. (ed.) *Studies in Social Power*. Institute for Social Research, Ann Arbor, MI.

Gill, R. (2006) *Theory and Practice of Leadership*. Sage Publications, London.

Goode, C.J. and Blegen, M.A. (1993) Development and evaluation of a research-based management intervention: A recognition protocol. *Journal of Nursing Administration* **23**(4): 61–6.

Harris, K. (1995) *Collected Quotes from Albert Einstein*. http://rescomp.stanford.edu/~cheshire/EinsteinQuotes.html (accessed May 2009).

Herzberg, F. (1987). One more time: how do you motivate employees? *Harvard Business Review* **65** (Sep/Oct).

House, R.J. (1996) Path-goal theory of leadership: lessons, legacy and a reformulation. *Leadership Quarterly* **7**(3): 323–52.

House, R.J. and Mitchell, T.R. (1974) Path-goal theory of leadership. *Contemporary Business* **3**(2): 81–98.

Kennedy, I. (2001) *The Report of the Public Enquiry into Children's Heart Surgery at the Bristol Royal Infirmary 1984–1995: Learning from Bristol*. The Stationery Office, London.

Kotter, J. (1995) *The New Rules: How to Succeed in Today's Post-Corporate World*. Free Press, New York.

Kotter, J. and Cohen, D. (2002) *The Heart of Change: Real Life Stories of How People Change their Organizations*. Harvard Business School Press, Boston.

Lewin, K. and Lippitt, R. (1938) An experimental approach to the study of autocracy and democracy: a preliminary note. *Sociometry* **1**: 292–300.

Lewin, K., Lippitt, R. and White, R.K. (1939) Patterns of aggressive behaviour in experimentally created social climates. *Journal of Social Psychology* **10**: 271–301.

Maslow, A. (1970) *Motivation and Personality*, 2nd edn. Harper & Row, New York.

McGregor, D. (1960) *The Human Side of Enterprise*. McGraw-Hill, New York.

Mullins, L.J. (1996) *Management and Organisational Behaviour*. Pitman Publishing, London.

Mullins, L.J. (2005). *Management and Organisational Behaviour*, 7th edn. FT Prentice Hall, Harlow.

NMC (Nursing and Midwifery Council) (2008a) *Essential Skills Clusters*. Available at: http://www.nmc-uk.org/aArticle.aspx?ArticleID=2914 (accessed April 2010).

NMC (Nursing and Midwifery Council) (2008b) *The Code: Standards of Conduct, Performance and Ethics for Nurses and Midwives.* NMC, London. www.nmc-uk.org

Northouse, P.G. (2004) *Leadership Theory and Practice,* 3rd edn. SAGE Publications, Thousand Oaks, CA.

Nursing Times.Net (2007) *Giving Constructive Feedback.* http://www.nursingtimes.net/giving-constructive-feedback/215184.article (accessed June 2009).

Pike, J., Janssen, R. and Brooks, P. (2002) *Nursing Report Card for Acute Care.* American Nurses Publishing, Inc., Washington DC.

Stewart, R. (1967) *Managers and their Jobs.* Macmillan, London.

Stodgill, R.M. (1974). *Manual for the Leader Behaviour Description Questionnaire Form XII.* Bureau of Business Research, Ohio State University, Columbus.

Sullivan, E.J. and Decker, P.J. (2005) *Effective Leadership and Management in Nursing,* 6th edn. Pearson Prentice Hall, Upper Saddle River, NJ.

Sullivan, E.J. and Decker, P.J. (2009) *Effective Leadership and Management in Nursing,* 7th edn. Pearson Prentice Hall, Upper Saddle River, NJ.

Vroom, V.H. (1964). *Work and Motivation.* John Wiley, New York.

Yoder Wise, P.S. (1995). *Leading and Managing in Nursing.* Mosby, St Louis.

Yukl, G. (2006) *Leadership in Organizations,* 6th edn. Pearson Prentice Hall, London.

Answers to Test Yourself! Questions

Chapter 1

1. Assessment
   Diagnosis
   Planning
   Implementation
   Evaluation.

2. It enables the nurse to plan care for a client on an individual basis and to solve problems.

3. Physical health information
   Psychological information
   Social health information
   The activities of living.

4. Two: actual and potential.

5. Setting goals
   Identifying actions.

6. The MACROS criteria:
   Measurable and observable
   Achievable and time limited
   Client centred
   Realistic
   Outcome written
   Short.

7. Nursing handover
   Reflection
   Patient satisfaction or complaint
   Reviewing the nursing care plan.

Chapter 2

1. Empathic understanding; genuineness, or congruence; unconditional acceptance.

2. Confronting, informative, prescriptive, catalytic, supportive, cathartic.

3. Listening, simple and selective reflection, paraphrasing, open and closed questions, logical and empathic building, checking for understanding.

4. Setting, perception, invitation, knowledge, emotions, strategy and summary.

5. Could include: physiotherapists, nurses, doctors, social workers, occupational therapists, pharmacists and psychologists.

6. Primary groups tend to be closer and more intimate, all the members having face-to-face contact. Examples include: family, groups of friends, clubs, small work groups such as the ward team.
   Secondary groups are usually considered to be larger, and their members have less direct contact. Examples include: political party; nursing as a professional group.

7. Team, task and individual.

8. Forming, storming, norming and performing.

9. Aggressive, submissive/passive, assertive.

10. Listen carefully. Say what you think and feel. Say what you want to happen. Be persistent. Be prepared to compromise.

11. Open answer.

Chapter 3

1. Professional practice involves engagement in activities underpinned by a body of professional knowledge and exercising professional judgement in the application of this knowledge to situations encountered in practice.

2. The NMC Code is underpinned by the ethical principles of respect for the person (autonomy), the obligation to maximise benefit (beneficence), to avoid harm and keep people safe (non-maleficence) and the responsibility to treat everyone equally and ensure that they are informed of their rights (justice).

3. Professional accountability means being answerable for the decisions taken particularly when problems arise. Nurses may be accountable to several different bodies simultaneously: namely an employer, under a contract of employment, the patient under existing

legal provision and to the profession under the terms of the Nursing and Midwifery Order 2001.

4   Evidence-based practice involves having the skills to discern between good and poor quality evidence for practice and applying the evidence conscientiously and judiciously. The two key aspects of evidence include clinical expertise and systematic research.

5   To become more aware of own beliefs and values and how these impact on decisions taken, to understand the four ethical principles (autonomy, beneficence, non-maleficence, justice), to have knowledge of the personal accounts of clients through studies that explore people's experience of health problems and to be effective communicators to ensure that the values and evidence which inform care decisions are brought together.

6   The NHS Constitution outlines the purpose, principles and values of the NHS and brings together the rights, pledges and responsibilities for staff and patients. It can therefore provide important information to patients on such issues as access to health services, treatments and choice.

Chapter 4

1   Reflective practice is professional practice guided by structured reflection on feelings, experience and empathy in order to make practice robust and enhance learning.

2   Reflection-in-action is reflection on an event as it is being experienced. Reflection-on-action is in-depth reflection on an event after it has finished.

3   Some of the benefits of reflective practice include:
    • it can help to avoid mistakes and provides practitioners with an evidence base for future practice
    • it can identify learning needs
    • it can identify the ways we learn best
    • it encourages personal and professional development
    • it demonstrates your competence to others
    • it supports decision-making
    • it allows you to be aware of the consequences of your actions
    • it demonstrates your achievements to both yourself and others
    • it allows you to explore alternative ways of solving problems
    • it can be self-empowering
    • it allows you to build theory from practice
    • it is self-empowering

4   Stage one – selecting an event to reflect on
    Stage two – observing and describing the experience
    Stage three – analysing the experience
    Stage four – interpreting the experience
    Stage five – exploring alternatives
    Stage six – framing action

5   Models and frameworks can be helpful as they are specifically designed to draw you through the stages of the reflective processes.

6   When choosing a model of reflection, you must consider the desired outcome of the reflective activity, and whether you wish to use it: as a learning strategy; to identify your knowledge base, or deficit; to improve patient care; or to develop practice and practice theory.

7   There are several things that you can do to ensure that you make the most of learning opportunities in the clinical environment:
    • Prepare for your placement – review your last placement (if applicable), your practice assessment documents and your learning outcomes. Find out as much as you can about the placement area before your first shift and reflect on the opportunities the placement is likely to offer.
    • Take a positive-action approach to learning – you could keep some sort of clinical log or diary to record your activities for future reflection.
    • Use others to support your learning – ensure that you use your supervisor to maximum effect and take up any opportunities offered for reflective work. You can also learn through working reflectively with student colleagues, both in groups and in pairs.

8   Written reflection is different to mental or verbal reflection because of the particular features of reflective writing:
    • We always write for a purpose
    • Reflective writing always takes place in the first person
    • Writing requires us to order our thoughts
    • Writing creates a permanent record that we can return to again and again, and view differently each time
    • Writing helps us to develop our creativity
    • Writing enhances our analytical ability by helping us to break things down
    • Writing reflectively helps us to be critical thinkers
    • Writing can be used to develop new understanding and knowledge.

Chapter 5

1   Health-care associated infection.
2   Micro-organisms, portal of exit, mode of transmission, portal of entry, susceptible patient, infection.
3   Urinary tract, lungs, wound, blood.
4   Groups A, B, C, D, E. (See Table 5.1)

Chapter 6

1   The right medication
    The right amount
    The right time
    The right patient
    The right route.

2   The deltoid muscle in the upper arm
The dorsogluteal site in the buttocks
The ventrogluteal site in the hip area
The vastus lateralis in the thigh
The Rectus Femoris Site.

3   Unusual body movements
Feeling drowsy and sedated
Heart arrhythmia
Weight gain (Clozapine, olanzapine)
Diabetes
Excess salivation
Stroke
Dizziness
Blurred vision
Hormonal changes: increased levels of prolactin causing osteoporosis, reduced libido, impotence.

Chapter 7

1   33 per cent vegetables and fruit, 33 per cent complex carbohydrate, 12 per cent protein containing foods, 15 per cent dairy products or similar foods and 8 per cent fat and sugar containing foods.

2   A high intake of total fat, especially saturated fat, is associated with a high LDL cholesterol level whereas a relatively low intake of fat, with a high proportion in the form of unsaturated fat, is associated with a lower LDL cholesterol level.

3   Rich dietary sources include liver, meat, beans, nuts, dried fruit, fish, enriched cereals, soybean flour and dark leafy green vegetables.

4   Overweight.

5   Refeeding syndrome: In starvation, levels of electrolytes, particularly phosphate, in the cells are low. When a person who has been starved is given food containing carbohydrate, insulin release is stimulated leading to electrolytes in the extracellular fluid moving into the cells, which can result in abnormally low levels outside the cells. This results in metabolic changes in the body causing serious illness (Mehanna et al., 2008).

Chapter 8

1   The client's normal bowel habit
The frequency/time of faecal/urinary elimination
The presence of pain/discomfort when eliminating
The amount eliminated
Odour
Diet/fluid intake
Disease
Mobility.

2   Drugs, resulting in reduced motility of the intestine
Laxative abuse, resulting in a diminished normal reflex

Pregnancy, due to reduced abdominal space and progesterone slowing peristalsis
Disease processes, altering the time of passage of the faeces
Pain, causing the client to be reluctant to defaecate
Psychiatric problems, causing a lack of interest in the surroundings and diet, or an altered dietary intake
A diet low in fibre, or an inadequate intake
Fluids not sufficient for the patient's needs
Immobility, reducing intestinal motility
Ignoring the call to defaecate, allowing more fluid to be absorbed from the faeces, which therefore become harder and more difficult to eliminate
Psychological factors caused by unfavourable conditions, the client delaying the defaecation process until more favourable conditions exist.

3   Stress incontinence
Urge incontinence
Reflex incontinence
Overflow incontinence.

4   Ileostomy: an opening from the ileum; faecal material liquid
Colostomy: an opening from the colon; faecal material ranges from semisolid to more formed stools
Urostomy: the bladder is removed and urinary excretion is diverted via a stoma formed on the abdominal wall.

5   Embarrassment (the most common factor)
Depression
Anorexia nervosa
Chronic psychoses.

6   Calculated on a 30–35 ml/kg body weight, this equals 1950–2275 ml per 24 hours.

Chapter 9

1   25 breaths per minute.

2   A cycle of breathing characterised by episodes of decreasing rate and depth of breathing, followed by increasing rate and depth of breathing. Periods of apnoea may also be observed.

3   Mucoid (chronic inflammation), purulent (infection), tenacious (asthma, dehydration), frothy (pulmonary oedema).

4   94–98 per cent.

Chapter 10

1   Hypovolaemic, cardiogenic, distributive, obstructive, and dissociative.

2   Increased pulse rate, increased respiratory rate, narrowing in pulse pressure, restlessness/agitation.

3   60–100

4   Peripheral resistance, intravascular blood volume, and stroke volume.

5   Pallor of the limb, decreased/absent pulses, signs of pain, ulceration of the skin, shiny/hairless skin, increased capillary refill time.

6   2 seconds or less.

7   Infants = 2 mls/kg/hr
    Children = 1 ml/kg/hr
    Adults = 0.5 mls/kg/hr

8   Hypovolaemia, hypothermia, hypoxia, hypo/hyperkalaemia and other metabolic disorders, tension pneumothorax, cardiac tamponade, toxic/therapeutic disorders, thrombo-embolic and mechanical obstruction.

9   Verbal descriptor scales, visual analogue scales, pain behaviour tools, combined approaches, for example pain rulers.

10 Circulatory overload, haemolytic mismatch, allergic reactions, disease transmission, hypothermia.

Chapter 11

1   Pressure, shear and friction, moisture may exacerbate the problem.

2   Use a pressure ulcer risk assessment tool, use a pressure reducing foam mattress (alternating or low air loss mattress, depending on the patient's level of risk), encourage regular movement and use 30 degree tilt to reposition if appropriate, limit sitting times and assist with mobility. Encourage a balanced diet.

3   Haemostasis, inflammatory phase, proliferation and maturation.

4   See Figure 11.1.

5   Moist, free from excess exudate, protected from bacterial, particulate and toxic contamination, thermally insulated, well perfused, protected from mechanical trauma and undisturbed.

6   Location and dimensions of the wound, appearance of the wound, wound bed status, type and level of exudate, signs of infection, presence of odour, wound edge, state of surrounding skin and mode of healing.

Chapter 12

1   Environment: space constraints, ventilation, lighting, floor type etc.
    Load: weight, stability of the load, sharp, hot or cold etc.
    Individual: education, training, fitness, ability to assist etc.
    Other factors: resources, equipment, clothing, catheters, IVs etc.
    Task: Clearly defined? What does it involve? Consider your options. Has informed consent been obtained? Etc.

2   LOLER (1998): Lifting Operations and Lifting Equipment Regulations
    PUWER (1999): Provision and Use of Work Equipment Regulations.

3   Repetitive and heavy lifting
    Bending and twisting
    Repeating an action too frequently

Uncomfortable working/sitting position
Exerting too much force
Working too long without breaks
Exerting a force in a static position for extended periods of time
Adverse working environment (for example hot, cold)
Psychosocial factors (for example high job demands, time pressures and lack of control)
Not receiving and acting upon reports of symptoms quick enough.

4   Building a therapeutic relationship
    Client involvement
    Gaining consent
    Education
    Comprehensive assessment
    Recognising client and staff beliefs and values.

5   Use of bed sheets to drag client up the bed
    Non-completion of risk assessments
    No assessment of client's abilities
    Lifting/using condemned techniques
    Supporting the patient's weight
    Poor communication
    Poor management of equipment
    Non-completion of equipment safety checks
    (Cornish and Jones, 2009).

6   We all have a base of support and running through that base of support is the line of gravity (which runs through the centre of gravity). This line of gravity needs to fall within an object's base of support to ensure that the object or person is stable and balanced.

Chapter 13

1   Cessation of breathing, a lack of a palpable heart beat and fixed dilated pupils.

2   Finding meaning, preserving integrity, connecting, doing for, empowering, valuing.

3   Social, spiritual and emotional as well as physical.

4   It is a three-step process for managing pain. It begins with non-opioid drugs and then gradually increases to use opioids, and adjuvant treatment until the pain is controlled.

5   Pain, nausea and vomiting, constipation, diarrhoea, anorexia, fatigue, breathlessness, confusion, insomnia, anxiety, depression.

6   Last offices is the term used to describe the care carried out for the person when they have died.

7   For euthanasia it is someone other than the person themselves that brings about the death. In physician assisted suicide it must be by the person's own hand that their life is ended.

8   Loss-oriented and restoration-oriented.

9   Listening, being with silence, encouraging them to talk about the deceased, being present.

10   Religious, situational, moral and biographical.

11   Open answer.

Chapter 14

1   Physiological dependence occurs when a substance is repeatedly taken that has reinforcing properties causing the body to physiologically adapt to the use of the substance (Wilbourn and Prosser, 2003, p. 179). The substance needs to be taken regularly to avoid withdrawal symptoms. Psychological dependence could be described as a compulsion or a craving to continue to take a substance for its effects; for example, its hallucinatory or stimulatory properties.

A description of dependency should include:

- Increased tolerance to the substance
- Repeated withdrawal symptoms
- Compulsion to use the substance (craving)
- Salience of substance-seeking behaviour (seen as more important than anything or anyone else)
- Relief of avoidance of withdrawal symptoms
- Narrowing of the repertoire of substance taking (drug use becomes an everyday activity)
- A return to the substance use after a period of abstinence
- Important social, occupational or recreational activities or interests are given up or reduced because of substance use
- The substance use is continued despite knowledge of having a persistent or recurrent physical or psychological problem that is likely to have been caused or exacerbated by the substance (for example continued drinking despite recognition that an ulcer was made worse by alcohol consumption).

2   The definition of harm reduction:

Harm reduction is a strategy which accepts that some substance users choose to carry on using their substance of choice and want contact with services and nurses for information, support and guidance on reducing the harm and risks associated with their substance use.

Examples of harm reduction strategies include:

- Substitute prescribing – methadone, buprenorphine (see Table 14.4)
- Outreach working
- Needle and syringe exchange services (which may be linked with local pharmacies or substance misuse services in some areas)
- Health-care checks (which may be available through local substance misuse services)
- Harm reduction teams – who offer support and guidance to substance users and health-care professionals working with substance users. This can include advice on safer injecting, teaching cleaning techniques, and encouraging other routes of administration – for example smoking heroin as opposed to injecting it.

- Homeless services
- Sexual health clinics
- Websites which offer advice on safe drinking.

3   • Class A – heroin, cocaine and ecstasy
- Class B – cannabis, codeine and amphetamine (not injected)
- Class C – Ketamine, buprenorphine and benzodiazipines

4   • Oesophagitis
- Gastritis
- Fatty liver
- Cirrhosis of the liver
- Korsokoff's syndrome
- Peripheral neuropathy.

Chapter 15

1   Read the section on body image (pg 349-50) and pick out the main words used.

2   Body reality, body presentation and body ideal.

3   Circumcision, caesarean section, oopherectomy, lumpectomy, termination.

4   A high incidence of sexually abusive experiences; Multiple experiences of bereavement and loss; Difficulties in talking about emotions; Limited sex education; Limited expectations and low self-esteem; A lack of assertiveness about sex and relationships; A lack of privacy.

5   Permission, Limited Information, Specific Suggestions, Intensive Therapy.

6   Intimacy; antidiscriminatory practice; empowerment and partnership.

Chapter 16

1   Principles of: privacy, consent, confidentially, non-discrimination.

2   Adenine, thymine, cytosine and guanine.

3   A with T, and C with G - Adenine paired with thymine, and cytosine paired with guanine.

4   (a) 47, XY+21 is a male individual with Down's syndrome, so has an extra chromosome at pair 21. It is classified as a chromosomal numerical condition – a trisomy, caused by an error in cell division.

(b) 47, XXY is a male individual with Klinefelter syndrome, so has an extra X chromosome. It is classified as a chromosomal numerical condition – a trisomy, caused by an error in cell division. In this condition it is an extra sex chromosome.

(c) 45, XO is a female individual with Turner syndrome, so only has one X chromosome rather than the expected XX. It is classified as a chromosomal numerical condition – a monosomy, caused by an error in cell division.

(d) 12q24.1 is the karyotype for the condition Phenylketonuria (PKu). It is a condition inherited in an autosomal recessive manner. This karyotype indicates that the condition is inherited on an autosome (number 12) and the locus (location) for the gene is at banding 24.1 and located on the q arm (long arm).

(e) Xq28 is the karyotype for the condition Major Affective Disorder (2). This karyotype indicates that the condition is inherited on the X chromosome and the locus (location) for the gene is at banding 28 and located on the q arm (long arm).

5   (a) Autosomes: Pairs 1 to 22 of the chromosomes. The final pair (pair 23) is called the sex chromosomes (XX in the female and XY in the male).

(b) Trisomy: the presence of a complete chromosome, so gives the karyotype of 47 rather than the expected of 46.

(c) Monosomy: the absence of a complete chromosome, so gives the karyotype of 45 rather than the expected 46.

(d) Non-disjunction: failure of the chromosomes to split at the centromere, during mitosis or meiosis.

6   (a) Inheritance of a dominant condition is 1:2 (50 per cent) risk/chance of an offspring being affected.

(b) Inheritance of a recessive condition is 1:4 (25 per cent) risk/chance of an offspring being affected.1:2 (50 per cent) risk/chance of an offspring being of carrier status. 1:4 (25 per cent) chance of an offspring not being affected.

(c) Risk from affected father and unaffected mother is 1:2 (50 per cent) risk/chance an offspring will be a carrier daughter and 1:2 (50 per cent) risk/chance an offspring will be an unaffected son. Risk from carrier mother and unaffected father is 1:4 (25 per cent) risk/chance an offspring will be an affected son; 1:4 (25 per cent) risk/chance an offspring will be a carrier daughter; 1:4 (25 per cent) risk/chance an offspring will be a unaffected son; 1:4 (25 per cent) risk/chance an offspring will be an unaffected daughter.

Chapter 17

1   'Interprofessional practice' is one of the terms used to describe a group of professionals working together to achieve mutually agreed goals. These goals should involve the service user and the carer. Other terms are often used in place of interprofessional, for example interdisciplinary, multiprofessional and multidisciplinary. Interprofessional practice has been most common in primary care and community care settings, and more recently it has become an element of acute care practice.

2   Open answer.

3   With the establishment of primary care groups, the role of many professionals may change. Practice nurses, district nurses and health visitors, for example, may be involved in the management of primary care groups, bringing together the work of GPs and other professions. Social workers may also be represented, especially in child protection and mental health issues. In the hospital setting, nurses will be involved in the care-planning process for discharge in elderly care, as well as in working alongside physiotherapists

and occupational therapists in the field of stroke rehabilitation. Ensuring that the client's or patient's needs are met by the person with the appropriate skill and knowledge is the most significant role that all professionals bring to teamwork. Equally, the ongoing evaluation and review of practice intervention will mean that the most effective use of resources is being made.

4   Ensuring that the specific skills and knowledge held by the nurse are recognised by others in the team. If the nurse is employed by the GP, he or she may have limited involvement in the allocation of resources for the particular area of practice. Equally, a difference in payment can lead to differing levels of status within a team. Status may play a major part in the decision-making process, and nurses may have to work proactively to ensure that their views on good practice are heard and evaluated.

5   Personalised services mean that the service user will manage his or her care in the health or social care setting. This means that collaboration will involve the service user and/or his carer in all stages of decision making. The needs of the service user will be driving all care delivery and professionals will need to work actively together to make this happen giving full informed rationale for action.

Chapter 18

1   Table 18.1.

2   Table 18.6.

3   See core activity 3 and 4 page.

4   See Table 18.3.

5   Table 18.6 and Leadership and management skills, ability to base public health activity on evidence, understand, analyse and work with government policies on health, understand health and the influences on health (Table 18.4).

6   Maintain strict hygiene standards (handwashing, use of alcohol based handrub). Control of infectious diseases, prevention of transmission of communicable.

Chapter 19

1   Data is a symbol (or series of symbols) usually representing a fact but without any explanation of how it might relate to other things.
Information is data interpreted into understanding of contextual meaning.
Knowledge is the level of understanding required in order to use information constructively and purposefully.

2   Data is in abundance within all clinical settings. The interpretation of data into information occurs when there is need, providing there is a level of understanding of contextual meaning. This information will be acted on, communicated or effectively discarded depending on an interpretation of its value. Value of information is related to

an understanding of how the information may be used; in other words the knowledge of the user.

3   Please see Figure 19.3.

4   An electronic care record is a virtual record; this means instead of storing the specifics of any one patient in a paper file the information is stored in an electronic file located within a central computer system. However, access to electronic care records may be limited by the imposed controls of any one health organisation. For example, a GP may not have access to a hospital's electronic care records for the patients within his care. Integrated care records seek to move the ownership of the electronic record from the individual organisation to the patient. In so doing, all the separately held records of health organisations would be combined into one *integrated* health record, allowing access to any patient's file at the point of care.

5   Resources used to inform practice can be diverse and of variable quality. Consider the following list: word of mouth; visible practice; a guideline; a protocol; a care pathway/bundle; a website; a book; a discussion within a journal; research reported within a journal. Each of these sources can be argued to be of variable quality, and hence variable benefit to the provision of evidence-based practice. Obviously word of mouth and visible practice can be relatively dubious sources of information on which to base practice. Both may as easily relate to very poor care practices borne from tradition or misinterpretation as well as best practice. The use of guideline, protocols and care pathways represent a better source of information. However, questions should be asked in regard to how current the guidelines are. When they were last reviewed against the evidence base? Also, in what circumstances the guidelines should be applied. The internet is a massive potential information source, but the limitations identified for source earlier apply, for example, what assurances do you have as to the quality of the information provided? Books and journals often provide quality information on which to base care; however it remains important to consider the source critically. How recent is the information presented and how relevant is the information to the situation you are in? In regard to research, how can you be assured that the research is of value and may be generalised?

6   Evidence, clinical judgement, patient preference.

7   Efficiency relates to processes which avoid wasted time and expense.
     Effectiveness relates to processes that achieve a set purpose.

8   HORUS is an acronym associated to information governance and relates specifically to how information is:
     ● Held
     ● Obtained
     ● Recorded
     ● Used
     ● Shared.

9   Yes. The Data Protection Act 1998 provides individuals with the right to access any information stored about them on computer records and some manual records. Remember with integrated care records the owner of the record is the patient.

10   A concise answer to this question is difficult to achieve given it implicates both codes of confidentiality and legislation. For example, the Code of Professional Conduct 2004 and the Data Protection Act 1998 or the Freedom of Information Act 2000. In terms of specific advice it is worth considering if you have answers to the following questions before divulging information:
     ● Do you have the patient's permission, or the legal right to share the information?
     ● Does the patient know that you intend to divulge information? If so, do they know who to?
     ● Have you got consent – can you prove this?
     ● What legal rights does the person(s) requesting the information have to the information requested?
     ● Is it absolutely necessary to share the information?
     ● What are the implications of sharing the information?
     ● What are the consequences of retaining the information?

Chapter 20

1   Planning
     Organising
     Directing
     Controlling.

2   Intellectual stimulation
     Inspirational motivation
     Idealised influence
     Individualised consideration.

3   Identifying what has to be done
     Dividing the work up between members of the team
     Assigning authority for the work (delegating) and ensuring the team know who to report to regarding the work they are undertaking.
     Reviewing the use of human and material resources in achieving the work.

4   Ensure they know what they have to do (give clear instructions as to what you want them to do)
     Develop their knowledge and skills (teach them how to do the job)
     Provide the necessary tools, equipment, information and other resources required to do the job.

5   Observing to see what is/has happened
     Comparing what has happened to what was planned
     Deciding what actions need to be taken in view of the results and making longer-term plans to overcome problems which have arisen.

Index

Contents

Introduction

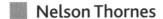

Nelson Thornes

Nelson Thornes has worked hard to ensure that this book offers you excellent support for your AS level course. You can be confident that the range of learning, teaching and assessment practice materials has been checked, and provides useful support for your course.

How to use this book

The features in this book include:

Timeline

Key events are outlined at the beginning of the book. The events are colour-coded so you can clearly see the categories of change.

Learning objectives

At the beginning of each section you will find a list of learning objectives that contain targets linked to the requirements of the specification.

Key chronology

A short list of dates usually with a focus on a specific event or legislation.

Key profile

The profile of a key person you should be aware of to fully understand the period in question.

Key terms

A term that you will need to be able to define and understand.

Did you know?

Interesting information to bring the subject under discussion to life.

Exploring the detail

Information to put further context around the subject under discussion.

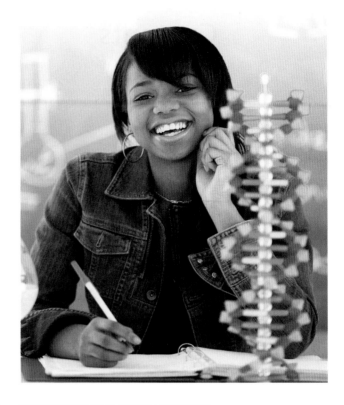

A closer look

An in-depth look at a theme, person or event to deepen your understanding. Activities around the extra information may be included.

Sources

Sources to reinforce topics or themes and may provide fact or opinion. They may be quotations from historical works, contemporaries of the period or photographs.

Cross-reference

Links to related content within the book which may offer more detail on the subject in question.

Activity

Various activity types to provide you with different challenges and opportunities to demonstrate both the content and skills you are learning. Some can be worked on individually, some as part of group work and some are designed to specifically 'stretch and challenge'.

Question

Questions to prompt further discussion on the topic under consideration and are an aid to revision.

Summary questions

Summary questions at the end of each chapter to test your knowledge and allow you to demonstrate your understanding.

Study tip

Hints to help you with your study and to prepare for your exam.

Practice questions

Questions at the end of each section in the style that you may encounter in your exam.

Learning outcomes

Learning outcomes at the end of each section remind you what you should know having completed the chapters in that section.

Introduction to the History series

When Bruce Bogtrotter in Roald Dahl's *Matilda* was challenged to eat a huge chocolate cake, he just opened his mouth and ploughed in, taking bite after bite and lump after lump until the cake was gone and he was feeling decidedly sick. The picture is not dissimilar to that of some A level History students. They are attracted to History because of its inherent appeal, but when faced with a bulging file and a forthcoming examination, their enjoyment evaporates. They try desperately to cram their brains with an assortment of random facts and subsequently prove unable to control the outpouring of their ill-digested material in the examination.

The books in this series are designed to help students and teachers avoid this feeling of overload by breaking down the AQA History specification in such a way that it is easily absorbed. Above all they are designed to retain and promote pupils' enthusiasm for History by avoiding a dreary rehash of dates and events. Each book is divided into sections, closely matched to those given in the specification itself, and the content is further broken down into chapters which present the historical material in a lively and attractive form. Each book offers guidance on the key terms, events and issues and blends thought-provoking activities and questions in a way designed to advance students' understanding. The series encourages students to think for themselves and to share their ideas with others as well as helping them to develop the knowledge and skills they need. This book should ensure that students' learning remains a pleasure rather than an endurance test.

To make the most of what this book provides, students will need to develop efficient study skills from the outset and it is worth spending some time considering what these involve:

▓ **Good organisation of material in a subject specific file.** Organised notes help develop an organised brain and sensible filing ensures time is not wasted hunting for misplaced material. This book uses cross-references to indicate where material in one chapter has relevance to that in another. Students would be advised to employ the same technique.

▓ **A sensible approach to note-making.** Students are often too ready to copy large chunks of material from printed books or to download sheaves of print from the internet. These books are designed to encourage students to think about the notes they collect and to undertake research with a particular purpose in mind. The activities given here will encourage students to pick out that which is relevant to the issue being addressed and to avoid making notes on material that is improperly understood.

▓ **By far the most important component of study is taking time to 'think'.** By encouraging students to '*think*' before they write or speak, be it for a written answer, presentation or class debate, students should learn to form opinions and make judgements based on their accumulation of evidence. These are the skills the examiner will be looking for in the final examination and the beauty of History is that there is rarely a right or wrong answer, so, with sufficient evidence, one student's view will count for as much as the next!

▓ Unit 2

Unit 2 promotes the study of significant periods of history in depth. Although the span of years may appear short, the chosen topics are centred on periods of change that raise specific historical issues and they therefore provide an opportunity for students to study in some depth the interrelationships between ideas, individuals, circumstances and other factors that lead to major developments. Appreciating the dynamics of change, and balancing the degree of change against elements of continuity, make for a fascinating and worthwhile study. Students are also required to analyse consequences and draw conclusions about the issues these studies raise. Such themes are, of course, relevant to an understanding of the present and, through such an historical investigation, students will be guided towards a greater appreciation of the world around them today, as well as develop their understanding of the past.

Unit 2 is tested by a 1 hour 30 minute paper containing three questions. The first question is compulsory and based on sources, while the remaining two, of which students will need to choose one, are two-part questions as described in Table 1. Plentiful sources are included throughout this book to give students some familiarity with contemporary and historiographical material, and activities and suggestions are provided to enable students to develop the required examination skills. Students should familiarise themselves with the question breakdown, additional hints and marking criteria given below before attempting any of the practice questions at the end of each section.

Answers will be marked according to a scheme based on 'levels of response'. This means that the answer will be assessed according to which level best matches the historical skills displayed, taking both knowledge and understanding into account. All students should have a copy of these criteria and need to use them wisely.

Table 1 *Unit 2: style of questions and marks available*

Unit 2	Question	Marks	Question type	Question stem	Hints for students
Question 1 based on three sources of c.300–350 words in total	(a)	12	This question involves the comparison of two sources	Explain how far the views in Source B differ from those in Source A in relation to…	Take pains to avoid simply writing out what each source says with limited direct comment. Instead, you should try to find two or three points of comparison and illustrate these with reference to the sources. You should also look for any underlying similarities. In your conclusion, you will need to make it clear exactly 'how far' the views differ
Question 1	(b)	24	This requires use of the sources and own knowledge and asks for an explanation that shows awareness that issues and events can provoke differing views and explanations	How far… How important was…How successful…	This answer needs to be planned as you will need to develop an argument in your answer and show balanced judgement. Try to set out your argument in the introduction and, as you develop your ideas through your paragraphs, support your opinions with detailed evidence. Your conclusion should flow naturally and provide supported judgement. The sources should be used as 'evidence' throughout your answer. Do ensure you refer to them all
Question 2 and 3	(a)	12	This question is focused on a narrow issue within the period studied and requires an explanation	Explain why…	Make sure you explain 'why', not 'how', and try to order your answer in a way that shows you understand the inter-linkage of factors and which are the most important. You should try to reach an overall judgement/conclusion
Question 2 and 3	(b)	24	This question is broader and asks for analysis and explanation with appropriate judgement. The question requires an awareness of debate over issues	A quotation in the form of a judgement on a key development or issue will be given and candidates asked: Explain why you agree or disagree with this view	This answer needs to be planned as you will need to show balanced judgement. Try to think of points that agree and disagree and decide which way you will argue. Set out your argument in the introduction and support it through your paragraphs, giving the alternative picture too but showing why your view is the more convincing. Your conclusion should flow naturally from what you have written

Marking criteria

Question 1(a)

Level 1 Answers either briefly paraphrase/describe the content of the two sources or identify simple comparison(s) between the sources. Skills of written communication will be weak. *(0–2 marks)*

Level 2 Responses will compare the views expressed in the two sources and identify some differences and/or similarities. There may be some limited own knowledge. Answers will be coherent but weakly expressed. *(3–6 marks)*

Level 3 Responses will compare the views expressed in the two sources, identifying differences **and** similarities and using own knowledge to explain and evaluate these. Answers will, for the most part, be clearly expressed. *(7–9 marks)*

Level 4 Responses will make a developed comparison between the views expressed in the two sources

and own knowledge will apply to evaluate and to demonstrate a good contextual understanding. Answers will, for the most part, show good skills of written communication. *(10–12 marks)*

Question 1(b)

Level 1 Answers may be based on sources or on own knowledge alone, or they may comprise an undeveloped mixture of the two. They may contain some descriptive material which is only loosely linked to the focus of the question or they may address only a part of the question. Alternatively, there may be some explicit comment with little, if any, appropriate support. Answers are likely to be generalised and assertive. There will be little, if any, awareness of differing historical interpretations. The response will be limited in development and skills of written communication will be weak. *(0–6 marks)*

Level 2 Answers may be based on sources or on own knowledge alone, or they may contain a mixture of the two. They may be almost entirely descriptive with few explicit links to the focus of the question. Alternatively, they may contain some explicit comment with relevant but limited support. They will display limited understanding of differing historical interpretations. Answers will be coherent but weakly expressed and/or poorly structured. *(7–11 marks)*

Level 3 Answers will show a developed understanding of the demands of the question using evidence from **both** the sources **and** own knowledge. They will provide some assessment backed by relevant and appropriately selected evidence, but they will lack depth and/or balance. There will be some understanding of varying historical interpretations. Answers will, for the most part, be clearly expressed and show some organisation in the presentation of material. *(12–16 marks)*

Level 4 Answers will show explicit understanding of the demands of the question. They will develop a balanced argument backed by a good range of appropriately selected evidence from the sources and own knowledge, and a good understanding of historical interpretations. Answers will, for the most part, show organisation and good skills of written communication. *(17–21 marks)*

Level 5 Answers will be well focused and closely argued. The arguments will be supported by precisely selected evidence from the sources and own knowledge, incorporating well-developed understanding of historical interpretations and debate. Answers will, for the most part, be carefully organised and fluently written, using appropriate vocabulary. *(22–24 marks)*

Question 2(a) and 3(a)

Level 1 Answers will contain either some descriptive material which is only loosely linked to the focus of the question or some explicit comment with little, if any, appropriate support. Answers are likely to be generalised and assertive. The response will be limited in development and skills of written communication will be weak. *(0–2 marks)*

Level 2 Answers will demonstrate some knowledge and understanding of the demands of the question. They will either be almost entirely descriptive with few explicit links to the question **or** they provide some explanations backed by evidence that is limited in range and/or depth. Answers will be coherent but weakly expressed and/or poorly structured. *(3–6 marks)*

Level 3 Answers will demonstrate good understanding of the demands of the question providing relevant explanations backed by appropriately selected information, although this may not be full or comprehensive. Answers will, for the most part, be

clearly expressed and show some organisation in the presentation of material. *(7–9 marks)*

Level 4 Answers will be well focused, identifying a range of specific explanations backed by precise evidence and demonstrating good understanding of the connections and links between events/issues. Answers will, for the most part, be well written and organised. *(10–12 marks)*

Question 2(b) and 3(b)

Level 1 Answers may **either** contain some descriptive material which is only loosely linked to the focus of the question **or** they may address only a limited part of the period of the question. Alternatively, there may be some explicit comment with little, if any, appropriate support. Answers are likely to be generalised and assertive. There will be little, if any, awareness of different historical interpretations. The response will be limited in development and skills of written communication will be weak. *(0–6 marks)*

Level 2 Answers will show some understanding of the demands of the question. They will either be almost entirely descriptive with few explicit links to the question **or** they contain some explicit comment with relevant but limited support. They will display limited understanding of differing historical interpretations. Answers will be coherent but weakly expressed and/or poorly structured. *(7–11 marks)*

Level 3 Answers will show a developed understanding of the demands of the question. They will provide some assessment, backed by relevant and appropriately selected evidence, but they will lack depth and/or balance. There will be some understanding of varying historical interpretations. Answers will, for the most part, be clearly expressed and show some organisation in the presentation of material. *(12–16 marks)*

Level 4 Answers will show explicit understanding of the demands of the question. They will develop a balanced argument backed by a good range of appropriately selected evidence and a good understanding of historical interpretations. Answers will, for the most part, show organisation and good skills of written communication. *(17–21 marks)*

Level 5 Answers will be well focused and closely argued. The arguments will be supported by precisely selected evidence leading to a relevant conclusion/judgement, incorporating well-developed understanding of historical interpretations and debate. Answers will, for the most part, be carefully organised and fluently written, using appropriate vocabulary. *(22–24 marks)*

Introduction to this book

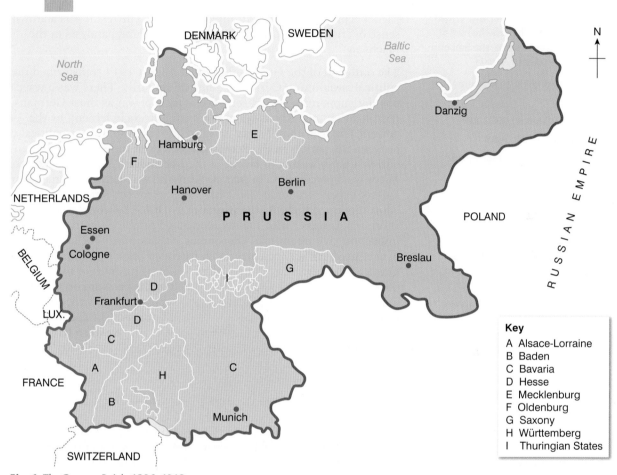

Fig. 1 *The German Reich, 1890–1918*

In 1890, the German *Reich* (empire) was governed by the *Kaiser* (emperor), Wilhelm II, who in many ways exercised autocratic power. He alone could appoint and dismiss ministers and his ministers alone could propose any changes in the law. Supporting the **autocracy** were the *Junkers*, the powerful aristocratic landowning class. Junkers dominated the upper ranks in the army, the civil service and the justice system. The *Reichstag* (parliament) was elected by universal male suffrage, but this had very little real power. Nevertheless, the Reichstag increasingly became the focus for opposition parties to develop and challenge the autocratic system of government. The economy of the German Reich had grown rapidly since 1871 and Germany had become, by 1900, a leading industrial nation. Industrialisation transformed German society in many ways, leading to the emergence of a wealthy middle class and an increasingly discontented working class. Many of Germany's leading industrialists saw political stability as the best guarantee of their future prosperity and formed an alliance with the **Junker** landowners to support

Exploring the detail

The German Reich

The German Reich which was established in 1871 was referred to as the Second Reich. The First Reich, the Holy Roman Empire which lasted from 962 until 1806, was a loose confederation of mainly German states ruled over by the Holy Roman Emperor. For much of the history of the Holy Roman Empire, the emperor was also the ruler of Austria.

In the Second Reich, there were three Kaisers:

- Kaiser Wilhelm I, 1871–88
- Kaiser Frederick, 1888
- Kaiser Wilhelm II, 1888–1918

Key terms

Eastern front: the line along which Germany and its main ally, Austria-Hungary, were fighting against Russia, mainly in Poland, in the First World War.

Western front: the line which stretched from the Belgian coastline, across northern France as far as the border with Switzerland, along which Germany fought against Britain and France in the First World War.

Exploring the detail

The Weimar Republic

The republic which was established in Germany after the First World War has become known as the Weimar Republic because its first government was temporarily based in the small town of Weimar in 1919. This was because the situation in Berlin was too unstable for a capital city.

the autocratic system of government. Workers, on the other hand, formed trade unions to put pressure on employers for higher wages and better conditions. They also, in increasing numbers, voted in Reichstag elections for the Social Democratic Party (*Sozialdemokratische Partei Deutschlands* or SPD), a party which campaigned for greater democracy and social change. By 1912, the SPD had become the largest single party in the Reichstag and Germany had become an increasingly divided nation, socially and politically. No political party was genuinely national or broadly based, and politics became fragmented, with many different parties representing different interest groups. The result was a growing sense of crisis in the German political system and paralysis in the Reichstag.

The outbreak of the First World War in August 1914 transformed the political situation in Germany, albeit temporarily. There was a wave of popular support for the Kaiser's declaration of war as most Germans regarded their country as being the victim of 'encirclement' by the Allied powers, Great Britain, France and Russia. The result was a political truce between the parties in the Reichstag, with even the SPD, hitherto an anti-war party, voting in favour of the war budget. As long as German forces were perceived to be successful in the war, and German civilians did not experience undue hardship, support for the Kaiser and the war effort remained high. By the winter of 1916–17, however, severe food shortages, together with rapidly rising food prices, began to have an impact on civilian morale. Discontent increased in 1917 after the passing of the Auxiliary Service Law, which extended conscription into the armed forces and industry to all males aged 17–60. The entry of the USA into the war on the Allied side in 1917 added to the pressure on Germany. On the other hand, the conclusion of a separate peace treaty between Germany and Russia in March 1918 freed many of the German forces on the **eastern front** for a major offensive on the **western front**. In the early stages of this spring offensive, German forces in France and Belgium almost succeeded in breaking through the Allied lines before the German advance petered out.

By the autumn of 1918, German forces were in retreat along the whole length of the western front. There was also growing unrest on the home front and there were signs of mutiny in the German navy. Knowing that Germany faced certain defeat, the two most senior commanders in the Germany army, Hindenburg and Ludendorff, informed the government that an armistice was necessary. These two men had effectively taken over the government of Germany since 1916. They realised, however, that the Allies would only agree to a negotiated peace settlement if Germany was ruled by a democratic government. In November 1918, therefore, they brought civilian politicians into the government, including SPD politicians, and advised the Kaiser to abdicate. It was this provisional civilian government of a new German republic which signed the armistice terms and brought the fighting to an end in November 1918. The majority of German soldiers and civilians knew nothing about the true position of Germany's forces at the end of the war and the news of the armistice, on Allied terms, came as a complete shock. Ludendorff and Hindenburg had managed to shift the blame for this defeat onto the politicians who formed the new government. This was the basis of the myth that the German forces had been 'stabbed in the back' by the so-called 'November criminals'. This myth, exploited by right-wing nationalist parties to undermine the new republic, poisoned post-war German politics for years to come.

■ Key profiles

Field Marshal Paul von Hindenburg

An aristocratic landowner and professional soldier, Hindenburg (1847–1934) became a hero after defeating a large Russian army at the battle of Tannenberg. In 1916, he became chief of the general staff. After Germany's defeat in 1918, Hindenburg shifted the blame for this humiliation onto the politicians by inventing the 'stab in the back' myth. He was elected president of the Weimar Republic in 1925 and re-elected in 1932. A strong believer in authoritarian rule, he disliked the democratic values of the republic but, at least until the early 1930s, he strictly observed the constitution.

General Erich Ludendorff

Ludendorff (1865–1937) was a key figure, alongside Hindenburg, in the German victories at Tannenberg and the Masurian Lakes. In 1916, he joined with Hindenburg in engineering the overthrow of the Chancellor, Theobald von Bethmann-Hollweg, and became a member of the military committee which effectively ruled Germany until the end of the war. He was reactionary in his politics and an implacable opponent of the new republic. He took part in Hitler's Munich Putsch of 1923 and sat as a Nazi deputy in the Reichstag from 1924–28.

The new republic was beset with problems from the beginning. Apart from being associated in many eyes with defeat and national humiliation, the politicians who now ruled Germany had to deal with a severe economic crisis, the polarisation of German society and the growth of extremist parties which aimed to overthrow the republic. Price inflation was a hangover from the First World War when the Kaiser's governments had borrowed heavily to pay for the war and had failed to control price increases. After the war, inflation spiralled out of control and reached its peak in the autumn of 1923. Economic problems, which led to workers losing their jobs, wages becoming worthless and savings being wiped out, caused a severe loss of confidence in the governments of the day. These governments were, in any case, inherently unstable because the constitution of the new republic introduced a system of Reichstag elections based on **proportional representation.** This enabled Germany's many small political parties to gain seats in the Reichstag but prevented the larger parties, such as the SPD, the **Centre Party** and the Democratic Party (DDP) from winning majorities. All governments in this period were, therefore, coalition governments and there were frequent changes of government as coalition parties fell out amongst themselves.

Political extremism was another problem which dogged the early years of the new republic. There were many on the left of German politics who believed that Germany was ripe for the kind of revolutionary change that had recently occurred in Russia. In January 1919, a revolutionary break-away group from the SPD, the **Spartacists**, had attempted to seize power in Berlin in a communist uprising. They were defeated, but only after the army had intervened to support the new government. Throughout the history of the Weimar Republic, the army continued to play a key role in German politics. On the right of the political spectrum there were many German nationalists who believed that the new republic was responsible for a national humiliation and should be overthrown. Some on the right wished to see a return of the Kaiser, others favoured a dictatorship. Their support came mainly from ex-soldiers who had been released from the army but returned to civilian life to face unemployment. Many of these ex-servicemen

■ Key terms

Proportional representation: a system of allocating seats in the Reichstag to the political parties in direct proportion to the percentage of the votes they received in the election. This guaranteed that the smaller parties gained some seats in the Reichstag, but it also meant that it was virtually impossible for any political party to win an outright majority.

Centre Party: the political party which represented the interests of Germany's large Roman Catholic minority. The Centre Party was pro-democracy and prepared to work with other parties in coalition governments.

Spartacists: the Spartacist League was an extreme left-wing revolutionary group led by Rosa Luxemburg and Karl Liebknecht. Inspired by the Russian Bolshevik revolution of October 1917, the Spartacists attempted to stage a similar uprising in Germany in January 1919. Luxemburg and Liebknecht were shot by the army and over 100 workers were killed.

Key terms

Freikorps: the Free Corps, a paramilitary organisation of ex-soldiers, which was armed and financed by the army and used to support right-wing groups in German politics before 1933.

Cross-reference

For a definition of Bolshevism see page 66.

Did you know?

The SA, or *Sturmabteilung* (Storm Division) of the Nazi Party, had been set up in 1921 as the fighting force of the party. Members wore brown shirts and swastika insignia, hence they were also known as the 'Brownshirts'. Their role was to intimidate the Nazis' political opponents, especially the communists, by breaking up their meetings and street parades. The SA attracted unemployed young men to its ranks, especially ex-soldiers and men who were looking for excitement and violence. They were provided with a uniform, meals and accommodation in SA hostels. They also staged orderly, disciplined marches which served a useful 'propaganda by deed' purpose for the Nazi Party in conveying an impression of a strong, determined and disciplined organisation.

Cross-reference

For details of the Young Plan, see pages 12.

joined paramilitary organisations such as the ***Freikorps*** which were funded by the army and used street violence to attack and undermine the parties of the left. Among the right-wing groups which were founded in the chaos of post-war Germany was the National Socialist German Workers' Party (NSDAP) which, in 1920, came under the leadership of Adolf Hitler. Right-wing violence was a serious challenge to the republic. In 1920, there was an unsuccessful attempt to overthrow the government by Wolfgang Kapp and his Freikorps supporters. There were also many assassinations of prominent left-wing politicians. Finally, in 1923, Adolf Hitler and his paramilitary supporters, the SA, attempted to stage a coup in Munich. This so-called Beer Hall Putsch was defeated when the local police and army commanders decided to put down the revolt and arrest Hitler. He was tried and convicted but served only nine months of a five-year prison sentence, largely because the judges supported his aims, if not his methods.

The association of the new republic with defeat and humiliation was made worse in 1919 when the Allied powers imposed the Versailles Peace Treaty on Germany. Germany was forced to accept responsibility for starting the First World War and was punished accordingly.

The main terms of the treaty were:

- Germany lost land in the east to Poland, Alsace and Lorraine in the south-west to France, Eupen and Malmedy to Belgium and Northern Schleswig to Denmark. As a result of these territorial losses, East Prussia became separated from the rest of Germany by the so-called 'Polish corridor'. Germany thus lost 13% of its territory and 12% of its population.
- Germany's army was reduced to a small defence force of 100,000 men. Germany was not allowed to have an airforce and its navy was not allowed to have submarines or large battleships.
- No German forces were allowed in the Rhineland, a part of Germany adjacent to the French and Belgian borders.
- Germany had to accept responsibility for causing the war.
- Germany had to pay reparations to the Allies for the damage and destruction caused by the war. In 1921, the amount of reparations was fixed at 132 billion gold marks, to be paid over 30 years.

Reparations became a running sore in the relations between Germany and its former enemies and also a focus for German nationalist resentment. When Germany failed to make reparations payments to France and Belgium in 1923, troops from these countries occupied the industrial area of the Ruhr and began to take German coal and manufactured goods in lieu of reparations payments. This crisis temporarily united the nation in opposition to the occupation but, when the government called off its campaign of passive resistance to the occupiers, nationalist opinion was outraged. This was the background to Hitler's attempted coup in Munich. The reparations issue had been partially defused by an agreement in 1924 under which Germany would receive American loans to rebuild its economy and pay reparations. Another attempt in 1929 to settle the reparations issue, with a plan drawn up by the American banker, Owen D. Young, provoked a right-wing backlash in Germany which enabled Hitler and the Nazi Party, with skilful propaganda and backing from wealthy industrialists, to make a breakthrough in national politics.

The years 1924 to 1928 had been a period of relative stability and prosperity in the history of the Weimar Republic. Inflation was finally brought under control with the issue of a new currency, trade improved and unemployment decreased. Coalition governments became more stable as support for the anti-democratic extremist parties of the right

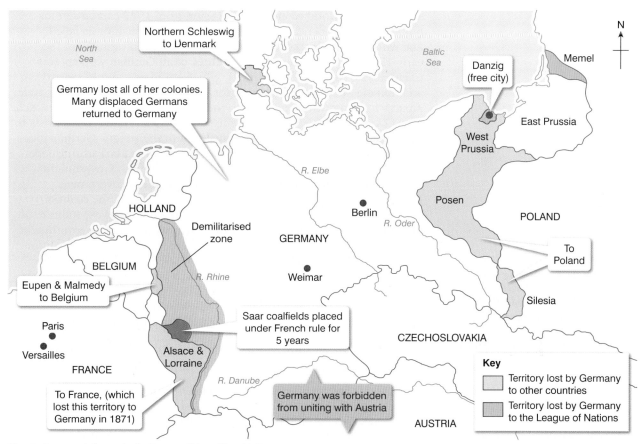

Northern Schleswig
to Denmark

Germany lost all of her colonies.
Many displaced Germans
returned to Germany

Danzig
(free city)

Memel

East Prussia

West
Prussia

Posen

POLAND

To
Poland

Silesia

CZECHOSLOVAKIA

Berlin

GERMANY

Demilitarised
zone

Weimar

HOLLAND

BELGIUM

Eupen & Malmedy
to Belgium

Saar coalfields placed
under French rule for
5 years

Paris

Versailles

FRANCE

Alsace &
Lorraine

To France, (which
lost this territory to
Germany in 1871)

Germany was forbidden
from uniting with Austria

AUSTRIA

Key

☐ Territory lost by Germany
to other countries

☐ Territory lost by Germany
to the League of Nations

*North
Sea*

*Baltic
Sea*

R. Elbe

R. Oder

R. Rhine

R. Danube

N

Fig. 2 *Germany's losses in the Treaty of Versailles, 1919*

and left declined. This was also a period of experimentation in the arts
as painters, architects, musicians, film-makers and actors took advantage
of the newly won freedom to explore modern ideas and trends. For many
traditionally minded Germans, however, this was just another example of
the weakness and degeneracy of the new Germany.

Key profile

Adolf Hitler

Hitler (1889–1945) was born in Austria. As a young man he had
ambitions to be an artist but was twice rejected by the Academy
of Arts in Vienna. During the years 1906–13, he lived as a vagrant
in Vienna before he moved to Bavaria in Germany in 1913. He
volunteered to serve in a Bavarian regiment in the German army
shortly before the outbreak of war in 1914. He served on the western
front in France where he was wounded twice and decorated for
bravery. On returning to civilian life in Munich in 1919, Hitler was
one of the many ex-soldiers who blamed the politicians in Berlin
for Germany's defeat and humiliation. In 1919, he started working
for the army's political department in Munich, which brought him
into contact with the German Workers' Party, a small radical right-
wing group. The party later became the National Socialist German
Workers' Party (NSDAP) and Hitler became its chairman in 1921.
After his unsuccessful attempt to overthrow the government in
1923, he was sent to prison, where he worked on his book, *Mein
Kampf* (my struggle), in which he set out his political philosophy.

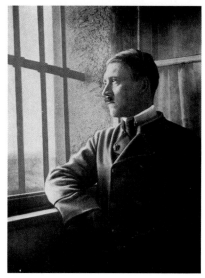

Fig. 3 *Hitler in Landsberg Prison in 1924,
after the failure of the Beer Hall
Putsch*

The onset of a world economic depression from 1929 caused serious problems for democracy in Germany. As German businesses failed and workers were laid off, unemployment climbed inexorably in the early 1930s. By 1932, nearly one in three of all German workers was unemployed. Mass unemployment, which led to widespread poverty and homelessness, caused despair for those who had lost their jobs and anxiety for those who hadn't. Both the communist party (*Kommunistiche Partei Deutschlands* or KPD) and the Nazi NSDAP exploited the crisis to build their support and took their rivalry onto the streets. German cities in the early 1930s became political battlegrounds as Nazi stormtroopers battled for control of the streets with the communists. Governments were overwhelmed by the crisis. In 1930, a coalition government led by the SPD leader, Hermann Müller, collapsed after the coalition partners could not agree on how to finance the increased expenditure on unemployment benefits. This was the last truly democratic government in the history of the Weimar Republic. There were three more coalition cabinets between March 1930 and January 1933, none of which had majority support in the Reichstag and which were sustained in power by presidential decrees, under **Article 48** of the constitution. The President, Hindenburg, was surrounded by advisers who favoured an authoritarian style of government but who were engaged in political in-fighting and intrigue between themselves. The result was a period of political instability, with governments which were incapable of rising to the challenges facing Germany.

There were three main coalition governments in the period between the fall of the Müller coalition in 1930 and the appointment of Adolf Hitler as chancellor in January 1933. Between March 1930 and May 1932, Heinrich Bruning, a leading member of the Centre Party, led a coalition of centre and right-wing parties. After he lost Hindenburg's support in May 1932, Bruning was forced to resign and was replaced by Franz von Papen, also a member of the Centre Party. His government, which was known as the 'cabinet of the barons' because it consisted of members of the elite, relied on Hindenburg's support since he did not have a Reichstag majority. He was, however, dismissed after General Schleicher intrigued against him and won the support of Hindenburg. Schleicher, who had been one of Hindenburg's chief advisers, now formed a government of his own and tried to persuade elements in the Nazi Party to join him. Papen gained revenge for his dismissal by conspiring with Hitler and Hindenburg to form a new coalition, with Hitler as chancellor.

In elections, support drained away from the moderate, democratic parties to the extremes. The KPD's vote in Reichstag elections increased from 10.6% of the electorate in 1928 to 14.3% in July 1932. This caused serious alarm among Germany's middle and upper classes who feared a communist revolution in Germany. The Nazi Party played on these fears, and also exploited the weakness of the democratic system in Germany, to attract support for their anti-communist, anti-democratic political programme. The Nazis took advantage of three Reichstag elections and one presidential election in the years 1930 to 1932 to boost their vote. They became the largest party in the Reichstag but were unable to win a majority of the seats; they were, however, able to frustrate the efforts of other parties to form coalition governments with majority support and so undermined the whole democratic political process. Even though the Nazis' share of the vote slipped back in the Reichstag election of November 1932, Hitler was still in a very strong position to negotiate with Franz von Papen in January 1933 to form a coalition government with himself as chancellor.

Key terms

Article 48: The constitution granted the president emergency powers to issue presidential decrees which had the force of law and which did not have to be approved by the Reichstag. This power was only supposed to be used in exceptional circumstances.

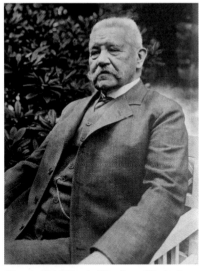

Fig. 4 *Field Marshal Paul von Hindenburg was president of the German Republic between 1925 and 1934*

Key profile

Franz von Papen

A former army officer from an aristocratic Catholic background, Papen (1879–1969) had a wide network of influence within political circles. Although a member of the Centre Party, he was thoroughly anti-democratic and believed in the restoration of the powers and privileges of the old elite and the re-establishment of an authoritarian state. Despite not being a member of the Reichstag (he was minister-president of Prussia), he was appointed chancellor in May 1932 and headed a 'cabinet of the barons' selected from the industrial and landowning elite. He was brought down by the intrigues of Schleicher in December 1932.

Timeline

The colours represent different types of events as follows: political, economic, social, international.

1914	1917	1918	1919	1920
Germany enters First World War in alliance with Austria-Hungary, fighting against Great Britain, France and Russia	USA enters war on side of Great Britain, France and Russia	Germany defeats Russia but defeated on western front Kaiser Wilhelm II abdicates and a new republic established **November** New German government signs armistice to end fighting on western front	**January** Communist (Spartacist) uprising in Berlin, suppressed by army and Freikorps **June** Germany forced to accept Treaty of Versailles	Kapp Putsch in Berlin attempts to overthrow government NSDAP established

1929	1930	1932	1933
June Young Plan introduced to reorganise reparations payments **October** Wall Street Crash leads to collapse of German economy and mass unemployment	**March** Collapse of coalition government led by Müller. Replaced by Bruning who needs to rule by presidential decree **September** NSDAP gain support in Reichstag election	**April** Hitler challenges Hindenburg in presidential election and achieves second place **July** NSDAP becomes largest party in Reichstag after election **November** NSDAP loses votes and seats	**January** Hindenburg appoints Hitler chancellor, in coalition with other parties **February** Reichstag fire leads to Decree for Protection of the People and the State which suspends basic freedoms **March** NSDAP gain 44% of vote in election to Reichstag **March** Enabling Act gives Hitler dictatorial power

1937	1938	1939	1940
Encyclical letter from the Pope criticises repression of Catholic Church in Germany	**February** Hitler purges army leadership to increase his control over military **March** Germany annexes Austria in the Anschluss **September** Germany gains control over Sudeten area of Czechoslovakia after negotiations with Britain, France and Italy at Munich **November** Jewish property and synagogues attacked on Kristallnacht	**March** Germany occupies the rest of Czechoslovakia RSHA established to bring all police forces under SS control Membership of Hitler Youth becomes compulsory **August** Nazi-Soviet Pact agreed with USSR to divide Poland between the two powers **August** Rationing of some key foodstuffs begins **September** German forces invade Poland, leading to start of Second World War	**April** Germany invades Denmark and Norway **May** Germany invades Holland, Belgium and France **June** France defeated

1921	1923	1924	1926	1925
Adolf Hitler becomes leader of NSDAP SA established	German economy hit by hyperinflation **January** French and Belgian troops occupy the Ruhr industrial area to force Germany to pay reparations **November** Hitler and Nazis attempt to seize power in Beer Hall Putsch in Munich	**February** Hitler sentenced to five years imprisonment for leading the Beer Hall Putsch **April** Dawes Plan introduced to ease reparations payments **December** Hitler released from prison	SS established	General Hindenburg elected president of German Republic

1933	1934	1935	1936
Law for the Re-establishment of a Professional Civil Service leads to purge of Jews from public employment **May** Trade unions banned and replaced with German Labour Front **July** All non-Nazi parties either banned or voluntarily disbanded Nazi regime and Catholic Church sign a concordat	Protestant Confessional Church established as breakaway group from official Evangelical Church **June** SA purged in Night of Long Knives **August** Death of Hindenburg allows Hitler to become president and chancellor with title of Führer	**March** Hitler announces start of rearmament programme	**March** German troops enter the demilitarised Rhineland Law for the Incorporation of German Youth makes the Hitler Youth an official education movement Olympic Games held in Berlin **September** Four Year Plan introduced to prepare country for war Himmler placed in charge of SS, SD and Gestapo

1941	1942	1943	1944	1945
June German forces invade the USSR	'Total war' measures implemented in Germany	**January** Defeat of German army at Stalingrad marks the decisive turning point in the war Start of sustained bombing campaign against German cities by British and Americans	**June** Allied forces open 'second front' in west with D-Day landings **July** Attempt to assassinate Hitler by army officers in Bomb Plot fails	**April** Hitler commits suicide **May** Germany defeated

1 Hitler and the Nazis in 1933

In this chapter you will learn about:

- how Hitler came to power in Germany in January 1933
- the ideology of the Nazi Party.

> That is the miracle of our age, that you have found me, that you have found me among so many millions. And I have found you. That is Germany's good fortune.
>
> **1** *Adolf Hitler, quoted in Fest, J. C., **The Face of the Third Reich**, 1970*

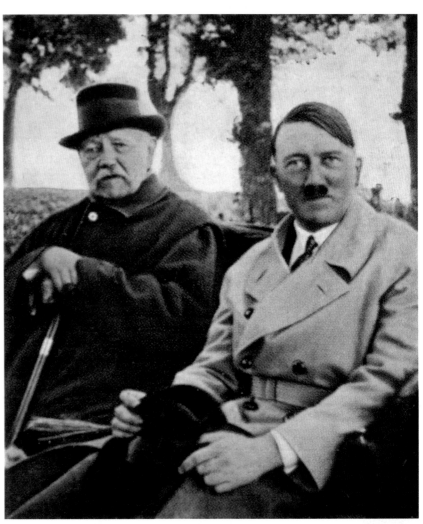

Fig. 1 *Field Marshal Paul von Hindenburg was president of the German Republic between 1925 and 1934. He appointed Adolf Hitler chancellor in 1933*

Hitler and the Nazis come to power

On the morning of 30 January 1933, Adolf Hitler, leader of the National Socialist Party, was summoned to the office of the president of the German Republic, Field Marshal Hindenburg. At this short but momentous meeting Hitler was invited by Hindenburg to lead a new 'government of national concentration', a coalition government in which the National Socialist Party would share power with the

DNVP (*Deutschnationale Volkspartei*) and others, including Franz von Papen. When he left the meeting to return to his party headquarters, Hitler had been appointed chancellor of the new government, a process which was conducted in accordance with the constitution. Although Hitler was the leader of the largest party in the Reichstag, Hindenburg and Papen believed his inexperience meant that he could be easily manipulated by the more experienced politicians in his cabinet. *'We have hired him,'* declared Papen. *'Within two months we will have pushed Hitler so far into a corner that he'll be squeaking.'*

Later that day, Hitler held his first cabinet meeting. It was a cabinet in which the Nazi Party held only three posts out of a total of twelve ministers. Franz von Papen, a close friend and confidante of the President, held the position of vice-chancellor and was also the minister-president of Prussia, Germany's largest state. He also had won the right to be present whenever Hitler met with President Hindenburg. The minority position of Hitler and the Nazis within the cabinet reinforced Papen's view that the inclusion of the Nazis in government would make no fundamental change to the political situation. The real decisions in cabinet would be taken by the non-Nazi majority, many of whom belonged, like Papen himself, to the old aristocratic elite. Papen believed that Hitler would not be able to dominate his own cabinet; still less would he be able to become the dictator he aspired to be.

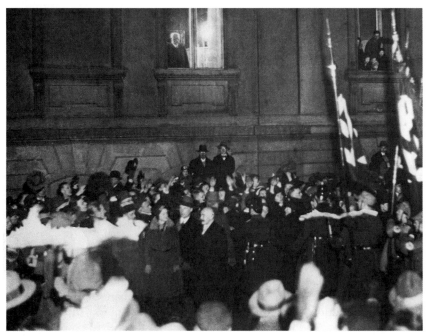

Fig. 2 *President Hindenburg watches the Nazi torchlight procession on the night of 30 January 1933*

Later that night Hitler stood on the balcony of the Reich Chancellery to review a torchlight procession by around 100,000 Nazi members which wound its way through the streets of the capital, Berlin. Organised by Hitler's propaganda chief, Josef Göbbels, this demonstration was designed to show that Hitler's appointment as chancellor was not going to be a normal change of government, one of the many that had been seen in the fourteen years since the German Republic had been established. It was a spectacular demonstration of

Key terms

DNVP (Deutschnationale Volkspartei): the German National People's Party, a conservative, nationalist party which shared some of the same aims as the Nazis, including hostility to the pre–1933 democratic system.

Stahlhelm: the Steel Helmets, a nationalist, right-wing paramilitary force which recruited ex-servicemen. It was a significant force in the politics of the Weimar Republic.

Activity

Revision exercise

Make a list of the strengths and weaknesses of Hitler's position when he became chancellor in January 1933.

Exploring the detail

Hitler's first cabinet

Apart from Hitler (Chancellor) and Papen (Vice-Chancellor), the cabinet contained two Nazi Party ministers; Wilhelm Frick was minister of the interior and Herman Göring was minister without portfolio (he was also minister of the interior in Prussia). Nazi ministers thus controlled the police forces and justice systems in key parts of Germany. General Blomberg, an aristocratic army officer, was defence minister. Alfred Hugenberg, the media tycoon and leader of the DNVP, was minister for economics. Freiherr von Neurath, an aristocratic, conservative, professional diplomat with wide experience of foreign affairs, was made foreign minister at Hindenburg's insistence. The cabinet also included Franz Seldte, the leader of the paramilitary *Stahlhelm* (Steel helmets), as minister of labour.

Cross-reference

For a more information about the Stahlhelm, see page 25.

Hitler's personal triumph and of the victory of the Nazi movement. Hitler and his Nazi Party were making clear that their accession to power would mark a historic break with the past and the start of their 'National Revolution'.

■ Key profiles

General Werner von Blomberg

Before becoming defence minister in Hitler's first cabinet, Blomberg (1878–1946) had been the army commander in East Prussia. Described as weak and easily influenced, Blomberg was persuaded by Hitler's promise of an aggressive foreign policy and rearmament to steer the army towards increasingly enthusiastic support for the regime. In 1938, however, Hitler removed Blomberg from the government.

Alfred Hugenberg

An ambitious and ruthless businessman who had become involved in politics during the Weimar Republic, Hugenberg (1865–1951) was nicknamed the 'silver fox' because of his cunning. As well as owning a vast newspaper and cinema business, Hugenberg was also the leader of the DNVP. He was a fervent German nationalist, an opponent of the Weimar Republic and an outspoken critic of the Versailles Treaty. He was a leading figure in organising a campaign against the **Young Plan** in 1929, through which he became closely associated with Hitler.

Franz Seldte

The leader of the paramilitary Stahlhelm, Seldte (1882–1947) was a conservative German nationalist who had been hostile to the Weimar Republic but retained his independence from the Nazis. In April 1933, however, he joined the Nazi Party and his Stahlhelm organisation was incorporated into the SA.

■ Key terms

Young Plan: a plan drawn up by an American banker, Owen D. Young, to reschedule Germany's reparations payments. Under the plan, the total reparations to be paid was reduced, payments were spread over 58 years, and Allied troops were to be removed from Germany. In the eyes of German nationalists, the reparations payments were viewed as unjust and the German government's agreement to the Young Plan was therefore denounced as a sell-out.

■ A closer look

The rise of the Nazi Party

In 1928, the Nazi Party had been a small, fringe party which could only gain 2.6% of the vote in that year's Reichstag election. Its support was largely confined to Bavaria in the south of Germany. After the failure of the Beer Hall Putsch in Munich in 1923, Hitler had abandoned his strategy of trying to achieve power through armed force and had opted instead for a legal route to power, fighting elections in order to secure a majority in the Reichstag. In 1928, this strategy appeared to have failed. Within five years, however, the position of Hitler and the Nazi Party had been dramatically transformed. In 1932, the Nazis had become the largest party in the Reichstag, although not yet with an overall majority, and Hitler had gained 13.4 million votes in the second round of the presidential election in April. The Nazis had attracted support from many different regions and different social groups. With the Weimar Republic undergoing a severe political crisis in the years 1930–32, Hitler had been in a position to undermine the efforts of other parties to form stable governments and demand that

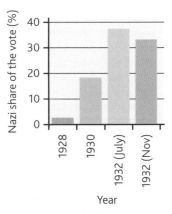

Fig. 3 *Support for the Nazi Party in Reichstag elections, 1928–32*

he be appointed chancellor. The success of the Nazi Party during these years was due to a range of different factors, some of which were the result of the serious economic and political crises which Germany was experiencing at this time, and some of which were due to Hitler and the Nazi Party's own efforts.

Nazi ideology in 1933

In their rise to power, Hitler and the Nazis put forward a wide ranging but loose collection of ideas which, when assembled, might be described as an ideology. Nazi policy was first put forward in their Twenty-five Point Programme of 1920, a programme which was still officially the statement of their aims in 1933. Hitler made many speeches and gave occasional interviews to journalists; these give an insight into Hitler's thinking. While he was in prison after the failed Beer Hall Putsch, Hitler wrote *Mein Kampf*, his most complete statement of his ideas and aims. Hitler's ideas were not original; he borrowed from nationalistic and racist writings of the 19th and early 20th centuries of the kind that could be found in the cheap pamphlets sold on the streets of German cities. Nor were his ideas coherent or consistent; he modified his policy statements according to the audience he was addressing. Although the 1920 Programme had contained a mixture of nationalistic, anti-Semitic and anti-capitalist policies, Hitler had refused to be bound by this programme and had abandoned its more radical economic policies in order to win the support of wealthy businessmen. Much of Hitler's speeches and writings contained superficial and simplistic statements, dressed up as being scientifically based but in fact little more than irrational prejudices. This did not amount to an ideology according to the normal definition of that word. Nevertheless part of the Nazis' appeal was based on their constant repetition of a number of simplistic ideas which found a receptive audience among many sections of German society.

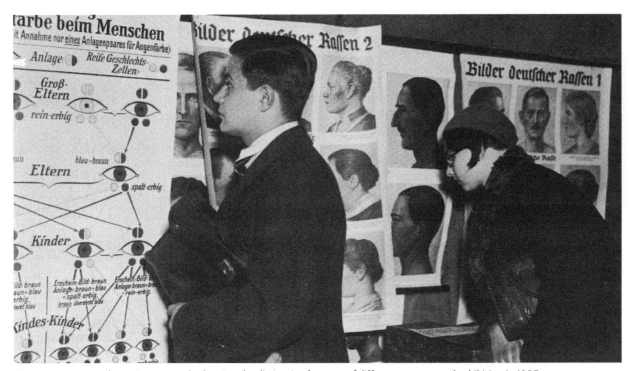

Fig. 4 *Germans study Nazi propaganda showing the distinctive features of different races at and exhibition in 1935*

Key profile

Alfred Rosenberg

One of the Nazi Party's leading ideologists was Alfred Rosenberg (1893–1946), the writer of many nationalistic, anti-Semitic pamphlets. His main work, *The Myth of the Twentieth Century*, published in 1930, drew on the theories of earlier 19th-century racial theorists and interpreted world history in terms of racial conflict. Rosenberg was also involved in the publication of a pamphlet, *The Protocols of the Elders of Zion*, which purported to expose a Jewish conspiracy to achieve world domination but which was, in fact, a forgery. Rosenberg originally came from Estonia in eastern Europe but claimed to have an ethnic German heritage. He moved to Germany in 1918 and became involved in a number of nationalist groups in Munich before joining the Nazi Party. He had ambitions to become a senior figure in Nazi ranks but his rigid ideological beliefs were his undoing. In the rise to power, and in the exercise of power after 1933, it was tactical flexibility, not ideological purity which was valued most highly in the Nazi Party.

Activity

Revision exercise

Use this section to construct your own table of Nazi beliefs.

The power of the will

> If one has realised a truth, that truth is valueless so long as there is lacking the indomitable will to turn this realisation into action.
>
> Power, in the last resort, is only possible where there is strength, and that strength lies not in the dead weight of numbers but solely in energy. Even the smallest minority can achieve a mighty result if it is inspired by the most fiery, the most passionate will to act. World history has always been made by minorities.

2 *From speech by Adolf Hitler, April 1922*

In his speeches and in his writing, Hitler presented himself and the Nazi movement as being a force for change in Germany. Power, strength and determination to succeed were qualities which Nazi propaganda claimed were personified by Hitler. The movement which he led, with its parades of stormtroopers, presented an image of discipline, unity and coordination which would sweep all opponents aside. 'The People's State', wrote Hitler, '*will never be created by compromise but only by the iron will of a single movement which has successfully come through in the struggle with all others.*'

Struggle, violence and war

> Those who want to live, let them fight and those who do not want to fight in this world of eternal struggle do not deserve to live.

3 *From Hitler, A., **Mein Kampf**, 1925*

Struggle, violence and war were at the heart of Nazi thinking and also of their actions. Hitler defined his **Weltanschauung** in terms of struggle and he claimed scientific justification for his view that struggle and conflict between races was inevitable, part of the natural order of things. War, he believed, was the means to reconstruct German society and to create a

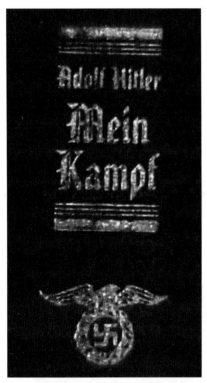

Fig. 5 *The cover from the 1933 edition of Mein Kampf*

Key terms

Weltanschauung: a term meaning 'world outlook', used to refer to the beliefs and attitudes through which an individual perceives the world. It can be used as another term for ideology.

new German Reich through conquest and the subjugation of other races. Nazi propaganda, therefore, glorified the military virtues of courage, loyalty and self-sacrifice and the SA was projected as an organisation which gave German males the chance to demonstrate their manliness.

Social Darwinism and the master race

> In the struggle for daily bread all those who are weak and sickly or less determined succumb, while the struggle of the males for the female grants the right or opportunity to propagate only to the healthiest. And struggle is always a means for improving a species' health and power of resistance and, therefore, a cause of its higher development.

4 ───────────────── *From Hitler, A.,* **Mein Kampf**, *1925*

Hitler saw human life as little more than a Darwinian struggle for survival, in which only the fittest would prevail. He viewed humanity as consisting of a hierarchy of races, with races such as the Jews, black people and Slavs being inferior races, while the *Herrenvolk* (master race) were the **Aryan** peoples of northern Europe. Hitler believed that struggles between the races over resources were inevitable and that it was the destiny of the Aryans to rule over the inferior races. In order to ensure their success in the racial struggle, it was vital for the Aryans to maintain their racial purity; intermarriage and the mixing of the races would undermine the Aryans by polluting their blood with that of inferior races.

'All the human culture,' wrote Hitler, *'all the results of art, science and technology that we see before us today, are almost exclusively the creative product of the Aryan. He alone was the founder of all higher humanity.'* The Jews, on the other hand, were *'the ferment of decomposition among nations, the wreckers of human civilisation'*.

Exploring the detail

Social Darwinism

Charles Darwin, in his book, *The Origin of Species*, put forward the view that plants and animals have evolved through a process of 'natural selection'. This biological concept has been adapted by some social theorists to explain how societies have evolved. Social Darwinism is based on the belief that competition between individuals, groups, nations and races leads to a process of natural selection in which only the fittest will survive.

Key terms

Aryan: the term used by racial theorists, including the Nazis, to describe the race to which non-Jewish Germans belonged.

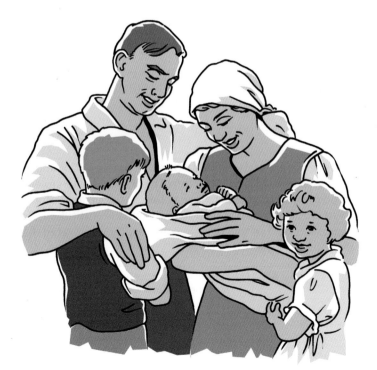

Fig. 6 *The Aryan ideal: blond hair, blue eyes and fair skin*

■ **Key terms**

Volkisch: concerning the distinct identity of the German people.

People's community

The supreme purpose of the **Volkisch** state is to guard and preserve those original racial elements which create that beauty and dignity which are characteristic of a higher mankind.

It will be the task of the People's State to make the race the centre of the community. It must make sure that the purity of the race will be preserved.

5 *From Hitler, A., **Mein Kampf**, 1925*

The concept of a 'people's community', or *Volksgemeinschaft*, was a key element in Nazi ideology although it was never defined very clearly. Hitler saw the State in racial terms. Only Aryans could be citizens of the State; all others were to be denied the rights of citizenship and the benefits that accrued from it and would be treated as mere 'subjects' of the State. Within the 'real community of the people' there would be no social classes and all Germans would have equal chances to find their own level in society. All would work together for the good of the nation, thereby demonstrating their commitment to common 'German values', and in return would benefit from access to employment and to welfare benefits. Every individual would know his place within the larger community and in every aspect of his or her life would strive for the good of the community.

Nazism thus aimed for a cultural and social revolution in Germany. The objective was to create a 'new man' and a 'new woman', individuals who would have awareness of the importance of race and soil, the strength of character to work unselfishly for the common good, and the willingness to follow the leadersip in the pursuit of their aims. Yet this revolutionary ideology was essentially reactionary and backward looking. When the Nazis talked of a 'people's community' they in fact wanted to return to a romanticised, mythical German past before the race had become 'polluted' with alien blood and before industrialisation had divided society along class lines. Their *Volksgemeinschaft* would be based on 'blood and soil'; it would be based on the German peasants who they believed had retained their racial purity and their traditional values more than city dwellers.

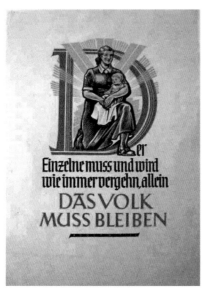

Fig. 7 *Nazi propaganda image of a single mother. The slogan reads 'Single mothers will always be alone'*

A national socialism

Socialism is the science of dealing with the common weal. Communism is not Socialism. Marxism is not Socialism. The Marxians have stolen the term and confused its meaning. I shall take Socialism away from the Socialists. Socialism is an ancient Aryan, Germanic institution. Our German ancestors held certain lands in common. They cultivated the idea of the common weal.

6 *Adolf Hitler, in an interview with George Viereck in 1932, published in **Guardian News and Media**, 2007*

The Nazis adopted the title 'National Socialist German Workers Party' in an attempt to gain working-class support, but at the same time to differentiate themselves from the international socialism of the Communist Party. The 1920 Programme contained a number of points

■ **Exploring the detail**

International socialism

The German Communist Party (KPD), following the political theories of Karl Marx, believed that socialism needed to be a truly international movement. Marx taught that workers in different countries had more in common with each other than they did with the capitalist rulers of their own countries. Marx expressed this idea in his famous slogan: *'Workers of the world unite. You have nothing to lose but your chains.'*

which were economically radical and were similar to many of the anti-capitalist policies of the communists and the socialists. They called, for example, for the confiscation of war profits, the nationalisation of large monopoly companies and the expropriation of land without compensation to the landowners. Hitler, however, never fully committed to these radical aims and modified his message according to the audience he was addressing. Increasingly after 1929 Hitler sought the support of wealthy businessmen such as Hugenberg and Thyssen and was at pains to reassure them that a Nazi government would not threaten their interests.

Key profile

Fritz Thyssen

Chairman of the United Steelworks Company, Thyssen (1873–1951) was a wealthy businessman and one of the early financial backers of the Nazi Party. He joined the Nazi Party in 1931 and acted as a link between the party and big business interests. By the late 1930s, however, he had become highly critical of the regime's economic policies. He opposed the outbreak of war and fled the country in 1939. He was captured in France and spent the rest of the war in Sachsenhausen and Dachau concentration camps. His wife Amelie instead of escaping France, voluntarily joined her husband in the camps.

Hitler used the word socialism loosely in a way that might appeal to working-class voters. In his view, socialism and the *Volksgemeinschaft* were one and the same thing: *'To be national means to act with a boundless, all-embracing love for the people and, if necessary, even to die for it. And similarly to be social means to build up the state and the community of the people so that every individual acts in the interest of the community of the people.'*

Anti-democracy and a belief in dictatorship

A government needs power, it needs strength. It must, with brutal ruthlessness press through the ideas which it has recognised to be right. But even with the most ruthless brutality it can ultimately prevail only if what it seeks to restore does truly correspond to the welfare of the people.

7   *From Hitler, A., **Mein Kampf**, 1925*

Hitler set out to destroy the Weimar Republic because it was a parliamentary democracy, a system which he viewed as weak and ineffective and entirely at odds with Germany's traditions of strong, authoritarian government. He also believed that parliamentary democracy encouraged the growth of communism, an even greater evil. *'Democracy'* he argued in a speech in April 1922, *'is fundamentally not German; it is Jewish. This Jewish democracy, with its majority decisions, has always been only a means towards the destruction of any existing Aryan leadership.'* Weimar democracy, established at the end of the First World War, was regarded by the Nazis as being based on a betrayal, in which the 'November criminals' had stabbed the German army in the back. As such it should be destroyed and replaced by a dictatorship, a one-party state run on the basis of the *Führerprinzip* (the principle of leadership).

Exploring the detail

The Strasser brothers

There were some radicals within the Nazi Party who believed in greater equality and State ownership of the main industries (i.e. national socialism). These included Otto and Gregor Strasser, who had built up Nazi support in industrialised northern Germany by supporting strikes and establishing the Nazi Factory Cell Organisation, rivalling the socialist and communist trades unions. Both brothers became disillusioned, however, with Hitler's courting of big business; Otto was expelled from the Nazi Party in 1930 while Gregor hung on until 1932. Gregor was murdered during the Night of the Long Knives in 1934. Otto went into exile after 1933.

Exploring the detail

Führerprinzip

The *Führerprinzip* was the basis on which the Nazi Party had been run since 1925; within the Party, Hitler had supreme control over policy and strategy and Party members became subordinated to Hitler's will. Hitler frequently praised *'the dominant significance of personality in every sphere of human life'*, and contrasted this with democracy which undermines and destroys natural leadership. *'The best form of government'*, he wrote, *'is that which makes it quite natural for the best brains to reach a position of dominant importance and influence in the community. The People's State will not have any body of representatives which makes its decisions through the majority vote'*.

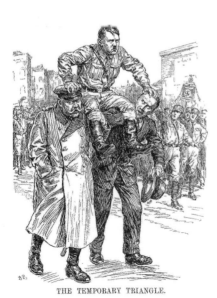

THE TEMPORARY TRIANGLE.

Fig. 8 *This British cartoon shows how foreign observers viewed the deal which brought Hitler to power in 1933*

Key terms

Lebensraum: 'living space', a concept by which Hitler justified his plans to take over teritory to the east of Germany.

Slav peoples: a very diverse ethnic group which includes Czechs, Slovaks, Poles, Russians, Ukrainians, Croats, Serbs and Slovenes. They live mainly in Central and Eastern Europe.

Anti-Semitism: hatred and fear of Jews (Semites).

Did you know?

Anti-Semitism has a long history in Europe and Hitler had developed his own bitter hostility to the Jews in pre-war Vienna. There were anti-Semitic parties in Germany during the Second Reich and, in Weimar Germany, parties other than the Nazis (e.g. the DNVP) were also anti-Semitic. Hitler, however, played down the Nazis' anti-Semitism in his election campaigns between 1930 and 1932 because he realised that this would not win many votes.

Aggressive nationalism

> As a state the German Reich shall include all Germans. Its task is not only to gather in and foster the most valuable sections of our people, but to lead them slowly and surely to a dominant position in the world.
>
> We National Socialists must hold unflinchingly to our aim in foreign policy; namely, to secure for the German people the land and soil to which they are entitled on this earth. If we speak of soil in Europe today, we can primarily have in mind only Russia and her border states.

8 *From Hitler, A., **Mein Kampf**, 1925*

As a German nationalist, Hitler's three basic aims were:

- to reverse the humiliation of the Treaty of Versailles – which Hitler described as an instrument of *'unlimited blackmail and shameful humiliation'* – and restore to Germany those lands taken from it
- to establish a 'Greater German Reich' in which all Germans would live within the borders of the State
- to secure for Germany its **Lebensraum** to settle its people and provide Germany with the food and raw materials needed to sustain it as a great power, since *'only an adequately large space on this earth assures a nation its freedom of existence'*.

This was an aggressive form of nationalism. Hitler did not merely want to restore Germany to its borders of 1914 but also to expand the territory of the Reich. The justification for a policy which would involve a war of conquest to secure for Germany its Lebensraum in the east came from Hitler's racial theories and from his belief in the necessity of violence and struggle. The **Slav peoples** who inhabited Poland, the Ukraine and Russia were, in Hitler's eyes, racially inferior to the Aryans and therefore had no right to occupy fertile farmland and vast reserves of raw materials. The struggle for control of these lands was but another stage in the inevitable struggle for mastery between races and, in the course of this struggle, the German people would rediscover its sense of national purpose and the people's community would be strengthened.

Activity

Thinking point

'To describe Hitler's thinking as an ideology is to flatter it.' What is your response to this statement?

Positive and negative stereotypes

Nazi ideology was based on crude stereotypes, both positive and negative. The identification of the groups which, in Hitler's eyes, had undermined Germany in the past and would have no part in the people's community of the future, was a constant theme in Hitler's speeches and his writing. The Nazis did not invent these stereotypes, just as they did not invent **anti-Semitism** or extreme German nationalism, but in their hands the promotion of positive and negatives images of different groups of people became a deliberate and consistent endeavour. By exaggerating and over-simplifying the observable characteristics of particular groups, they were able to demonise them and establish a justification for prejudice and discrimination against them.

The division of social groups into positive and negative stereotypes was based on three main criteria:

- **Ideological:** Those whose ideology threatened to undermine the political unity of the people's community were classified as threats and presented in a negative light. The main group in this category was the communists, but the Nazis also portrayed the socialist SPD, other bourgeois parties and any political party which had taken part in coalition governments during the Weimar Republic as having collaborated with communism and Jewish democracy.

- **Biological:** Any group which represented a threat to the racial purity and the health of the nation was presented in a negative light. This included not only the Jews but also gypsies and the mentally and physically unfit. Since the aim of Nazi racial policy was to improve the race through selective breeding, those who suffered from hereditary defects were candidates for compulsory sterilisation. The Nazis based this part of their ideology on the science of **eugenics**.

- **Social:** Groups whose values or behaviour conflicted with Nazi social norms were portrayed as 'asocial', meaning that they existed on the fringes of society. These included vagrants, alcoholics, criminals, juvenile delinquents, prostitutes and homosexuals. Many of these asocial behaviours were attributed to heredity which could therefore be eradicated through a programme of compulsory sterilisation.

Positive stereotypes

Racially pure Aryans

Hitler defined the Aryans as the superior, or master race, that which had been the creator of human culture in the past. In stereotypical terms, it was the physical characteristics of the race which were highlighted in Nazi ideology and propaganda, as the following makes clear:

> The Aryan race is tall, long-legged, slim. The race is narrow-faced, with a narrow forehead, a narrow, high-built nose and a prominent chin. The skin is rosy bright and the blood shines through. The hair is smooth, straight or wavy. The colour is blond.

9

From a Nazi leaflet, 1929, quoted in the German Propaganda Archive

The ideal citizen of the people's community would be a person who combined *'a splendid physical beauty with nobility of mind and spirit'* (Hitler). Such a person would submit to the authority of the leadership and thus be part of a vast, disciplined mass of people that would move in perfect coordination at the leader's direction. Women would accept their role as child-bearers while men would be warriors and providers.

German farmers

Much of Nazi propaganda in the late 1920s and early 1930s was aimed at farmers, largely on the grounds that they were a group which was experiencing severe economic hardship and was largely overlooked by the mainstream parties. But in Nazi ideology, the German peasant occupied a special place. With their romaniticised view of Germany's past, the Nazis believed that a people's community had existed in rural areas before the start of industrialisation and that German farmers had retained their traditional values of attachment to the soil and respect for authority. The Nazis also believed that German farmers had retained their racial purity. They would therefore be a key part of the Nazi *Volksgemeinschaft* (People's community) of the future.

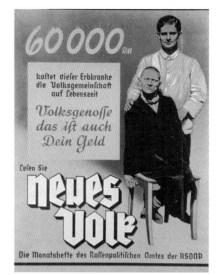

Fig. 9 *A propaganda poster showing Nazi attitudes to the mentally and physically disabled. The slogan reads 'These sick people cost 60,000RM to the National Community during their lifetimes. Comrades, this is also your money'*

Key terms

Eugenics: the science of racial improvement through such methods as selective breeding.

Did you know?

Eugenics became a subject for academic study in the late 19th and early 20th centuries and was very influential with politicians in many countries and from many different ideological standpoints. Eugenicists advocated intervention of many kinds to improve the hereditary traits of a nation or a race. These could include birth control, sterilisation and euthanasia to select out those who were considered to be unfit, either mentally or physically.

German workers

> Without the help of the German working man, you will never regain a German Reich. Not in our political salons lies the strength of the nation, but in the hand, in the brain and in the will of the great masses.

10 *From a speech by Adolf Hitler, April 1923*

The Nazis rejected the Marxist ideology of class conflict as a divisive force which would undermine their concept of a people's community. Nevertheless, Hitler tried to appeal to the 'German working man' to win the votes necessary to achieve power. In Nazi ideology, however, the working class was defined in much broader terms than the manual workers in heavy industry who were seen as the proletariat by Marxists. Hitler's reference to 'the hand' and 'the brain' reflects the fact that his definition of the German working man included office workers as well as artisans, self-employed craftsmen and small retailers. In other words, Hitler included elements of the lower middle class, or **Mittelstand**, in his notion of the 'great masses'. These groups were portrayed as the useful, productive and diligent members of society whose efforts had been undermined by the rapaciousness of big business and the divisive policies of Marxist politicians.

Key terms

Mittelstand: the lower middle class, a group which included artisans, farmers and shopkeepers.

Women

The Nazis put forward an idealised, traditional view of women and their role in society. Women should be homemakers and childbearers. They needed to be physically fit, with broad hips and should display the Aryan characteristics of blond hair and blue eyes. Women should be discouraged from pursuing professional careers because their main sphere was in the home. Motherhood was their vocation and they were therefore responsible for the *'success or ruin of the nation'*. Women should be discouraged from wearing make-up, wear only simple flat-soled shoes and should not wear trousers.

Negative stereotypes

Jews and communists

> All who are not of good race in this world are chaff.

11 *From Hitler, A., **Mein Kampf**, 1925*

Hitler saw the Jews as having been responsible for all of Germany's ills. Jews were represented in Nazi propaganda as greedy, cunning and motivated only by selfish motives. They were described as *'a parasite in the body of other nations'*, having no state of their own and working through a world-wide Jewish conspiracy to establish their dominance over other races. The Jews were held to be responsible for the evils of capitalism and, at the same time, for the growth of communism. They were therefore responsible for Germany's defeat in the First World War, the hated Treaty of Versailles and Germany's decline as a great power, together with the political weaknesses of the democratic system in the Weimar Republic. They were also to blame for all of Germany's economic and social problems, from the rampant inflation of the immediate post-war years to the mass unemployment of the depression years. Above all, Hitler regarded communism as a Jewish creed which had undermined the political and social cohesion of Germany and which should be eradicated.

Gypsies

Gypsies had long been the objects of suspicion in German society, as in other European countries, because they existed at the margins of society. Their appearance, their language and customs, their nomadic lifestyle and their lack of regular employment, marked them out as being different from other Germans. Racially they were seen as inferior and their presence in Germany (although there were only 30,000 of them) a threat to the purity of the German people. They were also regarded as being parasitic and a source of contagious diseases. In Nazi propaganda, they were often referred to as the 'Gypsy Plague'.

Intellectuals and pacifists

Hitler valued action over thought and regarded intellectuals with suspicion. His writings and speeches are peppered with references such as: *'Learned men who are physical weaklings'*, to the *'weak-willed and cowardly'* and to *'timid pacifists'*. The counterpart to this was the emphasis in Nazi propaganda on physical strength, unquestioning obedience and courage which was supposedly embodied in Nazi organisations such as the SA. *'To be a pacifist'* said Hitler in a speech in 1923, shows *'a lack of conviction, a lack of character'*.

Homosexuals

The behaviour of homosexuals was regarded as deeply offensive by traditionally minded Nazis, since it was seen as being against the laws of nature. Homosexuals were also seen as threatening Nazi policy for racial domination since they produced no children. In Nazi ideology, sexual behaviour was not simply a matter of individual preference but a matter of vital concern for the future of the race. Homosexuals were therefore demonised as being poisonous weeds which had to be eradicated for the health of the nation.

Vagrants, prostitutes and the workshy

Unwillingness to work was considered by the Nazis to *'give offence to the community'*. Since citizenship in a people's community was considered to be a privilege not a right, something which had to be earned, willingness to work for the good of the nation was one of the key criteria for admission. Beggars, prostitutes and vagrants were deemed unworthy to be granted the privileges of citizenship.

The physically and mentally unfit

> The People's State must see to it that only those who are healthy shall beget children. It is wrong for parents that are ill or show hereditary defects to bring children into the world.

12
*From Hitler, A., **Mein Kampf**, 1925*

For the Nazis, a healthy and pure race was essential if they were to achieve their goal of racial dominance. The passing on of hereditary diseases was considered to be a crime against the race and therefore the physically and mentally ill were demonised. Hitler identified syphilitics, tuberculosis sufferers, 'cripples' and 'imbeciles' as examples of the groups who threatened the racial hygiene of the people's community. The mentally and physically unfit were regarded as burdens on the community, unproductive and therefore *'unworthy of life'*.

Feminists

> The slogan 'Emancipation of Women' was invented by Jewish intellectuals. If the man's world is said to be the state, his struggle, his readiness to devote his powers to the service of the community, then it may perhaps be said that the woman's is a smaller world. For her the world is her husband, her family, her children and her home.

 From Hitler's speech to the 1934 Nuremberg Rally

Hitler saw female emancipation, and the feminists who promoted it, as unnatural and harmful to the State. The Nazis rejected the new freedoms given to women during the Weimar period, such as giving women the vote, the move towards equal pay with men and the breaking down of barriers to women entering the professions.

Activity

Revision exercise

Construct a table with two columns, one labelled for 'Positive stereotypes' and the other 'Negative stereotypes'. Use the information in this section to produce a summary of the way in which the Nazis either idolised or demonised various groups in German society. Against each entry, indicate whether they were singled out by the Nazis for ideological (I), biological (B) or social (S) reasons.

Summary questions

 1 Explain why Hindenburg appointed Hitler as chancellor in January 1933.

2 'Nazi ideology was nothing more than an incoherent collection of second-hand ideas'. Explain why you agree or disagree with this view.

2 How the Nazis consolidated their power, 1933–34

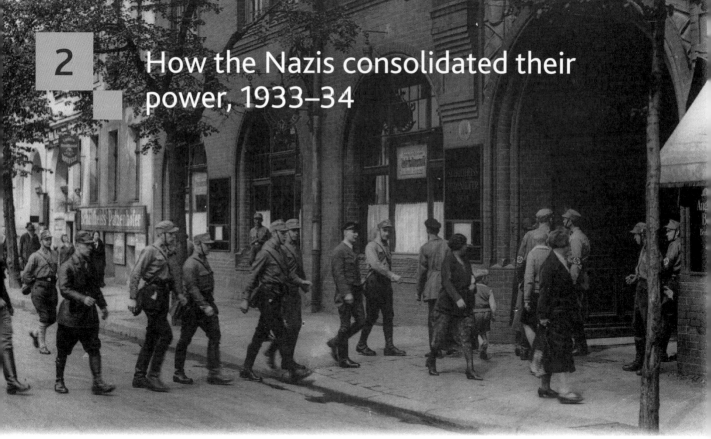

Fig. 1 *Members of the SA occupy the headquarters of the trade unions in Berlin on 2 May 1933*

In this chapter you will learn about:

- how Hitler and the Nazi Party consolidated their hold on power between January 1933 and August 1934

- how Hitler succeeded in establishing a dictatorship by means of terror, compromise, legal power, propaganda and policies.

Cross-reference

For a more detailed study of the process of *Gleichschaltung*, see pages 69–91.

Key terms

Führer: a title meaning 'leader' used by Hitler within the Nazi Party since the early days of his leadership. In 1934, he began to use the title to demonstrate his official role combining of the offices of chancellor and president of Germany.

When Hitler was appointed German chancellor at the end of January 1933 he was not yet the dictator he aspired to be. Although parliamentary democracy had been undermined by Hindenburg's use of presidential decrees since 1930, the Weimar constitution was still in force. Hitler headed a coalition government in which his own Nazi Party did not even have a majority in the cabinet. The Nazi Party was the largest party in the Reichstag but did not have an overall majority and was dependent on its coalition with the DNVP to win parliamentary votes. The German army, which wielded considerable political influence, was loyal to Hindenburg, not to Hitler. Although the Nazis effectively controlled the state government in Prussia, the largest of Germany's federal states, elected governments in most other German states were under the control of other parties.

By the summer of 1934, all this had changed and Hitler's dictatorship had been firmly established. Non-Nazi political parties had either been banned or had voluntarily disbanded themselves. Opponents of the Nazis had been divided, demoralised and, in many cases, thrown into prison. After Hindenburg's death in August 1934, Hitler became president as well as chancellor and had taken the title of **Führer**. He had the power to rule by decree as the constitution, with its guarantees of individual freedom, had been suspended. Through a process known as *Gleichschaltung* (coordination, or literally 'forcing into line'), key institutions in German society, such as the trade unions, had been brought under Nazi control. This process had been extended to the state governments. Finally, the army had sworn allegiance to the Führer.

This process of consolidation was achieved using a variety of methods, legal and illegal, peaceful and violent:

- the use of terror to beat down opponents
- compromise and concessions to powerful institutions
- the introduction of new laws to legitimise dictatorial rule

■ the use of propaganda to win the hearts and minds of the majority

■ the introduction of new policies to consolidate Nazi control.

■ Key chronology

Nazis' consolidation of power

1933	
1 February	Hitler dissolves the Reichstag and calls new elections
27 February	Reichstag building set on fire
28 February	Decree for the Protection of the People and the State
5 March	Reichstag elections; Nazis win 288 seats (43.9% of vote), still short of overall majority
6–7 March	Nazis begin takeover of state governments
8 March	First permanent concentration camp established
13 March	Ministry for Public Enlightenment and Propaganda established
24 March	Enabling Act passed
1 April	First one-day national boycott of Jewish-owned shops
7 April	Law for Restoration of a Professional Civil Service
1 May	International Labour Day declared a national holiday in Germany
2 May	Independent trade unions disbanded and their place taken by a new German Labour Front (DAF)
6–10 May	Ceremonial book burnings in Berlin and other university towns
10 June	Employment Law, set up new public works schemes to give work to unemployed
5 July	Centre Party voluntarily disbanded
14 July	Law against Formation of New Parties: Germany now a one-party state
20 July	Concordat with Catholic Church
12 November	Reichstag elections; Nazis won 92% of vote
30 November	Gestapo established
1934	
30 January	Law for Reconstruction of the Reich (elected state assemblies abolished, states to be run by appointed Reich Governors)
30 June	Night of the Long Knives
2 August	Death of President Hindenburg; Hitler becomes president and army swear oath of allegiance
19 August	Hitler becomes Reich chancellor and takes title of Führer

■ Activity

Thinking point

Construct a timeline for the period January 1933 to August 1934. Mark on the line the key events in the Nazis' consolidation of power. Alongside each event indicate whether it was a legal act (L), involved the use of force (F) or involved a compromise (C).

Select three or four events from this timeline which you consider to have been the most important turning points. For each point, write a paragraph explaining your choice.

■ The use of terror

The violence of Nazi stormtroopers had played a key role in Hitler's rise to power. Once he was in power and able to use the resources of the regime to consolidate his position, violence and terror were vital weapons in his struggle to eliminate opposition. The Nazi 'legal revolution' and the 'revolution from below', in which the SA unleashed a reign of terror against political opponents, were opposite sides of the same coin.

> Brownshirt violence was continuing all over the country, most notoriously in the 'Kopenick blood week' in June 1933 when a raiding party of stormtroopers had encountered resistance from a young Social Democrat in a Berlin suburb. After the Social Democrat shot three stormtroopers dead, the brownshirts mobilised en masse and arrested more than 500 local men, torturing them so brutally that 91 of them died. Amongst them were many well known Social Democrat politicians.

1

*From Evans, R., **The Third Reich in Power**, 2005*

In January 1933, the SA were the Nazis' main instrument of terror and violence. One of the immediate results of the Nazis coming to power was the rapid expansion of the SA. From a membership of around 500,000 in January 1933, the organisation grew to around 3,000,000-strong a year later. Another result of the Nazis being in power was that the activities of the SA gained legal authority. In late February 1933, the SA and the Stahlhelm were merged and became recognised as 'auxiliary police'; orders were issued to the regular police forces forbidding them from interfering with SA activities.

Using their new-found powers, the SA unleashed a sustained assault on their socialist and communist opponents. Thousands were rounded up and imprisoned in makeshift concentration camps set up in old factories or army barracks. By July 1933, 26,789 political prisoners had been arrested by the SA, or taken into 'protective custody' to use the official terminology of the Nazis, and imprisoned in some 70 camps. National and local leaders of the Communists and the SPD were arrested, their election meetings were broken up, their newspapers were suppressed and the distribution of election leaflets became virtually impossible. After the Reichstag fire and the issuing of the Decree for the Protection of the People and the State, violence and intimidation against the left intensified. During the election campaign for the March 1933 Reichstag elections, left-wing parties were virtually driven underground. Despite this, however, the Communist Party still managed to secure 12% of the votes, less than in the previous election of November 1932 but still a significant core of support. The SPD also gained 18% of the votes. The widespread use of violence and intimidation during the election campaign still could not deliver an outright majority in the polls for the Nazi Party. Clearly, terror alone could not guarantee that the Nazis would remain in power.

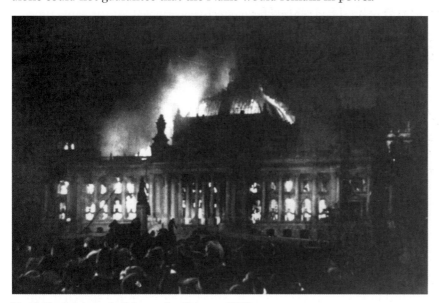

Fig. 2 *The Reichstag building on fire, February 1933*

After the elections, Hitler moved quickly to eliminate all remaining opposition to the Nazis and to gain legal sanction for his dictatorship. The Enabling Act, which granted Hitler's government emergency powers to rule by decree for four years, was passed by the Reichstag on 24 March. Since this was a fundamental change in the constitution, the Enabling Act required a two-thirds majority in the Reichstag vote in order to become law. The Nazis achieved this partly through the use of violence and intimidation. When Reichstag deputies arrived for the debate, held at the Kroll Opera House in Berlin, they had to pass through the massed ranks of Nazi supporters in the square outside; inside the building the

▪ **Exploring the detail**

The Stahlhelm

Taking its name from the steel helmets which were issued to German soldiers in the First World War, the Stahlhelm, or League of Frontline Soldiers, was a paramilitary organisation of ex-servicemen which was dedicated to the restoration of the monarchy and the revival of Germany as a military power. Founded in 1918 by Franz Seldte, the Stahlhelm grew rapidly and had 500,000 members by 1930, making it the largest paramilitary organisation in Weimar Germany.

▪ **Exploring the detail**

The Reichstag fire

On 27 February 1933, the Reichstag building was destroyed by fire. A young Dutch communist, Marinus van der Lubbe, was arrested and charged with causing the fire. The Nazis claimed that this was part of a communist plot to start a revolution in Germany and the event was used to justify the immediate suspension of civil liberties. There have been suspicions ever since that the Nazis deliberately set up van der Lubbe to set fire to the Reichstag in order to justify introducing repressive measures but no definitive evidence has ever emerged to show exactly who was responsible.

walls and corridors were lined by men from the SA and the SS (a Nazi special police force). Communist deputies were banned from taking their seats. Those of the Centre and DNVP were bought off with threats and promises. Only the SPD deputies had the courage to vote against the Act, which was duly passed and thereby gave Hitler the power to rule without the need for a Reichstag majority.

> The wide square in front was crowded with dark masses of people. We were received with wild choruses, 'We want the Enabling Act!' Youths with swastikas on their chests eyed us insolently, blocked our way, in fact made us run the gauntlet, calling us names like 'Centre pig', 'Marxist sow'. The Kroll Opera House was crawling with armed SA and SS men. The assembly hall was decorated with swastikas and similar ornaments. When we Social Democrats had taken our seats on the extreme left, SA and SS men lined along the walls behind us in a semi-circle.Their expression boded no good.

2 *A description of the scene at the Kroll Opera House by a Social Democrat, quoted in Layton, G.,* **Germany: The Third Reich**, *1992*

The next stage in the establishment of a dictatorship was to eliminate all other political parties and incorporate independent institutions into the Nazi regime. The trade unions, with their close links to the SPD, were a prime target and the Nazis set about destroying them. In town after town, trade union offices were raided by the SA; officials were arrested, their offices ransacked and their meetings broken up. By the time the trade unions were legally dissolved on 2 May, their organisation at grass-roots level had already been effectively crippled. At the same time, Nazi groups were seizing control over local government, forcing elected politicians to give up their posts in town halls and replacing them with Nazi Party officials. At all levels of local government, across the whole of Germany, the old guard were ruthlessly purged; those who would not leave office voluntarily were unceremoniously kicked out.

Hitler benefited from the violence of his supporters, but he was not always in control of events. Much of the violence of the SA against the Nazis' political opponents, and against the Jews, was unplanned, uncoordinated and piecemeal. In the period from February to June 1933, when the Nazis were eliminating opposition and establishing undisputed control, Hitler was prepared to go with the flow of SA violence. He was careful to ensure, however, that the SA did not attack the State itself; assaults on the police and the army were avoided, as Hitler was careful not to alienate those conservative forces which had shoe-horned him into power. Violence was a vital tool in the hands of the Nazi leadership but, in its uncontrolled and uncoordinated form, its usefulness was limited and at some point Hitler was bound to want to call a halt. This point was reached in the summer of 1933, as Hitler made clear in a speech in July.

> Revolution is not a permanent condition. The stream of revolution has been undammed, but it must be channelled into the secure bed of evolution. The slogan of the Second Revolution was justified as long as positions were still present in Germany that could serve as points for crystallisation for a counter-revolution. That is not the case any longer. We do not leave any doubt about the fact that if necessary we will drown such an attempt in blood.

3 *From a speech by Adolf Hitler, July 1933*

Cross-reference

For more information about the SS, see pages 95–96.

Activity

Source analysis

What can we learn from Sources 1 and 2 about the role played by terror in the Nazis' consolidation of power?

Activity

Source analysis

Read Source 3.

1 Who is Hitler threatening when he warns '*we will drown such an attempt in blood*'?

2 Who is Hitler trying to reassure when he states that '*Revolution is not a permanent condition*'?

Hitler's speech contained a warning that, in the future, the SA would become the targets for Nazi violence and terror. He did not, however, act on this warning for a further eleven months. In July 1933, Hitler was able to declare that the Nazi revolution was over. He had acquired dictatorial powers, all other parties had been banned or had voluntarily dissolved themselves and the process of *Gleichschaltung*, coordinating independent organisations into the Nazi regime had been completed. SA violence had served its purpose but was now increasingly an embarrassment for Hitler and the Nazi leadership. For Ernst Röhm, the leader of the SA, however, the Nazi revolution was far from complete and the SA were determined to continue with their violence until they had achieved their radical agenda, the Second Revolution. Chief among Röhm's aims was for the SA to become the nucleus of a new national militia which would, eventually, absorb and replace the existing army. With a combined SA and Stahlhelm membership of 4.5 million in January 1934, Röhm's forces already vastly outnumbered the army. However, since the summer of 1933 the role and importance of the SA had declined. In August 1933, they had lost their 'auxiliary police' status and were subject to stricter regulations over their powers of arrest. In the election campaign of November 1933, there was only one party, hence there was no longer a need for SA violence and intimidation. Lacking an 'official' outlet for their violence, and feeling resentment at the way that former conservative opponents of the Nazis were allowed to join the Nazi Party and take important jobs in local and central government, SA members became disillusioned and restless. Drunken brawls, always a feature of the SA, became increasingly common and, when police tried to intervene, they became the targets.

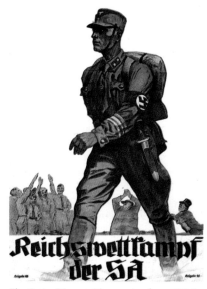

Fig. 3 *An SA recruiting poster from 1934. The slogan reads 'The National Struggle of the SA'*

■ Key profile

Ernst Röhm

Röhm (1887–1934) had been a soldier in the First World War and had risen to the rank of captain. After the war, he joined the Freikorps and was employed by the army to gather information on opposition groups. He met Hitler in 1919 and recruited him to infiltrate the small German Workers' Party. He later joined the renamed National Socialist German Workers' Party and helped to set up the SA. He took part in the Beer Hall Putsch and was briefly jailed after its failure. From 1925 to 1930, he worked in Bolivia as a military instructor but was recalled to Germany by Hitler in 1930 to take control of the SA. He turned the SA into a formidable fighting force but his radical views and his lifestyle – he drank heavily and was homosexual – proved a source of embarrassment to Hitler after the Nazis took power in 1933.

The Night of the Long Knives

The army remained the only institution which had the power to remove Hitler from office. Despite the fact that Blomberg, the Defence Minister, had brought the army closer to Nazi ideology, the army was not a Nazified institution and still retained some independence from Hitler. The ambitions of the SA and its leader Röhm were regarded as a serious threat by the army leaders, the more so when in the summer of 1934 SA units began stopping army convoys and confiscating weapons and supplies. When Blomberg, with Hindenburg's support, threatened to declare martial law and give the army power to deal with the SA, matters came to a head. Hitler had dithered since the spring of 1934, delaying taking decisive action against the SA, but in June he knew he could wait

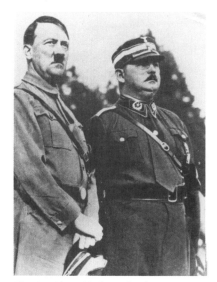

Fig. 4 *Hitler with the SA leader Ernst Röhm*

■ Activity

Thinking point

Explain why Röhm came into conflict with Hitler after the Nazis came to power.

■ **Exploring the detail**

The victims of the Night of the Long Knives

At least 84 were executed and another 1,000 or more were arrested. The victims included Röhm and other leaders of the SA, but Hitler took the opportunity to remove other opponents and settle some old scores. Among the victims were General Schleicher, Gregor Strasser and Gustav von Kahr who had played a key role in crushing the Beer Hall Putsch in 1923. Members of Papen's staff were executed and, although Papen himself was spared death, he was placed under house arrest and whatever power he still had was destroyed. Many leading conservative politicians were also targeted.

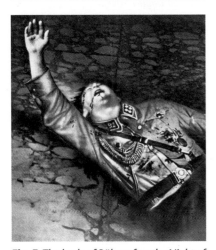

Fig. 5 *The body of Röhm after the Night of the Long Knives*

■ **Key terms**

Civil service: employees of central and local government. These are the people employed to advise politicians and to implement government policies.

no longer. A ruthless purge of the SA, known as the 'Night of the Long Knives', was launched on 30 June 1934 when the SS, acting on Hitler's orders, eliminated the leadership of the SA and many other political opponents of the Nazis.

■ **Key profile**

Gustav von Kahr

A conservative Bavarian nationalist, Kahr (1862–1934) was minister-president of Bavaria in 1923 at the time of the Beer Hall Putsch. Although he had initially been sympathetic to Hitler's aims of launching a march on Berlin to overthrow the government of the republic, he changed his mind after the putsch was launched and banned the Nazi Party. He also ordered the police and army to put down the revolt.

When Hitler addressed the Reichstag on 13 July he accepted full responsibility for the executions. He was acting, he said, as the *'supreme judge'* of the German people, and had been compelled to act in order to save the country from an SA coup. This secured the army's support and, when Hindenburg died in August, this support was vital in enabling Hitler to take on the role of president as well as chancellor. Hitler also gained public support for his apparently decisive actions. The SA declined sharply after the purge. By October 1935, its membership had declined to 1.6 million and, without Röhm as its leader, its political power was destroyed. Violence and terror remained vital weapons in the Nazi Party's efforts to retain political control but, after the Night of the Long Knives, it was the SS which controlled the terror machine. After June 1934, violence and terror were used more systematically and in a more controlled manner.

■ **Activity**

Discussion point

How might the Night of the Long Knives have affected the future development of the Nazi regime?

■ Compromise and concessions to powerful institutions

When Hitler took power in January 1933, there were three main conservative forces in German society which shared his anti-democratic values but were not fully in agreement with Nazi ideology. These were:

■ the army
■ the leaders of big business enterprises
■ the professional **civil service**.

The Nazi 'revolution from below' threatened to destroy Hitler's image of legality and to alienate these conservative forces. The army, in particular, was in a position to remove Hitler from power. Hitler, therefore, had to take care to reassure them that his regime would bring firm government, stability and the maintenance of order.

The army

Hitler's constitutional position in the weeks following his appointment by President Hindenburg was far from secure. He clearly understood that, even after he had gained dictatorial powers, the army was the one institution which could remove him from office. This could be done either by the army leaders appealing to Hindenburg to dismiss Hitler from office, or by the army using force to remove him. Hilter therefore had to take steps to secure the support of the army leaders. On 3 February, just days after taking power, Hitler attended a dinner organised by Hammerstein, the army's commander in chief, at which he outlined to the senior officers present his plans for rearmament. He also took care to reassure the army leaders that, despite pressure from the SA for a Second Revolution, Hitler would not undermine the army's role as the most important institution in the State. In return, the army leaders gave Hitler a free hand in establishing a dictatorship.

■ Key profile

General Kurt von Hammerstein

Hammerstein (1878–1943) had been the army's commander in chief since 1930. A conservative, aristocratic officer, Hammerstein was very close to Schleicher and Hindenburg. He was anti-Nazi and wished to preserve the independence of the army from the new regime.

In 1933 and 1934, as one German institution after another was subjected to the process of *Gleichschaltung*, the army remained immune. Although many younger and more junior officers were committed Nazis, the army high command remained thoroughly conservative and aristocratic, representative of the old Germany.

> The army breathed a sigh of relief. General Blomberg expressed his gratitude and assured Hitler of the complete devotion of the army. He congratulated Hitler on his 'soldierly decision' to deal with 'traitors and murderers'. Army officers uncorked bottles of champagne in the mess to celebrate.

4   *From Evans, R., **The Third Reich in Power**, 2005*

Big business

Hitler had been receiving support from some leading industrialists such as Hugenberg since 1929. After Hitler came to power, both he and business leaders were keen to develop the relationship. On 20 February, Hitler met a group of leading industrialists to ask for financial support for the Nazi election campaign and secured donations of three million Reichmarks. Big business would benefit from a government that was anti-communist but, as with the army, the anti-capitalist rhetoric of the SA and the more radical Nazi leaders worried the businessmen. Hitler, for his part, needed strong businesses to help him to achieve his aims of reviving the economy and rearmament. The price of business support for the Nazis, therefore, was that Hitler had to stop Nazi attacks on large capitalist enterprises. He also appointed Dr Kurt Schmitt, the managing director of Germany's largest insurance company, to replace Hugenberg as economics minister.

Dr Kurt Schmitt

A self made man, Schmitt (1886–1950) had risen to become the director-general of Germany's largest insurance company. He had first become associated with the Nazis in the early 1930s and became a party member in 1933. He also became an officer in the SS. He did not survive long as economics minister, resigning in January 1935 due to ill-health, although he had also become increasingly critical of the regime's spending on rearmament and *Autobahns* (motorways).

Business and industry did not entirely escape the Nazi process of *Gleichschaltung*. In June 1933, employers' associations were coordinated into the Estate of German Industry, while in January 1934, the whole of German business was grouped together in the Reich economic chamber. Individual businesses, however, were left to manage their own affairs with limited state intervention.

The civil service

In the *Kaiserreich* (empire), civil servants enjoyed a status almost on a par with that of soldiers. The higher ranks of the service were recruited almost exclusively from the aristocracy and civil servants closely identified with the authoritarian values of the State. Traditional, conservative-minded, civil servants could not embrace the democratic values of the Weimar Republic and welcomed the appointment of Hitler in 1933. Their support for the new regime was based, however, on a misunderstanding. They believed that the powerful state which would be created by the Nazis would be run by non-political, expert administrators. When Nazi activists at local level began, in March 1933, to take over the running of local and state governments, professional civil servants realised that the Nazi revolution heralded a very different kind of state. Hitler also realised that the 'revolution from below' threatened to place incompetent Nazi activists in charge of local government and undermine his attempts to build an alliance with the conservative forces in German society. He moved to regain control of the situation through the Law for the Re-establishment of a Professional Civil Service of April 1933, which led to a purge of Jews, communists and socialists from the civil service. There was, however, no concerted effort to appoint Nazis to key positions in the civil service. The German Foreign Ministry, for example, continued to be staffed by non-political, aristocratic civil servants and diplomats.

In one sense, this decision to leave the civil service largely untouched by *Gleichschaltung* represents a compromise by Hitler with conservative forces in German society. For the most part, the Nazi Party and the professional civil service remained separate in the new Reich, although career-minded civil servants quickly understood that membership of the Nazi Party would be beneficial to advancing their careers. On the other hand, the 'independence' of the civil service counted for less and less in the Third Reich once the Nazis began creating alternative power structures within the government machine. For example, a leading Nazi, Joachim von Ribbentrop increasingly took control over foreign policy while the Foreign Ministry was reduced to carrying out merely administrative functions.

Revision exercise

Construct a table with three columns, headed 'Conservative forces', 'Reasons for supporting the Nazi regime' and 'Reasons for disliking the Nazi regime'. In the first column, list 'The army', 'Big business' and 'The civil service'. Use this section to help you complete the other two columns.

Key profile

Joachim von Ribbentrop

Although coming from the middle class, Ribbentrop (1893–1946) styled himself as the aristocratic 'von' Ribbentrop by marrying into wealth and persuading a distant relative to give him an aristocratic title. An arrogant, egotistical man, he has been described as a 'self-important busybody'. He spoke several languages and had experience of commercial dealings with foreigners; this prompted him to take a special interest in foreign affairs. In 1933, he created his own Ribbentrop Bureau, with a staff of over 300, to push his own agenda in foreign policy and rival the influence of the Foreign Ministry. He was appointed ambassador to London in 1936 and became foreign minister in 1938.

Conclusion

In 1933, Hitler knew that, in order to successfully consolidate his power, he needed to compromise with powerful conservative forces in German society. His anti-democratic and anti-communist values were shared by the army, businessmen and the civil service. His aim of rearmament offered benefits to both the army and big business. The historian Kershaw has referred to the *'pact of 1933'* in which Hitler, the army leaders and big business agreed to cooperate; an earlier historian, Franz Neumann, has described this pact as a *'power **cartel**'*. Although there was no formal written agreement between Hitler and these conservative forces, it is clear that he needed their support in his efforts to consolidate his power and that the price of this support was that he had to leave these institutions largely untouched by the process of *Gleichschaltung*. He also had to restrain the more radical elements in the Nazi movement from attacking big business and the army, culminating in the Night of the Long Knives in June 1934.

■ Legal power

Hitler was appointed chancellor by Hindenburg in a way that was strictly legal, according to the constitution of the Weimar Republic. That constitution technically remained in force during the period of the Third Reich. The legal basis of the Nazi dictatorship was based on two key instruments:

■ **The Decree for the Protection of the People and the State:** Signed by Hindenburg on 28 February 1933 in the immediate aftermath of the Reichstag fire, this decree suspended important civil and political rights which had been guaranteed under the Weimar constitution. Thus the police were given increased powers to arrest and detain without charge those deemed to be a threat to the security of the State. The police also gained increased powers to enter and search private premises, while the government had the power to censor publications. In practice, these powers were used to arrest communists and socialists, to ban their leaflets and newspapers and to disrupt their organisations. The decree also gave the central government the power to take over state governments if they refused to act against the Nazis' political opponents.

■ **The Law for Removing the Distress of the People and the Reich (Enabling Act):** Passed by the Reichstag on 24 March 1933, this law gave Hitler the power to issue decrees, without the approval of the

■ Key terms

Cartel: an arrangement whereby a group establishes a monopoly position by agreement. It is usually applied to business where large companies work together to fix prices and control the market. Neumann's use of the phrase 'power cartel' refers to the understanding between the Nazis, the army and big business to work together.

■ Activity

Thinking point

'Without the support of traditional conservative forces, Hitler would not have succeeded in establishing his dictatorship in 1933–34'. What is your response to this statement?

Reichstag, for a period of four years. He was also given the power to make treaties with foreign states without the Reichstag's approval. Because this law was a change in the constitution it required a two-thirds majority of the Reichstag in order to be legally enforceable. With the Communist deputies unable to take their seats and the DNVP willing to collaborate with the Nazis in passing the bill, the Centre Party held the key to getting the necessary two-thirds majority. By offering the Centre Party deputies the reassurance that he would not use his powers without first consulting Hindenburg, Hitler won their support. Only the SPD deputies voted against the bill and the Enabling Act duly became law. With full executive and legislative powers, Hitler could rule without needing a Reichstag majority and after 1933 the Reichstag rarely met.

The legal basis of Nazi rule played a crucial role in convincing the civil service and the judiciary that they should cooperate fully with the new regime. It was also important in reassuring the majority of the population that Nazi rule was legitimate.

■ Activity

Discussion point

How 'legal' was Hitler's establishment of a dictatorship in Germany in 1933?

■ Cross-reference

Propaganda will be dealt with in more detail in Section 2.

A profile of Göbbels can be found on page 40.

■ The use of propaganda

Hitler had written in *Mein Kampf* about the crucial role that propaganda would play in the people's community that he aimed to create. On taking power in 1933, he and his propaganda chief Josef Göbbels set about using the resources and legal authority of the regime to extend their control over the media and make their propaganda more effective. On 13 March 1933, Hitler established a new Reich Ministry of Popular Enlightenment and Propaganda with Göbbels in charge.

> I view the first task of the new ministry as being to establish coordination between the government and the whole people. It is not enough for people to be more or less reconciled to our regime, to be persuaded to take a neutral attitude towards us; rather we want to work on people until they have capitulated to us.
>
> The new ministry has no other aim than to unite the nation behind the ideals of the national revolution.

Josef Göbbels, 15 March 1933, quoted in Noakes, J. and Pridham, G., **Nazism 1919–45, Vol. 2,** *1984*

Before coming to power, Nazi propaganda had developed effective techniques for demonising the opposition and for projecting the Nazi Party's own message. In power, Göbbels' new Propaganda Ministry could use the full legal powers of the State to control the media, which in 1933 consisted of radio broadcasting and the press.

Radio broadcasting

> We make no bones about the fact that the radio belongs to us and no one else. And we will place the radio in the service of our ideology. The radio must subordinate itself to the goals which the government of the national revolution has set itself.

Josef Göbbels, 25 March 1933, quoted in Noakes, J. and Pridham, G., **Nazism 1919–45,** *Vol. 2, 1984*

Hitler and Göbbels believed that the spoken word had much more impact than written communication and had used radio broadcasts effectively in the election campaigns of 1932 and 1933. Göbbels described radio as *'the most modern instrument in existence for influencing the masses'*. Already in 1933, some 4.5 million German households possessed a radio and this number would increase dramatically in the next few years. Radio broadcasts gave Hitler the opportunity to talk directly to German people in their own homes and in 1933 alone he made over 50 such broadcasts. In January 1933, however, radio stations in Germany were controlled by state governments, not the central government. Göbbels was determined to change this situation. His first step was to initiate a purge of those working in radio, as a result of which some 13% of staff were dismissed on racial or political grounds. Establishing central government control over radio stations took longer, however, mainly because Göbbels encountered resistance from Göring who, as Prussian minister of the interior, tried to keep control in the hands of state governments. It was not until April 1934 that all radio stations in Germany were brought together under the umbrella of the Reich Radio Company which was under the control of the Propaganda Ministry.

The press

> The press is not only there to inform but must also instruct. You will also recognise that it is an ideal situation for the press to be a tremendously important instrument for influencing the masses.

7 *Josef Göbbels, 15th March 1933, quoted in Noakes, J. and Pridham, G.,* **Nazism 1919–45, Vol. 2***, 1984*

Establishing control over the press proved more difficult for Göbbels since in January 1933 there were some 4,700 privately owned newspapers in Germany. These were mainly local and regional newspapers which reflected a wide variety of political opinions and religious allegiances. There were relatively few national newspapers. There were Nazi newspapers, particularly the *Volkischer Beobachter*, but the combined circulation of all Nazi-leaning papers amounted to no more than 2.5% of total newspaper sales. Göbbels, therefore, adopted a step-by-step strategy towards establishing control over the press:

1 Socialist and communist newspapers were closed using the powers of the Decree for the Protection of the People and State.

2 The Nazis began to buy up more newspapers; by the end of the year they had acquired 27 daily newspapers with a combined circulation of 2.4 million per day.

3 News agencies which supplied the press with information were all merged into a State-controlled organisation. Information had already been censored, therefore, before reaching the press.

4 Göbbels introduced a daily briefing for journalists at which he gave instructions on what they could and could not print.

5 An Editors' Law of October 1933 gave the responsibility for a newspaper's content to its editor alone. Editors had to follow the instructions of the Propaganda Ministry or they personally would have to take the consequences. In this way, editors became censors of their own newspapers.

Exploring the detail

The *Völkischer Beobachter*

This was the Nazis' own newspaper which the party had bought in 1921 with money supplied by wealthy patrons and the army. Originally a weekly newspaper edited by Dietrich Eckart, the newspaper became a daily in 1923 with Alfred Rosenberg as editor. The *Völkischer Beobachter* was suppressed after the failed Beer Hall Putsch of 1923 but was restarted in 1925. The English translation of the name is the 'Racial Observer'.

■ The use of policies to consolidate power

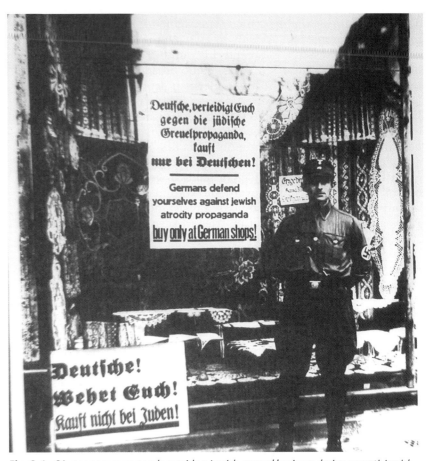

Fig. 6 *An SA stormtrooper stands outside a Jewish-owned business during an anti-Jewish boycott. The notice on the left reads 'Germans! Defend yourselves, do not buy from Jews'*

During the years 1930 to 1933, when the Nazi Party was competing for power with other political parties, the party built a broad base of support among people from different social classes. Through carefully targeted propaganda, the Nazis attracted support from key groups such as independent shopkeepers, artisans, white-collar workers and farmers. Recent studies have also revealed that the Nazis enjoyed some success in attracting working-class voters, particularly among those made unemployed by the depression. Nazi economic policies played an important role in attracting this wide range of support. The Nazis said that the economy should serve the needs of the State rather than individuals. They promised public investment in industry to boost employment, measures to protect those in debt, controls on prices to protect farmers and controls on imports to protect German industry against foreign competition.

Once in power the Nazi regime began taking steps, through legislation, to implement these economic policies and thereby consolidate support for the regime. The results were very mixed.

The Law for the Protection of the Retail Trade, May 1933

This law banned any further extension of large department stores. A series of decrees in July 1933 extended this policy by banning department stores from offering a range of services which included baking,

■ **Activity**

Revision exercise

Construct a table with three columns headed 'Policy', 'Target group' and 'Effectiveness'. Put the three laws outlined on pages 34–36 into the first column. Complete the other two columns using the information in this section.

hairdressing and shoe-repairing. The aim of these regulations was to protect the small shopkeepers from competition from the larger stores which, in Nazi eyes, were Jewish-owned.

A Nazi organisation for small shopkeepers and artisans, the Combat League of Middle-class Tradespeople, began to organise boycotts of department stores and began to try to take control over chambers of industry and commerce. Such actions appealed to the more radical elements within the Nazi Party, particularly in the SA; however, disruptions to business at a time of depression threatened to put thousands more employees out of work and also alienated the banks which had made big loans to the department stores. The regime therefore moved to control the activities of the Combat League and tried to stop attacks on department stores. Indeed, when the large retail firm of Tietz, which was Jewish-owned, ran into difficulties, the regime came to its aid with a large loan.

The Law to Reduce Unemployment, June 1933

Through this law, the Nazi regime began schemes of public works to provide work for the unemployed. The law also provided subsidies for private construction projects and offered tax rebates and loans to companies to encourage them to increase production. The law insisted that all projects should be carried out with manual labour, in order to maximise employment. It also included a scheme to persuade women to leave their jobs once they married, in order to give male workers priority in the labour market. Also, in June 1933, the regime began the construction of a network of Autobahns, although these were designed more for their propaganda impact than for their actual effect on the level of unemployment.

Cross-reference

For information about the creation of the Autobahns, see page 60.

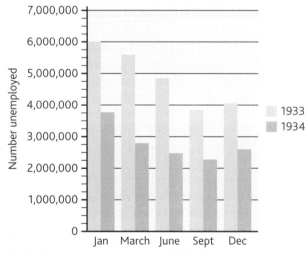

Fig. 7 *Unemployment in Germany, 1933–34*

Unemployment was already beginning to fall when the Nazis took power at the end of January 1933. The early job creation schemes of the Nazi regime appear to have made little difference to the rate of decline in the unemployment figures in the months immediately after June 1933. Once rearmament began to take effect in 1934, however, unemployment began to decline more rapidly.

The Reich Entailed Farm Law, September 1933

Under this law, all farms of between 7.5 and 125 hectares in size, were declared to be hereditary estates which were **entailed**, and therefore could not be sold or closed due to indebtedness on the part of the farmer. It

Key terms

Entailed: subject to a legal limitation which prevents future heirs from selling or dividing the property.

was also decreed that only 'Aryan German citizens' were allowed to own farms. Designed to be a measure to protect small peasant farmers from being forced to leave the land, this law actually deprived farmers of the freedom to sell or mortgage their properties. Small farmers subsequently found increasing difficulty in getting loans from banks which they needed when they wished to improve their farms.

There were also measures by the Nazi regime in 1933 to protect farmers against competition and control the market in food. Hugenberg, the Agriculture Minister, increased tariffs on imported food in February 1933. After he was replaced by the Nazi, Richard Darré, in the summer of 1933, a Reich Food Estate was established to control the distribution of agricultural produce. These early moves to protect German farmers and control the market pleased neither farmers nor consumers. Import controls led to price increases of commodities such as butter and margarine, while controls on the distribution of food actually resulted in lower prices being paid to the farmers.

■ **Key profile**

Richard Walther Darré

Darré (1895–1953) had risen to prominence as a leading Nazi ideologist. He was a firm believer in the 'blood and soil' racial theories of the Nazis and had established his own racial bureau in 1932. He was also thoroughly anti-Christian in his religious beliefs, arguing that medieval Germans had been weakened by their conversion from paganism to Christianity. As well as being minister of agriculture, he was also Reich peasant leader.

■ **Exploring the detail**

Sopade report

'Sopade' stands for the 'German Social Democratic Party (SPD) in exile'. Although some of the leaders of the party escaped into exile, initially to Prague, after the Nazi purge in 1933, many SPD members remained behind in Germany working undercover. These SPD agents sent regular reports on the state of public opinion in Germany to the leadership in exile.

Nazi policies towards agriculture had mixed results in terms of consolidating support for the regime. Many of their policies were highly unpopular and resulted in growing hostility towards the regime. A Sopade report on the mood among farmers in north-west Germany in the summer of 1934 reported that *'The medium-sized and big peasants of Oldenburg and West Friesland, who were once enthusiastic Nazis, are now virtually unanimous in rejecting the Nazis and in reaffirming their old Conservative traditions.'*

Learning outcomes

In this section, you have looked at the factors which enabled Hitler to consolidate power in the months after he was appointed chancellor in January 1933. In power, Hitler continued to rely, as he had done when he was attempting to become chancellor, on the old elite in the army, civil service and political system to help him consolidate his position. Propaganda also played a key role, as did the Nazi's willingness to use terror and repression to silence their opponents. This section has also given an introduction to Nazi ideology. After reading this section, you should be able to assess which factors were most important in helping the Nazis to consolidate power and to make links between the various factors.

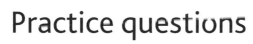

Practice questions

Read the following source material and answer the questions which follow.

The Nazi 'revolution' was hardly the peaceful, orderly affair that many claimed at the time. Violence was one of the key factors in turning the 'backstairs intrigue' which brought Hitler to power into one of the most brutal dictatorships the world has ever seen. While it was the machinations of the men of power and influence which put Hitler into the saddle in Berlin, it was the actions of the Nazi stormtroopers in cities and towns throughout the country which helped smash opposition to the 'new Germany'.

A *Adapted from Bessel, R., 'Political Violence and the Nazi Seizure of Power',* **History Today,** *1985*

In the spring and summer of 1933 Hitler established the apparatus of party dictatorship in Germany. Strengthened by the Enabling Act, he concentrated all power in the hands of the government, dissolved the trade unions and abolished all political parties except the Nazis. However, Germany had not yet become the brutal tyranny which was to appal the conscience of mankind within a very few years. Admittedly much violence had already occurred; thousands were put into hastily constructed concentration camps; discrimination against the Jews had begun; and police and courts were virtually powerless to deal with acts of lawlessness by gangs of SA men. But this was largely the work of over-enthusiastic or unscrupulous supporters at local level; at this stage terror and brutality had not been systematised into an instrument of government.

B *Adapted from Carr, W.,* **A History of Germany,** *1991*

Every one will know in future that if he lifts his hand against the State certain death is his fate, and every National Socialist will know that no rank and no position allows him to escape punishment.

If anyone reproaches me and asks why I did not resort to the regular courts of justice for conviction of the offenders, then all I can say to him is this; in this hour I was responsible for the fate of the German people, and thereby became the Supreme Judge of the German people. I gave the order to shoot those parties mainly responsible for this treason.

C *From Hitler's speech to the Reichstag, 13 July 1934, in which he justified the Night of the Long Knives, quoted in Evans, R.,* **The Third Reich in Power,** *2005*

(a) Use Sources A and B and your own knowledge. Explain how far the views in Source B differ from those in Source A in relation to the Nazis' use of violence to consolidate their power in the period January 1933 to July 1934.

(12 marks)

Study tip When answering this question it is important to remember that both sources have to be used and explicitly referred to. The question asks 'how far' the views in the sources differ. This requires you to identify both points of agreement and of disagreement. It is a good idea to make a simple table with two columns for agreement and disagreement and make notes from each source under these headings. There are clear differences between the sources on the role played by the Nazis' use of violence in consolidating their power. Source A identifies violence as being a key factor in turning the Nazi regime into a brutal dictatorship, especially in relation to smashing the opposition. Source B, on the other hand, highlights the role of the Enabling Act (i.e. legal power) in the consolidation process. There are also, however, similarities between the sources, and you will need to address these in order to answer the question 'how far?' Note that Source A states that violence was 'one of the key factors', so not necessarily the only one, while Source B also identifies violence as one of the methods used by the Nazis. The question also asks you to use your own knowledge. This does not have to be extensive, nor should it dominate your answer which must be mainly about the sources. Do try, however, to place the sources in their historical context – in this case, the process of the consolidation of power between January 1933 and July 1934.

(b) Use Sources A, B and C and your own knowledge. How successful was Hitler in keeping control over the SA in the period January 1933 to July 1934?

(24 marks)

Study tip This question requires you to use all three sources and your own knowledge. The omission of one or other of these elements in your answer will place a limit on the marks you can achieve. Source A refers to SA violence and implies that this was directed by Hitler and the Nazi leadership. Source B specifically states that SA violence was the result of over-enthusiastic actions by the SA at local level, thereby implying that Hitler was not controlling their actions. Source C, on the other hand, is taken from Hitler's own speech to the Reichstag after the purge of the SA in the Night of the Long Knives. This, therefore, shows that Hitler had not been fully in control of the SA before June 1933 but that, having purged Röhm and the SA leadership he was now firmly in control. These sources need to be placed in context which is where you should use your own knowledge. You could, for example, point out that the Nazi leadership had been prepared to allow the SA considerable freedom to use violence and intimidation against opponents in the period from January to June 1933, when political power had been concentrated in Nazi hands, but that from June 1933 until June 1934 the SA had become a potential threat to the Nazi regime. The examiner will be looking for a balanced answer in which you put forward two sides of an argument which leads to a conclusion in which you offer your own judgment on the degree of success.

Göbbels and the organisation of propaganda

As an experienced and proven master of the arts of propaganda, Göbbels was the automatic choice to head the new Ministry of Public Enlightenment and Propaganda in 1933. He also kept his post as the Nazi Party propaganda chief. Under the auspices of his new ministry, he was president of a Reich chamber of culture which oversaw the work of seven subsidiary chambers covering the work of the press, radio, film, literature, theatre, music and fine arts. He thus created a vast bureaucratic empire which gave him enormous power over the cultural life of the nation. All professionals working in each of the seven fields of culture were compelled to belong to their relevant chamber, giving Göbbels the power to control who could and could not be employed. Those deemed to be 'racially impure' or 'politically unreliable' were purged; those remaining in work quickly came to realise that any criticism of the regime would lead to the loss of their livelihoods.

As in other areas of the Nazi regime, however, there were overlapping organisations and jurisdictions and Göbbels' control over propaganda was never total. Ministers in other departments fought to retain control over propaganda within their own particular jurisdiction. There was also a party organisation, the Combat League for German Culture, led by Alfred Rosenberg, which competed for control over cultural policy. With a power-base in both the Reich government and in the party, however, Göbbels was the regime's chief propagandist although he could not take Hitler's support for granted.

Exploring the detail

The Combat League for German Culture

This was one of many specialist organisations within the Nazi Party which was set up in the 1920s. Its aim was to 'purify' German culture of alien and modernist 'contamination'. The Combat League was small but very active, being responsible for assaults on Jewish musicians, writers, and so on.

Methods of propaganda

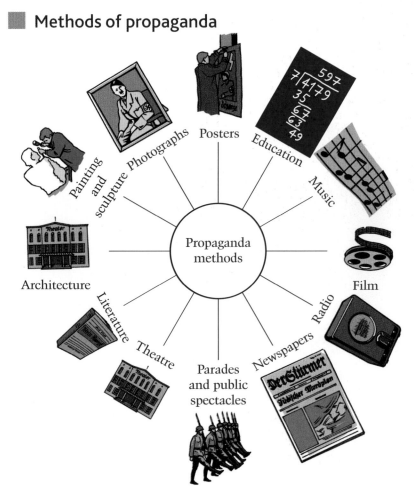

Fig. 3 *Methods used by Göbbels to spread Nazi propaganda*

The Horst Wessel song

Horst Wessel was a local SA commander in Berlin who was killed by communists in 1930 and thus became a martyr to the Nazi movement. In 1929, Wessel had composed a song which became one of the most popular marching songs for the SA after his death. The following verses are an extract from this song:

'The Flag is high! The ranks tightly closed!
SA marches with a brave firm pace.
Comrades whom Red Front and Reaction shot dead
March in spirit within our ranks.
Make the street free for the brown battalions;
Make the street free for the SA man!
Already millions are looking to the swastika, full of hope;
The day of freedom and bread is dawning.'

The use of parades and public spectacle

Propaganda marches by uniformed SA and SS units are a very effective method of propaganda when the number of participants, their organisation and appearance are in order. Bands and music increase the effectiveness of such marches.

 4

From a Nazi Party pamphlet, 1927, quoted in the German Propaganda Archive

Marches and parades had been a feature of Nazi Party activity since its formation. During the 1920s and early 1930s, military-style parades were used by the party to raise its profile, to intimidate opponents and to create the impression of a large, well-supported and disciplined organisation. In 1930, a Nazi Party pamphlet, *Modern Political Propaganda,* stated that *'good discipline is the best propaganda'* and this discipline was best displayed in marches and parades. In this way, the Nazis were able to convey the impression that they were a force for order and discipline in a society that was degenerating into chaos. The theatricality of these marches, and therefore their effect on passive onlookers, was heightened by the wearing of uniforms and medals, the carrying of banners and the choreographed singing of party songs. The carrying of lighted torches in night-time processions was particularly effective in capturing people's attention.

After taking power the Nazis lost no time in demonstrating their command of the streets by holding large processions. On the night of 30 January 1933, Hitler stood on the balcony of the Reich Chancellery to take the salute from 100,000 SA and SS men marching past in a torchlight procession, an event which symbolised the Nazi's power and the start of their 'national revolution'. Such events could also now be used to convey the impression that the nation was united behind

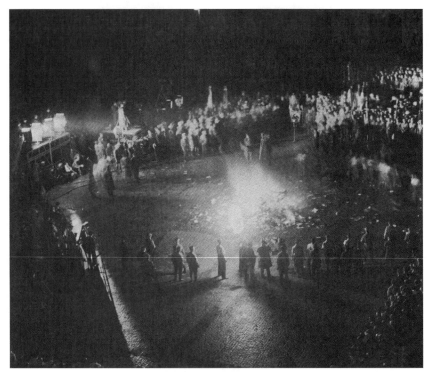

Fig. 4 *Nazi students burn books in Berlin, May 1933*

the new regime. Spectators were obliged to salute the flags of the SA and SS units as they marched past. On national holidays, when parades were held in towns and cities across Germany, householders were expected to show support by hanging out swastika flags from their windows. Compliance was monitored by Nazi Party 'block leaders' and failure to conform would be reported to the authorities; to be labelled 'politically unreliable' in this way could lead to a person being dismissed from his or her job or possibly more serious consequences. As Göbbels had said, '*On 30 January 1933, the era of individualism finally died. The individual will be replaced by the community of the people.*' Ritual parades and flag waving were the visual 'proof' that the German people were solidly behind the regime, even though this support was being manipulated by Göbbels and his Propaganda Ministry. '*All that goes on behind the backcloth*' said Göbbels, '*belongs to stage management.*'

As ritual was so important to the Nazis, the regime introduced twelve new national festivals, celebrating key dates in the Party's history and elements of its ideology.

Table 1 *Key celebration dates in the Nazi calendar*

30 January	Day of the seizing of power
24 February	Anniversary of the founding of the party
March (1st Sunday)	Day of the commemoration of heroes
20 April	Hitler's birthday
1 May	National day of labour
May (2nd Sunday)	Mother's day
21 June	Summer solstice
July (2nd Sunday)	Day of German culture
September	Nuremberg rally for Nazi Party
October	Harvest thanksgiving
9 November	Remembrance of Munich Putsch
21 December	Yuletide

These festivals were occasions for parades and rallies to be held across Germany. On Hitler's birthday, for example, elaborate initiation rites were performed to receive new entrants into the Nazi Party. Photographs of Hitler were displayed in shop windows and bunting and swastika flags decorated the streets.

> In the streets after January 1933 suddenly in every shop there were little swastika flags and pictures of Hitler. I heard that Hitler was at the Hotel Rosa. I was curious. I got there just at the end of Hitler's speech, so I didn't really hear him speak. There was a huge crowd singing the Deutschland anthem and the Horst Wessel song. Until then I had always laughed at the Hitler salute, but when they sang the Horst Wessel song, I suddenly realised I was raising my arm. Much later I thought that's what they call mass suggestion. In my youthful innocence I thought that if all these people were so enthralled and enthusiastic about it, then there must be something in it. So I tried to do something myself for this new movement.

5 *Liselotte Katscher recalls her conversion to Nazism; quoted in Haste, C., **Nazi Women**, 2001*

Exploring the detail

The Nuremberg rallies

The annual Party rallies at Nuremberg in September were stage-managed to achieve maximum theatrical effect. Vast numbers of Party members attended; the 1937 rally involved some 100,000 people. Floodlights shining into the sky at night created the effect of a vast 'cathedral of light', under which large columns of disciplined and well-drilled members raised their flags in salute. Stirring music accompanied the marching columns. Finally Hitler delivered a speech, at the end of which the Nazi members on parade raised their arms and gave the Hitler salute. Films made of these rallies were shown in cinemas across Germany so that even non-participants could be over-awed by the experience.

■ **Activity**

Source analysis

Read Sources 4, 5 and 6 and the main text in this section.

1 How did the Nazis use parades and spectacles to generate support for their regime?

2 What can we learn from Source 6 about the effectiveness of Nazi parades?

■ **Cross-reference**

Nazi efforts to control newspapers and radio in the early months of the regime have been dealt with in Chapter 2, pages 32–33.

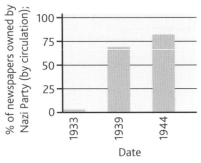

Fig. 5 *Nazi ownership of newspapers in Germany, 1933–44*

The rallies expressed power, order, solemnity. Hitler, the theatre fanatic, assisted by the mass orator Josef Goebbels [Göbbels] and the architect Albert Speer, who built the settings for these spectacles – created his ultimate stage productions. The mass became part of the set in a gigantic happening, a communal celebration that eliminated the brain and led to ecstasy. The timing of pauses and the stage management of climaxes were as important as the music and the banners.

 6   *From Adam, P.,* **The Arts of the Third Reich**, *1992*

Newspapers and radio

Newspapers

Göbbels had moved quickly during 1933, when the Nazi Party was consolidating its power, to establish control over the press. During the years 1933 to 1939, this control was extended and deepened by a variety of means:

■ The Reich press chamber was established and all those involved in the publishing of newspapers, including the owners, the editors and the journalists, had to be members of this body.

■ Applications for membership were vetted for 'racial and political reliability'. By 1935, 1,300 Jewish and Marxist journalists had been dismissed from their jobs.

■ The State-controlled news agency, the *Deutsches Nachrichtenbüro* (DNB), held daily press conferences and issued detailed directives on what newspapers could and could not print. Often the DNB provided newspapers with complete articles which they were obliged to print verbatim. By the late 1930s, about half of the content of daily newspapers was provided by the DNB.

■ The regime used its control over official advertising and over printing contracts to put pressure on the independent press to fall into line.

Control over newspapers by Göbbels' Propaganda Ministry was gradually tightened between 1933 and 1939. Socialist and communist publishing houses were closed down. The Nazi Party increased its direct ownership of newspapers while those which remained in private hands were obliged to comply with government directives. The result was that newspapers became bland, conformist and boring and the circulation figures of many newspapers declined.

■ **A closer look**

The *Frankfurter Zeitung*

The *Frankfurter Zeitung* was a long established, liberal-leaning newspaper which had acquired an international reputation for fair and objective reporting. Although it had a relatively small circulation, its readership included many among the well-educated political and professional elite in the Weimar period. Until the early 1930s, the newspaper took a firm anti-Nazi line. In 1932, however, the *Franfurter Zeitung* was taken over by the giant chemical company I.G. Farben and the editorial line began to be more sympathetic to the Nazis. Even though the newspaper supported the suppression of the Communist Party after January 1933, its offices were invaded by stormtroopers on 11 March 1933 and it was threatened with closure if it did not toe the

Nazi Party line. Editorial staff were forced to resign and Jews were dismissed.

Carl Bosch, the owner of I.G. Farben, was an old conservative who was sympathetic to the Nazis but not a member. He did not want to see the newspaper's traditional independence abandoned and the *Frankfurter Zeitung* continued to voice some criticism of the regime. The editor also occasionally refused to print stories which the Propaganda Ministry ordered him to carry. A Gestapo report stated that the newspaper contained articles that *'must be described as malicious agitation'*. In the early years of the regime, Hitler and Göbbels were careful not to alienate traditional conservative and international opinion and therefore tolerated this defiance while gradually increasing the pressure. A key turning point came in 1938 when I.G. Farben secretly sold the *Frankfurter Zeitung* to the Nazis' own publishing house. The circulation of the newspaper then declined to such an extent that it was forced to close in 1943.

Activity

Thinking point

Using all the evidence in this section, assess the effectiveness of Nazi efforts to control the German press in the years 1933–39.

Radio

> I consider radio to be the most modern and crucial instrument that exists for influencing the masses. I also believe that radio will in the end replace the press.
>
> **7** *Josef Göbbels, 25 March 1933, quoted in Noakes, J. and Pridham, G., **Nazism 1919–45, Vol. 2**, 1984*

Because radio enabled him to speak to people directly, in their own homes, Hitler regarded radio as one of the most powerful propaganda instruments at his disposal. This was a view shared by Göbbels and he moved quickly to establish control over the airwaves. He also took steps to make radios more widely available. In a deal with industrialists he promoted the mass production and sale of cheap radio sets. The first model, called the '30th January' went on sale in 1933 for 78 Reichsmarks. In 1938, a cheaper version, the 'people's receiver', costing 35 RM, was made available. As a result of this policy by 1939, 70% of German households possessed a radio set, the highest proportion anywhere in the world.

Political propaganda was given a high priority in Göbbels' directions to radio stations concerning their programming. In 1933, 50 speeches by Hitler were broadcast over the radio. In plays and talk shows, emphasis had to be placed on the themes of race, blood and the *Volksgemeinschaft*. Nevertheless, Göbbels was shrewd enough to realise that an overwhelming concentration on political propaganda, at the expense of entertainment, would alienate the majority of listeners. He therefore refused requests from leading Nazis other than Hitler to speak on the radio and he instructed radio stations to concentrate on music and light entertainment.

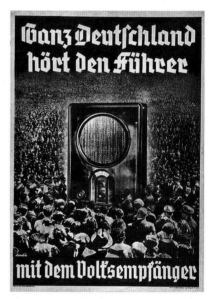

Fig. 6 *A propaganda poster enouraging people to listen to the Führer on the radio. The slogan reads 'The whole of Germany listens to the Führer on the People's Receiver'*

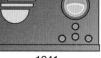

| 1933 | 1941 |
| 4.5 million | 15 million |

Fig. 7 *Radio sets in private ownership in Germany, 1933–41*

Exploring the detail

Communal radio listening

Göbbels also encouraged the spread of communal radio listening in factories, offices, cafes, shops and in town squares. The owners of workplaces, restaurants and pubs were ordered to install loudspeakers. German towns began to install loudspeaker columns in public spaces in 1938. When Hitler's speeches were being broadcast, sirens would sound as a signal to stop work and gather around the radio or loudspeaker. The regime inculcated the notion that citizens were under a political responsibility to listen to the radio regularly and local 'radio wardens' were recruited to monitor compliance.

Activity

Thinking point

1 Using all the information in this section, explain why the Nazis considered the radio to be such an important medium for spreading propaganda.

2 How did Göbbels show his skill as a propagandist in his use of the radio?

At all costs avoid being boring. You must help to bring forth a nationalist art and culture which is truly appropriate to the pace of modern life and to the mood of the times. You must use your imagination, an imagination which is based on sure foundations and which employs all means and methods to bring to the ears of the masses the new attitude, in a way which is modern, up-to-date, interesting and appealing.

8   *Göbbels' instructions to radio stations, quoted in Noakes, J. and Pridham, G.,* **Nazism 1919–45, Vol. 2,** *1984*

Popular culture

Of all modern regimes, that of the Third Reich defined itself most clearly by its art and mass culture.

9   *From Evans, R.,* **The Third Reich in Power,** *2005*

The Nazis believed that the modern culture of the Weimar period symbolised Germany's moral bankruptcy and its weakened position in the post-war world. The struggle against artistic 'degeneracy' went hand in hand with the Nazis' political struggle against democracy and communism. Artistic individualism was, for Hitler and Göbbels, the enemy of the official, mass Volkisch culture which they wished to establish in Germany. For Hitler, the arts were an expression of race. He believed that only the Aryan was capable of producing true art and that the 'degenerate art' of the Weimar period was evidence of racial decline. Nazi policy was to promote arts which glorified the healthy, the strong and the heroic, particularly heroes from Germany's past, whether real or mythical.

Music

The Weimar period was a time of experimentation and diversity in German music, both popular and classical. Foreign influences, such as American jazz music, were popular among young Germans in the 1920s. The Nazis, however, denounced foreign imports, especially jazz with its roots in black American culture. They disapproved also of modern, avant-garde experimental music such as the compositions of Schoenberg, but of all the arts music was the one which the Nazis found most difficulty in trying to control. A Reich music chamber was established by the Propaganda Ministry, with the leading German composer, Richard Strauss, as its president. The task of this chamber was to control musical production and to promote the kind of music of which the Nazis did approve. Under its direction, experimental music and jazz were banned from being performed, published or played on the radio. Works by the 19th-century German Jewish composer, Felix Mendelsohn, were also banned. The Nazis commissioned composers to write Volkisch operas which would arouse patriotic and nationalist feeling through the depiction of German heroes from the past. For example, Gottfried Müller's *Requiem for German Heroes,* first performed in 1934, honoured Germany's war dead.

■ Key profile

Richard Strauss

Strauss (1864–1949) was one of Germany's leading composers of the late 19th and early 20th centuries, noted for his operas and orchestral works. Although he accepted the post of president of the Reich music chamber, he tried to keep out of politics and was never himself a Nazi. Indeed, he was removed from the presidency in 1935 after he gave his support to a Jewish friend and fellow musician. He composed the official Olympic hymn for the Berlin Olympics of 1936.

The Nazis showed a consistent hostility to American popular music, especially jazz, but they had no clear policy on the kind of music they wished to promote. Hitler himself was an avid fan of the operas of Richard Wagner, based as they were on mythical tales of Germany's heroic past, but his enthusiasm was not shared by other leading Nazis. The performance of classical music by 18th and 19th century German composers such as Beethoven, Brahms and Bruckner was encouraged but Göbbels understood that the mass of the German people preferred popular styles of music. There was a long tradition in Germany of playing and singing music within the home; this form of musical expression was difficult, if not impossible, for the regime to control.

The cinema

Göbbels was a keen fan of cinema and recognised the potential of film as a propaganda medium. He understood that film could work on the subconscious, delivering subliminal messages and reinforcing prejudices. He also, however, saw film as a form of escapism, an opportunity to remove the film-goer, if only temporarily, from the pressures and strains of everyday life and make them more accepting of their lot. He therefore disapproved of blatantly political films which were too serious and risked boring the audience.

There were four major, privately owned film companies in Germany in 1933. These were allowed to continue in private ownership but the Propaganda Ministry gradually bought shares in these companies and increasingly became the main financial sponsor of new films; this indirect ownership of film making was made more direct in 1942 when the film companies were nationalised.

A Reich film chamber was established in July 1933 to regulate the content of films and employment within the industry. Göbbels, however, made himself personally responsible for approving every film made in Germany after 1933. Foreign films were not banned outright but were carefully checked by the ministry for political and racial content. Most American films were banned, although the popularity of Disney cartoons meant that many of these were still approved.

Between 1933 and 1945, over 1,000 feature films were produced in Germany and cinema attendances increased fourfold in the years 1933 to 1944. Of these films, only 14% had an overtly political theme. The most common types of films were historical dramas, comedies and musicals. All films, to some degree, contained political messages. Leadership was glorified, 'Blood and soil' (the close relationship of race and land) was a common theme, as was the demonising of Jews and communists. Films with a pacifist message were banned outright. Newsreels were more overtly political and often portrayed events which had been especially

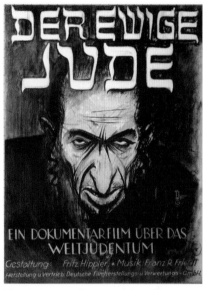

Fig. 8 *A poster for an anti-Semitic propaganda film from 1940 entitled 'The Eternal Jew'*

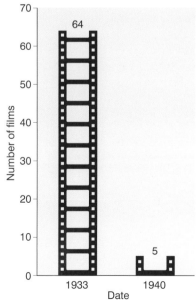

Fig. 9 *American films shown in German cinemas, 1933–40*

Cross-reference

A profile of Leni Riefenstahl can be found on page 60.

Activity

Thinking point

Explain why the Nazis considered film to be a particularly effective medium for propaganda.

staged for the camera. The planned invasion of Britain in the summer of 1940 was filmed in advance using actors and portrayed the surrender of British forces to the conquering German invaders, although needless to say this newsreel was never actually shown.

■ A closer look

The Triumph of the Will

The Triumph of the Will was a documentary film, made by the actress and film director Leni Riefenstahl, about the 1934 Nuremberg Rally. It was an explicitly propagandist film which set out to show the world the power, strength and determination of the German people under Hitler's leadership. Using skilful direction and camera work, Riefenstahl portrayed the Nuremberg rally as a monumental event in which a vast mass of disciplined Nazi SA and SS men moved in perfect coordination under Hitler's direction. The film was also a celebration of militarism, physical strength and struggle. Hitler was portrayed as a lone figure – for example, when he descended through the clouds in an aeroplane on his approach to Nuremberg – as the Führer who stands out from the mass and receives their adulation. *The Triumph of the Will* thus celebrated Hitler's will to lead the German people to regeneration and victory.

The film was actually made in the face of opposition from Göbbels who considered it to be too serious and too blatantly propagandist. Riefenstahl received her commission directly from Hitler, who ordered that she be provided with all the resources she needed.

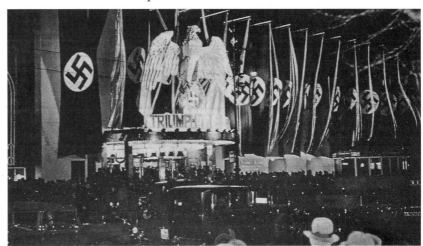

Fig. 10 *Crowds gather for the ceremonial opening of the film* The Triumph of the Will

The manipulation of education

The chief purpose of the school is to train human beings that the State is more important than the individual, that individuals must be willing and ready to sacrifice themselves for Nation and Führer.

 From a manual for teachers issued by Bernhard Rust, Education Minister, quoted in **Grunberger, R., A Social History of the Third Reich**, *1974*

Education was the primary means by which the Nazi regime could indoctrinate the nation's youth. In the Third Reich, all school textbooks had to be vetted for ideological correctness by the Education Ministry and new textbooks were produced. The National Socialist Teachers' League had been founded in 1927. After January 1933, there was a rapid increase in membership of the league as teachers tried to protect their career prospects by joining. Although membership was not compulsory, by 1936 around 97% of all schoolteachers were members. The league was responsible for the political indoctrination of teachers, a task which it achieved by sending teachers on political education courses. Teachers came under increasing pressure to conform and act as the regime's mouthpieces; those who voiced any criticism could find themselves reported to the *Gestapo* (the secret State police) by their pupils, the parents or by other members of staff. Teachers, as State employees, were also covered by the Law for the Re-establishment of a Professional Civil Service of April 1933 under which many Jewish teachers and those who were 'politically unreliable' were dismissed from their posts. Step by step, schools were pressured into promoting the ideology of the National Socialist State.

Cross-reference

For information about the Gestapo, see page 94.

> A picture of Adolf Hitler is hanging on the wall in almost every classroom. Teachers and pupils greet each other at the beginning and end of every lesson with the German greeting. The pupils listen to major political speeches on the radio in the school hall.

11   *Report from a German headmaster, 1934, quoted in Evans, R.,* ***The Third Reich in Power***, *2005*

Political indoctrination permeated every area of the curriculum:

- The Nazis' aim to promote 'racial health' led to an increasing emphasis on physical education. Military style drill became a feature of P.E. lessons.

- In German lessons, the aim was to inculcate a 'consciousness of being German' through the study of Nordic sagas and other traditional stories.

- Essay writing involved the regurgitation of propaganda handouts on themes such as 'The Reich Labour Service' or 'The Jews are our misfortune'.

- In biology, there was a stress on race and heredity. Pupils were taught to measure the size of their skulls and classify each other's racial types. There was also a strong emphasis on evolution and the survival of the fittest.

- Geography was used to develop awareness of the concepts of Lebensraum, 'blood and soil' and German racial superiority. Atlases implicitly supported the concept of 'one people, one Reich'.

- In mathematics, problems were set on the trajectories of artillery shells, or pupils were asked to calculate the relative costs of treating the mentally ill versus the cost of building workers' housing.

- Girls were obliged to study needlework and homecraft to prepare them for their role as homemakers.

- Sex education was banned. The emphasis in moral messages was that individuals had a duty to have as many children as possible.

Exploring the detail

Using mathematics lessons for political indoctrination

A mathematics problem from a textbook in the 1930s read: *'The proportion of Nordic blood in the German population is estimated as four fifths of the population. A third of these can be regarded as blond. According to these estimates, how many blond people must there be in the German population of 66 million?'*

Activity

Discussion point

'History lessons were the most effective means by which the Nazi regime was able to indoctrinate school pupils in Germany'. Explain why you agree or disagree with this view.

The purpose of history was to teach people that life was always dominated by struggle, that race and blood were central to everything that happened in the past, present and future, and that leadership determined the fate of peoples. Central themes in the new teaching included courage in battle, sacrifice for a greater cause, boundless admiration for the leader and hatred of Germany's enemies, the Jews.

*From Evans, R., **The Third Reich in Power**, 2005*

Key terms

Cultural autarky: a policy of attempting to isolate Germany from foreign and 'alien' influences in German culture. The Nazis' aim in cultural policy was to promote their own narrow view of what constituted a truly German culture. They set out to ban foreign and 'alien' influences such as jazz music from America and modern art which they associated with Jewish intellectuals.

Censorship

The totalitarian ideology of the Nazis did not permit the expression of any alternative viewpoints or any criticism of the regime. Free expression in any form was seen as a threat to the unity and coordination in the 'people's community' which the Nazis were attempting to build. They also aimed to impose a form of '**cultural autarky**' in which the German people would be sheltered from outside influences and in which only the Nazis' version of reality would be heard. Censorship was an essential tool for the Nazis in achieving these aims.

Censorship of the media and the arts was achieved in a variety of different ways:

- Outright bans were placed on the communist and socialist parties, preventing them from publishing any newspapers, books, pamphlets or posters.

- There was a purge of communists, socialists and Jews from their employment in the media and the arts.

- Göbbels' Propaganda Ministry issued detailed instructions to newspapers and the radio about what could and could not be reported.

- Newspaper editors were given responsibility for what their newspapers reported. With the threat of legal penalties hanging over them if they refused to toe the line, editors practised self-censorship.

- The Propaganda Ministry drew up a list of 'damaging and undesirable literature', and the police were given powers to seize books that *'tended to endanger public security and order'*.

- Film censorship was taken over by the Propaganda Ministry, which had the right to view scripts even before films could be made.

Göbbels' Propaganda Ministry, with its vast and growing bureaucracy, was at the hub of the system of censorship. In common with other aspects of the Nazi regime, however, there were many other State and Party organisations which had overlapping responsibilities in the field of censorship. These included:

- the Criminal Police, the SD intelligence agency and the Gestapo, which all had the power to search bookshops and libraries and confiscate banned publications
- the Interior Ministry and the justice system
- local authorities

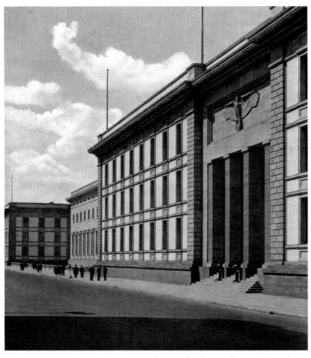

Fig. 11 *Nazi architecture, as in the Reich Chancellery pictured here, was monumental in scale, designed to show the power and permanence of the regime and the insignificance of the individual. The buildings were designed to make a propaganda statement*

Cross-reference

For more about the Nazi police system, see pages 93–94.

- the Supreme Censorship Authority for Dirty and Trashy Literature, based in Leipzig and separate from the Propaganda Ministry
- the Combat League for German Culture, led by Alfred Rosenberg, which grew rapidly in size after January 1933
- the Official Party Censorship Commission, which had responsibility for vetting Party publications
- the SA, Hitler Youth (HJ) and Nazi Students' Organisation, which all claimed the right to seek out, confiscate and destroy publications of which they disapproved. The ceremonial book-burning in Berlin in May 1933, for example, was instigated by the Nazi Students' Organisation.

Despite the confusion of overlapping authorities and rivalries within the party hierarchy for control of censorship, there was a gradual tightening of control and by 1935–36 the system of censorship had become very effective. Those who had opposed the Nazis had been dismissed from their employment and were either in prison, in exile or under surveillance. Those non-Nazis who continued working in the arts concentrated on themes they knew would be acceptable. Many leading writers, artists and musicians chose to leave Germany and live in exile. Some of their works were published abroad and smuggled back into Germany but the quantities of illicit material circulating in Germany were never sufficient to trouble the regime. On the whole, therefore, censorship worked but the result was to stifle creativity and impose a dull conformity on German cultural life.

The effectiveness of propaganda and indoctrination

The Nazi regime placed great emphasis on propaganda and the effort to indoctrinate the German population into the Nazi Weltanschauung. Undoubtedly Hitler and Göbbels were very skilled propagandists, but the effectiveness of their efforts is very difficult to gauge. The Nazis carried out occasional plebiscites to demonstrate the support of the people for the regime but since these were in no way free elections they cannot be regarded as evidence of genuine support. It is possible to conclude, from the many Gestapo reports on the state of public opinion, that there was at the very least scepticism among some sections of the population towards particular Nazi policies. Attitudes of Germans towards the regime depended on a range of factors – on age, on class, occupation, religion to name but a few. Attitudes could also change over time. It is therefore impossible to give a definitive judgment on whether the majority of Germans supported the regime, whether they did so consistently, and whether the support they did show was due to propaganda and indoctrination or to other influences such as fear of repression. Any judgments on the success of propaganda and indoctrination, therefore, can only be provisional and tentative.

Nazi propaganda and indoctrination appears to have been most successful when it was aimed at the young, whose opinions were not yet strongly formed. Their efforts also appear to have been effective when their messages overlapped with the traditional attitudes and values of particular groups. Aristocratic, old conservatives shared the Nazis' beliefs in the need for order and their anti-democratic sentiments, although even among this group there was a noticeable reluctance to swallow the more radical elements in Nazi ideology. Germany's middle class shared the Nazis' hostility to communism and socialism and were susceptible

Activity

Thinking point

Explain why censorship was so important to the Nazi regime.

Cross-reference

For more about the Combat League for German Culture, see page 41; for more about the Hitler Youth, see pages 72–76.

Exploring the detail

Plebiscites

A plebiscite, or referendum, was a vote in which people were asked to approve the regime's policies. Four main plebiscites were held in the years 1933–39:

November 1933	to approve the decision to leave the League of Nations
August 1934	to approve of Hitler becoming Führer
March 1936	to approve the remilitarisation of the Rhineland
April 1938	to approve the *Anschluss* (union) with Austria

Activity

Discussion point

Why is it difficult to assess the effectiveness of propaganda in a dictatorial regime?

to the propaganda message that the Nazis were the only credible alternative to a left-wing takeover in Germany. Anti-Semitism and nationalist resentment of the Treaty of Versailles ran through all classes and the Nazis were able to reinforce these attitudes through their propaganda. Thus propaganda and indoctrination in the Third Reich was most successful when it built upon existing beliefs and values; where, however, Nazi propaganda challenged deeply held beliefs, such as religion, it was less successful.

Summary questions

1 Explain why parades and spectacles were important to the Nazis in spreading their propaganda.

2 How successful was the Nazi regime in controlling the German people's access to alternative viewpoints and sources of information?

The Hitler myth and the content of propaganda

In this chapter you will learn about:

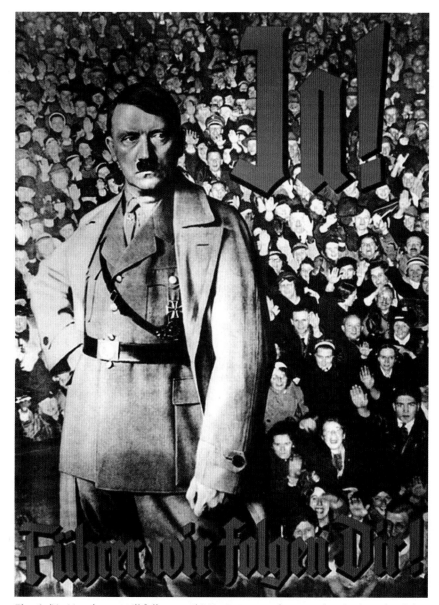

Fig. 1 *'Yes! Leader, we will follow you!' A Nazi propaganda poster showing how the Hitler myth was cultivated*

We see in him the symbol of the indestructible life-force of the German nation, which has taken living shape in Adolf Hitler.

1 *From a eulogy to Hitler on his birthday, 1935, by Otto Dietrich, quoted in Kershaw, I., **The Hitler Myth**, 1989*

▨ Göbbels and the Hitler myth

In 1941, Göbbels claimed that the creation of the 'Hitler myth' had been his greatest achievement. A personality cult surrounding Adolf Hitler had been gaining ground within the Nazi movement since the early 1920s, but, in 1933, the majority of the German population remained unconvinced by or hostile to the Nazi leader. In the March 1933 Reichstag election, the last in which the German people had been offered a genuine choice between the political parties, less than half of the electorate voted for Hitler and the Nazi Party. By the end of 1934, however, a powerful 'Hitler cult' had taken hold in the national consciousness. Hitler was being hailed as the 'symbol of the nation' and the 'leader for whom the nation had been waiting'. This image of Hitler, carefully constructed through propaganda to mask reality and to project him as an almost superhuman figure, became so powerful that in time Hitler himself came to believe in it.

Myth and reality

> The Führer is the bearer of the people's will; he is independent of all groups, associations and interests, but he is bound by laws which are inherent in the nature of his people. In his will the will of the people is realised. He shapes the collective will of the people within himself and he embodies the political unity and entirety of the people in opposition to individual interests.

2   *Ernst Huber, a Nazi ideologist, 1935, quoted in Kershaw, I.,* ***The Hitler Myth***, *1989*

> My Führer! I feel compelled to thank our creator daily for giving us and the entire German people such a wonderful Führer and in a time where our beautiful dear Fatherland was threatened with the most horrible destruction through Jewish **Bolshevism**. It does not bear thinking about what floods of tears, what blood after the scarcely healed wounds of the First World War, would have flowed, if you, my beloved Führer, in all your anguish for such a great people had not found the courage to win through as the saviour of 66 million Germans.

3   *A letter from a Nazi Party member to Hitler, 1936, quoted in Kershaw, I.,* ***The Hitler Myth***, *1989*

In Nazi propaganda, Hitler was portrayed as being unlike other politicians. He was presented as a 'man of the people' and the 'people's chancellor'; in other words, he symbolised the coming together of the Nazi Party and the people. He was presented as a man who:

- was tough, uncompromising and ruthless in fighting and defeating the nation's enemies, both internal and external
- was hard working, toiling unstintingly for his people while others slept
- was a political genius who had mastered the problems faced by Germany in 1933 and was responsible for Germany's 'national awakening', in which order had been restored, the economy revived and Germany had thrown off the humiliating shackles of the Treaty of Versailles
- was dynamic, energetic and forceful, in contrast with the weak politicians of the Weimar years
- lived a simple life and sacrificed personal happiness to devote himself to his people. He was invariably shown as being alone and removed from the Nazi Party
- was the guardian of traditional morality and popular justice
- was a man of peace and a statesman of true genius.

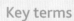

Activity

Source analysis

Study the images of Adolf Hitler in Sources 2 and 3, figures 1 and 2, and the main text. Make a list of the personal and leadership qualities that Hitler was shown to possess.

Key terms

Bolshevism: an alternative term for communism, derived from a name of the Russian Communist Party which seized power in 1917, the Bolshevik Party.

The reality was in many ways very different from these propaganda images:

■ Hitler, as Führer, was surrounded by officials who competed with each other to gain his attention and implement his wishes. Hitler supplied the vision, his ministers and officials interpreted this and turned it into detailed policies. He was actually very little involved in decision-making, still less in administrative matters.

■ Far from working hard, Hitler stayed up late watching films and would usually not get up until mid-day. His days were spent in eating, walking in the grounds of his mountain retreat and delivering long, rambling speeches to his subordinates. He disliked reading official documents and rarely got involved in detailed discussions on policy. His officials often had great difficulty in getting him to make decisions.

■ Although he was undoubtedly ruthless and unwavering in his determination to crush communism and socialism in Germany, when he faced problems with the radicals in his own movement, the SA, Hitler delayed making a decision for several months. Only when he came under pressure from the army leadership did he finally decide to purge Röhm and the SA in the 'Night of the Long Knives'. The genius of Hitler and Göbbels as propagandists was demonstrated in the aftermath of the purge when they presented this act of blatant and brutal illegality as a blow for law and order and traditional morality. In the wake of the Night of the Long Knives, Hitler's personal popularity rose to unprecedented heights. This event helped to separate him in the public mind from the Nazi Party and showed him as representing the national interest rather than a narrow party interest.

■ Even though the image of the Nazi Party, especially at local level, was tainted by the corruption, greed, arrogance and high-handedness of party officials, Hitler escaped the blame for the actions of his subordinates. Indeed, the Night of the Long Knives was presented in such a way that Hitler was defending the ordinary German against the petty despots – or 'Little Hitlers' – in the Nazi movement. The myth then took on a life of its own as many ordinary Germans convinced themselves that other petty despots would be removed from office 'if only the Führer knew' what they were doing.

The development of the Hitler myth, 1933–39

Every effort was made by Göbbels, during the decisive early months of the Nazi regime, to promote the image of Hitler as 'people's chancellor' and the saviour of the nation. Since the Hitler myth was a product of propaganda, Göbbels had to deploy all of his skills and his resources to achieve his objectives. Key events, such as the opening of the Reichstag after the March 1933 election and the Day of Potsdam, were carefully stage-managed to create a piece of pure political theatre with Hitler as the central character. Radio, the press, newsreels and posters were used to promote the cult of the Führer. Celebrations for Hitler's birthday on 20 April, when flags, bunting and photographs of the Führer were displayed in towns and villages across Germany, were orchestrated to project an impression of universal public acclaim for Hitler. The Nuremberg rallies, and the film *The Triumph of the Will*, in which Hitler was portrayed as showing enormous strength of will in overcoming major obstacles, were also instrumental in developing the Führer cult. This propaganda could only succeed, however, if there was a receptive audience.

There was a tradition of authoritarian leadership in Germany. In the Weimar period, the nationalist and conservative right-wing parties hankered

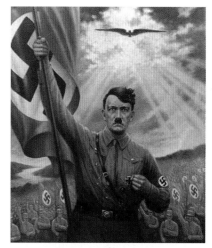

Fig. 2 *This propaganda poster showing Hitler holding the swastika flag of the Nazi Party contains many elements of the Hitler myth*

Activity

Revision exercise

Construct a table with two vertical columns headed 'Hitler myth' and 'Hitler reality'. Use the information in this section to complete the table.

Exploring the detail

The Day of Potsdam

On 21 March 1933, following their election victory, the Nazis staged the opening of the new Reichstag at the Garrison Church in Potsdam. The setting was deliberately chosen as being representative of the old, imperial Germany, as was the presence of President Hindenburg. The date, the official start of spring, was chosen to symbolise a new awakening. The Day of Potsdam, therefore, was a clever piece of theatre which was designed to emphasise the unity of old and new in Nazi Germany and the fact that the revered Hindenburg had conferred his blessing on the new Nazi regime.

for a return to Germany's traditional values, for order and for a heroic leader figure who would restore Germany's pride. Among a significant section of the German population, therefore, there was a political culture which was anti-democratic and receptive to Nazi propaganda in its projection of Hitler as a political giant. By ruthlessly suppressing left wing parties in the first weeks after taking power, Hitler won the approval of the middle and upper classes. His suppression of the SA in 1934 reinforced his image as a strong, determined and ruthless leader who would curb the excesses of the wilder, radical elements within his own party. The gradual reduction in unemployment and the actions taken to protect German farmers were trumpeted as evidence of the Führer getting to grips with Germany's economic problems. By the end of 1934, therefore, public support for Hitler had spread to all classes and all regions of Germany.

During 1935 and 1936, economic problems such as low wages, food shortages and the continuing high levels of unemployment led to a waning of enthusiasm for the regime. Successes in foreign and defence policy, however, increased popular support and helped to sustain the Hitler myth. Germans of all classes felt the Treaty of Versailles to have been a national humiliation that needed to be reversed; on the other hand, there was also a widespread fear of war. Hitler's successful step-by-step approach to challenging the Treaty of Versailles, which achieved 'triumph without bloodshed' in the years 1933–39, played well with the German people and bolstered his image as a statesman, man of peace and master tactician. There was strong public support for the reintroduction of conscription and the start of rearmament in 1935, great enthusiasm for the reoccupation of the Rhineland in 1936, while the Anschluss with Austria in March 1938 unleashed *'an elemental frenzy of enthusiasm'* (Kershaw). During the Sudeten crisis with Czechoslovakia in the autumn of 1938, when it appeared possible that Britain and France might go to war to resist German attempts to take over the **Sudetenland**, serious doubts began to be expressed about Hitler's policy. Fear of war outweighed

Key terms

The Sudetenland: the area of Czechoslovakia which bordered Germany and was inhabited by three million German speaking people. A Sudeten German Party, led by the Nazi Konrad Henlein, had been campaigning for the Sudetenland to be united with the German Reich, claiming that the German minority in Czechoslovakia suffered from discrimination.

Exploring the detail

The Munich Agreement

In the autumn of 1938, Hitler put pressure on Czechoslovakia for the Sudetenland area to be handed over to Germany. German forces were ordered to prepare for an invasion, which would almost certainly have led to Britain and France declaring war on Germany. Anxious to avoid war, however, the British prime minister, Neville Chamberlain, met Hitler on three occasions to try to find a peaceful settlement. Finally a four-power (Great Britain, France, Germany and Italy) conference was held in Munich on 29–30 September at which it was agreed to hand over the Sudetenland to Germany.

Key chronology

Nazi foreign and defence policy, 1933–39

October 1933	Germany withdraws from the League of Nations.
March 1935	Hitler announces reintroduction of compulsory military service (conscription) and beginning of rearmament.
March 1936	German forces march into the Rhineland area (officially demilitarised under the terms of the Treaty of Versailles).
March 1938	Anschluss with Austria breaks the Treaty of Versailles.
September/ October 1938	Sudeten crisis over German demands for the (mainly German-speaking) Sudetenland area of Czechoslovakia to be handed over to Germany. Resolved in Munich agreement giving Sudetenland to Germany.
March 1939	Germany annexes the remainder of Czechoslovakia.
September 1939	German attack on Poland leads Britain and France to declare war on Germany.

Note that a number of these events occurred during the month of March. This was also the month of the annual 'day of celebration of heroes' when Germans honoured their war dead, a patriotic festival which the Nazis turned into a celebration of militarism. There was an obvious propaganda value to the regime in linking its challenges to the Treaty of Versailles with the day of celebration of heroes, although the timing of some of these events was also influenced by other factors beyond the regime's control.

nationalist fervour at the start of the crisis, but the Munich settlement undermined Hitler's critics and boosted his image as a skilled statesman and a man who kept his nerve in a crisis. When war finally broke out in September 1939, after Hitler ordered German forces to invade Poland, Hitler's reputation was again enhanced. The success of Germany's forces in using *Blitzkrieg* (lightning war) tactics, especially in the summer of 1940 when France was defeated very quickly, enabled Nazi propagandists to present Hitler as a military genius.

By the late 1930s, an estimated 90% of the German people admired and supported Hitler. The Führer cult provided a focus for unity within the nation and helped to sustain the regime in power. It also helped to mask the regime's failings and its inconsistencies. Germans who might not have been wholehearted supporters of Nazi ideology were nevertheless drawn into admiration and adulation of the Führer. The success of Göbbels in generating and sustaining the Hitler myth was indeed one of his greatest achievements as a propagandist.

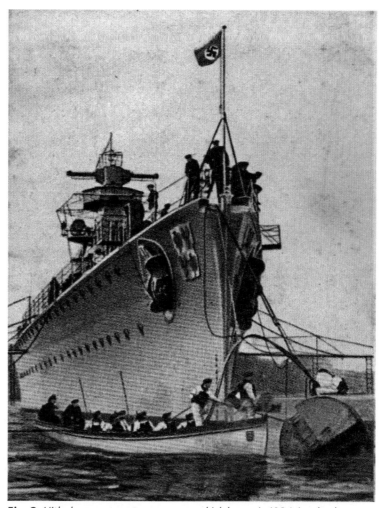

Fig. 3 *Hitler's rearmament programme, which began in 1934, involved building a new German navy, in defiance of the Treaty of Versailles. The ship shown here was the* Admiral Graf Spree, *a 'pocket-battleship' which sank many Allied ships before being sunk itself in December 1939*

Ideology and successes of the regime

In January 1933, the German economy was in the depths of depression, with nearly six million people out of work. Previous regimes had failed to make any significant impact on the unemployment problem and many people had voted for the Nazis during the depression years of 1930–32 because Hitler promised decisive action to get people back to work. By 1935, the official figures showed that unemployment had fallen to two million, while by 1939, there were labour shortages in key industries. This, in essence, was the basis on which Nazi propagandists hailed the success of the regime's policies as an 'economic miracle'. This section will explore the extent to which the claims of an economic miracle were more a propaganda myth than a reality.

Nazi economic policy

Aims

When Hitler was appointed chancellor on 30 January 1933, the Nazi Party did not have a coherent and carefully thought-out economic policy. Nevertheless, Hitler had some clear aims. In the short term, the priority was economic recovery from the depression and the reduction of unemployment. Achieving these aims would boost the regime's popularity and help the Nazis to consolidate their power. In the longer term, the Nazis aimed to create an economy capable of sustaining a major rearmament programme and geared to the needs of a future war. Such an economy would need to be self-sufficient in the production of food and vital raw materials – something the Nazis referred to as 'economic autarky' (self-sufficiency).

Activity

Thinking point

How far was Göbbels' success in promoting the Hitler myth due to the following?

- His skill as a propagandist
- Having a receptive audience
- The successes of the Nazi regime

■ Key profile

Hjalmar Schacht

Schacht (1877–1970) had been brought up in America before returning to Germany and becoming a banker. He became head of the Reichsbank in 1923 and was involved in the negotiations on both the Dawes and Young Plans. Originally a nationalist in his politics, Schacht had supported Hitler's appointment as chancellor in 1933 and was subsequently reappointed as head of the Reichsbank. He became economics minister in 1934 and was the mastermind behind the Nazi strategy for financing rearmament. After Göring took charge of the Four Year Plan in 1936, Schacht's influence declined. He was removed from the Economics Ministry in 1937 and lost his position as head of the Reichsbank in 1939.

Recovery

During the years 1933–36, Hjalmar Schacht, President of the Reichsbank and, from August 1934, Economics Minister, was the key figure in Nazi economic policy. Under his direction the regime stimulated economic recovery by:

- pumping money into the economy to build homes and Autobahns
- stimulating consumer demand by giving tax concessions and grants to particular groups
- giving subsidies to private firms to encourage them to take on more workers
- putting controls on wages and prices to control inflation
- introducing the 'New Plan' in 1934 to control Germany's foreign trade and improve the country's **balance of payments**
- taking the first steps towards rearmament.

■ Key profile

Hermann Göring

Göring (1893–1946) was a fighter pilot in the First World War and a member of the famous Baron Richtofen's squadron. He joined the Nazi Party in 1922 and took part in the Munich Putsch of 1923. He was elected to the Reichstag in 1928 and became the president (speaker) of the Reichstag in 1932. In 1933, he was appointed prime minister and interior minister of Prussia. He also became Reich aviation minister in 1933 and was responsible for the rebuilding of the **Luftwaffe**. As interior minister of Prussia, he established the Gestapo and the first concentration camps. In 1936, he was placed in charge of the Four Year Plan. After the failure of the Luftwaffe to defeat the RAF in the Battle of Britain, his influence declined and he was expelled from the party in 1945. He was captured by the Allies and put on trial but committed suicide in prison.

Rearmament and a war economy

Schacht's measures did succeed in reviving the German economy and reducing unemployment but the revival created a set of new problems. In addition to the balance of payments problems and shortage of foreign

---

■ Activity

Thinking point

What were the main aims of Nazi economic policy?

■ Key terms

Balance of payments: the difference between what a country earns by selling goods to other countries (exports) and what it has to pay to buy goods from other countries (imports).

Luftwaffe: the German air force.

■ Exploring the detail

The New Plan of 1934

As the economy began to revive in 1933 and 1934, foreign trade increased and this led to imports growing faster than exports. This in turn led to a shortage of foreign currencies which were needed to purchase imported goods. In order to rectify this situation, Schacht placed controls on imports and on access to foreign currency. He also initiated a series of trade agreements with foreign countries, especially states in the Balkans and South America, whereby Germany was supplied with food and raw materials which were paid for in German Reichsmarks. The supplying countries could then only use this money to buy German goods.

exchange, there were also food shortages, rising prices and lower living standards for ordinary Germans in 1935–36. Reports from around Germany at this time spoke of growing disillusionment with the regime. Moreover, from the point of view of the Nazis' long-term aim of creating a war economy, Schacht's approach was much too cautious and slow. The result of this was that, in 1936, Schacht was marginalised and a new Four Year Plan was introduced with Göring in charge. The aim of this plan was to make Germany ready for war within four years. Priority was given to rearmament and economic autarky. This was to be achieved by:

- creating a managed economy with controls on labour supply, prices, raw materials and foreign exchange
- setting production targets for private companies to meet
- establishing new State-owned industrial plants such as the Hermann Göring Steelworks
- increasing production of key commodities such as iron and steel and chemicals
- encouraging research and investment into the production of substitute products such as artificial rubber and extracting oil from coal, thereby reducing Germany's dependence on imports.

The Nazi economic miracle – myth and reality

Göbbels and the Nazi propaganda machine used all their resources and skills to project an image of the success of Nazi economic policies. Speeches and radio broadcasts by Hitler repeatedly claimed that the 'battle for work' had been won by 1936; indeed, the 'battle for work' was not even mentioned after 1936, reflecting the success of propaganda in convincing people that unemployment was no longer a problem. Advertising campaigns for products such as the 'people's receiver', the 'people's car' and for holidays on cruise ships gave the impression that Germans were experiencing an unprecedented rise in their living standards as a result of the regime's policies. Military parades showing off the latest equipment and patriotic campaigns to persuade Germans to buy only German goods were designed to show that Germany was achieving autarky and was ready for war. In each case, there was an element of truth in the claims but propaganda exaggerated the successes and covered up the failures in Nazi economic policies.

The reduction of unemployment

> The salvation of the German worker in an enormous and all-embracing attack on unemployment is a key aim of my government. Within four years, unemployment must be finally overcome.

4
 *From a radio broadcast by Adolf Hitler, February 1933, quoted in Evans, R., **The Third Reich in Power**, 2005*

Official unemployment figures show a dramatic reduction in the number of unemployed by 1934 and a continuing fall thereafter. This was the basis of the claim that the 'battle for work' had been won and that this victory was entirely due to Nazi economic policies. There were several flaws in these claims:

- Economic recovery had actually begun before the Nazis took power in January 1933. Many of the job creation schemes used by the regime to reduce unemployment were actually based on policies introduced by Bruning in the early 1930s.

Exploring the detail

The Hermann Göring Steelworks

This was an enormous enterprise established and owned by the State but partly financed by private companies. The company was given priority over private companies in the allocation of materials and labour and, by 1939, had become the largest industrial enterprise in Europe. It expanded its operations into coal mining and the manufacture of heavy machinery and synthetic fuels. Large, showpiece industrial plants like this had an obvious propaganda for the regime.

Activity

Revision exercise

Construct a table with three vertical columns headed 'Economic policy', 'Myth' and 'Reality'. In the first column, list 'Reduction of unemployment', 'Rising living standards' and 'Autarky'. Use the information in the following pages to complete the other two columns.

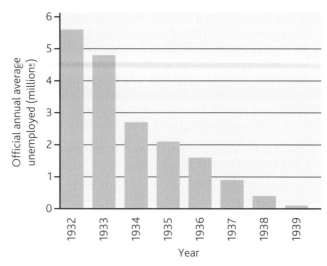

Fig. 4 *The reduction of unemployment in Germany, 1932–39*

■ Part of the reduction in the unemployment figures was achieved by persuading married women to give up their employment, through granting them marriage loans, thereby releasing jobs for unemployed male workers.

■ The reintroduction of conscription in 1935, for young men aged 18–25, took a large proportion of young males out of the labour market.

■ Official figures also showed a dramatic increase in the numbers of Germans in employment. This was partly achieved through various statistical devices to inflate the figures. Those who only had occasional employment, for example, were counted as permanently employed while those drafted into unpaid work in agriculture were also counted as employed.

Historian Richard Evans has estimated that 'invisible unemployment' (those who were out of work but were not counted in the official figures) was as high as 1.5 million workers. By this estimate, the official figure

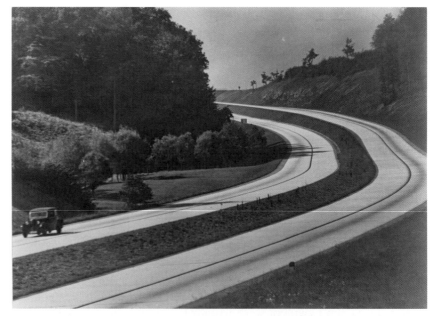

Fig. 5 *The Autobahns were a great propaganda success but of little practical value. The lack of vehicles on this new Autobahn relfects the fact that the volume of traffic did not justify the money spent on them*

of 1.6 million people out of work in 1936 should in fact be increased to over three million, far too many to support the claim that the 'battle for work' had been won. After 1936, rearmament led to a rapid expansion of employment and resulted in labour shortages appearing by 1939.

Rising living standards

Nazi propaganda emphasised the duty of all German citizens to make sacrifices on behalf of the 'people's community', by working harder and for longer hours and by accepting a squeeze on wages. At the same time, propaganda also stressed the benefits which the Nazi regime had bestowed on workers through improved working conditions, better social and welfare provision and access to goods and services which had previously only been available to the privileged few.

Despite official attempts to hold down money wages, incomes for many workers did increase during the years 1933–39. Some employers were prepared to pay bonuses and other benefits to get round the freeze on wage levels and so attract more skilled workers. Pay increased due to the longer hours being worked but, on the other hand, workers' wages were subject to increased deductions because of the compulsory contributions they had to make to the German Labour Front and to welfare organisations. It is, therefore, difficult to generalise about what happened to the standard of living of the majority of German workers in these years. Workers in key industries such as armaments were undoubtedly better off than previously, while those producing consumer goods were not.

> ■ **Cross-reference**
>
> The German Labour Front (DAF) is dealt with in more detail on pages 76–77.

Living standards depend as much on prices as they do on incomes. Prices rose during the 1930s and there were shortages of some key commodities, particularly fats. German consumers were able to buy enough food to feed their families but could afford few luxuries. The consumption of higher-value foods such as meat, fruit and eggs declined while the consumption of cheaper foods such as potatoes and rye bread increased. There was, then, pressure on living standards and Gestapo and Sopade reports occasionally show some discontent with the regime. On the other hand, the fact that the regime succeeded in persuading the population to shoulder the burden of the rearmament programme without triggering a wages explosion and without mass opposition indicates the success of propaganda campaigns such as the 'battle for production'.

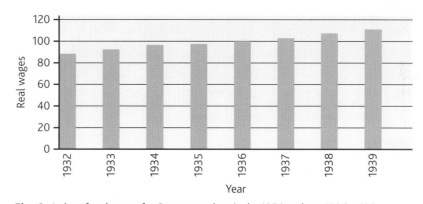

Fig. 6 *Index of real wages for German workers in the 1930s, where 1936 = 100*

Propaganda made much of the improved benefits which the regime's policies had brought to the majority of Germans. The 'Strength Through Joy' organisation gave workers access to cruises and holidays in Germany, taking advantage of the increase in paid holidays which most workers received. The 'Beauty of Labour' organisation improved working conditions and facilities in factories and other workplaces. Radio sets such as the 'people's receiver' and the Volkswagen car were heralded as evidence that the regime was providing goods for ordinary Germans that would only be available to a privileged few in other countries.

> ■ **Cross-reference**
>
> Strength Through Joy is dealt with more fully on pages 78–80 and the Beauty of Labour on pages 80–81.

The Volkswagen car

The idea of the *Volkswagen* (which translates literally as the 'people's car') had been taken up by Hitler in the 1920s and, after becoming chancellor in 1933, he enlisted the help of the racing car engineer Ferdinand Porsche to design it. The car's production was funded by the German Labour Front (DAF) and sales were promoted by Strength Through Joy (hence the Volkswagen was also known as the 'Strength Through Joy car'. A huge advertising campaign, under the slogan 'a car for everyone' was launched to persuade workers to pay into a savings scheme to purchase one. This scheme was very successful. A Sopade report from April 1939 told, *'The announcement of the people's car is a great and happy surprise. For a long time the car was the main topic of conversation in all sections of the population in Germany. All other pressing problems, whether of domestic or foreign policy, were pushed into the background for a while. The grey German everyday sank beneath notice under this impression of the music of the future. Wherever the test models of the new Strength Through Joy construction are seen in Germany, crowds gather around them. The politician who promises a car for everyone is the man of the masses if the masses believe his promises. And as far as the 'Strength Through Joy car' is concerned, the German people do believe Hitler's promises.'* The Volkswagen car, then, was one of the great success stories of Nazi propaganda, the more so since the car never went into full production during the Third Reich and only members of the Nazi elite were able to acquire the few preproduction models which were actually made.

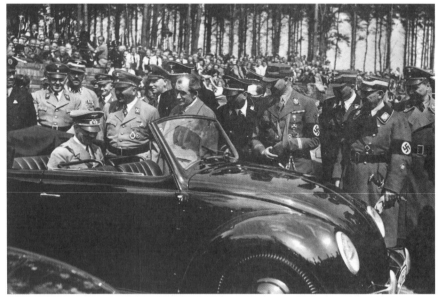

Fig. 7 *Hitler sits in the first prototype of the Strength Through Joy car, the Volkswagen, in 1938. The car was a propaganda success for the regime, even though no ordinary Germans ever had the chance to own one*

■ Activity

Thinking point

1 Explain how the Volkswagen car programme reflected Nazi ideology.

2 How far does the Volkswagen car programme show that Nazi propaganda was successful?

Autarky

The Four Year Plan aimed to achieve self-sufficiency, or autarky, in food production and vital raw materials in order to prepare the German economy for war. Autarky, with its links to national sovereignty and its embodiment of national pride and independence, fitted well with the Nazis' ideological aims. It would, according to the Nazi Party programme, *'free Germany from the chains of international capital'*. The effort to increase production was presented as a battle in which the whole 'people's community' had to participate. Propaganda campaigns to persuade people to buy only German goods, eat only German food and use only German raw materials in their work presented these targets as a patriotic duty on all German citizens. There were also propaganda campaigns to persuade Germans to save more, since savings would help to fund investment in new production facilities. In 1937, the regime launched a campaign to collect scrap metal from people's homes and gardens and from public spaces such as parks to make up for serious shortages in raw materials. Garden fences, park railings, iron lampposts were removed to be melted down. Pots and pans were collected from people's homes by the Hitler Youth and local committees were set up to coordinate collections.

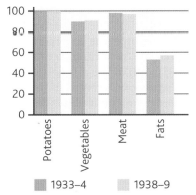

Fig. 8 *Percentage of food produced in Germany, 1933–39*

1933–4   1938–9

The results of the Four Year Plan did not match the propagandist claims. German industry, despite massive investment, did not meet the targets set by the regime and, in 1939, Germany still imported one third of its raw materials. In food production, there were similar failings.

The drive for rearmament and the target of achieving economic autarky placed considerable strains on the German people, including longer hours, higher prices and growing shortages. From time to time, there were serious shortages of eggs and meat, as well as wheat and rye for making bread. Price controls and the introduction of **rationing** on some key commodities in the late 1930s helped to alleviate the pressure. Despite these growing hardships, however, there were few signs of unrest or dissent. Nazi propaganda had succeeded in persuading the majority of the German people to accept these burdens.

> The people are suffering a great deal from the shortage of all kinds of foodstuffs and respectable, solid clothing. Still, this has not led to any kind of unrest apart from queuing in front of shops, which has become a daily occurrence.

5 *Sopade report from the Ruhr area, May 1939, quoted in Noakes, J.,* **Nazism 1919–45, Vol. 4**, *1998*

The Olympic Games of 1936

> For the Nazi regime, the Olympics are a through-and-through political undertaking. 'German Renaissance through Hitler', I read recently. People at home and abroad are constantly being told that they are witnessing the revival, the blossoming, the new mind, the unity, the steadfastness and glory and of course also the peacefulness of spirit of the Third Reich, that lovingly embraces the entire world. The slogan-chanting mobs are banned (for the duration of the Olympics), campaigns against the Jews, warlike speeches, everything disreputable has vanished from the newspapers until the end of the Games, and still, day and night, the swastika flags are flying everywhere.

6 *From Klemperer, V.,* **I Shall Bear Witness**, *1998*

Key terms

Rationing: controls on the supply and distribution of key commodities to ensure that all those eligible should receive their fair share. Shopkeepers were only allowed to sell these goods if a purchaser could produce the relevant ration book.

Cross-reference

For more about rationing, see page 117.

Activity

Thinking point

'The Nazi economic miracle was a propaganda myth which had no basis in reality.' What is your response to this statement?

Activity

Source analysis

Read Source 6 and the information in this section. Explain how the Berlin Olympics were used by the Nazis as a propaganda exercise.

Did you know?

The 1936 Berlin Olympics were the first Olympics to be televised; over 70 hours of Olympic competition was broadcast and 25 special viewing rooms were set up around Berlin to enable people to watch the games. Leni Riefenstahl was commissioned to make a documentary film about the games, entitled *Olympia*, which was released in 1938 and shown in cinemas across Germany and in other countries.

■ Activity

Thinking point

Explain why the Nazis placed so much emphasis on sport and physical fitness.

■ Exploring the detail

Snubbed by Hitler?

Jesse Owens (1913–80) won gold medals at the Berlin Olympics for the 100 metres, 200 metres, 4 x 100 metres relay and long jump events. It was reported that Hitler had deliberately snubbed him, because he was black, by refusing to shake his hand. In reality, Hitler had been advised by Olympics officials that he should either shake the hands of all winners or none at all, after he had only greeted the German winners. He opted to not shake any hands after this. As a black American, Owens faced constant discrimination in his own country and he said that it was not Hitler but Franklin Roosevelt (the American president) who had snubbed him by not inviting him to a White House reception.

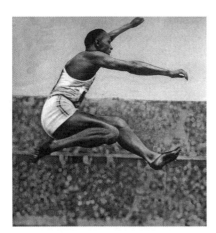

Fig. 10 *The black American athlete Jesse Owens was the star of the Berlin Olympics in 1936, winning four gold medals*

The Olympic Games of 1936 were held in Berlin. The regime saw the Berlin Olympics as an opportunity to present a positive image of the Third Reich to the rest of the world. No expense was spared in the building of an enormous Olympic stadium, capable of holding 100,000 spectators. Being at the centre of a large sporting complex with a swimming pool and other sporting venues, the stadium became a symbol of the revival and confidence of the German people under Hitler's leadership. During the opening ceremony the airship *Hindenburg* flew over the stadium trailing the Olympic flag, while a choir of thousands sang the Horst Wessel song. Around Berlin, Olympic flags were flown side by side with swastika flags. For the duration of the Olympics, anti-Semitic propaganda was pushed to one side and signs around Berlin saying 'Jews not welcome here' were removed. The police rounded up thousands of known criminals and the so-called 'workshy' and held them in detention while the games were in progress. Göbbels was quick to realise the propaganda potential of the games and all the modern technology at his disposal was used to project an image of the Third Reich as orderly, efficient and successful.

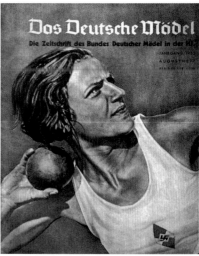

Fig. 9 *A poster for the 1936 Olympic Games, showing the Nazis' view that German women, living in the Third Reich, would prove themselves to be great athletes*

Sport and physical exercise played a very important role in achieving the Nazi ideals of racial purity and a 'people's community'. Participation in sporting competition would harden German youth and reinforce notions of struggle. Drilling for mass gymnastics displays would help to instill the idea that the individual could only achieve his or her full potential as part of a larger community. The regime, therefore, placed great emphasis on sport and Hitler appointed a Reich director of sport to coordinate all the various sporting organisations. Schools devoted a considerable amount of curriculum time to sport and physical education lessons while the Hitler Youth and the German Labour Front organised sports for millions of Germans. In Nazi ideology, the Aryan race was physically as well as mentally superior to all other races and sport provided an opportunity to demonstrate this. The Olympic Games, therefore, offered the chance to show the world the success of Nazi racial policies. No Jewish athletes were selected for the German team to compete at the Olympics. In heading the medals table with 89 medals, the German team did, to some extent, live up to expectations. However, the real star of the games was a black American athlete, Jesse Owens, who won four gold medals and the acclaim of the Berlin crowd.

I'm afraid the Nazis have succeeded with their propaganda. First, they have run the games on a lavish scale never before experienced, and this has appealed to the athletes. Second, they have put up a very good front for the general visitors, especially the businessmen.

7   *From Shirer, W., **Berlin Diary: The Journal of a Foreign Correspondent, 1933–41**, 1970*

Key profile

Leni Riefenstahl

Riefenstahl (1902–2003) had made her name as a dancer and actress in Berlin before being asked by Hitler, with whom she had a close personal relationship, to make propaganda films for the regime. She was responsible for *The Triumph of the Will* about the 1934 Nuremberg Rally and *Olympia* about the 1936 Olympic Games. As a pioneer of many film-making and photographic techniques, Riefenstahl had many admirers in the film world. She was captured by the Americans at the end of the war but never charged with any crime. She resumed her film-making career after the war.

The impact of war on Nazi propaganda

Overview of the war

War began on 1 September 1939 when German forces invaded Poland. Two days later the conflict became more widespread when Britain and France declared war on Germany. Over the course of the next two years, German forces achieved a series of victories and occupied countries in northern, western and southern Europe. By the summer of 1940, only Britain remained at war with Germany. After failing to defeat Britain during 1940, Hitler turned his attention to the east when, in June 1941, he ordered German forces to invade the Soviet Union. After initial successes which took German forces to the outskirts of Moscow, the Soviet Union's Red Army succeeded in halting the German advance in December 1941. This was also the month when the USA entered the war on the Allied side. During 1942, German forces in the USSR advanced to the south and east towards the oilfields in the Caucasus region but the attack was halted at Stalingrad. In a bitter struggle which lasted from November 1942 until January 1943, the Red Army inflicted a severe defeat on German forces which proved to be a decisive turning point in the war. After Stalingrad, German forces were on the defensive and the war became a struggle for survival. At this point, the Nazi regime adopted a '**total war**' strategy to try to stave off defeat.

The change to a total war strategy radicalised the Nazi regime. It also placed increasing burdens on the civilian population. Total war, therefore, had a considerable impact on Nazi propaganda.

The impact of total war on propaganda

> War is the father of all things; every generation has to go into war once.

 8   *From a speech by Adolf Hitler, 1938*

During the 1930s, one of the aims of Nazi propaganda had been to instill a 'military spirit' into the German people. While the majority of Germans undoubtedly supported the nationalist aim of Nazi foreign policy to overturn the Treaty of Versailles, the effort to arouse general enthusiasm for war met with limited success. There were no cheering crowds spontaneously welcoming the outbreak of war in September 1939, unlike in August 1914 when the First World War began. The easy victory over Poland, and the entry of German troops into the Polish capital Warsaw, was greeted by much flag-waving and rejoicing, but much of this was in response to directions from local Nazi Party offices.

 Activity

Discussion point

How far do you agree with Shirer in Source 7 that the Olympic Games were a propaganda success for the Nazis?

Cross-reference

The impact of war on the German people will be dealt with in more detail in Section 4, pages 114–143.

Key terms

Total war: the complete mobilisation of a country's resources, both economic and human, in order to maximise the war effort. It implies State control of industry and the conscription of labour as well as compulsory military service.

In honour of the impending entry of German troops into Warsaw there will be a general display of flags for the first time during this war. The exact time will be announced on the radio. The district propaganda leaders will ensure at once that there will be a unique display of flags. No house and no window must be without its swastika flag. Pictures of the Führer and swastika flags should be displayed in all shops in a dignified fashion.

> **9**   *Directive from propaganda department of the Nazi Party Gauleiter in Koblenz-Trier, 1 October 1939, quoted in Noakes, J.,* **Nazism 1919–45, Vol. 4,** *1998*

Activity

Thinking point

Research into Nazi propaganda posters from the early stages of the war (September 1939 to June 1941). Make a Powerpoint presentation of the ways in which the war was presented to the German people.

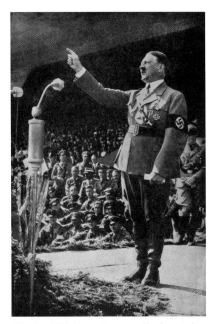

Fig. 11 *Hitler's oratory was the basis of his popular appeal. Here he is speaking at a Nazi Party rally*

In the early years of the war, 1939–41, the aims of Nazi propaganda were to maintain public morale and to mobilise the energies and commitment of the German people to the war effort. With a series of quick and seemingly easy victories, maintaining morale was not difficult to achieve. Nevertheless, Hitler showed that he did not take the commitment of the German people for granted by making sure that the war did not impose too great a strain on the civilian population. There was no major squeeze on civilian consumption of food and manufactured goods. The emphasis in propaganda was on the claim that Germany was fighting a defensive war and one that Germany itself had not chosen but could not avoid. *'Make clear'*, Göbbels directed party officials, *'that we are engaged in a fateful struggle of the German people which was imposed upon it by the English plutocracy. Germany is fighting for its freedom, for its honour, for its future.'*

The invasion of the Soviet Union in June 1941 did not bring an immediate change in the tone of Nazi propaganda. The success of German armies in the first weeks and months of the campaign led to a mood of confidence that the war would be over very soon. By December 1941, however, as the German advance was halted and the campaign became a long, bitter and costly war of attrition, through the depths of the Russian winter, Göbbels ordered a more sober and realistic tone in Nazi propaganda. Heavy air-raids and cuts in food rations also damaged civilian morale. The defeat of German armies at Stalingrad had a much more profound effect. It was also a disaster for Nazi propagandists. Having confidently predicted victory in the early stages of the battle, the propagandists had an almost impossible task in explaining away a devastating defeat. *'Stalingrad was the greatest single blow of the war'* wrote the historian Kershaw, *'Deep shock, dismay and depression were recorded everywhere.'*

In these circumstances Göbbels recognised the need to prepare the German people for a long, drawn-out struggle which had now become one for the survival of the German Reich. Göbbels used propaganda to justify the increasing sacrifices which were being demanded from the German people and to enlist their support for a strategy of total war. In this new climate, Nazi propaganda concentrated on a number of themes:

■ **Anti-Bolshevism.** Göbbels stated in February 1943 that *'the fight against Bolshevism must dominate all the propaganda instruments as the great and all-pervading propaganda theme'*. Germany was now engaged in a struggle for survival and the theme of anti-Bolshevism was used to frighten the German people with the threat of a Soviet invasion. Reports of atrocities carried out by Red Army troops in occupied territories, including the massacre of Polish officers at Katyn, were used to generate an atmosphere of fear and hatred towards the USSR.

■ **Anti-Semitism.** Anti-Semitism had always been a part of Nazi propaganda but, after the defeat of Stalingrad, the anti-Jewish campaign became a major preoccupation. Emphasis was placed on the *'war guilt of international Jewry which, through its Bolshevist-plutocratic satellites has imposed this struggle [on the German nation]'*.

■ **Strengthening resolve.** Göbbels was concerned that the cumulative effect of the air-raids and the high rates of casualties suffered by the civilian population would weaken the resolve of the German people to continue the war. *'The sole task of propaganda is to strengthen the will to resist, but on no account to antagonise the population,'* wrote Göbbels in 1943.

■ **Retaliation.** This became a major theme in the last two years of the war. Göbbels was at pains to reassure people of the strength of Germany's position and that the country still possessed the means, and the will, to strike back at the enemy. *'We know that against British-US bomb terror, there is only one effective remedy, counter-terror. One day, the hour of retribution will come,'* (Göbbels, 1943). Hopes were kept alive by claims that Germany possessed secret weapons of mass destruction which would be used at an appropriate moment. When the first flying bombs were launched against London in June 1944 this was hailed as the start of Germany's retaliation and the weapon was named the V1 to signify that this was the first in a series of such secret weapons.

Göbbels' task as propaganda minister in the final two years of the war was to sustain the morale of the German people. Despite all Göbbels' efforts, however, Nazi propaganda failed to prevent war-weariness and disillusionment with the regime developing among the German people. There was a growing gap between the realities of people's lives, especially those affected by the air-raids, and the images presented in Nazi propaganda. One of the main casualties in this climate of disillusionment and growing scepticism was the Hitler myth. The popular support for Hitler himself was still sufficient to sustain the myth as late as the beginning of 1943, but the defeat at Stalingrad gave a decisive boost to its decline. Hitler himself had assumed overall command of the German armed forces and it was his decisions which led the German army at Stalingrad to a catastrophic defeat. His aura of omniscience and omnipotence was fatally damaged by the defeat. After Stalingrad, direct criticism of Hitler himself became more common. Hitler increasingly withdrew from public life and was rarely seen or heard. By 1945, according to the historian Ian Kershaw, *'The potency of the Hitler myth had vanished. Silent bitterness replaced the earlier adulation of the Führer.'* In other words, the cult of the führer which had once exerted such a powerful influence over the German people had crumbled beneath feelings of disappointment and resentment, which most found difficult even speak of. It was still dangerous to openly criticise Hitler in 1945, and he was still held in awe by his own party, but it is unlikely that many Germans mourned his death at the end of April 1945. Nazi propaganda, which for so long had moulded the thinking of millions of Germans, had ultimately failed under the pressure of war and defeat.

Activity

Thinking point

How did the aims of Nazi propaganda change after the invasion of the Soviet Union in June 1941?

Exploring the detail

The Katyn massacre

At the same time as the Germans were invading Poland from the west in 1939, the Soviet Union invaded from the east as part of a division of Poland agreed in the Nazi-Soviet Pact. In an effort to eliminate the Polish officer class and other opponents of Soviet control in eastern Poland, the Russian secret police (NKVD) rounded up some 22,000 officers, policemen, intellectuals and civilian prisoners of war and executed them in the Katyn Forest on 5 March 1940. Their mass graves were discovered by the Germans in 1943.

Activity

Thinking point

How far did the realities of war undermine the effectiveness of Nazi propaganda in the years 1943–45?

Summary questions

1. Explain why the 'Hitler myth' was claimed by Göbbels to have been his greatest success as a propagandist.

2. How far did the aims of Nazi propaganda change during the course of World War Two?

Learning outcomes

In this section, you have looked at the aims, methods and successes and failures of Nazi propaganda. Propaganda was of vital importance to the Nazi regime in helping it to gain and to hold onto power. The Nazi propaganda chief, Josef Göbbels, therefore played a key role in the regime. The Nazis were very skilful at using modern technology and the power of the State to spread their propaganda and control the German people's access to information. After reading this section, you should be able to assess the strength of the Hitler myth in the Third Reich, the differences between appearance and reality in Nazi economic policy, and how the war had an impact on the success or failure of Nazi propaganda efforts.

Practice questions

(a) Explain why the the Nazi regime tried to control information in the years 1933 to 1939.

(12 marks)

Study tip This is a short, essay-style question which requires you to identify a range of factors which explain why the regime wanted to control information. You should try to identify a minimum of three factors and write a paragraph of explanation about each. Examiners will be looking for evidence that you have both knowledge and understanding of the issue and, in order for you to reach the higher levels in the mark scheme you will need to be able to show links between the factors and to differentiate between them (perhaps in terms of most important/least important, or in terms of political/ideological factors).

(b) 'Most Nazi propaganda was ineffective.' Explain why you agree or disagree with this view.

(24 marks)

Study tip This requires a longer answer as it is worth more marks. Remember that before you start you should identify the key words in the question. Focus on these key words in your answer. With questions of this type you need to consider points on which you agree and points on which you disagree with the quotation. Your answer will need to show balance between agreement and disagreement, although ultimately you should come down on one side or the other. You should aim to produce an answer that has a clear line of argument running through it, that looks at both sides of the debate and that has carefully selected factual information to support the points that you are making. Finally, end with a clear conclusion in which you make a judgment.

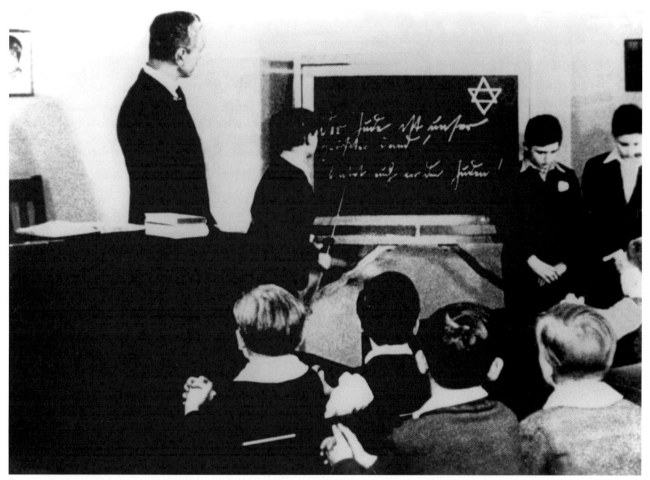

Fig. 1 *Jewish children were humiliated in school, as teachers became agents of Nazi propaganda. The words on the blackboard read, 'The Jew is our greatest enemy. Beware of the Jew'*

In this chapter you will learn about:

- why, how and with what success the Nazis tried to influence education and the German youth

- the impact of the Nazi regime on workers and peasants

- the relationship between the Nazi regime and the Churches.

Gleichschaltung – which literally means 'forcing into line' – was the process through which the Nazis attempted to control or 'coordinate' all aspects of German society. It was Hitler's intention that there should be no independent organisations standing between the State and the individual. Individuals would have no private space in which they could either think or act independently of the regime. All Germans must be made to conform to the norms of the regime in order that the Nazis could achieve their ultimate aim of creating a *Volksgemeinschaft*, or 'people's community'. The *Volksgemeinschaft* would be unified by blood, race and ideology, with a common bond of loyalty to the Führer. Through the coordination of German society, using propaganda and indoctrination, and through terror and repression, the Nazis aimed to eliminate all opposition and create a community in which all 'national comrades' would be loyal to the Führer, show self-discipline and a readiness to make personal sacrifices.

Men would be imbued with a fighting spirit and women would be willing to place their bodies at the service of the State by producing large numbers of children. In short, the Nazis aimed at nothing less than the creation of a new German man and a new German woman. The starting point for this experiment in social engineering was Germany's youth.

■ Youth

Schools and universities

In our eyes the German boy of the future must be slender and supple, swift as greyhounds, tough as leather and hard as Krupp steel. We must bring up a new type of human being, men and girls who are disciplined and healthy to the core. We have undertaken to give the German people an education that begins in youth and will never come to an end. It starts with the child and will end with the 'old fighter'. Nobody will be able to say that he has a time in which he is left entirely alone to himself.

| 1 | *From a speech by Adolf Hitler to the 1935 Nuremberg Rally* |

■ Cross-reference

The Nazis' use of the school curriculum for propaganda purposes has been dealt with above on pages 48–50.

■ Activity

Source analysis

Read Source 1. What were the aims of Nazi education policy?

Schools

Coordination of the education system in Germany was the responsibility of Bernhard Rust, the Education Minister. He did this in a variety of ways:

  Under the Law for the Re-establishment of a Professional Civil Service (1933), a number of teachers were dismissed on the grounds of political unreliability or because they were Jewish.

■ Teachers were pressurised into joining the National Socialist Teachers' League (NSLB). Only Catholic teachers retained their own Catholic Teachers' League but this was closed in 1937. By 1937, 97% of teachers had joined the NSLB and the majority had been sent on the one-month training course in which they were indoctrinated with Nazi ideology and obliged to participate in physical training. Most teachers were willing to comply with the regime's demands. The historian Fest has claimed that *'the teaching profession was one of the most politically reliable sections of the population.'*

■ Local Nazi officials kept an eye on what was happening in schools. Although there was no direct surveillance of lessons, teachers were aware that they could be denounced to the authorities by their pupils if they made any criticism of the regime.

■ Vetting of textbooks was undertaken by local Nazi committees after 1933. From 1935, central directives were issued by the Ministry of Education covering what could be taught and, by 1938, these rules covered every school year and most subjects.

■ Schools were run on the *Führerprinzip* (leadership principle). Headteachers were appointed from outside the schools and teaching staff were obliged to accept orders from above.

■ Cross-reference

The *Führerprinzip* is explained on page 17.

■ Key profile

Bernhard Rust

Rust (1883–1945) had worked as a schoolteacher before being sacked in 1930 for molesting a pupil. He had been a member of the Nazi Party since 1922 and was elected to the Reichstag in 1930. He became Reich minister of education in 1934. He committed suicide in 1945.

The Nazi regime did not make major changes to the structure of the school system but new Nazi institutions were created alongside the existing schools:

- Napola schools (National Political Institutes of Education) were created for boys between the ages of ten and eighteen. These were boarding schools which provided a military-style education. There was a heavy emphasis on physical education and drill, manual labour and political indoctrination. After 1936, these Napola schools came under the control of the SS. By 1938, 21 of these schools had been established across Germany.

- Adolf Hitler Schools, set up after 1937 by the leaders of the Hitler Youth and the German Labour Front (DAF), Baldur von Schirach and Robert Ley. These were for boys aged from twelve to eighteen and provided a military-style education but were more selective in their admissions policy than the Napolas, being intended purely for the future Nazi elite.

- *Ordensburgen* (Castles of Order) were large boarding schools, catering for one thousand students at a time from the 25–30 age group. Described by Fest as *'finishing schools for the future leadership'*, they were designed to complete the training of selected youths after school, army service and professional training.

Activity

Revision exercise

Construct a table with two vertical columns, under the heading 'Nazi control of education'. Put the headings 'Direct control' in the first column and 'Indirect control' in the second. Rearrange the information in this section into the two columns.

Key profile

Baldur von Schirach

Schirach (1907–74) joined the Nazi Party in 1924 while still a student and was head of the National Socialist German Students' League from 1929–31. He became Reich youth leader in 1933, continuing in this post until 1940. He was later governor of Vienna before he was arrested by the Allies and sentenced to 20 years imprisonment at the Nuremberg Trials.

Universities

With their stress on physical education and political indoctrination, the Nazis downgraded the importance of academic education and the number of students attending university decreased considerably between 1933 and 1939. Thereafter there was some expansion of university places. Access to higher education was therefore strictly rationed and selection was made on the basis of political reliability. Women were restricted to 10% of the available university places, while Jews were restricted to 1.5%, their proportion within the population as a whole.

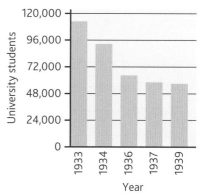

Fig. 2 *Numbers of students in German universities, 1933–39*

Coordination of universities followed much the same pattern as schools:

- Under the Law for the Re-establishment of a Professional Civil Service, about 1,200 university staff were dismissed on racial or political grounds. This amounted to around 15% of the total.

- In November 1933, all university teachers were made to sign a 'Declaration in support of Hitler and the National Socialist State'.

- University teachers were obliged to join the Nazi Lecturers' League and new teachers had to attend training courses where they were subjected to political indoctrination and physical training.
- Students had to join the German Students' League (DS), although some 25% managed to avoid doing this.
- Students had to attend twice-weekly political indoctrination and physical training sessions. They were also forced to do four months labour service and two months in an SA camp. Labour service would give students experience of real life, considered by the Nazis to be more important than academic learning.
- The university curriculum was modified, especially in history, geography, biology and German.

The Nazis encountered very little resistance to their policies of bringing the universities under their control. Indeed, coordination was made easier by the voluntary self-coordination of many faculties. Even in the Weimar period, the universities had been dominated by nationalist and anti-democratic attitudes and traditional student 'fraternities' were a breeding ground for reactionary politics. The Nazis were, therefore, able to tap into a pre-existing culture of extreme nationalism and infuse it with Nazi ideology. This was helped by the students' knowledge that their prospects of employment after graduating depended on showing outward support for the regime. The regime's efforts to coordinate universities were also aided by the fact that there was considerable support for its ideology among university teachers.

Activity

Thinking point

Explain why the Nazis were able 'coordinate' the universities with very little resistance.

The Hitler Youth

> What I liked about the Hitler Youth was the comradeship. I was full of enthusiasm when I joined the Jungvolk at the age of ten. What boy isn't fired by being presented with high ideas such as comradeship, loyalty and honour.

2 *Recollections of a former Hitler Youth member, quoted in Noakes, J. and Pridham, G., **Nazism 1919–45, Vol. 2**, 1984*

Before 1933, Germany had a thriving youth culture with many successful youth organisations. Some were linked to churches, others to political parties; there was also a flourishing 'free youth' movement which encouraged independence of mind and action among the young. The *Hitler Jugend* (HJ) or Hitler Youth was created in 1926 and in its early years was relatively unsuccessful. When the Nazis came to power in 1933, all other youth organisations, except those linked to the Catholic Church, were either banned or taken over by the Hitler Youth. Only then did the Nazis' own youth movement begin to flourish.

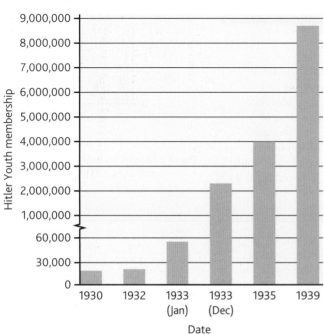

Fig. 3 *Membership of the Hitler Youth, 1930–39*

In 1936, a Law for the Incorporation of German Youth gave the Hitler Youth the status of an official education movement, equal in status to schools and the home. At the same time, Catholic youth organisations were banned and the Hitler Youth became the only officially permitted youth organisation. By 1936 also, the Hitler Youth had been granted a monopoly over all sports facilities and competitions for children under the age of 14. Membership of the Hitler Youth was made compulsory in 1939.

Table 1 *Divisions of the Hitler Youth*

Age	Division
6–10	*Pimpfen* (Cubs)
10–14	*Deutsches Jungvolk* (German Youth)
14–18	*Hitler Jugend* (Hitler Youth)

At the age of 18 boys who were not already in employment could be drafted into the Reich Labour Service (RAD), or they could be conscripted into the armed forces.

Cross-reference

For more information about the Reich Labour Service (RAD), see page 78.

In the Hitler Youth, there was a constant diet of political indoctrination and physical activity. Boys from the age of ten were taught the motto *'Live Faithfully, Fight Bravely and Die Laughing'*. The emphasis in youth activities was on competition, struggle, heroism and leadership, as boys were prepared for their future role as warriors. Hitler Youth members had to swear a personal oath of allegiance to the Führer. There was a set syllabus of political indoctrination which all members had to follow and a heavy emphasis on military drill. Boys were taught to sing Nazi songs and encouraged to read Nazi political pamphlets. They were taken on hikes and on camping trips. Ritual, ceremonies and the singing of songs reinforced their induction into Nazi ideology.

The opportunity to participate in sports and camping trips away from home made the organisation attractive to millions of German boys, many of whom grew up in the 1930s with no experience of any other system. For these boys, their growing up was shaped by the Hitler Youth and the Nazi emphasis on struggle, sacrifice, loyalty and discipline became accepted as the norm. Many children joined against the wishes of their parents who were not Nazi sympathisers and who had grown up in a different era. For these boys, the Hitler Youth offered an outlet for their teenage rebelliousness. By the late 1930s, however, as the organisation became more bureaucratic and there was a growing emphasis on military drill and training, there were signs that enthusiasm was beginning to wane. There were reports of poor attendance at weekly parades. Boys resented the harsh punishments imposed for minor infringements of the rules.

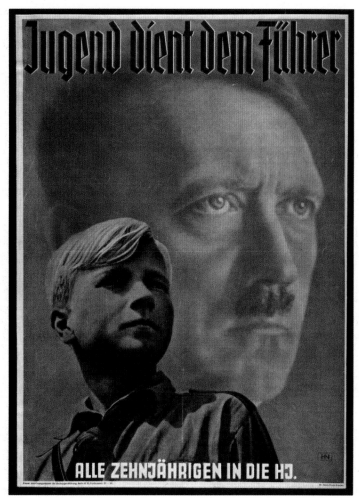

Fig. 4 *A recruiting poster for the Hitler Youth from 1936. The slogan reads, 'All ten-year-olds in the Hitler Youth'*

Activity

Source analysis

1. Sources 2 and 3 were written by the same author. What can we learn from these sources about the attitudes of young Germans towards the Hitler Youth?

2. How far did young people's attitudes towards the Hitler Youth change between 1933 and 1939?

3. Does the fact that membership of the Hitler Youth grew dramatically between 1933 and 1939 (see Figure 3) mean that we should doubt the reliability of these sources?

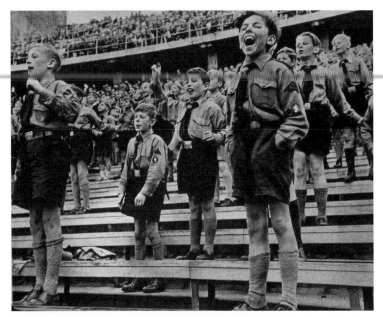

Fig. 5 *Members of the Hitler Youth at a rally in 1936*

Later, however, when I became a leader in the Jungvolk the negative aspects became very obvious. I found the compulsion and the requirement of absolute obedience unpleasant. I appreciated that there must be order and discipline in such a large group of boys, but it was exaggerated. It was preferred that people should not have a will of their own and should totally subordinate themselves.

*A former Hitler Youth member recounts his growing disillusionment, quoted in Noakes, J. and Pridham, G., **Nazism 1919–45, Vol. 2**, 1984*

The League of German Girls

We wanted the 'New German Woman' to be the bearer of German culture and moral standards for the whole people. Our aim was that they should achieve health, self-discipline, courage and, later on with the gymnastics, gracefulness – in the sense of beautiful harmonious movement which also reflects a healthy mind and body.

*Jutta Rüdiger, BDM leader, quoted in Haste, C., **Nazi Women**, 2001*

The *Bund Deutscher Mädel* (BDM) or League of German Girls was the female equivalent of the Hitler Youth. Its motto – *'Be Faithful, Be Pure, Be German'* – was part of a process of preparing girls for their future role as housewives and mothers in the *Volksgemeinschaft*. Membership became compulsory in 1939.

Table 2 *Divisions of the BDM*

Age	Division
10–14	*Jung Mädel* (Young Girls)
14–18	*Bund Deutscher Mädel* (League of German Girls)
18–21	*Glaube und Schönheit* (Faith and Beauty)

In the BDM, girls were taught that they had a duty to be healthy since their bodies belonged to the nation. They needed to be fit for their future role as childbearers. They were also instructed in matters of hygiene, cleanliness and healthy eating. Formation dancing and group gymnastics served the dual purpose of raising fitness and developing comradeship. At weekly 'home evenings', girls were taught handicrafts, sewing and cooking. There were also sessions for political education and racial awareness. Annual summer camps were highly structured, every minute being taken up with sports, physical exercise, route marches, as well as indoctrination, flag waving and saluting. In the Faith and Beauty groups, young women were instructed in baby care and social skills such as ballroom dancing.

> Your body belongs to your nation, to which you owe your existence and for which you are responsible.
>
> Always keep yourself clean, tend and exercise your body. Light, air and water can help you in this.
>
> Look after your teeth. Strong and healthy teeth are a source of pride.
>
> Eat plenty of raw fruit, uncooked greens and vegetables, first washing them thoroughly in clean water.
>
> Drink fruit juice. Leave coffee to the coffee addicts.
>
> Shun alcohol and nicotine; they are poisons which impair your development and capacity for work.
>
> Take physical exercise. It will make you healthy and hardy. Sleep at least nine hours every night.
>
> Practise first aid for use in accidents. It can help you save your comrades' lives.
>
> All your activities are governed by the slogan: 'Your duty is to be healthy'.

5   *Rules of the BDM, quoted in Haste, C.,* **Nazi Women***, 2001*

Many girls found their experiences in the BDM liberating. They were doing things which their mothers had not been allowed to do and they could escape from the constraints of the home. They also developed a sense of comradeship. Although strictly run on the leadership principle, the BDM groups were relatively classless, bringing together on an equal footing girls from a wide range of backgrounds. This was, of course, part of the strategy for capturing the minds of German youth and moulding them to the purposes of the Nazi regime. Racial awareness was an important element in this indoctrination. Jutta Rüdiger, the leader of the BDM, instructed girls on their future partners in marriage: *'Only the best German soldier is suitable for you, for it is your responsibility to keep the blood of the nation pure. German girl, your honour lies in being faithful to the blood of your race.'*

Key profile

Jutta Rüdiger

Rüdiger (1910–2001) was a psychologist who had been a committed Nazi since her days as a student in the 1920s. In 1937, she became the leader of the BDM but, as a woman, her position was subordinate to that of the overall youth leader, Baldur von Schirach. She continued to lead the BDM until 1945. At the end of the war, she was arrested by the Americans and spent two years in prison but was never charged with any specific offence.

Activity

Source analysis

What can we learn from Source 5 about the aims of the BDM?

Activity

Thinking point

1. In what ways were girls' lives regimented and controlled through their membership of the BDM?

2. In what ways was the BDM a 'liberating' experience for young girls?

After 1934, girls were expected to do a year's work on the land or in domestic service. The aim was to put girls in touch with their peasant roots and give them practical experience in child care. It also developed their sense of serving the community. This was very unpopular with girls from the cities and many tried to avoid it. In 1939, this scheme was made compulsory. All young women up to the age of 25 had to do a year's unpaid work with the Reich Labour Service before they could get paid employment. This was the female equivalent to compulsory military service for the boys and was part of the growing 'coordination' of all levels of German society under Nazi rule.

Workers

The working class and the Nazi Party

In 1933, the working class was the largest socio-economic group in German society, making up 46% of the economically active population. For this reason alone, their support was needed by political parties seeking to gain power in Weimar Germany. A large proportion of working-class voters in the 1920s and early 1930s had supported the socialist SPD, with a substantial minority voting for the communist KPD. Not all working-class voters, however, voted on the basis of class loyalty. In predominantly Catholic areas such as the Rhineland, workers tended to join Catholic trade unions and vote for the Catholic Centre Party. Trade unions were an important and powerful force in German industry and in politics. The Weimar constitution had recognised the legal right of workers to join trade unions and, during the Weimar period, workers had been able to participate in the running of their workplaces through elected Works' Councils. Mass unemployment in the early 1930s, however, had weakened trade unions and undermined the cohesion of working-class communities.

Attracting working-class support was important to the Nazi Party. By adopting the name National Socialist German Workers' Party, the Nazis had made a conscious effort to win working-class support away from socialism and communism. Many radical elements within the Nazi Party before 1934 were active in the National Socialist Factory Cell Organisation (NSBO) which used anti-capitalist, class war rhetoric to win working-class support. Nazism, however, relied mainly on support from peasant farmers, small craftsmen and small shopkeepers and the party did best in rural areas and small towns in predominantly Protestant areas of northern Germany, not in the main industrial areas. Recent studies, however, have indicated that in the early 1930s the Nazis were attracting growing support from industrial workers. According to Conan Fischer (*The Rise of the Nazis*, 1995), 40% of Nazi voters and party members were working class. It appears, therefore, that hostility towards the Nazis in many working-class communities was beginning to break down by 1933, although it must be remembered that the majority of working-class voters did not vote for the Nazi Party, even as late as March 1933.

The Nazis aimed to create a 'people's community' in which class differences, religious loyalties, regional, age and gender differences would all be put aside and replaced by an all-embracing national unity. Given their traditional ties to trade unions and non-Nazi political parties, industrial workers presented the greatest challenge to the process of *Gleichschaltung*. The Nazis could not ignore the working class, nor could they rely solely on repression to achieve their objective of 'coordinating' this very important part of German society.

Exploring the detail

Trade unions in the Weimar Republic

Before 1933, there were three main groups of trade unions in Germany:

- Free Trade Unions, which were linked to the socialist SPD. This was the largest trade union group.
- Catholic Christian trade unions, which were linked to the Centre Party.
- Hirsch-Duncker unions, which were linked to the Liberal Party. This was the smallest of the three groups.

Activity

Thinking point

1 Explain why Hitler was keen to win working-class support for the Nazi Party before 1933.

2 What were the main reasons why the majority of the working class did not support the Nazi Party before 1933?

Exploring the detail

The NSBO

The NSBO was involved in a number of strikes before 1933. While it was useful to Hitler to have a grass-roots Nazi organisation which was in direct competition with the socialist and the communists, the NSBO alienated the business leaders and conservative elite whom Hitler needed in order to achieve and retain power. The leader of the NSBO, Richard Muchow, wanted his organisation to become a gigantic trade union, representing every worker in the country. In 1934, the NSBO was purged of its radical leadership by Hitler and it was subordinated to the German Labour Front (DAF).

The German Labour Front (DAF)

The *Deutsches Arbeitsfront* (DAF), or German Labour Front, was established on 6 May 1933, under the leadership of Robert Ley, to undertake the coordination of workers into the National Socialist regime. With the Free Trade Unions having been banned on 2 May, and the Hirsch-Dunker unions voluntarily disbanding soon after, only the Catholic trade unions remained – albeit temporarily – as independent organisations of the working class. The DAF took over the assets of the banned trade unions and became the largest organisation in the Third Reich. Although membership of the DAF was not compulsory, its membership grew rapidly since it was the only officially recognised organisation representing workers.

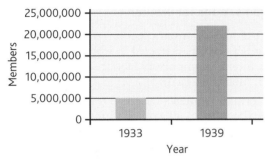

Fig. 6 *Membership of the DAF, 1933–39*

Key profile

Robert Ley

A former fighter pilot in the First World War, Ley (1890–1945) joined the Nazi Party in 1924. He was elected to the Reichstag in 1930, became Reich organisation leader in 1932 and leader of the DAF in 1933. He committed suicide in 1945.

The DAF had two main aims: to win the workers over to the *Volksgemeinschaft*, and to encourage workers to increase production. Because it was a symbol of the Nazi *Volksgemeinschaft*, the DAF included employers as well as workers. It was organised on the leadership principle, with Robert Ley giving instructions to his subordinates. The DAF replaced the trade unions but was not a trade union itself. It had no role in bargaining over wages and little influence over the regime's social and economic policies. It did, however, have its own propaganda department to spread Nazi ideology among working-class Germans. It also established a subsidiary organisation, Strength Through Joy, to organise workers' leisure time. In 1936, the DAF started to provide vocational training courses to improve workers' skills. The DAF also built up a large business empire of its own. This included banks and insurance companies, housing associations and construction companies, the Volkswagen car plant and its own travel company. By 1939, the DAF had 44,500 paid employees.

Relations between employers and employees in Nazi Germany were governed by two laws:

- the Law on the Trustees of Labour, issued on 19 May 1933, which gave the power to fix wages to appointed officials
- the Law for the Ordering of National Labour, issued on 20 January 1934, which established the basic principles on which workplaces would be run.

Key chronology

The Nazi coordination of labour

1933

4 April	Nazi takeover of works councils: socialists, communists and other non-Nazis purged
1 May	May Day parades taken over by Nazi regime as new national holiday
2 May	Free Trade Unions' offices occupied by Nazis; funds confiscated and leaders arrested. Hirsch-Dunker trade unions disbanded voluntarily. Catholic trade unions continued temporarily
6 May	German Labour Front established
19 May	Law on Trustees of Labour controls wage fixing

1934

20 January	Law for the Ordering of National Labour, governing the organisation of workplaces

Exploring the detail

Corruption in the DAF

The DAF gained a reputation as one of the most corrupt of all Nazi organisations. With its extensive business interests and vast funds to award contracts, there were many examples of local DAF officials using their positions to enrich themselves. DAF funds were embezzled by officials and bribes were offered to them to secure contracts. Local officials took their lead from Robert Ley. He used his position to acquire several houses, cars and valuable paintings. He was a serial womaniser and heavy drinker but, although Hitler was aware of Ley's many failings, he did not dismiss nor censure him.

Activity

Discussion point

1. What were the aims of the DAF?

2. How did the organisation of the DAF reflect Nazi ideology?

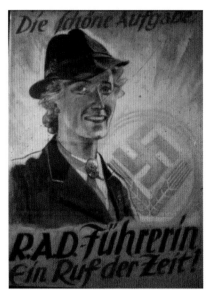

Fig. 7 *The Reich Labour Service recruited young women for various types of work. This poster from the 1930s carries the slogan, 'A job for today'*

Exploring the detail

The Reich Labour Service

The *Reichsarbeitsdienst* (RAD), or Reich Labour Service, was established in 1934 as a State labour organisation to combat unemployment. There had been voluntary labour schemes during the last years of the Weimar Republic under which the unemployed were sent to work camps to work in agriculture, forestry or public works. The Nazis extended the scheme and introduced an element of compulsion. During the war, the RAD became a civilian auxiliary organisation working with the army.

Cross-reference

For more information on Robert Ley, see page 77.

The Nazi system of labour relations was heavily weighted in favour of the employer and the State. Workers in the Third Reich came under increasing pressure to work harder and accept a squeeze on wages and living standards. Nazi propaganda tried to promote the message that the reward for working was not material gain but the knowledge that they were serving the community. Nevertheless, the Nazis were well aware that they could not take workers for granted and that there had to be some tangible compensation for the demands that were placed upon them. Improved leisure facilities and opportunities, provided by Strength Through Joy, were a key part of this strategy.

A closer look

Nazi organisations for women

- The DAF had a women's section, the *Frauenfront*. The Reich Labour Service was extended to women in 1939 and provided for six months compulsory labour service for young women aged 19–25, mostly on farms.

- The German Women's League (DFW) was set up in September 1933 to coordinate all women's groups under Nazi control. It had a domestic science department which gave advice to women on cooking and healthy eating. By 1939, the DFW had over six million members, 70% of whom were not members of the Nazi Party.

- The National Socialist Women's Organisation (NS-F) was an elite organisation to promote the nation's 'lovelife, marriage, the family, blood and race'. It was primarily an organisation for propaganda and indoctrination among women to promote the Nazi ideology that women should be child-rearers and home-makers.

- The Reich Mother's Service (RMD) was a branch of the DFW for training *physically and mentally able mothers, to make them convinced of the important duties of motherhood, experienced in the care and education of their children and competent to carry out their domestic tasks'*. By March 1939, 1.7 million women had attended its motherhood training services.

- The National Socialist Welfare Organisation (NS-V) catered for the welfare needs of both men and women. Its Mother and Child section established 25,000 advice centres to help women with child welfare. It also helped the unemployed and gave education grants to children. The scheme was financed by public collections and deductions from wages.

Strength Through Joy

The *Kraft durch Freude* (KdF), or Strength Through Joy, organisation was set up by Robert Ley and the DAF to organise workers' leisure time. The basic idea behind the scheme was w orkers would *'gain strength for their work by experiencing joy in their leisure'*. Workers who were refreshed by holidays, sports and cultural activities would be more efficient when they returned to work. The KdF also aimed:

- to submerge the individual in the mass and encourage workers to see themselves as part of a *Volksgemeinschaft*. With leisure time as well as work time regulated by the regime, there would be no time or space for workers to develop private lives. To this end, the KdF was a propagandist organisation which used its activities to indoctrinate workers and their families into Nazi ideology.

- to encourage a spirit of social equality. All KdF activities were organised on a one-class basis with no distinction between rich and poor.

- to bring Germans from the different regions of the country together and to break down regional and religious differences.

- to encourage participation in sport to improve the physical and mental health of the nation. Every youth in employment was obliged to undertake two hours each week of physical education at their workplace.

- to encourage competition and ambition. A KdF National Trades Competition was organised for apprentices to improve skills and standards of work.

Through the KdF, workers were offered subsidised holidays in Germany and abroad, sporting activities, hikes, and theatre and cinema visits at reduced prices. Classical music concerts were put on in lunch breaks in factories. There were KdF wardens in every factory and workplace employing more than 20 people. Supporting these were over 7,000 paid employees of the organisation by 1939. Membership of the KdF came automatically with membership of the DAF so that, by 1936, 35 million belonged to it.

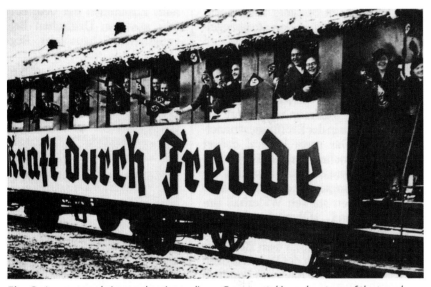

Fig. 8 *A propaganda image showing ordinary Germans taking advantage of the travel opportunites provided by Strength through Joy. This was a special KdF holiday train*

Exploring the detail

The KdF resort at Prora

The building of the model KdF resort at Prora, on the Baltic coast, was begun in 1936. It was planned to be eight kilometres long, with large residential blocks and communal refectories. The resort centred on a huge communal hall that could hold 20,000 people. It was designed for families and prices were low enough for working-class families to afford. Facilities were very modern, with central heating in the apartments, cinemas, a heated swimming pool and bowling alleys. The design, however, was soulless, with long featureless corridors in the residential blocks and large scale, monumental architecture dwarfing the people. Regimentation even extended to allocating a space for each family on the beach. Construction was halted in 1940 because of the war and the resort was never finished.

Mass tourism was one of the KdF's most successful activities, and cruises to foreign destinations opened up new opportunities for many Germans. By 1939, the KdF owned eight cruise ships and rented four more. Cruises took ordinary Germans to Madeira, Libya, Finland, Norway, Bulgaria and Turkey. Rail trips took Germans to Italy and countries in south-eastern Europe. KdF ships were built on a one-class basis to emphasise the unity and classlessness of the *Volksgemeinschaft*. Facilities on board ships included gyms, theatres, and swimming pools. Life on the cruise ships was regimented. Passengers were instructed to dress modestly, to avoid excessive drinking, not to have holiday affairs with other passengers and to obey the instructions of their tour leaders. In case any passengers might be tempted to voice critical opinions of the regime, Gestapo and SS agents travelled on the cruises to spy on them. The cruises were designed to demonstrate to the world how socially and technologically advanced Germans had become under the Nazi regime, and to remind Germans how superior they were to the inhabitants of the countries they visited.

Yet the reality of the cruise ships actually contradicted the ideological assumptions on which the whole enterprise was based. Tickets were too expensive for ordinary working-class wage earners and passengers were drawn mainly from the better-off middle classes. Only ten per cent of the passengers on one cruise to Norway were from the working class. The best cabins on the ships, those above the water-line, were allocated to party officials and civil servants. There was little mixing between classes on the ships and there were reports of fights between passengers from different regions of Germany. Gestapo agents reported mass drunkenness and riotous behaviour, especially from party officials. The worst offender was Robert Ley himself who frequently went on KdF cruises where he spent his time getting drunk and womanising. A popular nickname for the KdF was the 'big-wigs' knocking shop' (i.e. 'important persons' brothel').

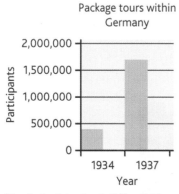
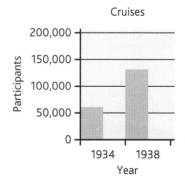
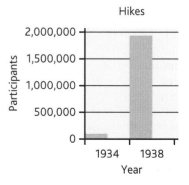

Fig. 9 *Participation in KdF activities*

Despite the gap between myth and reality in the KdF, it was one of the regime's most popular organisations. By offering opportunities that were not available to ordinary Germans before 1933, the KdF was valued by workers and thus helped to reconcile people, even former opponents, to the regime.

Activity

Discussion point

Did German workers in the 1930s view the KdF as a genuine benefit to themselves or as a cynical attempt by the regime to win their support?

Strength Through Joy is very popular. The events appeal to the yearning of the little man who wants an opportunity to get out and about himself and participate in the pleasures of the 'top people'. It's a clever appeal to the petty-bourgeois inclinations of the unpolitical worker. For such a man, it's really something if he goes on a Scandinavian cruise or even just travels to the Black Forest or the Harz Mountains. He imagines that this has moved him up a rung on the social ladder.

6   *From a Sopade report, Berlin, February 1938, quoted in Noakes, J., and Pridham, G.,* **Nazism 1919–45, Vol. 2,** *1984*

Beauty of Labour

The KdF department devoted to improving conditions at the workplace was *Schönheit der Arbeit*, or Beauty of Labour. Its aim was to get workers to work harder. Beauty of Labour campaigned for better washing facilities and toilets in factories. As with many Nazi social policies, there was a preoccupation with health and fitness which linked to the Nazi's ideological belief in racial health. Beauty of Labour encouraged the provision of sports and recreation facilities at the workplace, and campaigned for employers to provide canteens serving hot, nourishing meals. The regime claimed that, by 1938, 34,000 companies had improved their working conditions and facilities. Tax incentives were used to encourage employers to do this and

Beauty of Labour organized competitions and awarded prizes for the most improved firms. Winners were issued with certificates signed by Hitler stating that they were 'model firms'.

It was the workers, however, who had to bear the brunt of the cost of these improvements. Many firms expected their workers to paint the factory, clean up the working environment and build the new facilities in their own time and for no extra pay. 'Contributions' were taken from their wages to cover the costs and those who refused to 'volunteer' for these extra duties were threatened with dismissal.

The effectiveness of Nazi policies towards workers

The evidence from Sopade and Gestapo reports show that workers' reactions to these Nazi schemes to win their support were mixed. Many workers, of course, had been influenced by socialist and communist ideas before 1933 and would therefore have been resistant to Nazi ideology. The reports indicate that many workers were not impressed by Nazi propaganda but were nevertheless prepared to take advantage of what benefits were on offer. The KdF was popular not because people shared its ideological aims but because it offered workers a means of escaping the boredom and pressure of their working lives. German workers took advantage of the holidays and leisure activities because this was the only chance they would get to have some enjoyment and relaxation. A Sopade report from 1935 noted that KdF events *'offer cheap opportunities to find simple relaxation'*. An increase in paid holiday entitlement, from an average of three days per year in 1933 to an average of six to twelve days per year in 1939, was one of the few material benefits that workers gained from Nazi rule and enabled workers to take advantage of KdF opportunities. Many workers also concluded that, since they were paying for the DAF and KdF with compulsory deductions from their wages, they might as well get some benefits from this money.

■ Peasants

In Nazi ideology, the German peasants were regarded as special because they were seen as a racially pure group who had retained their traditional attachment to the German soil. They were portrayed as being free of the moral decline which the Nazis believed had taken root in the cities, especially in the Weimar years. It was the German peasants who would therefore become the nucleus of the *Volksgemeinschaft* which the Nazis attempted to build after January 1933. Nazi policy towards peasants and agriculture was to reverse the drift of population from the countryside to the cities, to relieve the farmers of the burden of debts they had incurred and to establish a harmonious and prosperous *Volksgemeinschaft* in the countryside.

The Reich Food Estate

Richard Darré, who became minister for food and agriculture in the summer of 1933, was in charge of Nazi policy towards farming and the countryside. His vehicle for ensuring the 'coordination' of peasants into the Nazi *Volksgemeinschaft* was the Reich Food Estate. This was a typically Nazi organisation based on the leadership principle. Darré himself was the Reich peasant leader; below him was a hierarchical structure of state, district and local peasant leaders who were all answerable to him. The Reich Food Estate was also similar to other Nazi organisations in that it was very bureaucratic: by 1939, it employed 20,000 full-time officials, working with 113,000 unpaid officials.

■ Activity

Thinking point

Explain why the Nazis gave a high priority to winning the support of the peasants.

 Cross-reference

For a profile of Darré, see page 36.

Darré's aim in establishing the Reich Food Estate was that producers, wholesalers and retailers of agricultural products would be linked together in a single chain, under the direction of his organisation. This, he believed, would eliminate profiteering by the 'middle-men' in the chain and ensure a fair deal for the farmers. All participants would benefit equally and would therefore feel themselves to be part of the wider 'people's community'. The sense of community would be reinforced by removing sources of conflict between the different interest groups and achieving mutual cooperation. In the view of Richard Evans, the Reich Food Estate was seen by Darré as *'the vehicle through which peasant farmers would strengthen their economic interests and claim their rightful place in the new Germany'*.

In practice, the Reich Food Estate, and Nazi policies on agriculture in general, brought mixed results for the peasants:

- The Nazi regime spent a total of 650,000,000 RM in the years 1933–36 to clear farmers' debts. Most of this money, however, went to the owners of large and medium-sized farms; only after 1935 did the smaller farmers benefit from this aid.
- Farmers' incomes increased by 41% between 1933 and 1938. This was a much higher increase than that received by industrial workers, but the profits of industry increased more than farmers' incomes.
- Price controls squeezed farmers' profits, which meant that they could not afford to pay higher wages to their labourers, nor could they afford to buy expensive labour-saving machinery.
- After 1936, the regime had the power to force the merger of smaller farms into larger, more efficient units. This angered many small farmers and conflicted with Nazi 'blood and soil' ideology, but was deemed economically justified in order to achieve higher agricultural production.
- The wages of agricultural labourers increased slowly and they benefited from being exempt from unemployment and health insurance contributions. Their wages were, however, far below those earned by industrial workers in the cities and they also suffered from poor social conditions, especially housing, in the countryside. The result was that the drift of population from the countryside to the towns actually increased during the Third Reich period and, by 1939, there were severe labour shortages in German agriculture.

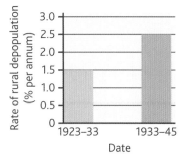

Fig. 10 *Rates of rural depopulation under Weimar and Nazi regimes*

Darré's problem was that the Nazi regime was trying to achieve rapid rearmament and autarky at the same time as he was trying to establish the *Volksgemeinschaft* in the countryside. When the military and economic interests of the Nazi regime clashed with its social objectives, the former took priority. Although farmers needed higher prices to improve their incomes, the interests of consumers in the wider *Volksgemeinschaft* dictated that prices should be held down. When German agriculture failed to achieve self-sufficiency in the production of animal fats, the regime's response was not to invest in agriculture to increase production but to ration consumption. Rearmament led to the need for more airfields, army camps and training grounds, which in turn led to the requisitioning of land from farmers. The building of the West Wall fortifications in the later 1930s, for example, led to the requisitioning of 5,600 farms, with a total of 130,000 hectares being taken out of production.

Did you know?

The West Wall was a line of fortifications, 390 miles long, which stretched from the Dutch border to the border with Switzerland. It was designed to counter a possible French attack on Germany and was placed opposite the French fortifications known as the Maginot Line. The West Wall was built between 1938 and 1940.

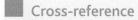

As far as we can observe the mood of the countryside, one must make a distinction between the older and younger generation of peasants. The older peasants are very critical, find it very difficult to get used to the new situation and can hardly get over the fact that their influence in the parish councils has been excluded by opposition forces. The younger generation, on the other hand, which now sits on the parish councils, appears National Socialist to a high degree.

7 *From a Sopade Report, Southern Bavaria, November/December 1934, quoted in Noakes, J., and Pridham, G., **Nazism 1919–45, Vol. 2**, 1984*

Many peasants were unhappy with the Entailed Farm Law. Older peasants were the most likely to be resentful of the regime's policies, whereas many younger farmers took advantage of the opportunities for social and economic advancement provided by the regime. Indeed, so marked was the generation gap in some areas that many villagers remembered the Third Reich as a time of 'war in every household'. Conflict between the generations did not lead to open resistance to the Nazi regime, but the fact that it occurred shows that the regime's aim of creating a *Volksgemeinschaft* in the countryside was far from being achieved.

As the Reich Food Estate faced mounting problems, a strong undercurrent of peasant discontent began to appear and Darré's influence began to wane. After 1936, the German Labour Front took over responsibility for the education and training of agricultural labourers. The social and cultural functions of the Reich Food Estate were taken over by the Nazi Party. Shortages of labour were addressed by drafting in members of the Hitler Youth and the RAD to work on farms. By 1939, the Reich Food Estate was widely regarded as a failure and Darré had been largely marginalised within the regime's hierarchy.

The Churches

Nazism and religion

Coordinating the Churches into the *Volksgemeinschaft* posed serious challenges for the Nazi regime for two main reasons. Firstly, Germans were divided by faith. Although the majority of Germans belonged to the Protestant faith, a significant and large minority were Roman Catholic. Secondly, religious loyalties were very strong and deep-rooted in some communities and were an obstacle to the Nazi aim of making the Führer the focus of loyalty for all Germans. Hitler realised that he could not trample over people's religious convictions and expect to win their wholesale support. He would have to proceed cautiously at first, with his initial objective being to gain control over the Churches before later trying to weaken their influence.

Cross-reference

For more information on the Entailed Farm Law, see pages 35–36.

Activity

Revision exercise

Draw up a balance sheet of the results of Nazi policies towards the peasants. On one side list the successes, on the other side list the failures.

Use this balance sheet to write a paragraph summarising the success/failure of Nazi policy towards the peasants.

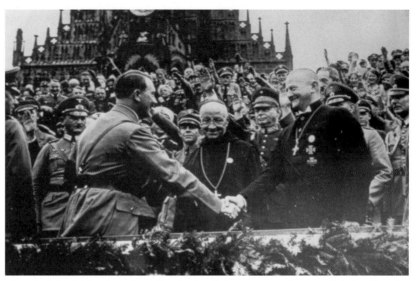

Fig. 11 *Reich Bishop Ludwig Müller, leader of the Protestant German Christian Church, shakes hands with Hitler at the Nuremberg, Rally in 1934*

Activity

Source analysis

Compare the two statements by Hitler in Sources 8 and 9 on his attitude to religion.

How do you explain the difference between the two statements?

Christianity is the unshakeable foundation of the moral life of our people.

> **8** *From a speech by Adolf Hitler to the Reichstag, March 1933, quoted in Hite, J., and Hinton, C., Weimar and Nazi Germany, 2000*

I will make peace with the Church. Why not? It won't stop me eradicating Christianity from Germany root and branch. You are either Christian or a German. You can't be both.

> **9** *Adolf Hitler, from a private conversation, 1933, quoted in Hite, J., and Hinton, C., **Weimar and Nazi Germany**, 2000*

Table 3 *Relative strengths of the two main Churches in Germany during the Weimar period*

	Protestant (German Evangelical Church)	Roman Catholic
Membership	40 million (58% of population)	22 million (32%)
Geographical spread	North and east	South (Bavaria) and west (Rhineland)
Social influence	Youth organisations (0.7 million members)	Youth organisations (1.5 million members), schools and charities
Political influence	Connected to DNVP and DVP	Close link with Centre Party

The Nazis did not have a coherent view towards religion and the Churches. Hitler himself had been raised a Catholic in Austria and he talked often of 'positive Christianity'. Yet at other times Hitler stated that he wanted to eradicate Christianity from Germany. Hitler was hostile to the Christian faith but, especially in the early months of his regime, he was careful not to alienate the Churches and incur their opposition and so tried to reassure Church leaders that Nazism posed no threat to their faith. Other Nazis, notably Alfred Rosenberg and Robert Ley, were atheists who wanted to replace the Christian Churches with a new Nazi faith. This lack of coherence in Nazi religious policy is evident in their dealings with the different Churches.

Activity

Thinking point

What were the main aims of Nazi policy towards the Christian Churches?

Protestants

The main Protestant Church in Germany was the German Evangelical Church, which was divided into 28 separate state Churches. Despite its organisational divisions, the Nazis saw in the Evangelical Church an opportunity for uniting the Germans into a single national Church. Evangelicals were politically very conservative and staunch nationalists, regarding Germany as a Protestant state. Within the German Evangelical Church, there was a strong tradition of respect for, and cooperation with, the State. Indeed, in the Second Reich the German emperor, who was also king of Prussia, was head of the Evangelical Church in his own state. Many Protestants were anti-Semitic and also vigorously anti-communist. There were, therefore, many points of convergence between Nazi ideology and the views of German Protestants and it was no coincidence that, before 1933, the strongest areas of Nazi support were in the Protestant north and east of Germany. In the early months of the Nazi regime, some Nazi-leaning Protestant pastors staged mass weddings of SA brownshirts and their brides. For their part the Nazis, in 1933, turned the 450th anniversary of the birth of Martin Luther into a major national celebration.

■ Key profile

Martin Luther

Luther (1483–1546) was a German Catholic monk who challenged the authority of the papacy in 1517 by nailing his 'theses' (criticisms) to a church door and set in train a process which started the Reformation and the beginnings of German Protestantism. His birthday was on 10 November.

The German Christians

The German Christians were a pressure group of Nazi supporters operating within the German Evangelical Church. First established in May 1932, the movement grew rapidly and by the mid-1930s it had some 600,000 supporters. Describing themselves as the 'SA of the Church', pastors who belonged to the German Christians wore SA or SS uniforms while conducting their services and hung swastika flags in their churches. German Christians fused Nazi racial ideology with their own religious faith and advocated a militant, aggressive, crusading form of Christianity. They regarded Church members as soldiers fighting for Christ and the Fatherland and their images of Christ portrayed him as a heroic figure, a role-model for German men. Hitler was portrayed as the national messiah. Swastika flags were hung in their churches.

The Reich Church

In the spring and summer of 1933 the Nazi regime began to 'coordinate' the 28 separate state churches in the Evangelical Church into a single, centralised Reich Church under Nazi control. In the Church elections of July 1933, the German Christians, with the support of Göbbels' Propaganda Ministry, won a sweeping victory and were now in a position to 'Nazify' the Church. Ludwig Müller, a Nazi nominee, was appointed as Reich bishop and took over the administrative headquarters of the Evangelical Church with the help of a squad of stormtroopers. Under the direction of these men, all elected bodies within the Church were abolished and the Church was reorganised on the leadership principle. In November 1933, the German Christians celebrated their triumph in taking over the Reich Church by holding a mass rally at the Sports Palace in Berlin. Here, they demanded that those pastors who had not declared their allegiance to the new regime should be dismissed, along with all non-Aryans. As a State institution, the Reich Church was forced to adopt this so-called 'Aryan paragraph' and eighteen pastors, mostly men who had converted to Christianity from Judaism, were dismissed. By the end of 1933, it appeared that the Reich Church had successfully been 'coordinated' into the *Volksgemeinschaft*.

■ Did you know?

The Aryan paragraph was the section of the Law for the Re-establishment of a Professional Civil Service which allowed for the dismissal of public servants on racial grounds.

The Confessional Church

Not all Protestant pastors, or their congregations, were willing to support these developments within the Church. In September 1933, a group of dissident pastors, led by Martin Niemöller and Dietrich Bonhoeffer, established a Pastors' Emergency League. This evolved

Cross-reference

For more information on Martin Niemöller and Dietrich Bonhoeffer, see pages 106–107.

into a breakaway Church known as the Confessional Church. With the support of about 5,000 pastors, the new Church was established to resist State interference in the Church and to re-establish a theology that was based purely on the Bible. The Confessional Church was thus in opposition to the official Reich Church and the Nazis' attempt to 'coordinate' religion under their control. Some rural congregations went over to the Confessional Church because, as the Gestapo reported on the Potsdam district, *'farming people seem to want to celebrate their Church festivals in the traditional form'*.

The very fact that the Confessional Church was established in defiance of the Nazi policy of *Gleichschaltung* shows that the regime's attempts to 'coordinate' the Protestant Church was a failure. In 1935, a new Ministry for Church Affairs was created and Reich bishop Müller was marginalised. The regime then switched to a policy of trying to weaken the Church through repression while at the same time trying to exploit the divisions that were beginning to appear within the Church. The regime also attempted to marginalise Christianity by focusing its attentions on young people. The abolition of Church schools in the late 1930s and the pressures on young people to join the Hitler Youth were attempts to drive a wedge between the Churches and young people. The regime also launched a campaign to persuade Party members to renounce their Church membership.

This Church Secession Campaign had some success:

- By 1939, 5% of the population were listed as 'god-believers', or people who retained some faith but had renounced formal membership of the Christian Churches.
- Party members were not allowed to hold any office in the Protestant or Catholic Churches.
- Stormtroopers were forbidden to wear uniforms at Church services.
- Priests and pastors were forbidden from playing any part in the Nazi Party.
- Pressure was also put on those whose employment depended on the regime; teachers and civil servants were particular targets.

By 1939, the Nazi Party had cut its links with organised religion.

Activity

Thinking point

What difficulties did the Nazis encounter in their efforts to coordinate the Protestant Church in Germany?

Activity

Source analysis

What can we learn from Source 10 about the success of Nazi efforts to reduce the influence of organised religion?

> In many areas the events put on by the State youth organization take less and less account of the Parish Church services and what would have been inconceivable in 1935 has become the norm in some places in 1939. Above all, youth is losing the habit of going to Church regularly. One need not fear that the village youth will be influenced by the German Faith Movement but rather will lose the habit of going to Church through being intentionally kept from Church services.

*From a report on Protestant Church visitations in Bavaria, 1937–38, quoted in Hite, J., and Hinton, C., **Weimar and Nazi Germany**, 2000*

The Roman Catholic Church

The Roman Catholic Church presented a far greater obstacle than the Protestants to the Nazi policy of *Gleichschaltung*. Catholics in Germany were part of an international Church and took their lead in religious matters from the pope. The Roman Catholic Church, therefore, was less susceptible to Nazi ideology than the wholly German Evangelical Church. The Nazis regarded the fact that the Roman Catholic Church demanded obedience to the pope from German Catholics as being subversive to Germany's unity as a nation. In the early 1930s, Catholic voters were among the least likely people to vote for the Nazi Party. On the other hand, Catholics as a group were keen to be seen and accepted as part of the German nation and, after Hitler came to power, the Church was prepared to compromise with the regime. There were also some points of convergence between Catholics and Nazism; the Catholic Church regarded communism as a far greater evil than Nazism and there were also many within the Church who shared the Nazis' anti-Semitism.

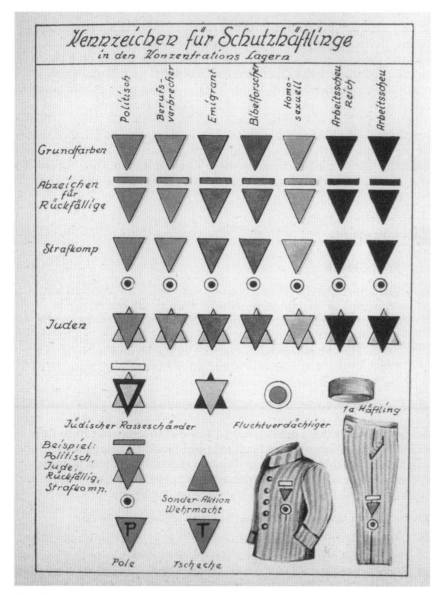

Fig. 12 *Labels for prisoners in Concentration Camps*

The concordat

After Hitler came to power in 1933, the Roman Catholic Church opted for cooperation and compromise with the new regime in the belief that this would preserve its autonomy. When the Free Trade Unions were taken over by the German Labour Front in May 1933, Catholic trade unions voluntarily disbanded. Rather than allow the Centre Party to be banned

Exploring the detail
Catholics in Germany

Since suffering repression at the hands of Bismarck in the 1870s, Catholics in Germany had developed a feeling of being outsiders within the Reich and had rallied around their Church as an assertion of their religious and cultural identity. Catholic children attended Catholic schools and Catholic youth groups. There were Catholic newspapers to promulgate a Catholic point of view on social and political issues and the Catholics had their own political party, the Centre Party to protect their interests.

Exploring the detail

The Nazis adopted an elaborate system of badges to identify the different categories of prisoners in the concentration camps. Figure 12, entitled 'Labels for prisoners in Concentration Camps', shows a series of colour-coded triangles, stars (for Jewish prisoners) and other shapes for prisoners to wear on their uniforms. The categories of prisoners (from left to right) were: political enemies; habitual criminals; foreign forced labourers; 'bible students' (e.g. Jehovah's Witnesses); homosexuals; asocials and the work-shy. The basic colours for each category are shown along the top line. Bars were placed above these triangles to denote repeat offenders and black, concentric circles identified members of penal battalions. Markings for Jews were the Star of David made up from a yellow base triangle overlaid with an inverted triangle of a different colour to identify Jewish political enemies etc. The yellow and black stars below showed special categories of 'Jewish race defilers' (e.g. Aryans who had converted to Judaism) and female race defilers (i.e. Aryan women who had had sexual relations with Jews). The triangles with the letters 'P' and 'T' at the bottom showed prisoners of Polish and Czech nationality.

Key terms

Concordat: an agreement or treaty. Since the Vatican was a sovereign state, this agreement was a treaty between it and the German Reich to clarify the relations between the Catholic Church and the State in Germany.

Activity

Thinking point

1. Why was it difficult for the Nazis to 'coordinate' the Catholic Church into the 'people's community'?

2. Why did the Catholic Church try to compromise with the regime?

by government decree, the Catholic authorities decided to abolish the party voluntarily. Then, in July 1933, the regime and the Vatican (the headquarters of the Catholic Church and the home of the pope) reached an agreement called a **concordat.**

Under the concordat:

- the Vatican recognised the Nazi regime and promised that the Church would not interfere in politics
- the regime promised that it would not interfere in the Catholic Church and that the Church would keep control of its schools, youth organisations and lay groups.

It was not long, however, before the Nazi regime was breaking the terms of this agreement. In the summer of 1933, the Nazis began to seize the property of Catholic lay organisations and forcing them to close. Catholic newspapers were also ordered to drop the word 'Catholic' from their names. The Gestapo and SS put Catholic priests under surveillance. In the Night of the Long Knives in August 1934, a number of leading Catholics were executed by the SS. Among them was Fritz Gerlich, the editor of a Catholic journal and a known critic of the regime. In the face of this mounting repression and blatant illegality, the Catholic hierarchy made no protest, believing instead that continued declarations of support for the regime would be the best way to protect the Catholic Church from the Nazis.

Key profile

Fritz Gerlich

Gerlich (1883–1934) had been brought up as a Protestant but converted to Catholicism in 1931. During the Nazis' rise to power he had been an outspoken opponent of the party and he was arrested and sent to Dachau concentration camp in March 1933. He was murdered in Dachau by the SS on the Night of the Long Knives. His wife was informed of his death by being given his blood-spattered glasses.

Some Catholic priests did begin, in 1935–36, to speak out from their pulpits about the dangers of Nazi religious ideas, especially those expounded by Alfred Rosenberg. Leading this criticism was Bishop Clemens von Galen, the Archbishop of Münster. In response, the regime increased the pressure on the Catholic Church:

- Permission to hold public meetings was severely restricted.
- Catholic newspapers and magazines were heavily censored and many publications had Nazi editors imposed upon them.
- Göbbels launched a propaganda campaign against financial corruption in Catholic lay organisations. Many had their funds seized and their offices closed by the SA.
- Membership of the Hitler Youth was made compulsory for all young people. Although Catholic youth organisations were still tolerated they experienced increasing difficulty in holding on to their members.

Key profile

Clemens von Galen

Galen (1878–1946) had become archbishop of Münster in 1933. His attitude to the Nazi regime was not one of outright opposition. He swore an oath of allegiance and supported Nazi foreign policy, especially the invasion of the Soviet Union, but he opposed the anti-Christian elements in Nazi ideology and he defended the interests of the Church. He is best known for speaking out against the euthanasia programme in 1940–41 when the Nazis tried to eliminate people with mental and physical handicaps. He became involved with opposition elements and was arrested in 1944. He spent the remainder of the war in Sachsenhausen concentration camp.

The papal encyclical, 1937

In 1937, the Pope, Pius XI, decided that the Church could no longer remain silent in the face of Nazi repression, He issued an **encyclical** entitled 'With Burning Grief' in which he condemned the hatred poured upon the Church by the Nazis. This was read out by priests at Church services across Germany. In response, the regime increased the pressure on the Church.

Key terms

Encyclical: a letter from the pope to Roman Catholic bishops.

■ Gestapo and SS agents were placed inside Church organisations to spy on the Church.

■ There was a tightening of restrictions on the Catholic press.

■ Pilgrimages and processions were restricted.

■ Youth groups were closed down.

■ The charity, Catholic Action, was banned in January 1938.

■ State subsidies to the Church were cut.

■ Many monasteries were closed down and their assets were seized.

■ Crucifixes were removed from Catholic schools.

■ Göbbels' Propaganda Ministry publicised many sex scandals involving Catholic priests, attempting to portray the Church as corrupt and immoral. Around 200 priests were arrested and tried on sex charges.

■ Finally, the Nazis began a campaign to close Church schools. By the summer of 1939, all Church schools had been converted into community schools.

By the summer of 1939, the power and influence of the Roman Catholic Church in Germany had been severely weakened. The Church and its priests had been intimidated and forced to retreat. The concordat had not been formally repudiated by the regime but the Nazis had ceased to honour the letter or the spirit of the agreement. The regime paid particular attention to young people of Catholic parents, denying them the opportunity to attend Church schools or belong to separate Catholic youth organisations. This was part of a long-term strategy to weaken the influence of the Church. Many older Catholics, however, were torn between their faith and their wish to be seen as 'good Germans'. With the Church under attack older Catholics, particularly in rural areas, reaffirmed their strong support for it by continuing to attend services. Although many had complaints about the treatment of their Church at the hands of the Nazis, they were careful not to place themselves in outright opposition to the regime. For Catholics, as for other Germans, the Hitler myth cast a powerful spell over them. Although individual Catholics did oppose many of the regime's policies, the Church as a whole did not mount any organised resistance to the Third Reich.

Cross-reference

The resistance of individual Catholics to the regime is dealt with in more detail on pages 107–108.

Activity

Source analysis

What can we learn from Source 11 about the success of the Nazis' efforts to 'coordinate' the Catholic Church?

Activity

Source analysis

What can we learn from Source 12 about the attitudes of the Catholic bishops towards the regime?

Key terms

Paganism: a general term referring to a range of pre-Christian religions. Pagans typically worship several gods, many of which are linked to natural phenomena such as the sun, the moon and the weather. Paganism was practised by Germanic tribes before their conversion to Christianity.

The more attempts are made to keep a watch on the Church, the more the peasantry support their priests. Catholic churchgoing, participation in various events such as processions, the blessing of the fields, pilgrimages, attendance at services during weekdays, and confession remain strong. For the time being the Party's propaganda is helpless in trying to resist this development. The mood is directed less against the State and much more against the Party. There are many peasants who make no bones about publicly declaring that their attitude to the Party is dependent on the Party's measures towards the Church.

 From a Bavarian district police report, June 1939, quoted in Hite, J., and Hinton, C., **Weimar and Nazi Germany**, *2000*

Nothing could be further from our intentions than to adopt a hostile attitude toward, or a renunciation of, the present form taken by our Government. For us, respect for authority, love of Fatherland, and the fulfilment of our duty to the State are matters not only of conscience but of divine ordinance. This command we will always require our faithful to follow. But we will never regard as an infringement of this duty our defence of God's laws and of His Church, or of ourselves against attacks on the Faith and the Church. The Führer can be certain that we Bishops are prepared to give all moral support to his historic struggle against Bolshevism. We will not criticize things which are purely political. What we do ask is that our holy Church be permitted to enjoy her God-given rights and freedom.

12 *From the Bavarian bishops' pastoral letter, December 1936, quoted in Hite, J., and Hinton, C.,* **Weimar and Nazi Germany**, *2000*

The German Faith Movement

Some leading Nazis, although by no means all, believed that the way to undermine the influence of the Churches in Germany was to create an alternative religion. Chief among the advocates of this was Robert Darré, the German peasants' leader. He was instrumental in establishing the German Faith Movement, which was a rejection of Christianity and based on pre-Christian **paganism**. Darré believed that paganism, in its Nordic version with gods such as Thor and Wotan, was more authentically Germanic (or Aryan) than Christianity. He believed that medieval German knights had been weakened by their conversion to Christianity under the influence of missionaries from southern Europe. In the German Faith Movement, Christian rituals surrounding baptism, marriage and death were replaced by pagan rites. Christmas was replaced by the celebration of the Winter Solstice. Morality was defined not in terms of conscience but in terms of service to the Aryan race.

The German Faith Movement was never more than a fringe cult within the Third Reich; it had only 40,000 adherents even at its height. Darre's ideas did, however, make a strong impression on the leader of the SS, Heinrich Himmler. Himmler adopted neo-pagan ideas, rites and symbols for the SS. An SS plan in 1937 stated that, *'We live in an age of the final confrontation with Christianity. It is part of the mission of the SS to give to the German people over the next fifty years the non-Christian ideological foundations for a way of life appropriate to their own character.'*

Key profile

Heinrich Himmler

Himmler (1900–1945) was born in Munich, the son of a strict, authoritarian schoolmaster. He became active in the Nazi Party in the early 1920s but was a marginal figure until Hitler appointed him head of the SS in 1929. In this role he displayed efficiency and organisational skill in building up the membership to over 50,000 by 1933. After the Nazis came to power, Himmler began to establish control over the police and, in 1936, his powerful position was confirmed when he was appointed chief of the German police as well as leader of the SS. This position was the springboard for him to extend his influence, and that of the SS, into the political, economic, military and ideological spheres of the Third Reich. His power was further extended in 1939 when he was given responsibility for the conquered territories in the east. At the end of the war he was captured by the Allies but committed suicide before he could be brought to trial.

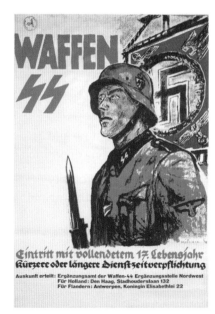

Fig. 13 *A recruiting poster for the Waffen-SS, showing the runic symbols used for the letters 'SS'*

Conclusion

By 1939, the Nazi Party had cut its links with organised religion but the religious policy of the regime was confused and inconsistent. Leading Nazis differed in their attitudes towards Christianity, ranging from Hitler and Göbbels who never formally renounced their Christian upbringing, through Rosenberg who was openly and unashamedly anti-Christian to Darré who was attempting to establish an alternative, pagan religion. The German Faith Movement was never more than a cult and did not even win wide acceptance within the Nazi Party. The Nazis had tried and failed to establish a single, unifying Protestant Church based on the German Christian Movement. With regard to the Catholic Church, the regime had initially shown a willingness to compromise through the concordat. By 1939, the concordat was effectively dead, yet Hitler held back from formally renouncing the agreement. He could still see some value, from a tactical point of view, in keeping the façade of cooperation with the Church while at the same time pursuing policies which were designed to weaken its hold over its congregations. It is clear that the Nazis had failed to 'coordinate' the Churches into the *Volksgemeinschaft* and that organised religion remained a powerful force within German society.

Exploring the detail

SS rituals

The SS had its own marriage service with runic symbols, a bowl of fire and symbols of the sun shining over the ceremony. The husband gave the wife his dagger as a token of her 'capability of bearing arms', while he received a replacement dagger from his SS commanding officer. At SS baptisms, the child was carried in by the father on his shield, wrapped in a blanket of undyed wool, which was embroidered with oak leaves, runes and swastikas.

Activity

Group activity

Divide the class into groups of four students. Each group should undertake a detailed study of one of the following: youth, workers, women, peasants and Churches, involving research from this book and other sources. In this study focus on:

■ the aims of Nazi policy

■ the organisations and methods for implementing their policy

■ the effectiveness of the policy.

When the research is complete, each group should present its findings to the rest of the class.

Summary questions

1 Explain why the indoctrination of youth was so important to the Nazi regime.

2 'The Nazi regime achieved great success in its policy towards the Churches.' Explain why you agree or disagree with this view.

Repression, conformity and resistance in Nazi Germany

In this chapter you will learn about:

■ the Nazi police state and its role in suppressing opposition

■ the extent of conformity and resistance to the regime by 1939.

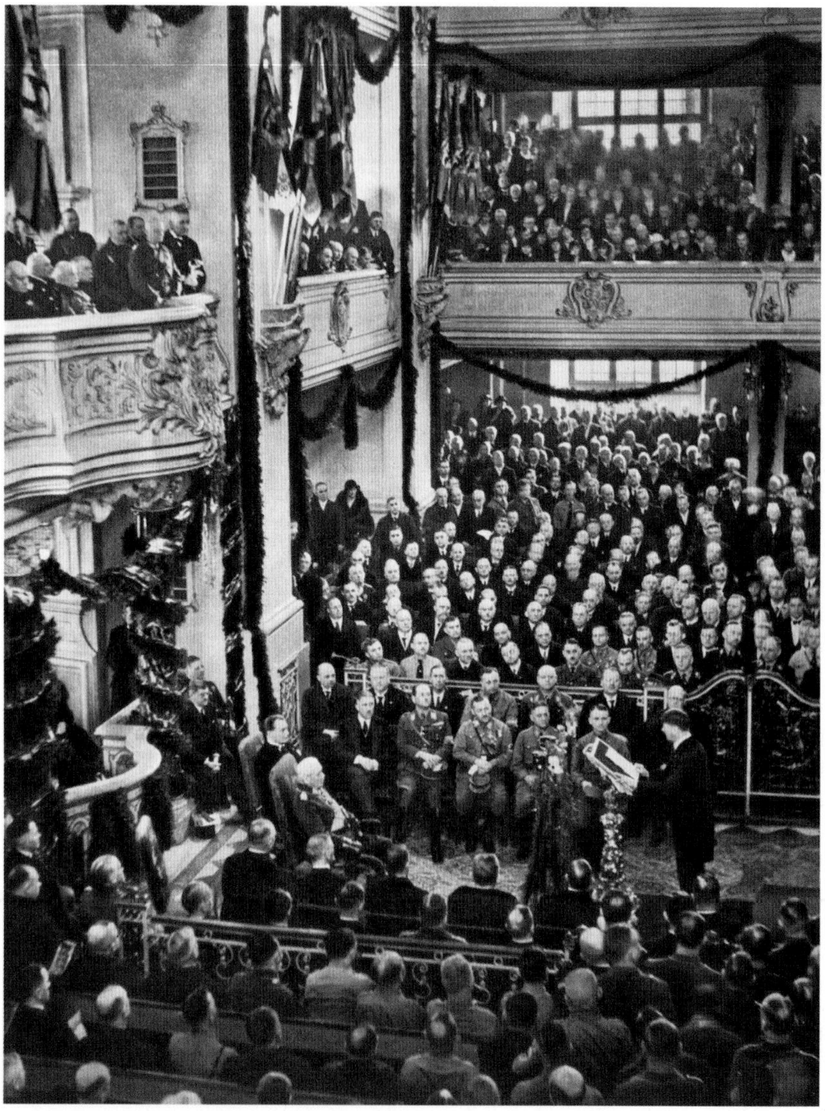

Fig. 1 *Hitler addresses the Reichstag at the Kroll Opera House, March 1933, on the occasion of the passing of the Enabling Act*

In politics there are only two possibilities: for Germany or not. Anyone who is not basically for Germany does not belong to us and will be eliminated. If he does not emigrate on his own initiative, then he will have to be locked up. If that does not help then we will have to make him a head shorter.

1   *From an article in an SS newspaper, 1939, quoted in Noakes, J. and Pridham, G.,* **Nazism 1919–45**, **Vol. 2**, *1984*

The police state

Nazism and the law

Hitler was determined that the Nazi regime would not be bound by the law and legal systems. The Nazi concept of authority was based on the leadership principle. As a 'man of destiny' who had been chosen to lead Germany and express the will of the people, Hitler refused to allow his freedom of action to be limited by a set of rules. *'There is only one kind of law,'* Hitler stated in 1928, *'and that lies in one's own strength.'* In other words, in the Third Reich Hitler's word was law. The Nazis did not introduce a new constitution or legal system after 1933. Instead they introduced some new laws to deal with political offences and forced the existing justice system – the police, the courts, the legal profession – to adapt and bend to their will. At the same time, they introduced new courts and new police organisations to ensure that political opponents were dealt with in accordance with the regime's priorities. The result was that in Nazi Germany the legal principles on which German law had been based in the Weimar period no longer applied. No longer were all citizens treated as equal before the law. The judges were not permitted to operate independently of the government. Individuals could be arrested and imprisoned without trial, without the police having to produce any evidence against them. The law was applied in an arbitrary and inconsistent fashion.

The courts

Alongside the existing criminal courts system the Nazis created new courts to deal with political offences. In April 1934, a People's Court was established in which two professional judges sat alongside three non-professional judges appointed by the Nazi Party. There were also new Special Courts which were created in every part of Germany. In these courts, there was no jury and defendants had no right of appeal against their sentence. Between 1934 and 1939, around 3,400 people were tried by the People's Court, most of whom were former members of the Communist and SPD parties. Many of those brought before the courts were given the death penalty which was used increasingly in the Third Reich and was applied to women as well as to men. Executions were carried out by beheading; this was done in the traditional way with a hand-held axe until 1936, when it was replaced by the guillotine.

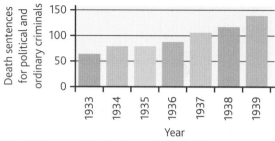

Fig. 2 *The use of the death penalty in Nazi Germany*

Criminality

Criminality in the Third Reich was defined according to the ideology of the Nazi Party. In Nazi Germany, a criminal was not necessarily someone who had offended against a specific law but someone who was outside the 'people's community'. This was based on the following criteria:

- **Racial:** Non-Aryans were automatically excluded and therefore considered to be enemies of the *Volksgemeinschaft*.

- **Ideological:** Marxists and Social Democrats were considered to be beyond the pale of Nazi coordination and had to be taken into 'protective custody'; liberals, reactionaries and Christians were regarded with suspicion and their treatment would depend on the extent to which they were prepared to conform.

- **Moral:** Ordinary criminals, 'asocials' and homosexuals were people who had offended against the social norms of the *Volksgemeinschaft* and should be punished accordingly. All of these groups were treated as 'hereditary degenerates' and so, even when their sentences had been completed, they were not set free. They were placed in 'security confinement' from which some were never released.

The police system in the Third Reich

Enforcement of the law was the responsibility of the police. In the Weimar Republic, it was the separate state authorities which controlled the police forces across Germany. The Nazis did not abolish these separate police forces but created a system of party-controlled, political police forces which were answerable to Hitler and which gradually gained control over the entire police system. This proliferation of police forces created confusion and competition between the forces and the powerful men who controlled them. The following forces existed:

Activity

Revision exercise

Read the information in this section. Summarise the Nazi attitude towards the law.

■ Cross-reference

For more information about the SA, see page 4.

■ **The SS:** controlled by Himmler

■ **The SD:** an intelligence gathering offshoot of the SS

■ **The SA:** controlled by Röhm, in 1933, the SA also acquired police powers to arrest and detain political prisoners

■ **The Gestapo:** the secret State police force in Prussia, of which Göring was the minister-president. During 1933, the remit of the Gestapo was extended to cover the whole country.

Between 1933 and 1936, there was competition and rivalry between Himmler, Röhm and Göring for control over the police. Himmler's hand was strengthened by the Night of the Long Knives in 1934 in which Röhm was eliminated and the SA's powers were reduced. Himmler was also able to exploit the rivalry between Göring and the Minister of the Interior, Wilhelm Frick. The situation was partially resolved in 1936 when the SS, SD and Gestapo were placed under the command of Himmler. Himmler's victory was sealed in 1939 with the creation of the Reich Security Department Headquarters (RHSA), which placed all party and State police organisations under one umbrella organisation, supervised by the SS.

■ Cross-reference

For more information on Göring, see above page 58. There are key profiles on Röhm on page 27, Himmler on page 90 and Heydrich on page 97.

Gestapo: Geheime Staatspolizei
Kripo: Kriminalpolizei
Orpo: Ordnungspolizei ('order' police), including Schutzpolizei and the gendarmerie
SD: Sicherheitsdienst (Security Service)
Sipo: Sicherheitspolizei (Security Police)
SS: Schutzstaffel (defence echelon)

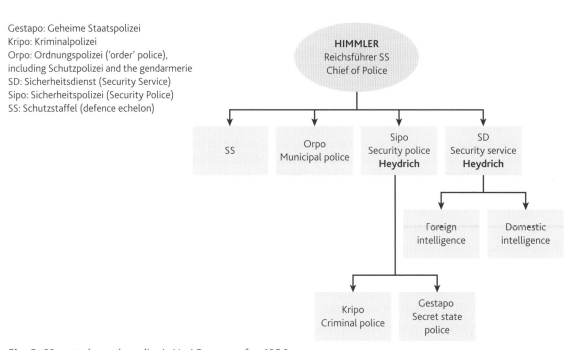

Fig. 3 *SS control over the police in Nazi Germany after 1936*

■ Activity

Thinking point

Read the information on the following pages. Explain the different roles of the SS, SD and Gestapo in the police system of the Third Reich. To what extent were their roles clearly separated?

■ **Key profile**

Wilhelm Frick

Frick (1877–1946) was interior minister from 1933 to 1943. He had studied law before working for the Munich police 1904–24. He joined the Nazi Party and was elected to the Reichstag in 1924. He was tried and executed by the Allies after the war.

The SS

The SS (*Schutzstaffel*) had been created in 1926 as Hitler's personal bodyguard. Heinrich Himmler had taken charge of the SS in 1929. Under Himmler's leadership, and especially after the Nazis came to power in 1933, the SS grew rapidly and expanded its role.

As Hitler's bodyguard, the SS had certain police functions from its inception. Once the Nazis came to power, and especially after the Night of the Long Knives, the police role of the SS was expanded and it became the main Nazi Party organisation involved in the identification, arrest and detention of political prisoners. By 1936, after Himmler had been appointed chief of the German police, the SS controlled the entire police system in the Third Reich. It was the SS which ran the concentration camps. Under SS control, the police system in Germany was an instrument of the Führer and the Nazi Party.

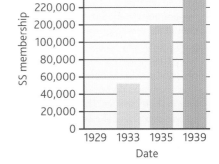

Fig. 4 *Membership of the SS, 1933–39*

The SS also took on other roles:

- **Ideological:** The SS was an elite force within the Nazi Party and its members were held up as role models for the racially based 'people's community' which the Party was trying to create. The SS ran its own elite schools for ideological indoctrination and had its own research institute to investigate heredity.

- **Military:** SS concentration camp guards were given paramilitary training for their jobs. Out of this grew the *Waffen-SS* (armed SS) which was a military organisation, with its own *Panzer* units (armed military units). Waffen-SS units were considered to be elite forces and were intended to give the party more control over the army.

- **Economic:** The SS owned several companies and, during the war, employed slave labour in the concentration camps to work for these companies. SS enterprises included a mineral water company and a publishing company.

- **Conquest:** After 1939, the SS was given responsibility for administering conquered territories. Himmler was appointed 'Reich commissioner for strengthening German nationhood'.

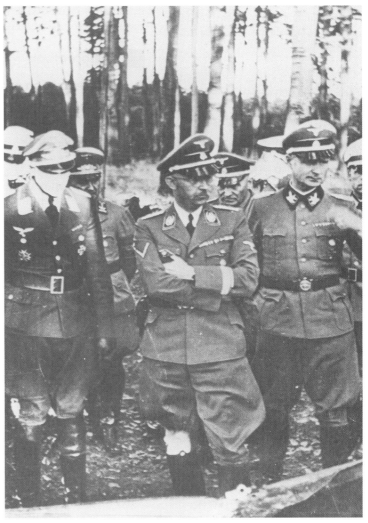

Himmler intended the SS to be strictly disciplined, racially pure, and unquestioningly obedient. The key values for an SS member were loyalty and honour, although honour was defined strictly in terms of adherence to Nazi ideology. Himmler described himself as a '*merciless sword of justice*'. A colourless personality, with no obvious leadership qualities, Himmler won Hitler's trust through his fanatical loyalty and will to carry out the Führer's bidding. A capable organiser and administrator, he approached the SS's main role as an instrument of State terror as a matter of bureaucratic necessity.

Fig. 5 *Heinrich Himmler, leader of the SS, pictured here with his officials during the Second World War*

Activity

Thinking point

What effect did the growing importance of Himmler and the SS have on the policing system in Nazi Germany?

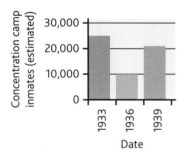

Fig. 6 *Prisoners in concentration camps, 1933–39*

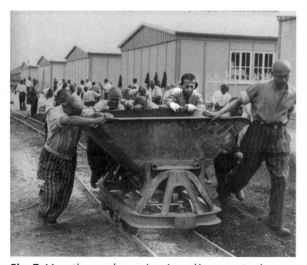

Fig. 7 *Many thousands were imprisoned in concentration camps after the Nazis came to power in 1933*

We swear to you Adolf Hitler as Führer and Chancellor of the German Reich to be loyal and brave. We vow to you, and the superiors appointed by you, obedience unto death. So help us God.

2 *The SS oath, quoted in Noakes, J. and Pridham, G., Nazism 1919–45, Vol. 2, 1984*

As the SS grew rapidly after 1933, Himmler took steps to ensure that its racial purity and its ideological cohesion were not diluted. Many of the new officers were men who were seeking career advancement and who placed administrative efficiency above ideological commitment. Himmler expelled 60,000 men from the SS between 1933 and 1935 on the grounds that they were homosexuals, alcoholics or opportunists.

After Himmler became chief of the German police in 1936, there was a noticeable tightening of control and an increase in repression, as can be seen in the increase in the numbers of concentration camp inmates. Whereas the SA had engaged in violence and terror on an emotional level, acting without close control and engaging in undisciplined street and bar brawls, the SS operated in a far more systematic and dispassionate way. Violence and murder were instruments of State power, to be employed ruthlessly and without reference to moral standards. SS concentration camp guards were deliberately brutalised to remove any feelings of humanity they might feel towards their prisoners. For Himmler and the SS, the end justified the means.

A closer look

Concentration camps

Concentration camps were essentially prisons in which the inmates were forced to work. They should not be confused with the extermination camps which were established in occupied countries after 1942. The first concentration camp was set up at Dachau, near Munich, in 1933, although there were also around 70 temporary camps. Following the SS takeover of the police and security system in 1936, six more camps were opened before September 1939. These included Sachsenhausen, Buchenwald, Mauthausen (in Austria) and Ravensbruck (a women's camp). The vast majority of prisoners in the early months of the regime were communists, socialists and trade unionists. Many of the temporary camps were closed down and, by May 1934, there were only a quarter as many prisoners as there had been a year before. Torture and brutality had rendered the majority of the prisoners unwilling to continue resistance against the Nazis and many were released.

All concentration camps came under SS control after 1934 with the result that the treatment of prisoners became systematised. After 1936, having crushed the communists and socialists, the regime reoriented the concentration camp system to deal with 'undesirables'. Habitual criminals, asocials and non-Aryans made up the majority of concentration camp inmates as the regime tried to purify the race. This change also coincided with an increase in violence and brutality in the camps. In Dachau, for example, there were 69 deaths among 2,200 camp inmates in 1937. In 1938, this figure increased to 370 out of a camp population of 8,000. Camp guards had been given immunity from prosecution by Himmler.

The SD

The SD (*Sicherheitsdienst*) was established in 1931 as the internal security service of the Nazi Party. An offshoot of the SS, it was set up to investigate claims that the party had been infiltrated by its political enemies. The SD was led by Reinhardt Heydrich.

■ Key profile

Reinhardt Heydrich

Heydrich (1904–42) came from a conservative middle-class family and had served in the navy during the 1920s, reaching the rank of lieutenant. He joined the Nazi Party and the SS in 1931 and became head of the SD in 1932. From 1933, he was Himmler's deputy in the SS leadership. In 1939, he became head of the *Reichssicherheitshauptamt* (RSHA), the Reich security head office, and also head of the Reich central office for Jewish emigration. In this capacity, he was responsible for the deportation of the Jews and, after 1941, for the mass murder of Jews. In 1941, he was made Reich protector of Bohemia and Moravia (Czechoslovakia) and was assassinated by the Czech resistance in 1942.

After 1933, the SD's role was intelligence gathering. It did not have police powers to arrest and detain suspects. One of its important roles was to monitor public opinion and to report on this to Hitler. By 1939, the SD had 50,000 officers, a sign of how important its role was considered to be, and also of how successful Heydrich had been in establishing his own power base.

The SD, as a Nazi Party organisation, worked independently of the Gestapo which was a State organisation. This could and did lead to overlap and confusion between the two organisations. The SD was staffed not by professional police officers but by amateurs who were committed Nazis and saw their role as to wage an ideological struggle. One of its tasks was to identify those who voted 'no' in plebiscites.

The Gestapo

The Gestapo, short for *Geheime Staatspolizei* (secret State police), was originally set up in Prussia but after the establishment of the Third Reich its operations were extended to cover the whole country. It was headed by Heinrich Müller who was a fanatical anti-communist but not a member of the Nazi Party. He was tolerated by the regime because of his efficiency and because he was dedicated to serving the State, whichever political party was in charge.

The Gestapo developed a reputation for being all-seeing and all-knowing. Ordinary Germans believed that the Gestapo had agents in every workplace, pub and neighbourhood. The reality was very different. It was actually a relatively small organisation, which in 1939 had only 20,000 officers to cover the whole country. In 1934, the Gestapo had only 41 officers in the major city of Frankfurt, 44 in Bremen and 42 in Hanover. Most of its agents were office workers, not field agents, and they were generally not members of the Nazi Party. Instead they were professional police officers who, like Müller, saw their role as being to serve the State. Of the 20,000 officers in 1939, only 3,000 were also members of the SS.

The Gestapo depended on information supplied by informers. Nazi Party activists, who were asked to spy on neighbours and workmates, were one important source of information. Every block of flats and every residential

■ Activity

Thinking point

Read this section on the Gestapo.

1 How far did the Gestapo succeed in its task of keeping German society under surveillance?

2 What can we learn from this about the relationship between the regime and its citizens?

3

Exploring the detail

Block leaders

In the Nazi Party's hierarchical organisation, the *Blockleiter*, or block leader, was on the lowest rung of the ladder, being responsible for a street block with about 40 to 60 households. Their role was to act as the eyes and ears of the party at local level, reporting on their neighbours to the State authorities. They were also expected to be a 'preacher and defender of National Socialist ideas'. Their job was to ensure that the people in their block became members of the various Nazi organisations (Hitler Youth, DAF, and so on) and that they should attend party rallies and display swastika flags during Nazi festivals. Above the block leader there were officials at cell level (around 160 to 480 households), town, district and regional (Gau) levels.

Exploring the detail

The use of torture

Many people were arrested by the Gestapo to extract information from them, with torture being carried out by the SS. One communist who was arrested, Richard Krebs, later wrote that for several weeks he was beaten and whipped while being questioned. In his cell he was chained to a cot and not allowed to wash. He suffered a broken thumb, kidney damage and the loss of hearing in one ear but the Gestapo were unable to break him until they arrested his wife and threatened to torture her. He then agreed to provide information but in fact he became a double agent, working for the communists while providing information of little value to the Gestapo.

Did you know?

The Law on Malicious Gossip was introduced on 21 March 1933 (the day of Potsdam) to clamp down on any expressions of dissent. It was used, for example, against those who told jokes about Hitler. It was used extensively. In 1937 alone, 17,168 contraventions of this law were reported by the Gestapo.

street had its 'block leader' who would report suspicious activity to the Gestapo. Still more information came from voluntary denunciations of workmates and neighbours by ordinary Germans. Most of these informers were motivated not by political commitment but by personal grudges. So overwhelming was the volume of information received that it was impossible to investigate all alleged crimes and the Gestapo therefore resorted more and more to arbitrary arrest and preventive custody.

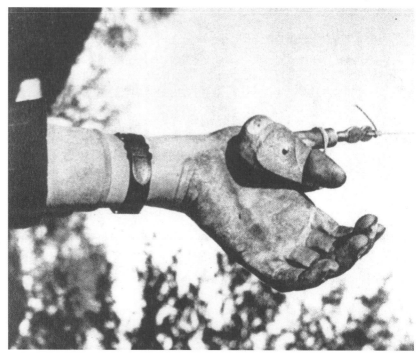

Fig. 8 *This thumbscrew was one of the instruments of torture used by the Gestapo*

The Law on Malicious Gossip of 1933 was used to prosecute those who were reported for making any statement which could be construed as being critical of the regime, including making jokes about the Nazi Party leadership. The Special Courts set up to deal with these offences sentenced over 3,700 people in 1933 alone. The majority were sent to prison for an average of six months. Many of those denounced under this law, who were mostly working class, had been reported by fellow drinkers in bars or by the innkeepers. Most of the 'offenders' were grumblers who did not oppose the regime in any organised way.

Despite its small size, therefore, the Gestapo was very successful in instilling an atmosphere of fear and suspicion in the German population. Political debate was stifled and criticism was driven underground. People believed that there were Gestapo agents and informers everywhere and adjusted their behaviour accordingly.

The extent of State terror in Nazi Germany

Violence and intimidation rarely touched the lives of most ordinary Germans. After 1933, at least, terror was highly selective, concentrating on small and marginal groups whose persecution not only met with the approval of the vast majority of Germans, but was actually carried out with the cooperation and often voluntary participation at the local level of the broad mass of ordinary German citizens. German society under the Nazis was, in this view, a society engaged in self-surveillance.

From Evans, R., **The Third Reich in Power***, 2005*

Thinking point

To what extent do you agree with Evans' view in Source 3 that *'German society under the Nazis was ... a society engaged in self-surveillance'*?

When assessing the nature and extent of State terror in Nazi Germany, it is important to acknowledge that there was a strong base of support for the regime. Through the use of propaganda to demonise political opponents and social and racial 'misfits', and through the policy of *Gleichschaltung*, the regime was able to gain acceptance from the majority of the people. The Nazi SS police system was presented as an instrument to protect the majority against the corrupting influence and threats from minorities. The use of the terms 'Peoples' Court' and 'popular justice' was designed to portray repression and persecution as something which reflected the will of the people. To a large extent this propaganda appears to have been effective. The Gestapo, with its limited resources, could not have instilled fear and suspicion to the extent that it achieved without the cooperation of many ordinary citizens.

Nevertheless, Nazi Germany was a society which lived under an oppressive and ruthless regime. In the final analysis, it was the Gestapo, SS and SD, along with the other police agencies, which kept society under surveillance and removed those identified as threats. In 1933, Nazi violence, carried out by the SA, was highly visible, but also rather wild and uncontrolled. By 1935, political opposition from the left had been crushed and the SA had been neutralised as a political force. From the mid-1930s, Nazi terror became more institutionalised, more bureaucratic and more systematic. Moreover, the main targets of persecution from 1936 onwards were the 'asocials', those who avoided work, habitual criminals, Jews and homosexuals. In other words, repression and persecution were no longer aimed at crushing political opponents but at purifying the race.

A closer look

The Nazi persecution of homosexuals

In common with most other European countries at the time, homosexuality was outlawed in Germany before 1933. In the relatively liberal climate of the Weimar Republic, however, homosexuality flourished in Berlin and other large cities. Most Nazis regarded homosexuals as degenerate and perverted and a threat to racial health of the German people. Himmler, who had a *'pathological fear of homosexuality'* (Evans), was particularly outraged that homosexuality was rife within the SA. The murder of Röhm and other leading members of the SA in the Night of the Long Knives was justified by Hitler and Himmler partly on the grounds of their homosexuality. Following the Night of the Long Knives, there was a widespread crackdown on homosexuals and a separate department of the Gestapo was established to deal exclusively with homosexuality. The law on homosexuality was amended in 1935 to widen the definition of what constituted a homosexual act and to prescribe harsher penalties. About 4,000 men were convicted under the old law between 1933 and 1935. After the law was changed, over 22,000 men were arrested and imprisoned between 1936 and 1938. In the whole period of the Third Reich, 1933–45, about 50,000 men were imprisoned for homosexual 'crime'. Even when the men arrested had served their sentences, they were immediately rearrested by the Gestapo or SS and held in concentration camps under 'preventive custody'. In the camps, they had to wear a pink triangle to distinguish them from other prisoners and they were subjected to particularly brutal treatment by the guards. The death rate for homosexuals in concentration camps was particularly high; about 50% of prisoners died during the period 1933–45. Many of those who survived were subjected to 'voluntary castration' to 'cure' them of their 'perversion'.

Although the activities of the Gestapo, SS and SD were carried on behind closed doors, the Nazis made a point of advertising the sentences handed down to offenders. The knowledge that long prison sentences and the death penalty were regularly handed down by the People's Courts and the Special Courts had a deterrent effect. The many prosecutions conducted under the Law on Malicious Gossip added to the climate of fear and helped create what Evans has described as a 'spiral of silence'. Kershaw has estimated that 225,000 people were imprisoned for 'political crimes' between 1933 and 1939. Although this was a small percentage of the total population of Germany, the numbers were sufficiently large to engender an atmosphere of fear in the general population. In a society where all basic civil rights had been abolished the law offered no protection for the individual in the face of State repression. Indeed, the law had become an instrument for imposing the ideology of the Nazi Party and ensuring that any resistance was stamped out.

Activity

Thinking point

1. How far did the nature of Nazi repression change between 1933 and 1939?

2. How far did the Nazis succeed in creating an atmosphere of fear in the general population by 1939?

The extent of conformity and resistance by 1939

Propaganda and indoctrination, repression and 'coordination' were all designed to ensure that the German population did not resist the Nazi regime. On the whole, there was very little active opposition and there was evidence of Hitler's increasing popularity. Life in Nazi Germany became depoliticised; there was no open and free debate about the regime or its policies, and people were given no official outlets for any complaints or criticisms they might wish to voice. Historians generally agree that there was a widespread acceptance of the regime and most Germans subscribed to the view that the Third Reich was preferable to the disorder and economic weakness of the final years of the Weimar Republic. Nevertheless, various individuals and groups did, from time to time, voice opinions which were critical of the regime or attempted to resist Nazi attempts to 'coordinate' them into the *Volksgemeinschaft*. The task of the historian in attempting to assess the extent of opposition to the Nazi regime has been made difficult by two main problems: the problem of sources and the problem of definitions.

The problem of sources

In Nazi Germany, there were no free elections and no opinion polls. Therefore, the tests of public opinion which exist within a democratic society were not available in Nazi Germany. There were elections to the Reichstag in 1934, 1936 and 1938, but since the Nazi Party was the only party permitted to put up candidates for election, and since the elections took place against a background of unremitting propaganda and underlying repression, the 99% of the vote achieved by Nazi candidates in most elections cannot be a reliable indicator of public opinion. There were also plebiscites which were held to put the seal of public approval on important policies. Since these were held under the same conditions as Reichstag elections, plebiscites also were not reliable indicators of public support for the regime.

Cross-reference

For more information on plebiscites, see page 51.

The Gestapo and the SD were given the task of reporting on the state of public opinion. Gestapo reports are therefore very valuable in providing an insight into the state of public opinion at different times. However, the reports were very subjective, reflecting the views of the writers, and were also compiled by people who had to be careful not to offend their superiors. There is at least a possibility that Gestapo agents were telling their superiors what they wanted to hear. They were also reporting only what they had been able to learn from their networks of informers; since people had learned to be cautious about expressing critical views, it is impossible to treat these reports as a reliable indicator of public attitudes.

The SPD leadership in exile (Sopade) received monthly reports from its agents in different parts of Germany. Naturally Sopade agents would report any expression of anti-Nazi sentiment and reliance on these sources could therefore lead a historian to exaggerate the extent of opposition. Nevertheless, Sopade reports also confirmed the strength of support for the regime and for the Führer, thereby corroborating some of the evidence from the Gestapo reports.

Historians base their judgements on a wide variety of sources in order to counteract the inbuilt bias of these reports. In researching the extent of conformity and resistance in Nazi Germany, however, historians have also proceeded from different starting points. The way in which a historian defines resistance has a major effect on the conclusions that are reached.

Cross-reference

For more information on Sopade, see page 36.

The problem of definition

Historians have taken different approaches to the question of what constituted resistance in Nazi Germany. Some have focused on the efforts of heroic individuals, motivated by religious convictions, to take a stand against the cruel and oppressive policies of the regime. Other historians have emphasised the organised, underground left-wing political opposition which continued to operate in Germany for some time after Hitler came to power. There was also opposition from elements within the German elites, particularly among high-ranking army officers and senior figures within the civil service. These groups and individuals were undoubtedly important elments in what may be termed a German resistance to Hitler, but to focus exclusively on their motives and activities has led to the view that opposition in Nazi Germany made no impact on the German people as a whole. In other words, this strand of historiography has been based on an assumption that the vast majority of the German people were at least compliant with, if not enthusiastic supporters of, the Nazi regime.

In the 1960s, some historians began to develop an alternative approach to resistance in Nazi Germany in which they focused more on actions rather than on motives. These historians therefore used a much broader definition of resistance to include any action or behaviour which did not conform to the social norms laid down by the Nazi regime. Any nonconformist behaviour – listening to jazz music, refusal to fly swastika flags from windows or a refusal to join a boycott of Jewish-owned businesses – was defined by the regime as an antisocial act and was liable to lead to punishment. Therefore it was the Nazi regime itself which defined behaviour which would be perfectly normal and acceptable within a free society as acts of resistance. Nonconformist behaviour did not amount to a fundamental challenge to the regime, but it was a way for ordinary Germans to retain some independence of thought and behaviour in a society where total conformity was demanded. The majority of those who acted in nonconformist ways were, in fact, people who broadly supported the Nazi regime but who felt unable to comply with all of its demands all of the time.

Both definitions of resistance in Nazi Germany are valid. There were many ways in which groups and individuals could register their dissent in Nazi Germany. It is, perhaps, useful to view dissent as a pyramid of behaviours and actions, with a broad base of nonconformity, rising through an unwillingness to cooperate and then criticism and protest. Outright resistance of a more fundamental kind occupied the narrow peak of the pyramid. There is a danger with this approach of attaching equal value to resistance which took the form of occasional grumbling at economic hardship with the more open and courageous challenges to the regime which led to individuals being executed. On the other hand, it is important to acknowledge that nonconformist behaviour was not confined to a few heroic individuals.

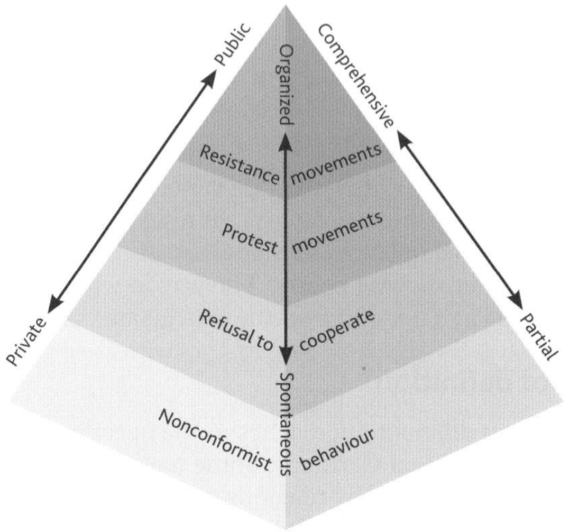

Based on the work of Detlev Peukert

Fig. 9 *The pyramid of dissenting behaviour in Nazi Germany*

Activity

Thinking point

Make an enlarged copy of the pyramid of dissenting behaviour. Place each of the following dissenting behaviours on the pyramid:

- Communists setting up an underground cell
- Workers going on strike for higher wages
- Priests criticising the regime's religious policies
- Young people failing to attend Hitler Youth meetings
- Army officers plotting to overthrow Hitler to prevent him leading Germany into a disastrous war

Political resistance

Within six months of taking power in 1933, Hitler had secured one-party rule in Germany. Those parties which did not disband voluntarily were banned and their assets seized. It was the parties of the left – the SPD and the KPD – which were expected to mount the stiffest resistance to Hitler; indeed, Hitler himself feared that the unions which were linked to the SPD would stage a general strike to thwart the Nazi takeover in 1933, just as they had done in Berlin in 1920 to defeat the Kapp Putsch. In the event, resistance from the left did not pose a serious threat to the Nazi regime. Partly this was due to the fact that the left was bitterly divided, with the KPD attacking the much larger and more moderate SPD as 'social-fascists'. A united front against Nazism was never a realistic possibility for the two main parties of the left.

The SPD

In January 1933, the SPD was unprepared for the Nazi takeover. As a constitutional party, committed to working within the legal framework of the State, the SPD did not have any means of organising resistance to a regime that did not respect the law. SPD activists continued to organise openly for the election campaign in March 1933 and were subjected to SA violence and repression as a result. SPD deputies bravely defied SA and SS intimidation to vote against the Enabling Act in the Reichstag but, once the regime had acquired legal powers to establish a dictatorship and began to crush the SPD, the party was unprepared for underground, illegal activity.

By the end of 1933, thousands of SPD activists had been murdered or placed into 'preventive custody' and the SPD leadership had fled into exile.

Gradually, the SPD adapted to the changed conditions in Germany. Organised by Ernst Schumacher from the SPD base in Prague, the party established small, secret cells of supporters in factories. There were also some city-based groups such as the Berlin Red Patrol and the Hanover Socialist Front. Propaganda pamphlets were smuggled across the border from Czechoslovakia but most of the contact between these cells was by word of mouth. The constant fear of exposure and the threat of arrest by the Gestapo limited the scope of these illegal activities. The priority for those involved was to survive and be prepared for a future collapse of the regime rather than to mount a serious challenge.

The KPD

With its background in revolutionary politics, the KPD was much better prepared than the SPD for engaging in underground activity. The KPD was, however, devastated by the wave of repression unleashed upon communists in Germany after Hitler came to power. It was the first party to be banned and its leader, Ernst Thälmann, was arrested at an early stage. It has been estimated that about 10% of the KPD's membership were killed by the Nazis during 1933. Nevertheless, the KPD succeeded in establishing an underground network in some industrial centres in Germany. Revolutionary unions were established in Berlin and in Hamburg which were able to recruit members and publish newspapers. A communist cell network in the Ruhr was able to publish two newspapers, while there was also a cell network in Mannheim. All these networks were, however, broken up by the Gestapo. Those in Berlin, Hamburg and the Ruhr were all destroyed in 1934, while the one in Mannheim managed to survive until 1935.

Secret communist activity was not completely eradicated by the successes of the Gestapo in 1934–35. Factory cells were established and contact between members was confined to word of mouth to reduce the risk of discovery. As with the SPD, however, the priority of communist cells was very much on survival since the party had ceased to exist and no serious challenge to the regime was possible.

Neither the SPD nor the KPD had any significant success in attracting working-class Germans to their cause after the summer of 1933. Quite apart from the fact that the Nazi regime had reduced unemployment, any workers associated with an illegal cell were risking their own lives and those of their families.

Resistance by workers

> It became clear that the effects of the economic crisis on the inward resistance of the workers were more appalling than had previously been thought. We see it time and time again: the most courageous illegal fighter, the most relentless antagonist of the regime, is usually the unemployed man who has no more to lose. Whereas if a worker gets a job after years out of work then – however bad his pay and conditions – he at once becomes apprehensive. Now he does have something to lose, however little, and the fear of the renewed misery of unemployment is worse than the misery itself. The National Socialists have not conquered the factories. But the National Socialists have destroyed the workers' self-confidence; they have crushed the forces of solidarity and crippled their will to resist.

4   *From a Sopade report, 1935, quoted in Noakes, J. and Pridham, G.,* **Nazism 1919–45, Vol. 2,** *1984*

 Activity
Revision exercise

Explain why the SPD and KPD were unable to mount an effective resistance to the Nazi regime.

 Activity
Group activity

Divide the class into groups of around four students. Each group should undertake detailed research, using this book and other sources, into one of the following: political resistance; resistance by workers; resistance by the Churches; reistance by young people; resistance by the elite.

In their research, groups should focus on

- the aims and motives of those who resisted
- the extent of resistance
- the effectiveness of their actions.

When the research is completed, each group should report their findings to the rest of the class.

Before 1933, the German working class was the largest and most unionised workforce in Europe. The largest unions in Germany were linked to the SPD and had been consistent in their opposition to the Nazi Party. After January 1933, however, union resistance crumbled surprisingly quickly. The ideology of class conflict and working class solidarity had sustained the trade union movement before 1933. After the Nazis came to power, the trade unions were absorbed into the DAF and Nazi propaganda emphasised the importance of national as opposed to class solidarity. Working-class Germans became depoliticised and working-class organisations were broken up. Nazi propaganda did not necessarily succeed in convincing workers that their interests were being protected by the DAF, nor that the interests of workers and employers were the same. Workers had many causes for complaint but few outlets to express their discontent and no independent organisation to press their case.

Nevertheless, there were means by which workers could express their dissatisfaction even under the conditions of a dictatorship. The most obvious and effective weapon at the disposal of workers was to withdraw their labour. Taking strike action was a very risky business but strikes did occur, for example among Autobahn workers in 1935. In September 1935, 37 strikes were reported in the Rhineland-Westphalia, Silesia and Württemberg regions. Gestapo records for 1935, which are by no means comprehensive, show that there were a total of 25,000 strikers in 1935 out of a total workforce of 16,000,000. In the last quarter of 1936, 100 strikes were reported to the authorities while, in the whole of 1937, a total of 250 strikes were recorded.

Most of these strikes were reactions to poor working conditions or low wages. Significantly, there was increased strike activity in 1935–36 at a time when then was widespread discontent over food prices. On the other hand, the DAF reported that there was some political content in 40 of the 250 stoppages in 1937. From the point of view of the regime, however, any expression of dissent in this way was regarded as a challenge and was dealt with accordingly. Of the 25,000 workers who participated in strikes in 1935, 4,000 spent short periods in prison. After the 17-minute stoppage at the Opel works in 1936, seven ringleaders were arrested by the Gestapo and imprisoned.

Strikes were dangerous for the participants because they could easily be identified. There were also less overt, but nonetheless effective, means by which workers could express their dissatisfaction. One of these was absenteeism, which was often resorted to by workers as a reaction against the pressure to work longer hours. The regime was so concerned about the level of absenteeism in 1938 that new labour regulations were introduced which laid down severe penalties for 'slackers'. In 1938, for example, the Gestapo arrested 114 workers at a munitions plant in Gleiwitz for absenteeism and slow working. Another tactic resorted to by some workers was to deliberately damage their machinery. Again the regime was concerned enough about this tactic to make 'sabotage' a criminal offence and there were an increasing number of prosecutions in 1938–39.

The evidence suggests that there was a widespread unwillingness to tolerate low wages, long hours and poor working conditions. None of this, however, amounts to any more than passive resistance. Without independent union organisation linking workers across industries, workers' resistance to Nazism could not amount to any more than sporadic and spontaneous protest. German workers did remain

Exploring the detail

Strikes

The vast majority of stoppages were small scale and short-lived. They were always limited to a single plant, or part of a plant, and lasted only a few hours. Typical examples were a six-hour strike at an Alte Union plant in Berlin and a seventeen-minute stoppage at the Opel works in Rüsselsheim in 1936. As such, these interruptions to production were an inconvenience rather than a major problem for the regime.

resistant to Nazi attempts at 'coordination' but most workers were resigned to Nazi rule and unable to offer any serious challenge to the regime.

Resistance by the Churches

The Christian Churches were the only organisations in Nazi Germany which retained an alternative ideology, independent of the regime. The Churches also retained some organisational autonomy. This placed the Churches in a powerful position within Nazi Germany. The influence of the pastor or the priest in many communities was at least as important as that of the Nazi Party. On the other hand, the Churches were well aware that, in a sustained and fundamental conflict with the regime, it was they who were likely to be the losers. The Churches' leaderships recognised that they needed to protect their organisations if they were to survive at all, and this led them into making compromises with the regime. Moreover, there was much common ground between the Churches and the Nazi regime, such as the determination to fight against communism and, for many, a shared anti-Semitism. Compromise and cooperation between the regime and the Churches was a realistic option for both sides. There were inevitably, however, issues on which the Churches were not prepared to compromise; at times, Protestants and Catholics felt it necessary to draw a line under Nazi efforts to force them into conformity and this led them into resistance. The response of the Christian Churches to the Nazi regime, therefore, was both complex and fluid, and varied not only over time but even from one priest or pastor to another.

Activity

Thinking point

1 What methods were used by German workers to register their dissatisfaction with the regime?

2 What were the dangers associated with each method for the workers involved?

Cross-reference

For more information about Sophie Scholl and the White Rose group, see page 137.

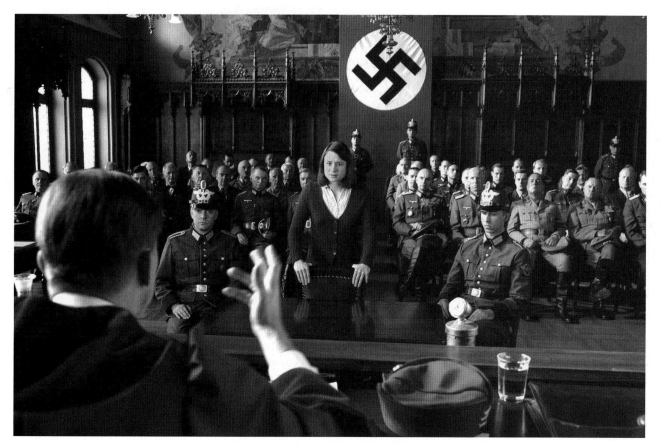

Fig. 10 *The 1943 trial of Sophie Scholl, one of the leaders of the Catholic-influenced White Rose protest group, from the German film Sophie Scholl – The Final Days*

Cross-reference

For more detailed information on the clash between the Reich Church and the dissenting Confessional Church, see pages 85–86.

Protestants

We have seen above how the efforts of the Nazi regime to coordinate the Protestant Church into the *Volksgemeinschaft* led to division within the Protestant congregation and to conflict between some Protestants and the Nazi regime. The establishment of the Pastors' Emergency League in 1933 and its development into the Confessional Church in 1934 were, in themselves, acts of resistance. The resistance in this case was led by pastors who were not members of the Nazi Party and who came largely from academic backgrounds. Their refusal to accept being part of a 'coordinated' Reich Church was due to three main factors:

- They were trying to protect the independence of the Protestant Church from the Nazi regime.
- They were resisting the attempt to impose the Aryan paragraph onto the Church. This involved purging from the Church any pastor who had converted from Judaism.
- They were trying to defend orthodox Lutheran theology which was based purely on the Bible. German Christians wanted to remove the 'Jewish' Old Testament from the Bible.

During 1934, there was a growing struggle between the dissenting pastors, who founded the Confessional Church, and the Nazi regime. Pastors spoke out against the 'Nazified Christ' from their pulpits. Many Churches refused to display swastika flags on festival days. When two Confessional Church bishops were arrested, there were mass demonstrations in their support. The Nazi regime responded with increased repression. Dissenting pastors had their salaries stopped, they were banned from teaching in schools and many were arrested. By the end of 1937, over 700 pastors had been imprisoned.

Key profile

Martin Niemöller

Martin Niemöller (1892–1984) was a Protestant pastor working in Berlin in 1933. He had been a U-boat commander during the First World War and continued to hold strong nationalist views during the Weimar Republic. He had been active in far right nationalist and anti-communist groups in the 1920s and had supported the Kapp Putsch. Although he initially welcomed Hitler's appointment as chancellor in January 1933, he was never himself a member of the Nazi Party and, by the end of 1933, he had begun to oppose Nazi efforts to politicise the Evangelical Church. Although he was anti-Semitic himself, he opposed the adoption of the Aryan paragraph by the Church on the grounds that it was God's will that Jews should be welcomed into the Christian faith. He was a co-founder of the Pastor's Emergency League and later of the Confessional Church. He became an outspoken opponent of Nazi efforts to control the Evangelical Church and was arrested and put on trial. Although acquitted on all charges, he was immediately rearrested by the Gestapo and sent to Sachsenhausen concentration camp. In prison, he was treated as Hitler's personal prisoner and allowed certain privileges, such as receiving visits from his wife. Within the Confessional Church, he was held up as a martyr and remembered daily in prayers. His experiences in prison led him to identify with other prisoners, including Jews, and he repudiated his anti-Semitic views.

Key profile

Dietrich Bonhoeffer

Dietrich Bonhoeffer (1906–45) was co-founder of the Pastors' Emergency League and joined the Confessional Church. He was an outspoken opponent of the Aryan paragraph and of Nazi attempts to take over the Church. Unlike Niemöller, he retained his freedom and became involved with other anti-Nazi elements among army officers. He was finally arrested in 1943 and murdered by the Gestapo in 1945.

Despite the repression, the Nazi regime failed to silence or crush the Confessional Church. Although harassment and repression continued, the regime had to accept the existence of the independent Church. For its part, the Confessional Church never became the focus of a more generalised opposition to the regime. The majority of its members professed their loyalty to Hitler and the Third Reich. Much of their energies were expended in fighting the bitter internal struggle against the official Reich Church, with the result that the Protestant Churches became rather inward looking. Although individual pastors risked their lives and liberty in speaking out against the barbarities of the regime, the Churches as a whole remained silent. There was no sustained defence of human and civil rights and no official condemnation of atrocities such as Kristallnacht in 1938, issues on which the Churches might have been expected to give a moral lead.

> In Germany, they came first for the communists, And I didn't speak up because I wasn't a communist;
>
> And then they came for the trade unionists, And I didn't speak up because I wasn't a trade unionist;
>
> And then they came for the Jews, And I didn't speak up because I wasn't a Jew;
>
> And then . . . they came for me . . . And by that time there was no one left to speak up.

 5   *From a statement by Martin Niemöller, quoted by Neuhaus, R. in an article in* **First Things***, November 2001*

Catholics

The Catholic Church was, in some ways, in a stronger position to retain its independence than the Evangelical Church. This was because the Catholic Church was more united, more centralised and had more of a tradition of independence from the State. Nevertheless, the Catholic Church leadership in both Rome and in Germany tried to come to terms with the Nazi regime rather than adopt an oppositional stance. It was when the privileges granted to the Catholic Church in the concordat of 1933 came under attack that the Church found itself increasingly at odds with the regime.

Activity

Thinking point

1. In what ways was the Catholic Church better placed than the Protestants for resisting the Nazi regime?

2. Why did the Catholic Church increasingly come into conflict with the regime between 1933 and 1939?

Exploring the detail

Kristallnacht

Kristallnacht (the night of broken glass) was a wave of anti-Jewish violence, mainly perpetrated by the SA, which took place on the night of 9–10 November 1938. Following the murder of a German embassy official in Paris by a Jew, the Nazis unleashed attacks on Jews and their property across Germany. 91 Jews were murdered and 20,000 were sent to concentration camps. Following these events, the Nazi regime forced the Jewish population of Germany to pay a fine of 1 billion Reichsmarks.

Activity

Source analysis

Read Source 5. What can we learn from this source about the weaknesses of the opposition to the Nazi regime?

Exploring the detail

Catholic protests in Oldenburg

In Oldenburg in 1937, the Education Minister ordered the removal of religious symbols such as crucifixes from all schools. Local priests used their pulpits to denounce this policy. Church bells were rung as a sign of protest and petitions were handed in to the Education Ministry. Crosses on houses, schools and church towers were illuminated to emphasise their significance to the Catholic faithful. Some Catholics began to resign from the Nazi Party and the Party's regional leader was forced to withdraw the decree. This victory was celebrated throughout the Catholic community in Germany and in Oldenburg itself the standing of the Nazi Party was damaged. In the Reichstag election of 1938, the party achieved 92% of the vote, whereas in 1936 it had received 99%.

Exploring the detail

The Jehovah's Witnesses

The Jehovah's Witnesses were *'alone amongst religious groups in their uncompromising hostility to the Nazi State'* (Evans). With around 30,000 adherents in Germany in 1933, the Jehovah's Witnesses were a small but closely knit sect. Their belief that they could only obey Jehovah (God) led them into conflict with the Nazi regime because they refused to take an oath of loyalty to Hitler. They refused to give the Hitler salute, participate in Nazi parades or accept conscription into the armed forces. They regarded persecution as a test of their faith and became more resistant under pressure from the regime. Many were arrested. In prison, they refused to obey orders, to attend parades or remove their caps. By 1945, around 10,000 Jehovah's Witnesses had been imprisoned but the regime failed to break their resistance.

The opposition of the Catholic Church to Nazi policies was piecemeal and concerned with protecting the independence and influence of the Church, rather than with mounting a more general attack on the immorality and inhumanity of Nazi policies. One cause of conflict was the decision of Clemens von Galen, the Bishop of Münster, to speak out against the atheistic views of one of the leading Nazi ideologists, Alfred Rosenberg. In 1935, Galen issued a pamphlet and an Easter message refuting Rosenberg's views, particularly his concept of the 'racial soul'. In response, 19,000 Catholics – double the usual number – turned out for the annual July procession through Münster to show support for their bishop. Local Nazi Party officials complained to Berlin that Galen was meddling in politics, but Galen was considered to be too important to be arrested. Controversies such as this, which drew thousands of ordinary Catholics into demonstrating their support for the Church, helped to build up Catholic resistance to the regime.

The 1937 papal encyclical 'With Burning Concern' was issued by the Pope against the background of mounting pressure on the Catholic Church in Germany. The document was smuggled into Germany, secretly printed in twelve separate places, distributed by messengers on bicycle or on foot and read out from almost every Church pulpit in March 1937. This was the one and only time that the Catholic Church as a whole had placed itself in open conflict with the regime. The regime's response was to increase repression, resulting in Catholic youth groups being closed down and other Catholic organisations coming under severe pressure. Charges against priests for 'abuse of the pulpit' became regular occurrences. Again there was some resistance. The arrest of one priest led to noisy public demonstrations at his trial. Intimidation and harassment of priests, however, had the desired effect. A local government official reported in 1937 that the clergy were beginning to show *'cautious restraint'*.

Many individual Catholic priests, and members of their congregations, showed great courage in opposing aspects of the Nazi regime's religious policies. The Church did not, however, move beyond a narrow defence of its independence to a wider opposition to Nazism. Although some individual priests criticised Nazi racial ideology, there was no formal protest against policies such as the Nuremberg Laws or events such as Kristallnacht. Resistance to the Nazis from the Catholic Church was, therefore, partial, spasmodic and ineffective.

Activity

Thinking point

What can we learn from the example of the Jehovah's Witnesses about the possibilities of mounting an effective resistance to the Nazi regime?

Resistance by young people

In many ways, the Hitler Youth, in the early years of the Nazi regime, was able to channel the energies and the rebelliousness of youth into officially approved activities. This was especially true for teenage Germans whose parents were opposed to them joining the Hitler Youth or BDM. By the mid-1930s, however, there were growing signs of disillusionment among young people with the official youth movements. This was partly because membership was made compulsory in 1936 and partly because of the growing regimentation of activities in the youth movements. Membership of the HJ and BDM made great demands on a teenager's free time. Indeed, this was the intention since the Nazi policy of *Gleichschaltung* was based on the premise that individuals should have no free time and no independent activity. Activities in the HJ which were particularly unpopular were compulsory gymnastics sessions on Wednesday evenings, all-day hikes on Sundays and the endless military drilling. The response of many young people was to opt out, either by failing to pay their dues so that their membership lapsed or by simply not attending the weekly parades. There was a growing rate of absenteeism from HJ activities in the late 1930s. Those who did attend sometimes demonstrated their independence by humming the tunes to songs that had been banned by the Nazis. There was also a growing problem of indiscipline within the Hitler Youth. This nonconformist behaviour amounted to little more than normal teenage rebelliousness but under the Nazis any assertion of independence was considered to be a threat.

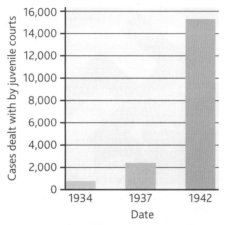

Fig. 11 *Cases dealt with in juvenile courts in Nazi Germany*

Some young people formed cliques, or gangs, to show their independence. Some were little more than criminal gangs, such as the Stauber of Danzig who waylaid and robbed soldiers home on leave from the war. Others were more overtly political, such as the Meuten gangs which flourished in old communist strongholds in Leipzig in the late 1930s. Youth resistance to the Nazis peaked during the war years.

Resistance by the elites

There were many within the conservative, traditional elites in Germany who had serious misgivings about the Nazi Party in general and Hitler in particular. Some aristocratic generals in the army and senior civil servants regarded Hitler with disdain and regarded him as a threat to the old Germany of monarchy and landowners. Even after the more radical Nazis in the SA had been ruthlessly purged in the Night of the Long Knives, many senior figures in the army and civil service continued to have misgivings about the Nazi regime. This was significant because, after the death of Hindenburg there was no longer any legal means for removing Hitler from power and a military coup was the only way to get rid of the regime. The conservative elites were, however, fatally compromised in their dealings with Hitler. Senior figures in the army had been instrumental in bringing Hitler to power in January 1933. The regime was sustained through the crucial period of the consolidation of power by an alliance with the army, big business and conservative politicians. The conservative elites broadly shared Hitler's aims for Germany, even if they sometimes disapproved of his methods. Both the civil service and the army had a strong tradition of serving the State, whoever was in charge, and active opposition to the Nazi leadership, therefore, would involve a major intellectual and emotional shift on their part. The number of those within the army and civil service who opposed the Nazis was actually very small and, because of their disdain for democracy, they had no plans for, or any prospect of, leading a mass movement in opposition to the regime.

Exploring the detail

Youth offending

There were other indicators which showed that Nazi indoctrination of youth was not wholly effective. There was, for example, a growing problem of youth offending.

Activity

Discussion point

To what extent can we describe the rebelliousness of young people in Germany in the 1930s as a form of resistance to the regime?

Cross-reference

For more information on youth resistance to the Nazis in the war years, see pages 136–137.

Activity

Thinking point

1 On what issues did members of the old elites agree with the Nazis?

2 On what issues did many members of the old elites disagree with Hitler?

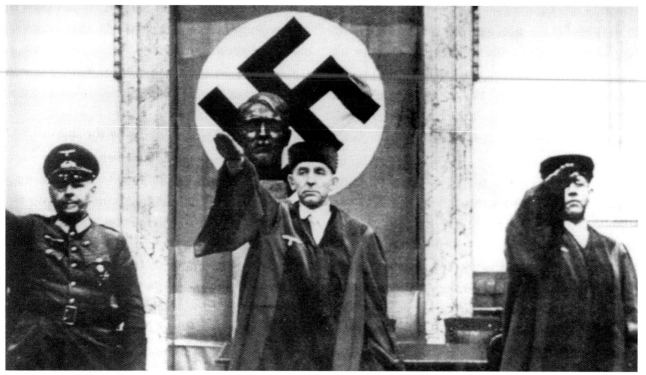

Fig. 12 *German judges give the Nazi salute at the opening of court procedings. The man in the centre is Roland Freisler, a leading Nazi judge who was made president of the People's Court*

Exploring the detail

The purge of Blomberg and Fritsch

Blomberg and Fritsch were purged in February 1938. Blomberg had recently married a younger woman who was shown to be an ex-prostitute. Fritsch was accused of being homosexual and, although he was able to disprove all the charges against him, Hitler was determined to remove him from office. In the wake of this purge, fourteen other generals were dismissed, 46 senior officers were moved to other jobs and Hitler made himself commander in chief of all Germany's armed forces.

Opposition to Hitler within the army and civil service came to a head in the autumn of 1938. For some time there had been growing unease within the elites about the rapid rearmament programme and the drift of Nazi foreign policy. It was not that the opposition disagreed with Hitler's long-term aims of rebuilding Germany's military strength and expanding to the east. The objection of those who opposed Hitler was that he was forcing the pace and leading Germany into a war for which the country was not yet prepared. In November 1937, Hitler outlined his secret thoughts to senior army commanders and leading Nazis such as Göring, making it clear that he envisaged a union with Austria and an invasion of Czechoslovakia within a year. At this meeting, the Defence Minister, General Blomberg, and the Commander in Chief of the army, General Fritsch, expressed their doubts to Hitler. Within three months, Hitler had purged them from the army leadership and replaced them with more compliant generals.

Hitler had decisively demonstrated his political mastery over the army but there were still senior figures who opposed his plans and were prepared to act in order, as they saw it, to save Germany from military disaster. In late September 1938, Hitler put pressure on Czechoslovakia and ordered the army to prepare plans for an invasion. Had the invasion been launched, it seemed likely that Britain and France would support Czechoslovakia and a general European war would result. The imminent threat of war prompted General Beck to plot against Hitler to remove him from power in a military coup. Detailed plans were made for a march on Berlin if war was declared, but the whole enterprise depended on Britain and France standing by Czechoslovakia and making the threat of war credible. An envoy was sent to London and Paris to inform the British and French governments of the plans but, although the plotters were listened to sympathetically, they were not given any assurances that these governments would be prepared to risk war. When the British prime minister, Neville Chamberlain, and the French prime minister, Édouard Daladier, met with Hitler at the end of September in Munich and agreed to a peaceful German takeover of the Sudetenland area of Czechoslovakia, the threat of war receded. This cut the ground from under the conspirators' feet. Hitler had achieved another 'victory without bloodshed' – although he himself felt cheated out of the war that he been planning – and the conspiracy to overthrow him receded quietly into the background. There would be further plots against Hitler from within the armed forces during the war but, for the time being Hitler's authority had been strengthened by the events of 1938.

Conclusion

Dissent within Nazi Germany was expressed in a variety of ways and was motivated by different factors. Grumbling about economic hardship appears to have been widespread at times. This was essentially non-political and not intended to be a threat to the regime but, in a society in which the regime demanded total subservience and conformity, even a moan about the shortage of essential foodstuffs could lead to arrest and criminal charges. Propaganda, indoctrination and repression had created an atmosphere in which the vast majority of Germans were prepared to support the regime. There was no basis for an organised and sustained resistance in Nazi Germany, certainly not one which could command mass support. Opposition to the Nazi regime, therefore, was fragmented and hampered by the fact that, even among those who were prepared on occasion to speak or act against the regime, there was a belief that the Nazi regime should be credited with having restored order, prosperity and national pride and had rid Germany of its internal enemies.

Summary questions

1. Explain why some groups in German society suffered more persecution than others.

2. 'Opposition to the Nazi regime made very little impact on the German people as a whole.' Explain why you agree or disagree with this view.

Learning outcomes

In this section, you have looked at the ways in which policies affected young people, workers, peasants and the Churches. You have also studied the Nazi police state and its methods of attempting to suppress opposition to the regime. Finally, you have studied the extent to which Germans from different social groups and different generations accepted or resisted the Nazis' efforts to make them conform. After reading this section, you should be able to assess to what extent the Nazis were successful in their attempts to build a *Volksgemeinschaft* and the extent of resistance to the Nazis.

Exploring the detail

The conspirators against Hitler in 1938

The plot to remove Hitler involved a number of senior figures in the armed forces, including Admiral Wilhelm Canaris, the head of military intelligence, and his assistant Brigadier-General Hans Oster. General Ludwig Beck had been head of the army general staff until August 1938, when he resigned in protest against Hitler's plans to invade Czechoslovakia. Also involved were General Erwin von Witzleben and General Erich Höpner. In the civil service, the conspiracy had the support of Ulrich von Hassell, who had been ambassador to Rome until February 1938, and Ernst von Weizsäcker from the foreign office. A key figure in the conspiracy was Carl Goerdeler, Mayor of Leipzig until 1937 and a member of the government until 1935, when he resigned over doubts about the speed of the rearmament programme. Goerdeler was one of the envoys who visited London and Paris on behalf of the conspiracy.

Practice questions

Study the following sources and answer the questions which follow.

My friend and I went to every American film going, no matter how bad it was. And there were shops where, if they knew you, you could buy jazz records in the back room. And, of course, they were THE things to have. What you did NOT do was to live up to the Nazi ideal of beauty, sex and culture. A woman's life under Hitler was completely dreadful. A German woman did not wear make-up, she did not smoke, she should have a thousand children – all that rubbish still brings a chill to my spine even now.

*From an interview with Karma Rauhut about her experiences growing up in Nazi Germany, quoted in Owings, A., **Frauen; German Women Recall the Third Reich**, 1993*

Most of the German students I and other non-Germans came into contact with at Marburg were only too anxious to show their Nazi leanings. They took us to Party demonstrations, to propaganda films and they taught us songs with a Nazi message. They talked a lot about team spirit, all-out endeavour and achievement. They defended the concentration camps. They lent us books glorifying the Nordic race. And yet at the same time they were pleasant companions, whose efforts to convert us were made sincerely, for our own good.

*The view of a visitor to Germany in the 1930s, adapted from Goodbody, M., **A Bristolian in the Third Reich**, 1991*

Even though father hated everything connected with the Nazis, I loved being in the Hitler Youth. I liked the comradeship, the marching, the sport and the war games. We were brought up to love our Führer who to me was like a second God. There was no law to join the Hitler Youth; even so, only one of my classmates managed to stay out of it. Early one morning my neighbour, a trade union secretary, was taken away by the SS and the police. My mother was too scared to be seen talking to his wife. Father became very quiet. He begged me not to repeat what he had said about the whole Nazi set-up.

*Adapted from Metelmann, H., **Through Hell for Hitler**, 1990*

(a) Use Sources A and B and your own knowledge to explain how far the views in Source B differ from those in Source A in relation to the attitudes of German youth towards Nazi ideology.

(12 marks)

Study tip When answering this question, it is important to remember that both sources have to be used and explicitly referred to. The question asks 'how far' the views in the sources differ. This requires you to identify both points of agreement and of disagreement. It is a good idea to make a simple table with two columns for agreement and disagreement and make notes from each source under these headings. There are clear differences between the sources on attitudes of young Germans towards Nazi ideology. Source A, for example, describes how young women rejected the Nazi ideal of beauty, sex and culture, whereas Source B describes how young Germans had enthusiastically embraced Nazi ideas. Source A, therefore, shows the rebellious side of German youth while Source B describes more conformist attitudes. There are less obvious similarities but the references to the Nazi ideal of beauty and so on in Source A and the reference to the glorification of the Nordic race in Source B do overlap to some extent. The question also asks you to use your own knowledge. This does not have to be extensive, nor should it dominate your answer which must be mainly about the sources. Do try, however, to place the sources in their historical context – in this case, the Nazi efforts to indoctrinate youth and their effectiveness.

(b) Using Sources A, B and C and your own knowledge, how successful was the use of fear and repression by the Nazi regime in securing conformity from German youth?

(24 marks)

Study tip This question requires you to use all three sources and your own knowledge. The omission of one or other of these elements in your answer will place a limit on the marks you can achieve. Source A suggests that the Nazis' efforts were not successful since it is evidence of rebelliousness. Source B shows the conformity of German youth but there is no suggestion that this was due to fear and repression. The tone of the source suggests that the students referred to had willingly adopted Nazi ideology. Source C, on the other hand, does refer to the fear of repression felt by parents and, indirectly, by the author. Once again the tone suggests that the young Henry Metelmann was a willing participant in the Hitler Youth. These sources need to be placed in context which is where you should use your own knowledge. You could, for example, point out that terror and repression were indispensable weapons in the Nazis' arsenal but that control over the German people was also achieved through propaganda and indoctrination. The examiner will be looking for a balanced answer in which you put forward two sides of an argument which leads to a conclusion in which you offer your own judgment on the degree of success.

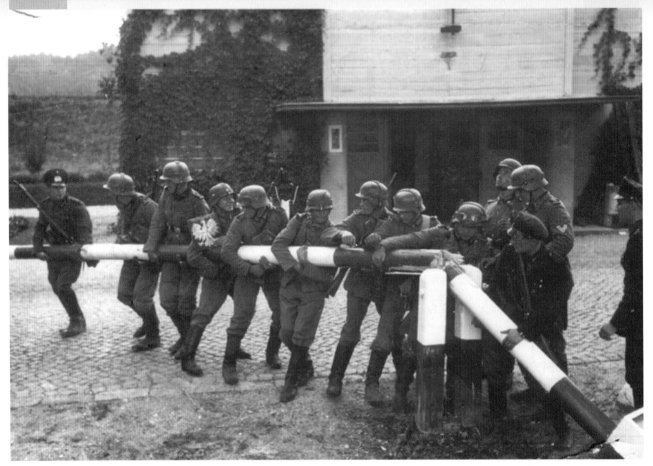

Fig. 1 *German soldiers dismantle a barrier on the border with Poland, prior to the invasion of Poland on 1 September 1939*

In this chapter you will learn about:

- the impact on the Nazi regime and the German people of the Second World War

- the ways in which 'total war' and the Allied bombing of Germany affected the regime and the people

- the state of Germany in 1945.

It has been a lovely September day, the sun shining, the air balmy, the sort of day the Berliner loves to spend in the woods or on the lakes nearby. I walked in the streets. On the faces of the people astonishment, depression. Until today they had been going about their business pretty much as usual. There were food cards and soap cards and you couldn't get any petrol and at night it was difficult stumbling around in the black-out. But the war in the east has seemed a bit far away to them. Few believed that Britain and France would move [against Germany].

In 1914, I believe, the excitement in Berlin on the first day of the world war was tremendous. Today, no excitement, no hurrahs, no cheering, no throwing of flowers, no war fever, no war hysteria.

1

*Description of the mood in Berlin on the day Britain and France declared war on Germany, from Shirer, W., **Berlin Diary; The Journal of a Foreign Correspondent, 1933–41**, 1970*

Changes in attitudes and daily lives, 1939–41

The morale of the German people

The experience of the First World War had left Hitler and the Nazis with two key points of reference in their approach to public opinion: in August 1914, Hitler was a member of a cheering crowd in the streets of Munich which greeted the declaration of war on Russia and France with patriotic enthusiasm, whereas at the end of the war in 1918, Hitler was one of many German soldiers who believed that their bravery and sacrifices had been undermined by a mood of defeatism and war-weariness on the home front. The aims of Nazi policy and propaganda were to recreate the patriotic enthusiasm and national unity of August 1914 and to avoid the despair and defeatism of November 1918.

When war started in September 1939, there were no cheering crowds in Berlin or other German cities. Although loyalty to the Führer was very strong, and his foreign policy triumphs between 1933 and 1939 had been very popular, the mood of the German public at the news of the start of hostilities with Poland was one of reluctant loyalty. In terms of public opinion, therefore, the start of the Second World War in Germany did not match Hitler's expectations. Moreover, the experience of the First World War had taught Hitler that public opinion can change. It was, therefore, a principal aim of Nazi domestic policy in the early years of the war to sustain the morale of the home front and eliminate any elements of weakness in the public mood. The SD was given the task of preparing regular reports on the state of public opinion.

Activity

Source analysis

Read Source 1 and the information in this section.

1 What was the reaction of the German people to the outbreak of war in September 1939?

2 How did this compare with the reaction to the outbreak of the First World War in 1914?

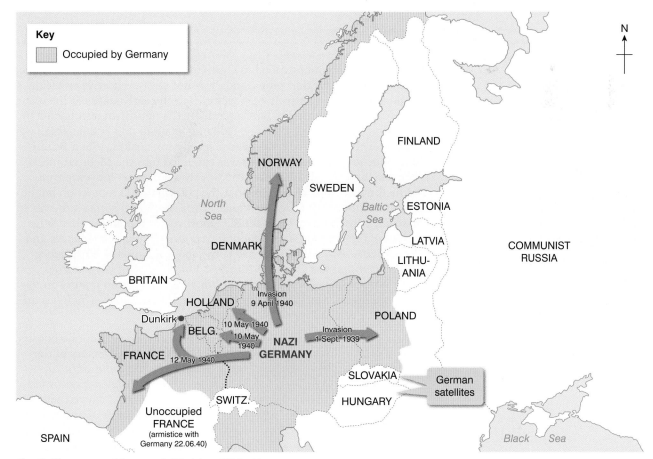

Fig. 2 *The success of Germany's Blitzkrieg, 1939–41*

Table 1 *Public mood in Germany in response to the progress of Germany's armed forces in the conflict*

Date	Events in the war	Public mood
Sept 1939	Invasion of Poland (1 Sept) Britain and France declare war on Germany (3 Sept)	Reluctant loyalty and a sense of foreboding
Oct 1939–April 1940	Rapid defeat of Poland, followed by period of 'phoney war' when the two sides consider their next moves	Growing hostility to Britain as the main cause of the war and a hope that the war will be over soon Growing discontent in the exceptionally severe winter of 1939–40 due to coal shortages and a partial breakdown of the railway network
May–June 1940	Rapid victories over Norway and Denmark Victories over Holland, Belgium	Euphoria and celebration of the speedy victories SD reports speak of unity and optimism
July–Sept 1940	Refusal of Great Britain to make peace Abandonment of German plans for invasion of Britain First large-scale bombing of Berlin by RAF (August)	Euphoria subsides; replaced by growing disillusionment Start of British air-raids adds to the sense of frustration, especially as Nazi propaganda claimed that this could not happen Göbbels launches a propaganda offensive against the 'mean and pathetic warmongers' in the British government
Oct 1940–May 1941	German advances in the Balkans and North Africa Start of blitz on British cities and U-boat campaign in North Atlantic	Disillusionment persists as Britain no nearer to defeat Second winter of the war marked by shortages of coal and shoes and rising prices At the end of 1940, Göbbels describes the public mood as one of 'light depression'
June 1941	Invasion of the USSR Early German successes force Red Army to retreat	Public mood mixed and uncertain

It is clear that the public mood in Germany in the first 21 months of the war was volatile and that propaganda was not always effective in lifting morale. Quick and relatively easy victories in the early stages of the war were a cause for celebration but, underlying the optimism engendered by the reports from Poland, Norway, Holland, Belgium and France, there was a desire for the war to be brought to a speedy conclusion. When Britain did not sue for peace and the war was extended into the Mediterranean, it became increasingly clear that the war would drag on for some time. The historian Craig has written that the optimistic SD reports on public opinion in June 1940 were the *'the last time that the reports were ever so reassuring'*. By October 1940, an SD report was complaining that *'large sections of the population are adopting a completely unappreciative and uncooperative attitude'* which had come about because of *'impatience with the fact that the "big blow" against Britain has not yet occurred'*. This SD report also complained that *'the oral and written reports on the effects of English bomb attacks have generated a psychosis which has an extremely adverse effect on our propaganda.'*

In these circumstances, Hitler had a vital role to play as a morale-booster. A speech Hitler made on 8 November 1940, on the anniversary of the Beer Hall Putsch, was reported by the SD to have *'lifted the spirits of large numbers of people once more who have recently been disgruntled and sceptical as a result of personal or economic worries'*. Nevertheless, the effect of such speeches was only temporary. The onset of another harsh winter and the realities of living under wartime conditions soon dissipated the optimism which Hitler had been able to generate. Even before the invasion of the Soviet Union there were growing fears that

Activity

Thinking point

To what extent did German public opinion towards the war change between September 1939 and June 1941?

'an expansion of the war will gradually weaken Germany'. By the summer of 1941 the SD was reporting people's fears that *'The war is going to go on for years. It is harder than we thought it would be.'*

Rationing

One of the critical factors in maintaining civilian morale was the availability of vital foodstuffs and other commodities. Shortages and the inadequacies of the rationing system during the First World War were one of the main causes of growing war-weariness in 1917 and 1918, and the Nazi regime was determined not to make the same mistakes as the Kaiser's government. Decrees establishing a rationing system were issued even before the war began. On 28 August 1939, rationing of bread and cereal products, meat, fats and dairy products, and sugar began. Clothing was not initially included in the rationing scheme but permits were needed to purchase clothes. This caused panic buying before the regulations took effect and led to the inclusion of clothing in the rationing scheme in November 1939.

The allocation of food rations was based on age, occupation and race. Those who were employed in manual labour received more than those who had more sedentary occupations. Jews received smaller rations. There were special allocations for groups such as pregnant women and nursing mothers and for the sick. The allocations which were established at the beginning of the war remained largely unchanged during the first two years of the war.

The Nazi regime was reluctant to ask the civilian population to make significant reductions in their consumption at the beginning of the war for fear that this might provoke anti-war feelings. The production of consumer goods did not decline significantly in the early stages of the war. The regime was able to exploit the newly occupied countries for food supplies for the German people and, while the Nazi-Soviet Pact was in force, there were also imports of grain from the Soviet Union. On the whole, therefore, the rationing system worked efficiently and there were no serious food shortages between 1939 and 1941. Shortages of coal, of shoes and of soap and washing powder, however, did cause discontent from time to time.

Workers

The outbreak of war led to an increase in the number of men who were conscripted into the armed forces. At the same time, there was a need to increase the production of armaments. With a limited supply of male labour in Germany, these two demands could only be achieved by using the available labour force in the most efficient way possible and by using foreign labour. Large numbers of non-essential workers were released for military service. There was also a reduction of workers employed in consumer goods industries with a consequent rise in the numbers employed in munitions. The full scale conscription of labour into essential war work, however, was not implemented in the first two years of the war.

In his 'Decree on the Conversion of the Whole German Economy onto a War Footing' of 3 September 1939, Hitler imposed wage reductions and a ban on the payment of bonuses for overtime, Sunday work and night-shift working. This caused widespread discontent among the labour force which was reflected in an increased level of absenteeism. Consequently, in October 1939, the regime relented. Wage levels were restored to their pre-war levels and the payment of bonuses was reintroduced.

 Activity

Thinking point

How effective was Nazi propaganda between September 1939 and June 1941 in sustaining the morale of the German people?

 Activity

Discussion point

What effect might the rationing system have had on the morale of the German people?

 Did you know?

In August 1939, Nazi Germany and the Soviet Union concluded the Nazi-Soviet Pact under which they agreed to divide Poland between them. When German forces entered Poland on 1 September 1939 the Soviet Union did not attempt to stop the invasion.

 Exploring the detail

The use of foreign labour

After the defeat of Poland, the German occupying authorities recruited Polish workers to work in Germany to fill some of the gaps in the labour market. Most of these workers were employed in agriculture, especially in the east of Germany. After May 1940, the German authorities began to coerce Poles to work in Germany and also began to use prisoners of war to undertake war work.

The German wartime economy

Despite Hitler's decree of 3 September 1939, the German economy was only partially mobilised for war and Germany's armed forces suffered from shortages of weapons and equipment. Hitler was determined that the civilian population should not suffer serious hardship as a result of the war, fearing that this would cause a loss of morale. As a result, vital raw materials were not reserved for the production of munitions. The Nazis were also the victims of their own early successes in the war. The quick victories against Poland, Norway, Holland, Belgium and France led to a belief that there was no need for a full-scale mobilisation for war, even when the invasion of the Soviet Union was launched. There was also a lack of coherent planning and organisation within the Nazi regime. Competing agencies and rivalries between leading figures led to chaotic decision making and wasteful duplication of effort.

Women

Women bore the brunt of the hardships endured on the home front. As housewives, married women were obliged to spend time queuing for supplies of vital foodstuffs when shortages occurred. As mothers, women had to shoulder even more of the task of childcare when their husbands were away in the armed forces. As workers, women played an increasingly vital role in the German war economy.

The Nazis placed great emphasis on the woman's role as a child-bearer. Measures were taken during the period 1933–39 to encourage couples to marry and have children. There was also pressure on married women, particularly in the early years of the Nazi regime, to give up paid employment and concentrate on their role as home-makers and child-rearers. This policy, however, was not followed consistently. When a severe labour shortage threatened to undermine the rearmament programme in 1936–37, the Nazi regime modified its position. By September 1939, the number of women in paid employment had increased; there were 6,400,000 married women in employment and women as a whole made up 27% of the industrial labour force. The need to increase armaments production after war had broken out and more male workers had been conscripted into the armed forces led to pressure for more women to be employed in industry. There was, however, tension between Nazi ideology and the needs of the war economy. When Hitler was advised, in the summer of 1940, that industry needed more women workers, he refused to sanction this on ideological grounds. Although the regime had taken powers to conscript workers into essential war work, these powers were used very sparingly in relation to women. By June 1940, only 250,000 women had been conscripted and those who were conscripted were merely transferred from the production of consumer goods to war work. The regime also provided generous benefits for the families of conscripted soldiers, thus removing one of the incentives for married women to seek work. With working hours in factories increasing due to the pressures of wartime production, there was even more pressure for married women with children to give up employment. The result was that the number of women workers in industry actually declined between 1939 and 1941.

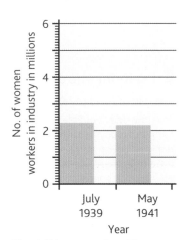

Fig. 4 *Women employed in industry, 1939–41*

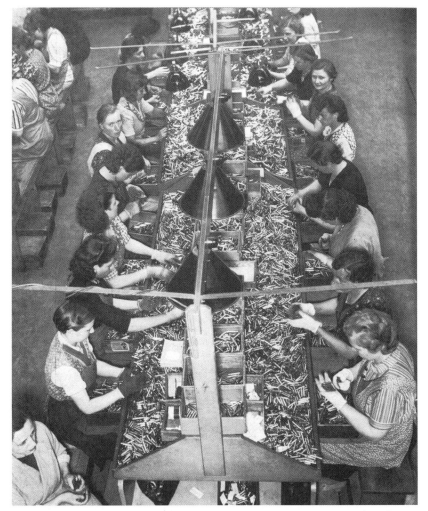

Fig. 3 *By 1942, despite Hitler's objections, many German women were employed in armaments factories*

The National Socialist Women organisation, the NS-F, organised classes to teach women how to cope with wartime conditions. There were cookery classes to teach housewives how to make the most economical use of the available food supplies and sewing classes to teach them how to repair worn clothing. Women were also mobilised by the NS-F to help with the harvest, to prepare parcels of food and clothing for soldiers at the front and to help with evacuated children from the cities. Community evenings were organised to sustain morale and also for the purpose of indoctrination.

Youth

Membership of the Hitler Youth and BDM had become compulsory for all young people in 1939. The Nazis treated the welfare and indoctrination of youth as a high priority and there was a recognition that young people were capable of contributing to the war effort. The regime did not, however, consider it necessary in the early stages of the war to conscript the young into helping with essential war work or military service. Hitler Youth activities continued much as in peacetime with a greater emphasis on preparing boys for their future role as soldiers. Training exercises in fieldcraft and shooting practice were part of the military training for boys. Hitler Youth members were also sent to help with the harvest, and all young people were expected to participate in collecting money for the Winter Aid programme.

Cross-reference

For more detail on the NS-F see page 78.

Cross-reference

For more detail on the Hitler Youth and the BDM see pages 72–75.

Exploring the detail

The Winter Aid Programme

The Winter Aid programme was established in September 1933 as a short-term relief programme for the unemployed. 4,000 paid workers and 1.5 million volunteers provided soup, food parcels and clothing to the destitute. Nazi propaganda presented the Winter Aid programme not as a form of welfare or charity, both of which were regarded by the Nazis as cossetting the weak and feeble members of the race, but as a form of racial self-help, aid given by the German people for the German people. Contributions to the programme were virtually compulsory since anyone who refused was branded as an enemy of the regime.

The evacuation of children from cities coming under bombing attack was begun in September 1940. This initially involved only children from Berlin and Hamburg but, as more cities came under aerial bombardment, the scheme was later extended. The evacuation organisation set up its own camps to receive evacuees and also requisitioned hotels and guest houses. Other evacuees were accommodated in foster families. Although the evacuation scheme was supposed to be voluntary, it was hard for children to opt out since whole schools were evacuated together and there was strong social pressure to participate.

Summary

The policy of the Nazi regime towards industrial production and sustaining morale on the home front in the first 21 months of the war was confused, inconsistent and, at times, contradictory. Although Hitler and other leading Nazis recognised the need to increase production of munitions and release young men for service in the armed forces, their policies did not always reflect these priorities. In many cases, Nazi ideology got in the way of implementing the measures that were needed to maximise production. The war effort was also hampered by lack of effective, centralised planning and coordination, a problem that was rooted in the systemic weaknesses of the Nazi regime. Finally, the speed and the ease of the victories over Poland in 1939 and Norway, Holland, Belgium and France in 1940 lulled the regime into a false sense of security. There appeared to be no pressing need to change direction and reorder priorities when Germany's success in the war appeared to be unstoppable. With the invasion of the Soviet Union in June 1941, however, the inadequacies of Germany's preparedness for war quickly became apparent and the pressure for a radical change of direction increased.

Activity

Thinking point

1. What was the impact of the war on workers, women and young people?

2. To what extent did the demands of the war effort force the Nazi regime to compromise its ideological beliefs?

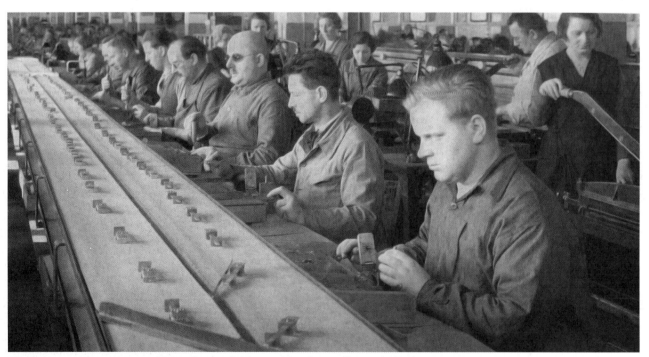

Fig. 5 *Men and women engaged in wartime production work in a German factory in 1942*

The impact of the invasion of the USSR and the start of total war

The morale of the German people

In domestic politics the mood and bearing of the population is still depressed, worried, full of mistrust, annoyance and frustration, although the food supply situation has improved somewhat. There is no lack of loud expressions of indignation and bitter complaints from the population. These continue to be about illicit trading, hoarding, 'good contacts', the behaviour of the better-off and of Party comrades.

2   *From an SD report from Stuttgart, July 1941, quoted in Noakes, J.,*
Nazism 1919–45, Vol. 4, *1998*

The events in the east are causing people a great deal of concern. While nobody doubts that the Soviets will be defeated, they had not reckoned with such a tough opponent. People are anticipating heavy losses, including on our side. And expecting the exhaustion of our reserves of human material, which for months will make it impossible to achieve our real war aim of finishing off England. There is concern about a new wartime winter involving very hard work with minimum food.

3   *From an SD report from Leipzig, August 1941, quoted in Noakes, J.,*
Nazism 1919–45, Vol. 4, *1998*

Activity

Source analysis

What can we learn from Sources 2 and 3 about the mood of the German people in the summer of 1941?

The invasion of the Soviet Union in June 1941, and the failure of German forces to achieve a quick and decisive victory in the east, led to a growing realisation among the German people that the war would drag on for some time to come and that the civilian population would be subjected to increasing strain. It was not until the winter of 1941–42, however, that the full extent of Germany's problems became apparent. Indeed, in November 1941, when the German army had pushed Soviet forces back to within twenty miles of Moscow and was besieging Leningrad, Reich Press Chief, Otto Dietrich, announced confidently that the Red Army was broken and victory would follow within weeks. This announcement induced a temporary mood of optimism among the civilian population.

By the end of the year, however, a series of setbacks had led to a perceptible change in the public mood:

- On 5 December 1941, the Red Army had launched a counter-offensive outside Moscow which had forced the German army to fall back onto defensive positions.

- On 11 December 1941, Hitler had declared war on the United States, after Germany's ally Japan had attacked the American Pacific Fleet at Pearl Harbour.

- On 19 December 1941, the army Commander in Chief, General Brauchitsch, had been dismissed by Hitler for the failures of the German army at Moscow.

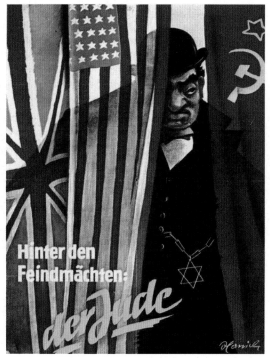

Fig. 6 *German wartime propaganda attempted to strengthen the resolve of the German people by showing Germany as the victim of a Jewish world conspiracy. The slogan reads, 'Behind the enemies, the Jew'*

Rising casualty figures and letters home from soldiers serving on the eastern front gradually awakened the civilian population to the realities of the war they were engaged in. When Göbbels broadcast an appeal for people to collect winter clothing for soldiers on the eastern front, the mood of disillusionment deepened.

> The announcement of the collection of winter things has produced a great response among all sections of the population and is still at the forefront of people's concern. It is unanimously reported that the announcement aroused great astonishment in view of the fact that recently the good and adequate provision of winter clothing for our soldiers has been repeatedly reported in the press and in various newsreels. The announcement was clear confirmation of the fact that the accounts of men on leave from the front about the lack of equipment capable of coping with the Russian cold were accurate and were not, as one would have assumed from the propaganda to the contrary, long out of date.

4 *From an SD report, January 1942, quoted in Noakes, J.,*
Nazism 1919–45, Vol. 4, 1998

The SD report in January 1942, however, stated that '*Faith in the Führer is unshakeable*'. Nevertheless, the scepticism about propaganda which was remarked upon in this report became a regular theme of SD reports for the rest of the war and was an early sign that confidence in the regime was beginning to erode.

The summer of 1942 brought better news about the progress of the war from a German point of view. There were victories for German and Italian forces against the British in North Africa while, in the Soviet Union, German forces advanced through the southern Ukraine towards the Caucasus and the vital Soviet oilfields in the Baku region. The autumn of 1942, however, brought a series of bad news reports. In October, German and Italian forces were defeated at El Alamein in North Africa and began a long retreat across the desert. More significantly, the German Sixth Army had been surrounded by Soviet forces at Stalingrad at the end of November. Having been ordered by Hitler not to retreat, the Sixth Army became trapped and was finally forced to surrender at the end of January 1943. Even before this shattering defeat, however, there was a growing mood of apprehension, demoralisation and scepticism among the German population, as the following source shows:

Exploring the detail

El Alamein

The battle of El Alamein on 23 October 1942 was a turning point in the war in North Africa. Rommel's Afrika Korps was decisively defeated by the British Eighth Army led by Field Marshal Montgomery, following which Rommel retreated westwards across the desert. He was trapped by another Anglo-American force which was advancing eastwards from Algeria and, in May 1943, German and Italian forces in North Africa surrendered.

Activity

Source analysis

What can we learn from Sources 4 and 5 about the following?

1 The effectiveness of Nazi propaganda

2 Attitudes towards the regime, at this crucial stage in the war

> At the moment the whole nation is deeply shaken by the impression that the fate of the Sixth Army is already sealed and by concern about the further development of the war situation. Among the many questions arising from the changed situation, people ask above all why Stalingrad was not evacuated or relieved, and how it was possible, only a few months ago, to describe the military situation as secure and as not unfavourable. In particular, people discuss, with a marked undertone of criticism, the underestimate of the Russian combat forces through which now for the second time a severe crisis has been triggered. Despite their readiness to subject themselves to the introduction of total war, many compatriots say that this step was taken very late.
>
> Fearing that an unfavourable end to the war is now possible, many compatriots are seriously thinking about the consequences of defeat.

5 *From an SD report, 28 January 1943, quoted in Noakes, J.,*
Nazism 1919–45, Vol. 4, 1998

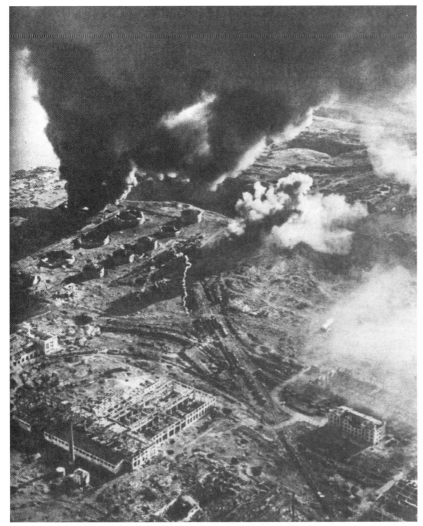

Fig. 7 *An aerial photograph taken during the Battle of Stalingrad, showing German fuel stores on fire*

The defeat at Stalingrad was a major turning point in the war, both militarily and on the home front. War-weariness, which had been growing since the end of 1941, now became much more evident. Criticism of the propaganda emanating from the regime increased and the Hilter myth began to lose some its potency. On the other hand, there was undoubtedly a deep well of patriotism and willingness to endure hardship and sacrifice on which the regime could draw as it, albeit belatedly, attempted to gear the nation up for total war.

Workers

The German reverse outside Moscow in December 1941 brought the labour supply issue to a head. Efforts to take labour away from civilian work to concentrate on armaments production had been frustrated by opposition from local Gauleiters, anxious to keep employment within their own areas. Since Hitler was opposed to the increased use of women in industry, the shortage of labour posed a serious threat to the plans to increase production of vital war materials. Part of the answer to this problem was found in the increase use of foreign labour. From June 1940 until the spring of 1942, foreign workers in German industry were mainly recruited from occupied countries in western Europe. After the invasion of the USSR, however, there was a dramatic increase in the number of prisoners of war and, in October 1941, Hitler agreed that Russian prisoners of war could be used as slave labour. By December 1941, there were some four million foreign workers employed in Germany. In March 1942, Hitler established the Plenipotentiary General for Labour Allocation to organise centralised control over the procurement and allocation of foreign labour. This department was headed by Fritz Sauckel, a Gauleiter, who used ruthless force to increase the number of foreign workers.

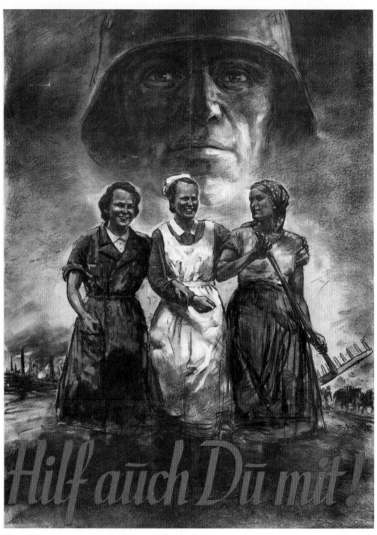

Fig. 8 *German wartime propaganda attempted to persude women to support the fighting men. This 1941 poster carries the slogan, 'You help with it too'*

The defeat at Stalingrad in January 1943 led to even more drastic measures to increase the labour supply. Even before the surrender of German forces, Hitler had issued, on 13 January 1943, a Decree for the Comprehensive Deployment of Men and Women for Reich Defence Tasks. This established a small committee to oversee the mobilisation of labour for the war effort. Under this decree, all men aged 16–65 and women aged 17–45 had to register for work with their local labour office. It was also decreed that small businesses which were not essential for the war effort should be closed and their employees transferred to more essential work. In terms of labour, this was the point at which the demands of total war began to have a significant impact. A rigorous 'comb-through' exercise was conducted to identify men who could be released from employment for military service and conscription of labour began to become a reality. Ideological considerations, however, still prevented the Nazi regime from treating women workers the same as males.

Key profile

Albert Speer

Speer (1905–81) was an architect who had joined the Nazi Party in 1931. He was responsible for the stage management of the Nuremberg rallies and for designing key public buildings in the Third Reich. In 1942, he was appointed armaments minister, with responsibility for increasing the production of armaments. After the war, he was tried at Nuremberg and sentenced to twenty years imprisonment.

Women

> I went to Sauckel with the proposition that we should recruit our labour from the ranks of German women. He replied brusquely that where to obtain workers was his business. Moreover, he said, as Gauleiter he was Hitler's subordinate and responsible to the Führer alone. Sauckel laid great weight on the danger that factory work might inflict moral harm on German womanhood; not only might their 'psychic and emotional life' be affected but also their ability to bear children. Göring totally concurred. But to be absolutely sure Sauckel went immediately to Hitler and had him confirm the decision. All my good arguments were therefore blown to the wind.

6   *From Speer, S., **Inside the Third Reich**, 1970*

The issue of the employment of women went to the heart of the weaknesses of the Nazi regime. Hitler and other leading Nazis had a deep-seated ideological objection to the employment of married women outside the home and their propaganda and policies reflected this. The needs of the rearmament programme in the 1930s, and total war after the invasion of the Soviet Union, however, required the maximum deployment of Germany's labour force. Although there had been some concessions to pragmatism in allowing some women to undertake industrial employment, there was an unwillingness to compel women to work in industry. Voluntary campaigns to persuade women to register for work in the early stages of the war had failed.

In June 1941, Göring issued a decree that all female workers who were in receipt of **family allowance** and had given up paid employment but had not produced children should be forced to register for work or lose their allowance. This was the first tentative step towards the conscription of female labour but in practice had only limited effect since it only applied to those women who had been employed previously. It did not apply to married women who had never worked outside the home. Since this group of women was overwhelmingly middle class, whereas those who had been previously employed were mainly from the working class,

Did you know?

Hitler was confident of victory against the Soviet Union and believed that gaining access to its vast reserves of raw materials and its fertile farmlands would solve the problems of the German economy. When the German advance, however, was halted outside Moscow in December 1941, Hitler realised that Germany had to prepare for a long struggle. In early 1942, Hitler took the first steps towards implementing a total war strategy. In February 1942, he appointed Albert Speer minister for armaments and munitions and gave him power to control the allocation of raw materials and the construction of new factories. Even then, however, Speer did not have total control over all aspects of armaments production although he did succeed in raising the production levels of vital weapons and equipment.

Key terms

Family allowance: a financial benefit paid to families to encourage them to have more children. It was based on the number of children in the family.

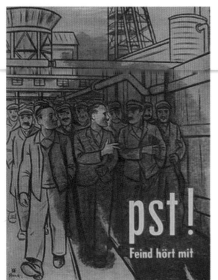

Fig. 9 *A propaganda poster warning German people to be aware of spies. The slogan reads, 'Shush! The enemy is listening to you'*

Activity

Source analysis

Read Source 7. What aspects of this report would have been particularly worrying for the Nazi regime?

Activity

Discussion point

How far is it true to say that the German people were increasingly reluctant to support the Nazi regime between September 1939 and early 1943?

Cross-reference

For more detail on the Waffen-SS, see page 95.

Key terms

Auxiliaries: people who supported the frontline troops or replaced them in non-combat roles. Air defence duties would include the operating of searchlights and anti-aircraft guns.

Göring's decree stoked up class resentments. As a result of this decree, only 130,000 extra women were sent to the armaments factories.

The defeat at Stalingrad meant that demands for the total mobilisation of labour had become irresistible. The decree of January 1943 which forced all women between the ages of 17 and 45 to register for work appeared to show that Hitler had abandoned his ideological objection to the employment of married women. In fact, Hitler had merely been persuaded to modify his views. It was at his insistence that older women were exempted from labour registration and that there were many other exemptions. Pregnant women, mothers with two or more children and farmers' wives were not obliged to register. Once again, working-class women resented the number of exemptions and the lack of consistency in implementing the decree. By June 1943, fewer than half a million extra women had joined the industrial labour force.

> The reports note that, in particular, those national comrades who have long been employed in important war work had expected tough regulations. However, after the publication of the details of the decree they were astonished that so many exemptions had been given. The disapproval of this manifested itself in some cases in quite drastic remarks such as 'rubber decree' etc. The question was frequently raised as to whether all those groups who up to now had succeeded in 'avoiding all work' would be caught.
>
> Already women and girls from every social class have been contacting numerous Labour Offices to try to prove that they are not available for labour mobilization.

7   *From an SD report, February 1943, quoted in Noakes, J.,* **Nazism 1919–45,** *Vol. 4, 1998*

Youth

The transition towards total war also had an impact on young people. Even before 1942, the age at which young men became subject to military conscription had been reduced. In 1940, a youth was liable to be called up into the armed forces at the age of 19; in 1941 the age was reduced to 18 and in 1943 to 17. There was also an increase in the demands placed upon younger teenagers. In 1942, 600,000 boys and 1,400,000 girls had been organised through their youth organisations to help with the gathering in of the harvest. The Hitler Youth placed more emphasis on military training for youths. Military training camps were set up at which 17-year-old youths would attend three-week courses under army and Waffen-SS instructors. By November 1942, 120 of these camps had been established.

In January 1943, as part of the implementation of total war policies, 16- and 17-year-old schoolboys were conscripted as Luftwaffe and naval **auxiliaries** and were deployed on air defence duties. Whole school classes were conscripted en bloc and the boys continued their education under visiting teachers.

The start of total war

The invasion of the Soviet Union, and the reverses suffered by German forces after December 1941, placed the regime and the German nation under severe strain. By December 1941, it was clear that Germany was engaged in a long struggle and by January 1943 it had become clear that

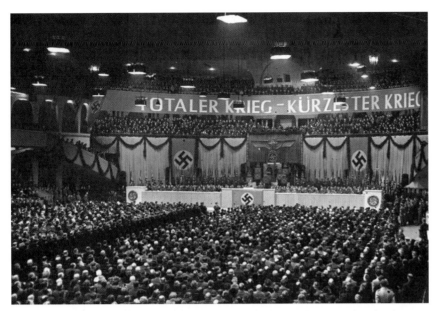

Fig. 10 *Göbbels delivering his total war speech at the Sports Palace in Berlin. The slogan reads, 'Total War – Shorter War'*

this was a struggle for survival. Göbbels made an important speech at the Sports Palace in Berlin in February 1943 in which he called for the nation to engage in total war. The regime, however, had been slow to adjust to the demands of total war and even those measures implemented in January 1943 fell far short of a strategy that would achieve the total mobilisation of Germany's population.

> The measures which we have already taken and which we must take will be animated by the spirit of National Socialist justice. We respect neither station in life nor occupation. Poor and rich, exalted and lowly must be made use of in equal measure. Every man will, in this serious phase of our fateful struggle, be induced to fulfil his duty to the nation; if necessary, he will be forced to do so.

8   *Göbbels' total war speech, February 1943, quoted in Noakes, J.,*
Nazism 1919–45, Vol. 4*, 1998*

> According to the reports we have received, a large section of the population listened to the speech of Dr Göbbels. Its effect – and the reports were unanimous on this – was unusually great and on the whole very favourable. The morale of the population had reached a low point on account of the most recent developments on the eastern front, and they were longing for a clear explanation of the situation. Dr Göbbels' speech, despite its frank description of the seriousness of the situation, had the effect of easing tensions and strengthening confidence and trust in the war leadership.
>
> The theme of 'imminent danger' confirmed the fear of many people that as yet there was no question of stabilizing the eastern front, that the series of setbacks was not yet at an end, and that the war could still take a serious turn. But, though they were shaken, they were not despairing. The population was grateful to the leadership for speaking frankly at last and for telling the plain unvarnished truth.

9   *From an SD report, February 1943, quoted in Noakes, J.,*
Nazism 1919–45, Vol. 4*, 1998*

Activity

Source analysis

To what extent can historians regard Source 9 as reliable evidence of the effects of Göbbels' speech on the German people?

Göbbels' total war speech does appear to have struck a chord with many people, although the main evidence for this comes from SD reports. His call for radical measures to mobilise the population and the economy were, according to the SD report, generally welcomed and the main criticism was that these measures were being introduced too late. Other reports, from Gauleiters, at around the same time said that *'People have become distrustful of National Socialist propaganda because, within a matter of a few weeks, it has been possible to go from one extreme to another, and so they have become mistrustful of every new regulation.'* The aftermath of the defeat at Stalingrad, therefore, was a crucial time for the Nazi regime. Although the total war measures were generally welcomed, and there was a positive response to Göbbels' speech, the military situation continued to deteriorate and there was a growing distrust of Nazi propaganda. With Hitler appearing less frequently in public and making only rare radio broadcasts, the Hitler myth also began to decline.

Summary questions

1 Explain why rationing of some essential foods was introduced in August 1939.

2 How successful was Nazi propaganda in maintaining support for the Nazi regime between September 1939 and early 1943?

The collapse of Hitler's Reich

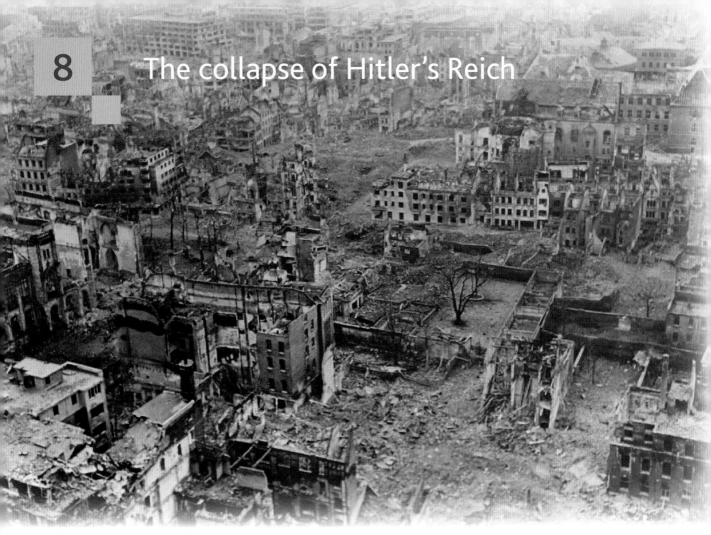

Fig. 1 *The major city of Cologne in ruins on 6 March 1945, as American troops enter the city*

The reports which have come in from all over the Reich are unanimous in the view that the urban and rural populations are increasingly concerned about the state of the air war and the effects of the latest terror raids. Almost all the reports state that in those areas which are not affected, in particular in central, south and east Germany, exaggerated descriptions and, in particular, figures of those killed are circulating and being believed and, as a result, the fear of air raids is spreading to even the most remote villages.

After the attacks the population appeared completely exhausted and apathetic. Most of the compatriots who had been completely bombed out were, however, cheerful and glad to have got away with their lives. While the population of the affected areas in general demonstrated an exemplary attitude and calmly accepted the fate that had befallen them, there were on a small scale signs of a pragmatic attitude. A few opponents who emerged made hostile remarks about the State, the Party and the leadership.

1	*From an SD report, June 1943, quoted in Noakes, J., **Nazism 1919–45, Vol. 4**, 1998*

The effects of mass bombing and military defeats from 1943

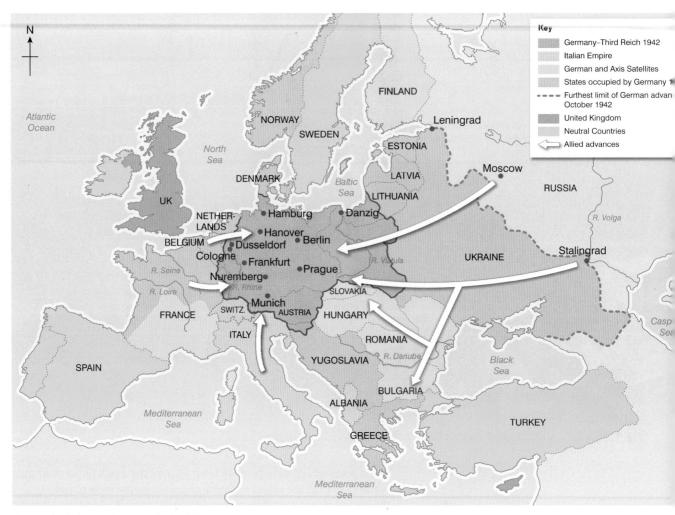

Fig. 2 *The defeat of Germany, 1944–45*

Morale

By the spring of 1944, morale had declined even further. News of almost continuous retreat by German forces on the eastern front, the failure of the U-boat campaign to bring Britain to its knees, and heavy Allied bombing raids on German cities had led to a *'a downbeat mood among the population'* (SD report, March 1944).

> At the moment large sections of the population are intimidated by the military situation. People do not know 'what they should believe'. The 'inexorable advance' of the Bolsheviks, the lack of any prospect of a foreseeable end to the air war, the noticeable increase in tension because of the numerous air raid warnings by day and night, and the thought that, almost like in the First World War, we are being forced to fight against a group of powerful enemies, together with the destruction caused by the air terror, and the deaths in many families reduce the belief that a change for the better can occur, which will bring about final victory, and instead concentrates people's thoughts on the question – what is the point of it all?

The majority of compatriots hold to the belief that whatever happens they have to keep going and 'grit their teeth'. One does it simply because one has to and because there is no alternative left. But there is a feeling of impatience that 'something has got to happen soon'.

2   *From an SD report, March 1944, quoted in Noakes, J., **Nazism 1919–45, Vol. 4**, 1998*

The Allied landings in Normandy on D-Day in June 1944 was a further serious blow to Germany. Paradoxically, events in June 1944 brought an, albeit temporary, lifting of morale. Partly this was due to the feeling that the final settling of accounts with the British and Americans was now at hand, and partly it was due to the reports that finally the Germans had begun their retaliation against the Allied bombing by using their new V1 flying bombs. The rapid advance of British and American forces through France, however, dampened the mood still further. By the end of August 1944, after Paris had been liberated and German forces had suffered further reverses in the east, defeat began to be accepted as inevitable. An SD report from Stuttgart in August 1944 stated that, *'The vast majority are convinced the enemy powers will win.'* Equally seriously, for the regime, was the report that, *'Most compatriots, even those whose belief has hitherto been unshakeable, have lost all faith in the Führer.'* The final months of the war saw growing cynicism about Nazi propaganda and the collapse of the Hitler myth as Germany headed inexorably towards final defeat.

The impact of bombing on morale

Since 1939, the RAF had bombed German cities with mixed results. A new phase in the air war began at the end of March 1942 when the British Royal Air Force (RAF) carried out a major bombing raid on the city of Lübeck. This was the start of the Allied mass bombing campaign in which the RAF attacked German cities by night and the United States Army Air Forces (USAAF) attacked by day, often with 1,000 aircraft at a time. In 1943, the bombing campaign reached an even greater intensity, with 43 German cities being attacked between March and July. Hamburg was bombed seven times between 25 July and 3 August. All of Germany's main industrial and port cities were attacked but there was a high concentration of raids on cities in the Rhineland and Ruhr areas.

Official reports on the impact of the bombing on morale, while detailing the horrific scenes of death and destruction, spoke of the resilience of the civilian population and their continuing support for the regime. The police report from Hamburg, after the raid of 27–28 July 1943, stated that, *'The behaviour of the population at no time and nowhere displayed signs of panic and was worthy of the greatness of this sacrifice.'* An SD report on the impact of the raid on Lübeck in March 1942 noted that, *'The population of Lübeck showed a really remarkable composure, despite the extreme destruction and loss of life.'* This report went on to say that, *'It was a sign of the calm, determined attitude and the unbroken spirit of the people of Lübeck that on the very next day numerous tradespeople demonstrated their unbroken spirit by opening their shops.'* Personal reminiscences of people who experienced at first hand the horrors of the bombing raids paint a rather different picture.

Activity

Source analysis

Read Source 2. What can we learn from this source about the morale of the civilian population in March 1944?

Exploring the detail

The Allied landings in Normandy

The D-Day landings on 6 June 1944, by British, Canadian and American forces, opened up a second front in Europe. Despite fierce resistance from German forces, the Allies succeeded in establishing a foothold in Normandy and, by July 1944, the Allied armies began their advance across France towards the German frontier.

Exploring the detail

The bombing of German cities

There were especially heavy and destructive raids on Cologne, Essen, Düsseldorf and Duisburg. There were also attacks on Munich, Berlin and other towns and cities across the whole of Germany. The raid on Hamburg on 27–28 July 1943 created a firestorm which killed 35–40,000 people and destroyed much of the city. Perhaps the most devastating raid of all was that on Dresden in February 1945. Overall, the Allied bombing campaign killed 305,000 people, injured another 780,000 and destroyed nearly 2,000,000 homes.

The following morning Maria reported that all women and children had to be evacuated from the city within six hours. There was no gas, no electricity, not a drop of water, neither the lift nor the telephone was working. It is hard to imagine the panic and chaos. Each one for himself, only one idea: flight. Since nobody could cook, communal kitchens were organized. But wherever people gathered together, more unrest ensued. People wearing Party badges had them torn off their coats and there were screams of 'Let's get that murderer'. The police did nothing.

3   *Mathilde Wolff-Mecklenburg, in Hamburg, quoted in Noakes, J.,*
Nazism 1919–45, Vol. 4, 1998

Activity

Source analysis

Read Sources 3 and 4.

What insights do these personal accounts of the bombing raids give us into the following?

1 The impact of the bombing on civilians

2 The effects of the bombing on people's support for the regime

At first I looked in the bunker where the children went during an alarm, but I didn't find them. I saw other children, but I could not find my own two. Later I heard that a whole group of people had been buried in a house in Nibelung St., including children from the kindergarten. My two children were pulled out dead. You could hardly see any injuries on them. They had only a small drop of blood on their noses and large bloody scrapes on the backs of their heads. I was in a state of total shock. I wanted to scream, right then and there I wanted to scream, 'You Nazis, you murderers!' A neighbour, who had only been released from a concentration camp a few days before, grabbed my arm and pulled me aside. He said, 'Do you want to get yourself arrested too?'

4   *Kathe Schlechter-Bonnesen, in Cologne, quoted in Haste, C.,* ***Nazi Women, 2001***

The evacuation of children and some women from towns and cities was stepped up in 1942. Although the rationale of this policy was generally accepted, the practicalities often caused friction and resentment. Class tensions increased as it appeared that there was unequal treatment of people from the working and middle classes. Working-class women complained of having to take in children, or live in overcrowded conditions, while middle-class women and those married to Nazi officials were given preferential treatment. There were also religious tensions as children from Protestant areas were often lodged with Catholic parents, or vice versa. Husbands who were working in vital war industries were obliged to remain in the cities while many of their wives and children were evacuated. The disgruntlement of the men at being left to fend for themselves posed a threat to productivity in the factories. Wives who defied official instructions and returned to the cities voluntarily could have their ration books withdrawn. This led to further tensions. In Dortmund in October 1943, for example, about 300 women demonstrated against the withdrawal of their ration books. SD reports in November 1943 recounted how miners refused to work in the pits until their families' ration cards had been restored.

As morale fell, the regime took an increasingly repressive line with those who expressed 'defeatist' remarks. The definition of defeatist included any remark which was critical of the leadership or which showed a loss of faith in Germany's ability to win the war. The maximum penalty for 'malicious denigration' was the death sentence. There were also increased penalties for listening to foreign radio broadcasts.

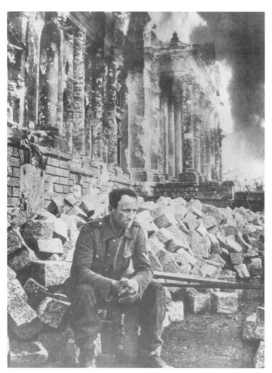

Fig. 4 *A German soldier sits among the ruins of Berlin during the final stages of the war*

Alongside increased repression, the regime also attempted to maintain morale by dealing with the practical problems caused by air raids. The NSV (*Nationalsozialistische Volkswohlfahrt*), a Nazi social welfare organisation, was given the task of providing food and drink, from mobile canteens, for survivors of air raids. There was an elaborate system of compensation payments for survivors to enable them to replace lost belongings. The provision of housing was a major problem. There had been a shortfall of 1,500,000 houses even before the war and the destruction of nearly 2,000,000 homes exacerbated the situation. Hitler came under pressure as early as 1941 to requisition empty homes for those made homeless by the bombing but, believing that this would be unpopular with property owners, he refused. It was not until June 1943, therefore, that Hitler would finally agree to the requisitioning of empty homes. Even this measure did not relieve the housing shortage which remained a cause of discontent until the end of the war.

Göbbels attempted to keep up morale in the face of the air raids with talk of retaliation using the secret weapons which were being developed. Germany's civilian population did display resilience and solidarity in defiance of the bombing but, as the raids continued, there was a serious erosion of civilian morale. The experience of sheer terror as many of Germany's cities were consumed by firestorms, the growing shortages and lengthening queues, the loss of sleep as nights were disrupted by air raid warnings, all contributed to a growing sense of exhaustion and war-weariness.

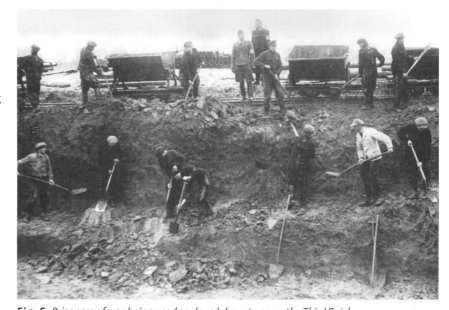

Fig. 5 *Prisoners of war being used as slave labour to serve the Third Reich*

The mass bombing of German cities was designed by the Allies to break the will of the civilian population to carry on supporting the war. Despite the growing war-weariness, workers continued to turn up for work and, at least until the end of 1944, production was maintained. There was undoubtedly pressure from a repressive regime for civilians to keep their heads down and not openly oppose the war. There was also, however, a need for people whose lives were being disrupted on a daily basis to try to find some stability in whatever way they could. Maintaining a daily routine of working was undoubtedly one way of achieving this. Bombing wore down the civilian population but it did not break their will completely.

Workers

Total war measures began to impact on workers during 1943 and 1944. In August 1944, a total ban on holidays was imposed, the working week was increased to 60 hours and extra payments for working overtime were abolished. This increased pressure did result in some rise in absenteeism but employers had a number of disciplinary measures at their disposal. Workers could have their reserved status removed, which would result in conscription into the armed forces and, possibly, a posting to the eastern front. Employers could also allot extra food rations to those employees

Exploring the detail

Help for workers

Through Beauty of Labour, more works canteens were set up and local traders were allowed to sell goods within factories so that workers did not have to spend time shopping. Welfare offices were set up within factories to help workers whose homes had been bombed with replacement ration cards, and an Emergency Homes Scheme provided temporary accommodation within reach of the factory for workers who had lost their homes in bombing raids.

who had good attendance records, and their fines for absenteeism and bad time-keeping. The regime also had at its disposal the DAF factory cell system, in which workers were divided into groups under a loyal Nazi Party member who acted as foreman, and it was the foreman who ~~was responsible for the attendance of workers in his cell. The regime also~~ used incentives to encourage workers to raise productivity. Many plants switched from an hourly paid system to a system of piecework under which workers could earn more if they produced more.

Women

> It has always been our chief article of faith that woman's place is in the home – but since the whole of Germany is our home, we must serve her wherever we can best do so.

5 *Statement by a Nazi Women's League official, quoted in Haste, C., Nazi Women, 2001*

The total war measures implemented in the early months of 1943 led to an extension in the conscription of female labour. The regime, however, remained reluctant to regard women as a vast reserve labour force and its approach to the industrial employment of women was still confused and inconsistent. In November 1943, Hitler was asked to approve the raising of the upper age limit for women to register for work to 50 years of age. He refused, but, by the summer of 1944, the situation had become so grave that Hitler was eventually persuaded to agree to this measure. More and more women were recruited into the industrial labour force and, by 1945, women comprised 60% of the labour force.

Women were also increasingly assigned to auxiliary roles within the armed forces, despite misgivings on the part of Hitler and other leading Nazis. In 1943, women were recruited to replace males in servicing anti-aircraft guns and, in 1944, women began to operate searchlights. By the end of the war, some 50,000 women were involved in anti-aircaft operations and another 30,000 worked on searchlights. In the summer of 1944, the army established an Auxiliary Corps for women serving with the armed forces and, by January 1945, there were 470,000 female auxiliaries serving with this corps. Many of them had been conscripted. Their duties were mainly secretarial and working on radio and telephone communications, but in many cases this involved serving at the front line. The militarisation of women was taken a stage further in the final stages of the war when women's battalions of the army were established and women were trained for combat roles.

Youth

Young people were also increasingly militarised in the final stages of the war. The age at which youths could be conscripted into the armed forces, which had been progressively reduced since 1939, was further reduced to 16 in 1945. Conscription into the *Volkssturm* (home guard) was also introduced, in September 1944, for 16- to 60-year-olds who were not fit for active service. The young men were used to dig anti-tank ditches and trained to use anti-tank weapons. By the end of the war, boys as young as 12 were being conscripted into the Volkssturm.

In 1943, a special Hitler Youth division of the Waffen-SS was set up and recruited boys in the 16–18 age group. Those who joined this group were selected by Hitler Youth group leaders. This division was sent to France in 1944 and saw action in the Battle of Normandy.

Exploring the detail

The Volkssturm

Founded on Hitler's orders, the Volkssturm was intended to be a force of six million members, although this was never achieved. Local units were under the control of Gauleiters to ensure that they showed the necessary ideolgical commitment to the struggle to defend Germany. Many units were sent to the front line, especially in the Battle of Berlin.

Resistance

Communist

The underground communist resistance had been severely weakened by the Gestapo in the 1930s but had managed to survive in some areas. The 1939 Nazi-Soviet Pact had undermined communist resistance to the regime as the KPD struggled to explain and justify this cynical arrangement. The invasion of the USSR in June 1941, however, had galvanised communist resistance to the regime. At the time of the invasion, the KPD had 89 underground cells operating in Berlin, with other cells in Hamburg, Mannheim and central Germany. Their main means of spreading their ideas and attempting to recruit was through issuing leaflets attacking the regime. Infiltration by the Gestapo was always a problem for these cells and, in 1942–43, the Gestapo had considerable success in destroying the communist underground network. Twenty-two of the communist cells in Berlin had been destroyed by the end of 1943. The communist underground did cling to life in some areas but, under pressure from the Gestapo and linked to the power which most Germans considered to be their main enemy, the movement had no prospect of attracting widespread support.

The Churches

As in the 1930s, the Christian Churches were influenced in their response to the regime by their desire to protect their organisations and by their support for many of the regime's policies. The Roman Catholic Church, for example, supported Germany's war aims in 1939 and gave wholehearted support to the invasion of the USSR in 1941. It was again left to individual churchmen to raise their voices in protest at some aspects of Nazi policies. Bishop Galen spoke out in a sermon in 1940 to condemn the euthanasia programmme which had resulted in the killing of 70,000 mentally and physically handicapped people. His protest struck a chord with other Christians and led to the temporary halting of the programme by the regime. Galen was not himself persecuted by the regime for his outspoken opposition but other priests who distributed his sermon were. Three Catholic priests were executed. Apart from Galen, the other leading Catholic who spoke out against the regime was Archbishop Frings of Cologne who condemned the killing of prisoners of war.

 Key profile

Josef Frings

Archbishop Frings (1887–1978) was archbishop of Cologne from 1942 to 1969. He denounced the Nazi persecution of the Jews as a *'crime that calls out to heaven'*. Because of his criticism he was placed under surveillance by the Gestapo.

The Protestant Confessional Church of Prussia was the only Christian body in Germany to protest publicly about the treatment of the Jews. In 1943, a statement was read from the pulpits in Prussian churches. Dietrich Bonhoeffer, who had been an outspoken critic of the regime since 1933, also called for wider Christian resistance to the treatment of the Jews. Since 1940, however, Bonhoeffer had been banned from speaking in public and his criticisms were not able to reach a wide audience in Germany. Bonhoeffer had become involved in the late

 Activity

Thinking point

To what extent, and in what ways, had women and young people been drawn into the war effort by 1945?

■ Activity

Group activity

Divide the class into groups of about four students. Each group should undertake research, using this book and other sources, into resistance to the Nazi regime from one of the following: communists; Churches; youth; the elites.

When the research is completed, each group should present its findings to the rest of the class.

■ Did you know?

The euthanasia programme was introduced in 1939 as part of the Nazi policy of purifying the race. Beginning with children, but later being extended to adults, the mentally and physically disabled were put to death in a programme of so-called 'mercy-killing'. By 1944, some 200,000 people had been killed under this policy.

Key terms

Bundisch youth: autonomous youth groups set up in Germany before the First World War were called 'bundisch' because they were linked together in a *Bund* (league). These groups concentrated on giving young people the chance to experience nature outside of the confines of youth groups linked to political parties or Churches.

Exploring the detail

The activities of the Edelweiss Pirates

The Edelweiss Pirates consciously rejected the official, disciplined and militaristic culture of the Hitler Youth by organising independent expeditions into the countryside, where they sang songs which had been banned in the Hitler Youth. In the war years, there were an increasing number of clashes between Edelweiss Pirates and Hitler Youth groups. In 1944, the Cologne group became linked to an underground group which helped army deserters, escaped prisoners of war, forced labourers and prisoners from concentration camps. They obtained supplies by attacking military depots. The chaos and destruction caused by bombing provided the conditions in which such underground activity could develop.

1930s with critics of the Nazi regime among the elite and had extensive contacts abroad. He was arrested by the Gestapo in 1943 and held in prison until his execution in 1945.

Youth

> The problem of the threat to youth and juvenile criminality manifests itself in particular in the formation of youth gangs. For, since the beginning of the war, and above all since the start of the terror air raids, there has been an increasing number of reports about combinations of young people who are pursuing partly criminal, but also to some extent political and ideological goals.
>
> In Gelsenkirchen a gang of approximately fifty young people were involved in thefts and robberies. They called themselves 'Edelweiss Pirates', met together every evening and were opposed to the HJ. Similar observations have been made at Essen, Bochum and Wattenscheid. In Cologne the Edelweiss Pirates have also made an appearance. They carried out propaganda for the **bundisch** youth and printed leaflets.

6 *From a Reich Ministry of Justice report, 1944, quoted in Noakes, J.,* ***Nazism 1919–45, Vol. 4,*** *1998*

There were a number of youth groups which sprang up during the war years in opposition to the Hitler Youth.

The Edelweiss Pirates

These were groups of mostly working-class young people aged 14–18 who were mainly active in the Rhineland and Ruhr areas. Their name derived from their badge which showed an edelweiss flower. According to the Justice Ministry report, the main 'uniform' of the group consisted of *'short trousers, white socks, a check shirt, a white pullover and scarf and a windcheater. In addition they have very long hair.'* Although not overtly political, the Edelweiss Pirates were anti-Hitler Youth and tried to avoid conscription. From the point of view of the regime, their assertion of the right to establish independent youth gangs placed them in opposition. The report stated that, *'They hate all discipline and thereby place themselves in opposition to the community. However, they are not only politically hostile but, as a result of their composition, they are also criminal and antisocial.'*

The Gestapo and Hitler Youth used their powers to crush the Edelweiss Pirates. When arrests, shaving of heads and banishment to labour camps did not work, the Gestapo turned to more severe measures. On 7 December 1942, the Gestapo in Dusseldorf broke up 28 groups in Düsseldorf, Duisburg, Essen and Wuppertal. The leaders of the Cologne Edelweiss Pirates were publicly hanged in November 1944.

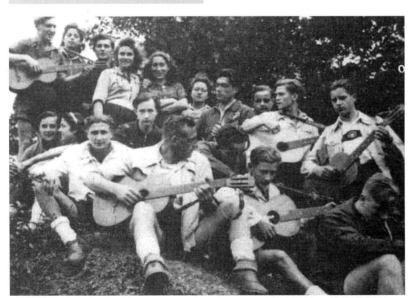

Fig. 6 *The Edelweiss Pirates adopted a lifestyle which was disapproved of by the Nazis. The activities of this group, from Cologne, Düsseldorf and Solingen, were harmless in themselves but did not conform to Nazi codes of behaviour for young people*

The Swing Youth

A different style of youth rebellion developed among young people from the prosperous middle class. The Swing Youth were motivated, according to the Ministry of Justice report, by *'the desire to have a good time'*. In a conscious rejection of Nazi values, the Swing Youth groups listened to American and British swing and jazz music and wore English-style clothes. Swing clubs sprang up in Hamburg, Kiel, Berlin, Stuttgart, Frankfurt, Dresden, Halle and Karlsruhe. By adopting jazz music – which the Nazis referred to as 'negro music' – as the emblem of an alternative youth culture, they were placing themselves in opposition to the regime, but they were not overtly political or attempting to overthrow the regime. Nevertheless their 'sleaziness' and unashamed pleasure-seeking offended the moral precepts of the Nazi regime and Himmler wanted to send the leaders of the movement to concentration camps for two to three years.

The White Rose group

Based in Munich, the White Rose group was a more consciously political movement. Led by Hans and Sophie Scholl, and supported by Professor Kurt Huber, the group was based at Munich University and its main target audience was the educated middle class. A religiously mixed body, the White Rose Group was influenced by Catholic theologians such as Bishop Galen and emphasised the importance of individual freedom and personal responsibility in questions of morality. This led the group to attack the Nazi treatment of the Jews and Slav peoples of Eastern Europe. During 1942–43, the White Rose group issued six pamphlets which were distributed mainly in Munich but were also taken further afield by sympathisers. In February 1943, the group became more daring when they painted anti-Nazi slogans, such as *'Hitler Mass Murderer'* on buildings. They were eventually caught by the Gestapo and executed.

■ Key profile

Hans and Sophie Scholl

Hans (1918–43) and Sophie (1921–43) were founder members and leading activists in the White Rose Movement. Hans had joined the Hitler Youth in his teens but had become disillusioned with the Nazi regime. They advocated passive resistance against the regime. They were arrested, tried and executed in February 1943.

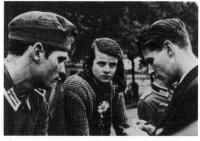

Fig. 7 *Sophie Scholl, wearing a white rose, with her brother Hans in 1943*

The growth of an alternative youth culture in some areas of Germany during the war years, particularly after the start of the mass bombing of the cities, showed that many young people had not been indoctrinated into Nazi ideology. It demonstrated that National Socialism was losing its grip on German society.

The elites

The plot to overthrow Hitler in 1938 by members of the army high command and senior civil servants was never activated and therefore remained undiscovered by the Gestapo. Those involved continued to oppose the regime. There was, however, no unity of purpose among those who opposed Hitler's policies. Some acted from a deeply felt moral conviction that the Nazi regime was evil, while others acted out of patriotism and the belief that Hitler was leading Germany to destruction. Some were democrats, while others were traditional, aristocratic conservatives who wanted a return to an authoritarian, non-Nazi style of government.

Exploring the detail

The Kreisau Circle

Many of the diverse views of the members of the elite who opposed Nazism could be found within the Kreisau Circle. Kreisau was the home of Count Helmut von Moltke, one of the leading figures within the group, which also included other aristocrats, lawyers, SPD politicians and churchmen such as Bonhoeffer. The common denominator which linked this diverse group was a belief in personal freedom and individual responsibility. Described as the *'intellectual power-house of the non-communist opposition'* in Nazi Germany, the Kreisau Circle held three meetings in 1942–43 before the group was broken up by the Gestapo.

Key profile

Count Helmut von Moltke

Moltke (1907–45) was a Prussian aristocratic landowner and a descendant of a Prussian military leader of the 19th century. A lawyer by training and a Christian by conviction, Moltke was critical of the atrocities committed by German forces in occupied countries and became an opponent of the regime. He did not believe that Hitler should be assassinated or overthrown by force, advocating only non-violent resistance. Nevertheless he was arrested by the Gestapo in January 1944 and tried and executed in January 1945.

Among those who had been involved in the 1938 plot, General Beck, Karl Goerdeler and Ulrich von Hassell continued to discuss acting against the regime. They had links to Dietrich Bonhoeffer and General Hans Oster. At first, Beck and Goerdeler concentrated on trying to persuade senior army generals to arrest Hitler. They also made contact, through a meeting between Bonhoeffer and Bishop Bell of Chichester, with the British government, hoping for a commitment to a negotiated peace if Hitler was removed. None of these moves were effective and, in 1943, the conspirators decided that their only option was to assassinate Hitler. The loss of the German army at Stalingrad, due largely to Hitler's refusal to allow a retreat, confirmed that Hitler was leading Germany to disaster. A first assassination attempt was made in March 1943 when a bomb was placed on Hitler's plane. This failed to explode. Although the plot was not discovered, the arrest of Bonhoeffer and other members of the Kreisau Circle in April 1943 was a warning that the Gestapo were getting close to uncovering the full extent of the conspiracy. In 1943, the conspiracy was joined by Colonel Claus von Stauffenberg, who actually succeeded in planting a bomb at Hitler's headquarters in East Prussia in July 1944. Plans were made for a military coup to take over Berlin after Hitler was assassinated. The bomb exploded but Hitler escaped with minor injuries. The planned coup did not materialise because of confusion among the conspirators, who failed to seize control of the radio stations. A broadcast by Hitler to prove that he was still alive was confirmation that the plot had failed. In the wake of this failed assassination, Himmler was placed in charge of rounding up the conspirators. The SS cast their net wide, arresting 7,000 people and executing 5,746. Beck committed suicide and Stauffenberg was shot. The failure of the plot led to the army losing the last vestiges of its independence from the regime as it was effectively placed under SS control.

Key profile

Bishop Bell of Chichester

George Kennedy Allen Bell (1883–1958) was a Church of England bishop who, in the 1930s, had supported the German Confessing Church and had thereby come into contact with Bonhoeffer and Niemöller. He also helped many Germans to emigrate in the late 1930s to escape Nazi persecution. During the war, he openly criticised the Allied policy of mass bombing of German cities. In June 1942, he met Dietrich Bonhoeffer in neutral Sweden.

The bomb plot gained very little sympathy among the majority of ordinary Germans. The plotters came from the old elite and made no attempt to arouse popular support. SD reports spoke of a widespread feeling of relief that the plotters had failed to kill Hitler, and there is no reason to doubt the general accuracy of these reports. The plotters were vilified as traitors, a judgment with which most Germans appear to have concurred.

Key profile

Claus von Stauffenberg

Stauffenberg (1907–44) was a professional soldier from an aristocratic background who had served in North Africa before being injured and sent back to Germany. Appalled by SS atrocities in the USSR and convinced that Germany was being led into a catastrophic defeat, he recruited supporters for an assassination plot against Hitler. He carried the bomb into Hitler's headquarters in July 1944 but it failed to kill Hitler. He was arrested and executed for his part in the plot.

The state of Germany in 1945

In his New Years' Eve radio broadcast at the end of 1944, Hitler told the German people of his *'unshakeable belief that the hour is near in which victory will finally come'*. It was reported that the broadcast did have some success in raising morale, although the reality was that Germany was facing certain defeat. Although the Allied forces in the west had not yet crossed the Rhine and Soviet forces in the east were still in Poland, the Allied bombing campaign had been intensified and the full force of the war was about to come to Germany itself. On 12 January, Soviet forces began their final offensive against Germany, unleashing what Bessel has described as a *'killing frenzy'*. *'During the last four months of the war'*, wrote Bessel, *'more Germans were killed than in 1942 and 1943 put together, and they were killed largely in Germany.'* In January alone, some 450,000 German troops were killed, more than had died at Stalingrad. By February, Soviet forces were advancing through eastern Germany towards Berlin. American forces crossed the Rhine on 23 March and continued their advance across southern and central Germany. British and Canadian forces were advancing across north-western Germany. On 20 April, Soviet forces entered Berlin and began fighting their way through the suburbs towards the heart of the city. Hitler and his mistress (and briefly wife) Eva Braun, committed suicide

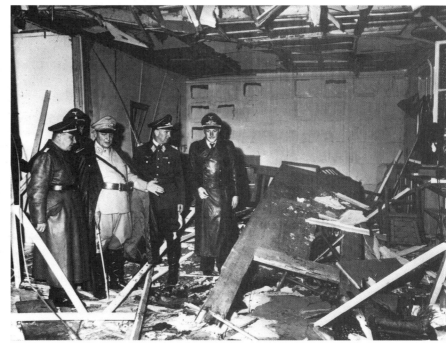

Fig. 8 *Hitler's headquarters after the unsuccessful attempt to assassinate him in July 1944. Göring and Martin Bormann are inspecting the damage*

in his underground bunker in the centre of Berlin on 30 April. Göbbels and his wife killed their children before committing suicide themselves. On 2 May, Berlin was captured by Soviet forces. Five days later, Admiral Dönitz, Hitler's successor, signed the instrument of unconditional surrender.

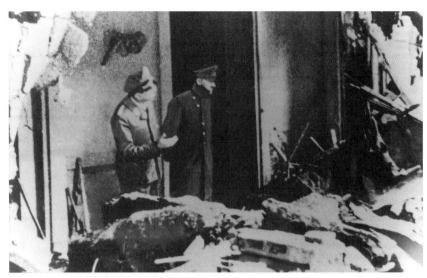

Fig. 9 *Allegedly the last photograph taken of Hitler before his death. Here he inspects the ruins of the Reich Chancellery in Berlin in late April 1945*

■ Key profile

Admiral Karl Dönitz

Dönitz (1891–1980) had joined the navy in 1910 and served in the First World War. He became a rear admiral in 1935 and had responsibility for the development of the German submarine fleet. In 1943, he became commander in chief of the German navy. After Hitler's suicide he was appointed chancellor of Germany and signed the unconditional surrender of German forces to the Allies in May 1945. He served ten years in prison after the war.

For the civilian population of Germany, the last months of the war brought unrelenting misery. Millions of Germans living in Poland, East Prussia and Czechoslovakia were driven out by hostile local people and forced to trek westwards in advance of the Soviet forces. As Soviet forces entered Germany itself, millions more Germans fled their homes to escape the fighting. In eastern Germany, some 3.5 million Germans were fleeing from the advancing Soviet troops. They could expect no help from the army as it too retreated, nor could the majority of them find berths on trains or ships, since priority was given to the transport of military supplies. Responsibility for the evacuations rested with local Gauleiters, many of whom delayed the order to leave until the very last minute. The result was that they were forced to walk hundreds of miles facing cold, hunger and disease and attacks by Allied forces. Estimates of the numbers who died on these marches vary from around 500,000 to over one million. When the survivors finally reached the western part of Germany, they found cities devastated by bombing and a civilian population facing severe hardships. Heavy bombing of cities and the added pressure of the evacuees from the east left at least a quarter of the civilian population homeless. Transport systems had ceased to function, electricity and gas supplies had been cut, water and sewage systems were seriously damaged and epidemic diseases were beginning to appear. Food supplies were running low and there was a serious risk of starvation in some areas. Unsurprisingly, civilian morale collapsed.

> A large part of the population has become accustomed to living only from day to day. They make the most of any comforts of life that present themselves. Suicides, due to real depression about the catastrophe which is expected with certainty, are an everyday occurrence.

7   *From an SD Report, March 1945, quoted in Bessel, R.,*
***Germany 1945**, 2009*

As morale collapsed, so too did the authority of the Nazi Party and Hitler. Defence ditches and gun emplacements, designed to slow down the Allied advance, were in many cases sabotaged by the local civilian population who wanted to avoid their homes being destroyed in a last-ditch struggle. Hitler ordered that all industrial plant, military equipment and transport installations in the line of the Allied advance should be destroyed to prevent them falling into Allied hands. This order was countermanded by Speer, who wanted to preserve something of Germany's industrial and transport infrastructure as a base on which to start rebuilding after the war.

Cross-reference

There is a profile of Speer on page 125.

This is not to say that the Nazi regime in any way relaxed its efforts to maintain a firm grip on Germany. The police, SS and armed forces were ordered to intensify the terror to prevent defeatist attitudes taking root. The spectre of 1918, with the collapse of civilian morale and mutinies in the armed forces contributing to Germany's defeat, hung over the Nazi regime. *'The year 1918 will not be repeated'*, Hitler declared on 11 March 1945. Summary executions of those unwilling to fight became the order of the day. Conditions in the concentration camps deteriorated and tens of thousands of inmates died from starvation, hypothermia and disease. Many camps were emptied and those inmates able to walk were forced to trek through appalling conditions. Those incapable of moving under their own steam were shot. Tens of thousands died on these 'death marches'. Foreign workers in Germany, of

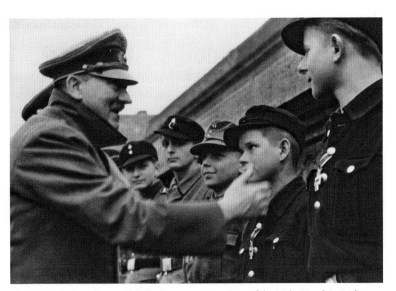

Fig. 10 *Hitler handing medals for bravery to members of the Hitler Youth in Berlin in 1945*

whom there were estimated to have been 7.6 million in August 1944, were especially vulnerable to Nazi terror. Many who were accused of lack of discipline were executed without trial.

The year 1918 was not repeated in Germany in 1945. Civilian morale collapsed, as did finally the resistance of Germany's armed forces. There were many desertions from the armed forces, but many of those who did so were captured by the SS and shot. The civilian population was exhausted and suffering severe hardship but there were few signs

Activity

Thinking point

'After twelve years of Nazi rule, violence had become second nature to the regime; in the end, violence was all that it had left to offer.' (Bessel, 2009) What is your opinion about this statement?

Exploring the detail

Freedom Action Bavaria

In contrast with 1918, there were few signs of revolutionary activity against the regime in 1945. There was one, isolated, attempted uprising in Munich on 28 April when a group calling itself 'Freedom Action Bavaria' took over the radio station and broadcast an appeal to soldiers to stop fighting and to civilians to resist the Nazis. It was led by Rupprecht Gerngross, the head of an army translation unit. Needless to say, this 'rebellion' was quickly crushed by the SS.

Activity

Group discussion

1. How far did the Allied bombing of German cities succeed in undermining the morale of the German people?

2. How successfully did the Nazi regime maintain control over the German people during the Second World War?

of outward resistance, still less of rebellion. On the whole, the German population reacted passively and with resignation to the final collapse of the regime and Germany's occupation by foreign forces, bound together in a 'community of fate'. Once Germany was defeated and occupied, however, the Nazi regime collapsed with remarkable speed.

> When it came, the collapse of the Nazi dictatorship was remarkable in its speed and thoroughness. Seemingly overnight the hold of the regime evaporated. Despite expectations to the contrary, despite the remarkable grip which National Socialism had had on the German people across twelve years of indoctrination in the schools, the media and public institutions of all kinds, despite police terror and widespread complicity in the crimes of the Nazi regime, when German towns and cities were occupied by Allied forces Nazism disappeared.

8   *From Bessel, R., **Germany 1945**, 2009*

The Third Reich had lasted just twelve years. In the wake of the Allied victory, Germany was occupied by foreign forces and divided into four zones – an eastern zone controlled by the Soviet Union and three western zones controlled by the USA, Great Britain and France. This division of Germany developed into a political division between the liberal-democratic German Federal Republic in the west and the communist German Democratic Republic in the east.

Learning outcomes

In this section, you have looked at the ways in which the Second World War had an impact on the lives of the German people and how this affected their attitudes towards the regime. After reading this section, you should have an understanding of the key events and turning points in the war and how the morale of the German people was affected by the changing fortunes of Germany's armed forces. The impact of the Allied bombing of German cities made unprecedented demands on the German people and the prospect of defeat undermined confidence in the regime. From your reading of this section you should be able to assess the extent of conformity and resistance among the German people at various stages in the war and, in particular, the extent of popular support for the Nazi regime in 1945.

Practice question

(a) Explain why Göbbels made his total war speech in February 1943.

(12 marks)

Study tip This is a short, essay-style question which requires you to identify a range of factors which explain why Göbbels made this speech. You should try to identify a minimum of three factors and write a paragraph of explanation about each. Examiners will be looking for evidence that you have both knowledge and understanding of the issue and, in order for you to reach the higher levels in the mark scheme you will need to be able to show links between the factors and to differentiate between them (perhaps in terms of most important or least important, or in terms of long-term or short-term factors).

(b) 'The defeat of the German army at Stalingrad in January 1943 led to a complete collapse of confidence in the Nazi regime.' Explain why you agree or disagree with this view.

(24 marks)

Study tip This requires a longer answer as it is worth more marks. Remember that before you start you should identify the key words in the question. Focus on these key words in your answer. With questions of this type, you need to consider points on which you agree and points on which you disagree with the quotation. Your answer will need to show balance between agreement and disagreement, although ultimately you should come down on one side or the other. You should aim to produce an answer that has a clear line of argument running through it, that looks at both sides of the debate and that has carefully selected factual information to support the points that you are making. Finally, end with a clear conclusion in which you make a judgment.

Conclusion

The Nazis aimed to transform German society. Their social policies aimed to persuade the German people to put aside their sectional interests in favour of an overarching loyalty to a greater national cause. The Nazi *Volksgemeinschaft* would be a society in which there would be social harmony based on a shared racial purity. No independent organisations or alternative ideologies would be allowed to divide German society; in the Third Reich, every individual of Aryan race who was sound in mind and body would totally identify with the regime and its aims.

Historians of the Third Reich have reached different conclusions about the impact of the Nazi regime on German society. This is partly because different historians have approached the subject from different perspectives. Whereas Marxist historians, for example, have concluded that Nazism was essentially a **reactionary** force which destroyed working-class organisations, held down living standards and strengthened capitalism in Germany, liberal-democratic historians have argued that Nazism produced a social revolution. According to Dahrendorf, Nazism *'finally abolished the German past as it was embodied in Imperial Germany'. Gleichschaltung*, it is argued, broke down the divisions in German society between religions, regions and sectional interests and paved the way for the liberal-democratic society which emerged in West Germany after the war.

The preconceptions of historians are only part of the reason why there is debate over the impact of the Nazi regime on society. Another problem is that it is difficult to define exactly what the Nazis' social aims were, since they were essentially contradictory. On the one hand, the Nazis looked back to a mythical German people's community in the middle ages that was based on the ties of 'blood and soil'. Nazism rejected 'modern' belief-systems such as Marxism, bourgeois democracy and feminism as being un-German and the products of a Jewish world conspiracy. In this sense, Nazism was essentially reactionary. On the other hand, Nazism was viewed by many of its adherents as a modernising force, dynamic and revolutionary. The Nazis placed great emphasis on the scientific basis of their racial theories and Nazi architecture reflected the fact that Nazism was not simply a rejection of modernism. Nazism attracted support from a wide range of social classes and many of its most committed adherents believed in wholesale social change. These contradictions were evident in Nazi policy. On the one hand, the Nazis promoted the image of the ideal Aryan woman and encouraged married women to leave employment in order to concentrate on home-building and child-rearing. On the other hand, the demands of the Nazi war economy dictated that more women should be employed in industry.

A final reason why historians cannot agree on the impact of the Nazi regime on German society is that it is difficult to distinguish between change that was brought about as a direct consequence of Nazi policies and that which was brought about by the disruption and chaos that resulted from the war and military defeat. Social change is a phenomenon in all countries during prolonged wars, especially total wars such as the

Second World War. Some of this change happens as a result of long-term factors which are accelerated by the impact of war, some are directly attributable to the strains placed on any society at war. Germany suffered so much destruction and social upheaval in the final stages of the war that social change would have occurred with or without the Nazi regime.

The Germany of 1945 was a very different place from that of 1933, but this does not mean that the Nazis succeeded in remoulding German society in their own image. Nor does it mean that there was no continuity with the past during the Third Reich period. The Nazi organisations, created under the policy of *Gleichschaltung* to unite German society, did not survive Germany's military defeat. Trade unions, which had been replaced in 1933 by the DAF, were quickly re-established in industrial areas during the allied occupation. Despite Nazi efforts to break down religious allegiances, according to Kershaw, '*The hold of the Churches and the clergy over the population, especially in country areas, was often strengthened rather than weakened by the Church struggle.*' The Nazis aimed to create a society in which traditional ties of 'blood and soil' were strengthened and to this end they attempted to protect the position of the peasant farmers. The over-riding need to maximise industrial production during the war, however, and the insatiable demands of the armed forces for male conscripts, took men away from agriculture. Women were supposed to accept their place as housewives and mothers within the Nazi scheme of things, but here again the demands of rearmament and the war effort meant that more women worked in industry in 1945 than in 1933. Finally, the Nazis placed great stress on social mobility and equal opportunities within their

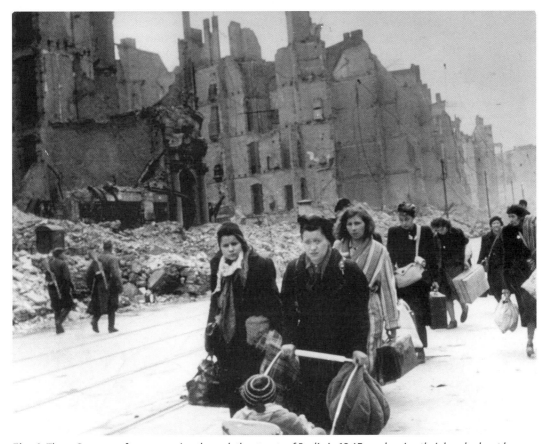

Fig. 1 *These German refugees, moving through the streets of Berlin in 1945, are leaving their bombed-out homes to escape the fierce fighting for control of the city*

Volksgemeinschaft. Every German would have an equal status, that of a 'national comrade'. In reality, the social position of the elite was largely unchanged, at least until the final stages of the war. There was social mobility in Nazi Germany, not least for the many senior Nazis who came from humble backgrounds. But this new political elite existed side by side with the old social elite and these two groups compromised and worked together. The higher ranks of big business, the civil service and the army were still, in the Nazi period, largely recruited from the same elite social classes as before. The old elite were, however, fatally compromised by their role in bringing the Nazis to power and sustaining them thereafter.

The Nazis did not create social institutions which survived the impact of defeat in war and the collapse of the Third Reich. In this sense, their impact was essentially destructive. The authoritarian structures and political dominance of the old elite, hangovers from the pre-1914 German Empire which had survived the 1918 revolution and the Weimar period, were finally swept away in the chaos and destruction of military defeat. Far from ensuring that a traditional way of life based on 'blood and soil' would endure, the Nazis unleashed forces which destroyed the traditional structures of German society and paved the way for a fresh start after 1945. What emerged from the ruins of defeat, in both liberal-democratic West Germany and the communist East Germany, were the very antithesis of what the Nazis were attempting to build.

Evans has written that, *'What Hitler and the Nazis wanted was a change in people's spirits, their way of thinking and behaving. They wanted a new man, and for that matter a new woman, to emerge out of the ashes of the Weimar Republic, recreating the fighting unity and commitment of the front in the First World War. Their revolution was, first and foremost, cultural rather than social.'* Much of what the Nazis wanted to achieve in social change was expressed in symbols, rituals and propaganda. There was very little real substance to Nazi social policy, certainly in terms of building lasting social structures. Great emphasis was placed on propaganda and indoctrination and in this respect the impact of Nazism for the vast majority of Germans was little more than temporary. For the millions who lost their lives as a result of the Nazis' experiments in social and racial engineering, however, the impact was rather more final.

Glossary

A

Anschluss: the union between Austria and Germany which occurred in March 1938.

Anti-Semitism: hatred and fear of Jews (Semites).

Aryan: the term used by racial theorists, including the Nazis, to describe the race to which non-Jewish Germans belonged.

Asocial: a person who, by virtue of his or her physical or mental characteristics, was deemed by the Nazis to be unfit to be included in the Volksgemeinschaft.

Autarky: a state of national self-sufficiency.

Authoritarian: the belief in government by a strong leader without any democratic limitations on his or her power.

Autocratic: with a ruler who has total power.

B

BDM (Bund Deutscher Mädel): the League of German Girls, a Nazi youth organisation.

Blitzkrieg: 'lightning war', a military doctrine used successfully by Germany 1939–41.

Bolshevism: an alternative term for communism, derived from a name of the Russian Communist Party which seized power in 1917, the Bolshevik Party.

C

Capitalism: an economic system based on private ownership, competition and the pursuit of profit.

Centre Party: the political party which represented the interests of Germany's large Roman Catholic minority. The Centre Party was pro-democracy and prepared to work with other parties in coalition governments.

Chancellor: the German title for prime minister.

Communist: a believer in a system based on public ownership of land and industry, where all are equal and people work for the common good.

Conservative: a person who resists change and tries to preserve social and political institutions in their current state.

Constitution: the basic laws which determine how a country should be run.

D

DAF (Deutsches Arbeitsfront): the German Labour Front, a Nazi organisation which replaced the trade unions which existed until May 1933.

Democracy: a system of government which allows people to choose their rulers through free elections and which guarantees to protect the human rights of individuals.

Dictatorship: rule by one person or by one party.

DNVP (Deutschesnationale Volkspartei): the German National People's Party, a conservative, nationalist party which shared some of the same aims as the Nazis, including hostility to the pre-1933 democratic system.

DVP (Deutsche Volkspartei): the German People's Party, a conservative group which was prepared to work with other parties in the pre-1933 system.

E

Encyclical: a letter from the pope to Roman Catholic bishops.

Eugenics: the science of racial improvement through such methods as selective breeding.

Euthanasia: killing a patient by painless means. The Nazis had a policy of euthanasia of those who were mentally or physically disabled.

Evangelical Church: the German Protestant Church.

F

Freikorps: the Free Corps, a paramilitary organisation of ex-soldiers, which was armed and financed by the army and used to support right-wing groups in German politics before 1933.

G

Gau(e): the regional units of the Nazi Party.

Gauleiter: the Nazi Party leader in each Gau (region). These men were responsible directly to Hitler.

German Labour Front: see DAF.

German National People's Party: see DNVP.

German People's Party: see DVP.

Gleichschaltung: the Nazi policy of 'coordination' by which all social, economic and political activities were brought under State control. It literally translates as 'forcing into line'.

H

HJ (Hitler Jugend): the Hitler Youth, the Nazi youth organisation for boys.

I

Ideology: a set of ideas and principles.

J

Junker: a landowning aristocrat from Prussia. This was the group from which most of the army officers, civil servants and government ministers were recruited in the Second Reich.

K

KdF (Kraft durch Freude): the Nazi 'Strength Through Joy' organisation which was part of the DAF. It organised leisure activities for workers and their families.

KPD (Kommunistiche Partei Deutschlands): the communist party of Germany which had a strong base of working-class support before 1933.

L

League of German Girls: see BDM.

Lebensraum: 'living space', a concept by which Hitler justified his plans to take over territory to the east of Germany.

Luftwaffe: the German air force.

M

Marxist: a follower of Karl Marx, the original communist theorist.

Mittelstand: the lower middle class, a group which included artisans, farmers and shopkeepers.

N

Nationalism: the belief that a nation should be independent and rule itself.

Nordic: the northern European sub-group of the Aryan race to which the Nazis believed the Germans belonged.

NSDAP (Nationalsozialistische Deutsche Arbeiterparte): the National Socialist German Workers' Party, or the Nazi Party.

NS-F (Nationalsozialistische Frauenschaft): the National Socialist Women's Organisation.

P

Plebiscite: a vote in which the government asks the electorate to approve of a particular policy.

Propaganda: the systematic spreading of ideas and information in order to influence the thinking and actions of the people at whom it is targeted, often through the use of media such as posters, film, radio and the press.

Putsch: an attempt to overthrow a government by force; sometimes referred to by the French phrase 'coup d'etat'.

R

RAD (Reichsarbeitsdienst): the Reich Labour Service, through which young men (and after 1939, young women also) were made to undertake compulsory labour service.

Reichstag: the German parliament.

Reparations: the payments demanded from Germany in the 1919 Treaty of Versailles to compensate the Allied nations for the damage caused by the First World War.

Republic: a country which has a president as head of state rather than a monarch.

S

SA (Sturmabteilung): the Storm Division, a Nazi paramilitary organisation which was set up to intimidate opponents. Their distinctive brown uniforms led to SA being referred to as the 'brownshirts'.

SD (Sicherheitsdienst): the German Security Service, under the control of the SS, which existed to collect information about opposition to the Nazis.

Socialism: the belief in a society based on collective ownership of land industry, equality and cooperation to benefit all. Socialism is similar to communism in many of its basic beliefs but socialists tend to believe in peaceful, gradual change rather than revolution.

Sopade: the German Social Democratic Party in exile, established after the Nazis banned all other political parties and arrested many SPD members.

SPD (Sozialdemokratische Partei Deutschlands): the German Social Democratic Party, the main socialist party and a leading political force in the Weimar Republic.

SS (Schutzstaffel): a special police force, originally formed as Hitler's bodyguard but which grew into the most powerful organisation in the Third Reich. They wore black uniforms.

Stahlhelm: the Steel Helmets, a nationalist, right-wing paramilitary force which recruited ex-servicemen. It was a significant force in the politics of the Weimar Republic.

Strength Through Joy: see KdF.

U

USSR: the Union of Soviet Socialist Republics, a large communist state with its capital in Moscow. From the late 1920s, the leader of the USSR was Joseph Stalin.

V

Vatican: the part of Rome ruled over by the pope; it was the government of the Roman Catholic Church.

Volkisch: concerning the distinct identity of the German people.

Volksgemeinschaft: the 'people's community', which the Nazis were attempting to build in the Third Reich.

W

Weltanschaung: a term meaning 'world outlook' used to refer to the beliefs and attitudes through which an individual perceives the world. It can be used as another term for ideology.

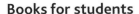

Bibliography

Books for students

Bessel, R. (1987) *Life in The Third Reich*, Oxford University Press.

Hite, J. and Hinton, C. (2000) *Weimar and Nazi Germany*, Hodder Murray.

Kirk, T. (1995) *Longman Companion to Nazi Germany*, Longman.

Layton, G. (1992) Germany, *The Third Reich 1933–45*, Hodder & Stoughton.

Lee, S. (1998) *Hitler and Germany*, Routledge.

Books for teachers and extension

Bessel, R. (2009) *Germany 1945*, Simon & Schuster.

Bullock, A. (1962) *Hitler, A Study in Tyranny*, Penguin.

Evans, R. (2005) *The Third Reich in Power*, Penguin.

Evans, R. (2008) *The Third Reich at War*, Penguin.

Grunberger, R. (1971) *A Social History of the Third Reich*, Penguin.

Haste, C. (2001) *Nazi Women*, Macmillan.

Kershaw, R. (1991) *Hitler*, Longman.

Kershaw, R. (1989) *The Hitler Myth*, Oxford.

Kershaw, R. (1993) *The Nazi Dictatorship*, Arnold.

Housden, M. (1996) *Resistance and Conformity in the Third Reich*, Routledge.

Noakes, J. and Pridham, G. (1984) *Nazism 1919–45, Vol. 2*, Exeter.

Noakes, J. (1998) *Nazism 1919–45, Vol 4*, Exeter.

Overy, R. (2004) *The Dictators*, Penguin.

Peukert, D. (1982) *Inside Nazi Germany; Conformity, Opposition and Resistance in Everyday Life*, Penguin.

Online resources

Hitler's *Mein Kampf* can be found at www.hitler.org/writings/Mein_Kampf

Hitler's speeches can be found at www.adolfhitlerspeeches.com

The Nazi propaganda archive can be found at www.calvin.edu/academic/cas/gpa

Acknowledgements

The author and publisher would also like to thank the following for permission to reproduce material:

Pages 10, 14, 20, 22, 26, 65, 70; from HITLER SPEECHES AND PROCLAMATIONS by Max Domarus, I. B. Tauris & Co. Ltd. Reprinted with permission.

Pages 14, 15, 16, 17, 18, 20, 21, 40; from MEIN KAMPF by Adolf Hitler, published by Hutchinson and Houghton Mifflin. Translated by Ralph Manheim. Copyright © 1943, renewed 1971 by Houghton Mifflin Company. Reprinted with permission of The Random House Group Limited and Houghton Mifflin Harcourt Company. All rights reserved.

Page 19; Short extract from George S. Viereck's interview with Adolf Hitler, Liberty Magazine, 1932. Reprinted with permission of Stephanie Viereck Gibbs Kamath.

Pages 24, 29, 49, 50, 59, 98; extracts from THE THIRD REICH IN POWER by Richard Evans (Penguin Books, 2005) Copyright © Richard Evans 2005. Reprinted with permission of Penguin Books UK and The Penguin Press, a division of Penguin Group (USA) Inc.

Page 26; extract from Germany: The Third Reich 1933–1945 by G. Layton, Hodder Arnold, 1992, Reprinted with permission of Edward Arnold (Publishers) Ltd.

Pages 32, 33, 45, 46, 63, 66, 72, 74, 80, 83, 92, 96, 103, 121, 122, 125, 126, 127, 129, 131, 132, 136; short extracts from NAZISM 1919–45 VOLUME 2, AND NAZISM 1919–45 VOLUME 4 by J. Noakes and G. Pridham, published by Exeter University Press 1984/1988. Reprinted with permission.

Page 37; Extract adapted from POLITICAL VIOLENCE AND THE NAZI SEIZURE OF POWER by Richard Bessel, History Today, October, 1985. Reprinted by permission of History Today Ltd.

Page 37; extract adapted from A HISTORY OF GERMANY 1815–1990 by William Carr, Hodder Arnold, 1991. Reprinted with permission of Edward Arnold (Publishers) Ltd.

Pages 37, 46; extracts from THE THIRD REICH IN POWER by Richard Evans (Penguin Books, 2005) Copyright © Richard Evans 2005. Reprinted with permission of Penguin Books UK and The Penguin Press, a division of Penguin Group (USA) Inc.

Pages 39, 40, 42,132, 134; from The German Propaganda Archive at www.calvin.edu/academic/gpa reprinted with kind permission.

Pages 43, 74, 75; from NAZI WOMEN by Cate Haste, Macmillan, 2001. Reprinted with permission of Macmillan.

Page 44; from THE ART OF THE THIRD REICH by Peter Adam, published by Harry N. Abrams Inc. © Peter Adam. Reprinted with the kind permission of the author.

Pages 53, 54; extracts from HITLER MYTH by I Kershaw, published by OUP 2001. Reprinted with permission of Oxford University Press.

Page 63; short extract from I SHALL BEAR WITNESS: THE DIARIES OF VICTOR KLEMPERER 1933–41 by Victor Klemperer, Reprinted with permission of The Orion Publishing Group and ….

Page 64; short extracts from BERLIN DIARY: THE JOURNAL OF A FOREIGN CORRESPONDENT 1933–41 by William Shirer © 1941 William Shirer.

Pages 84, 86, 89, 90; from WEIMAR AND NAZI GERMANY by J. Hite and C. Hinton, Hodder Murray 2000. Reprinted with permission.

Page 112; from FRAUEN: GERMAN WOMEN RECALL THE THIRD REICH by Alison Owings © 1993 by Alison Owings. Reprinted by permission of Rutgers University Press.

Page 112; short extract adapted from A BRISTOLIAN IN THE THIRD REICH by Margaret Goodbody.

Page 112; short extract from THROUGH HELL FOR HITLER by Henry Metelmann, History Press. Reprinted with permission.

Pages 141, 142; from GERMANY 1945 by Richard Bessel, published by Simon & Schuster 2009. Reprinted with permission of Simon & Schuster UK.

Photographs courtesy of:

Edimedia; 0.3, 1.7, 1.10, 2.6, 3.4, 3.8, 3.11, 4.2, 4.3, 5.4, 6.7, 7.1, 7.3, 7.7, 7.8, 7.10, 8.4, World History Archive; 1.9, 3.1, 3.2, 4.9, 4.10, 4.11, 5.5, 5.7, 6.12, Mary Evans Picture Library; 1.1, Photo 12; 1.2, 2.1, 2.3, 2.4, 3.10, 4.7, 5.8, 7.9, 8.1, 8.8, 8.9, 8.10, 9.1, Sante Archive; 1.4, Topfoto; 2.2, 2.5, 4.1, 5.1, 5.11, 5.12, 5.13, 6.1, 6.5, 6.8, 7.6, 8.5, 8.7, Ann Ronan Picture Library; 3.6, 4.5, 7.5, Public Domain; 1.5, 6.10, 8.6

Index